This book is to be returned on or before
the last date stamped below.

LIBREX

Schizophrenia
Second Edition

MEDICAL PSYCHIATRY

Series Editor Emeritus
William A. Frosch, M.D.
Weill Medical College of Cornell University,
New York, New York, U.S.A.

Advisory Board

Jonathan E. Alpert, M.D., Ph.D.
Massachusetts General Hospital and
Harvard University School of Medicine
Boston, Massachusetts, U.S.A.

Bennett Leventhal, M.D.
University of Chicago School of Medicine
Chicago, Illinois, U.S.A.

Siegfried Kasper, M.D.
Medical University of Vienna
Vienna, Austria

Mark H. Rapaport, M.D.
Cedars-Sinai Medical Center
Los Angeles, California, U.S.A.

Schizophrenia

Second Edition

Edited by

Siegfried Kasper, MD
Professor and Chairman
Department of Psychiatry and Psychotherapy
Medical University of Vienna
Vienna
Austria

and

George N Papadimitriou, MD
Professor and Chairman
First Department of Psychiatry
Athens University Medical School
Athens
Greece

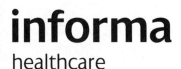

informa
healthcare

© 2009 Informa UK Ltd

First published in 2009 by Informa Healthcare, Telephone House, 69-77 Paul Street, London EC2A 4LQ. Informa Healthcare is a trading division of Informa UK Ltd. Registered Office: 37/41 Mortimer Street, London W1T 3JH. Registered in England and Wales number 1072954.

A CIP record for this book is available from the British Library.
Library of Congress Cataloging-in-Publication Data

Data available on application

ISBN-13: 978-1-4200-8004-9

Distributed in North and South America by

Taylor & Francis
6000 Broken Sound Parkway, NW (Suite 300)
Boca Raton, FL 33487, USA

Within Continental USA
Tel: 1 (800) 272 7737; Fax: 1 (800) 374 3401

Outside Continental USA
Tel: 1-859-727-5000
Fax: 1-859-647-4028
E-mail: orders@taylorandfrancis.com

Orders in the rest of the world
Informa Healthcare
Sheepen Place
Colchester
Essex CO3 3LP
UK

Telephone: +44 (0)20 7017 5540
Email: CSDhealthcarebooks@informa.com

Typeset by C&M Digitals (P) Ltd, Chennai, India
Printed and bound in Great Britain by MPG Books Ltd, Bodmin, Cornwall, UK

Contents

III Pharmacological Treatment Strategies

IV Nonpharmacological Treatment

V Schizophrenia and Society

Contributors

Elena Akimova
Department of Psychiatry and
    Psychotherapy
Medical University of Vienna
Vienna, Austria

Carlo A Altamura
Department of Clinical Psychiatry
University of Milan
Fondazione IRCCS
Ospedale Maggiore Policlinico,
    Mangiagalli e Regina Elena
Milan, Italy

Paul Amminger
ORYGEN Research Centre
University of Melbourne
Melbourne, Australia
and Department of Child and Adolescent
    Psychiatry
Medical University of Vienna
Vienna, Austria

Seyed M Assadi
Department of Psychiatry
Melbourne Neuropsychiatry Centre
The University of Melbourne and
    Melbourne Health
Melbourne, Victoria, Australia
and Department of Psychiatry
Psychiatry and Psychology Research Centre
Tehran University of Medical Sciences
Tehran, Iran

Hans-Gert Bernstein
Department of Psychiatry
University of Magdeburg
Magdeburg, Germany

Julio Bobes
Department of Psychiatry - CIBERSAM
University of Oviedo
Oviedo, Spain

Bernhard Bogerts
Department of Psychiatry
University of Magdeburg
Magdeburg, Germany

Manuel Bousoño
Department of Psychiatry - CIBERSAM
University of Oviedo
Oviedo, Spain

Susan Boyer
St. Louis Psychiatric Rehabilitation Center
Saint Louis, Missouri, USA

Raphael J Braga
Psychiatry Research Division
The Zucker Hillside Hospital
North Shore-LIJ Health System
Glen Oaks, New York, USA

Peter F Buckley
Department of Psychiatry and Health Behavior
Medical College of Georgia
Augusta, Georgia, USA

Jonathan Burns
Department of Psychiatry
Nelson R Mandela School of Medicine
University of KwaZulu-Natal
Durban, South Africa

Wiepke Cahn
Department of Psychiatry
University Medical Center
Utrecht, The Netherlands

Hun Soo Chang
Pharmacogenomic Research Center for
    Psychotropic Drugs
Depression Center
Department of Psychiatry
College of Medicine
Korea University
Seoul, Korea

Robert R Conley
US Medical Division
Eli Lilly and Company
and Department of Psychiatry and
    Pharmacy Science
University of Maryland
Baltimore, Maryland, USA

Caroline Corves
Department of Psychiatry and
    Psychotherapy
Technische Universität München
Klinikum rechts der Isar
Munich, Germany

John M Davis
Department of Psychiatry
University of Illinois at Chicago
Chicago, Illinois, USA

Evan G DeRenzo
Center for Ethics at the
    Washington Hospital Center
MedStar Health
Washington, DC, USA

Dimitris G Dikeos
First Department of Psychiatry
Athens University Medical School
Eginition Hospital
Athens, Greece

Filippo Dragogna
Department of Clinical Psychiatry
University of Milan
Fondazione IRCCS
Ospedale Maggiore Policlinico,
    Mangiagalli e Regina Elena
Milan, Italy

Marina P Economou
University Mental Health Research
    Institute
Athens, Greece

Martin Fink
Department of Psychiatry and
    Psychotherapy
Medical University of Vienna
Vienna, Austria

Marion Freidl
Department of Psychiatry and
    Psychotherapy
Medical University of Vienna
Vienna, Austria

Maria P Garcia-Portilla
Department of Psychiatry - CIBERSAM
University of Oviedo
Oviedo, Spain

Birte Yding Glenthoj
Center for Neuropsychiatric
    Schizophrenia Research
University of Copenhagen
Psychiatric Center Glostrup
Glostrup, Denmark

Eric Granholm
VA San Diego Healthcare System and
Department of Psychiatry
University of California, San Diego
San Diego, California, USA

Lisa H Guzik
Department of Psychiatry and Behavioural
    Sciences
University of California
Los Angeles, California, USA

Neeltje EM van Haren
Department of Psychiatry
University Medical Center
Utrecht, The Netherlands

Meredith G Harris
School of Population Health
The University of Queensland
Brisbane, Australia

Lisa P Henry
ORYGEN Research Centre
University of Melbourne
Melbourne, Australia

Alexis Jeannotte
Center for Ethics at the Washington
    Hospital Center
MedStar Health
Washington, DC, USA

Rene S Kahn
Department of Psychiatry
University Medical Center
Utrecht, The Netherlands

Siegfried Kasper
Department of Psychiatry and
    Psychotherapy
Medical University of Vienna
Vienna, Austria

Werner Kissling
Department of Psychiatry and
    Psychotherapy
Technische Universität München
Klinikum rechts der Isar
Munich, Germany

Martin Knapp
The London School of Economics and
    Political Science
London, UK

Lars V Kristiansen
Department of Psychiatry
Bispebjerg Hospital
Copenhagen, Denmark

Rupert Lanzenberger
Department of Psychiatry and
    Psychotherapy
Medical University of Vienna
Vienna, Austria

Min-Soo Lee
Pharmacogenomic Research Center for
    Psychotropic Drugs
Depression Center
Department of Psychiatry
College of Medicine
Korea University
Seoul, Korea

Stefan Leucht
Department of Psychiatry and
    Psychotherapy
Technische Universität München
Klinikum rechts der Isar
Munich, Germany

Catherine Loh
Department of Psychiatry
University of California, San Diego
San Diego, California, USA

Massimo C Mauri
Department of Clinical Psychiatry
University of Milan
Fondazione IRCCS
Ospedale Maggiore Policlinico,
    Mangiagalli e Regina Elena
Milan, Italy

Patrick D McGorry
ORYGEN Research Centre
Department of Psychiatry
The University of Melbourne, Australia

Peter McGuffin
MRC SGDP Centre
Institute of Psychiatry
King's College London
London, UK

Brian J Miller
Department of Psychiatry and Health
   Behavior
Medical College of Georgia
Augusta, Georgia, USA

Hans-Jürgen Möller
Department of Psychiatry
University of Munich
Munich, Germany

Ahmed Okasha
Institute of Psychiatry
Faculty of Medicine
Ain Shams University
Cairo, Egypt

Tarek Okasha
Institute of Psychiatry
Faculty of Medicine
Ain Shams University
Cairo, Egypt

Bob Oranje
Center for Neuropsychiatric Schizophrenia
   Research
University of Copenhagen
Psychiatric Center Glostrup
Glostrup, Denmark

Christos Pantelis
Melbourne Neuropsychiatry Centre
Department of Psychiatry
The University of Melbourne and
Melbourne Health
Melbourne, Victoria, Australia

George N Papadimitriou
First Department of Psychiatry
Athens University Medical School
Eginition Hospital
Athens, Greece

Steve Peterson
Center for Ethics at the Washington
   Hospital Center
MedStar Health
Washington, DC, USA

Georgios Petrides
Psychiatry Research Division
The Zucker Hillside Hospital
North Shore-LIJ Health System
Glen Oaks, New York, USA

Sara Pozzoli
Department of Clinical Psychiatry
University of Milan
Fondazione IRCCS
Ospedale Maggiore Policlinico,
   Mangiagalli e Regina Elena
Milan, Italy

John Rabun
St. Louis Psychiatric Rehabilitation Center
Saint Louis, Missouri, USA

Hans Rasmussen
Center for Neuropsychiatric Schizophrenia
   Research
University of Copenhagen
Psychiatric Center Glostrup
Glostrup, Denmark

Denise Razzouk
The London School of Economics and
   Political Science
London, UK

Michael Riedel
Department of Psychiatry
University of Munich
Munich, Germany

Gabriele Sachs
Department of Psychiatry and
    Psychotherapy
Medical University of Vienna
Vienna, Austria

Pilar A Saiz
Department of Psychiatry - CIBERSAM
University of Oviedo
Oviedo, Spain

Alexandra Schosser
MRC SGDP Centre
Institute of Psychiatry
King's College London
London, UK
and
Department of Psychiatry
Medical University of Vienna
Vienna, Austria

Jack Schwartz
Center for Ethics at the Washington
    Hospital Center
MedStar Health
Washington, DC, USA

Steve Selinger
Center for Ethics at the Washington
    Hospital Center
MedStar Health
Washington, DC, USA

Costas N Stefanis
University Mental Health Research
    Institute
Athens, Greece

Nick C Stefanis
University Mental Health Research
    Institute
and First Department
    of Psychiatry
Athens University Medical School
Eginition Hospital
Athens, Greece

Johann Steiner
Department of Psychiatry
University of Magdeburg
Magdeburg, Germany

Thomas Stompe
Department of Psychiatry and Psychotherapy
Medical University of Vienna
Vienna, Austria

Florence Thibaut
Department of Psychiatry
University Hospital Ch Nicolle
INSERM U 614
University of Medicine
Rouen, France

Annemarie Unger
Department of Psychiatry and
    Psychotherapy
Medical University of Vienna
Vienna, Austria

Evangelos Vassos
Division of Psychological Medicine and
    Psychiatry
Institute of Psychiatry
King's College Hospital
London, UK

Joseph Ventura
Department of Psychiatry and Behavioural
    Sciences
University of California Los Angeles
Los Angeles, California, USA

Johannes Wancata
Department of Psychiatry and
    Psychotherapy
Medical University of Vienna
Vienna, Austria

Murat Yücel
Department of Psychiatry
Melbourne Neuropsychiatry Centre
The University of Melbourne and
    Melbourne Health
Melbourne, Victoria, Australia

Introduction to Schizophrenia, 2nd edition

Schizophrenia, as a disease, and as a field of study, is shrouded with a large number of misunderstandings. However, patients and their relatives suffering from the disease have only one aim: to cure the disease as fast and efficient as possible. In general, patients with schizophrenia are overwhelmed by the complexity of the problems emerging with the disease, so are their relatives and caregivers. As the knowledge of the diagnosis, neurobiology, and pharmacological treatment strategies has expanded over the past years, we aim to summarize the current knowledge in this handbook.

The current edition covers the biopsychosocial approaches and current challenges of this disease. The chapters written by leading experts from all over the world cover diagnosis and psychopathology, neurobiology, pharmacological treatment strategies, nonpharmacological treatment, as well as the role of schizophrenia in the society.

Schizophrenia is a disease of the brain, and it is worthwhile to emphasize that it is a real (physical) disease like diabetes, epilepsy, or high blood pressure. However, in the medical community, schizophrenia is sometimes not viewed with the same methodological rigor like the latter diseases. In contrast to diabetes, epilepsy, or high blood pressure, there is less tolerance and understanding in the society when someone suffers from schizophrenia. Community studies revealed that a number of people think that schizophrenia is not a real disease and that it is more related to an irritable personality as a result of a trauma in early life or the result of an unfavorable social environment. However, intensive research in the field of neurobiology, including genetic and epigenetic factors, as well as brain abnormalities and biochemical alterations, provides us a different understanding, which will be dealt with in this handbook as well.

Since the first edition, pharmacological treatment strategies have expanded, and now, a number of more refined treatment strategies are available for both acute and long-term treatment of schizophrenia, including first episodes. The nonpharmacological treatment includes psychosocial and cognitive rehabilitation as well as specific psychotherapeutic approaches and aspects that need to be considered in transcultural psychiatry. How to overcome stigma as well as the role of violence and forensic issues in schizophrenia are discussed together with patient rights and ethical issues.

The chapters aim to reach an audience comprising of physicians and basic scientists in various psychiatric specialties as well as doctors of neurology and aim to be of importance in public health considerations. The book should also be of interest to policy makers who seek a comprehensive and current spectrum as well as treatment implications of this disorder. We sincerely believe our volume will prove to be attractive not only to individual practitioners but also to libraries/repositories of schizophrenia-related research knowledge around the world.

Siegfried Kasper and George N Papadimitriou

1 Schizophrenia: Historical roots and brief review of recent research developments

Costas N Stefanis and Nick C Stefanis

HISTORICAL ROOTS

The historiography of schizophrenia is built on rather shaky ground. The core problem is schizophrenia itself, which, even now, is defined operationally, is encroached by neighboring entities, and still lacks identity validation. True, some things are taken as certain: we know schizophrenia's god-father, and there is agreement on who should be regarded as its father. The father's kinship is also known (most of the German School of Psychiatry in the late 19th and early 20th century), as are their forebears (most of the early 19th century French School).

One imponderable issue is whether schizophrenia, as conceived now, had existed in antiquity or is a fairly recent phenomenon, caused by industrialization, urbanization and related socio-cultural factors since the 19th century. Answering the "persistency' versus 'recency" conundrum might shed light on the origins and nature of schizophrenia.

Methodological Issues—Limitations

Written records—fragmentary and incomplete at best—give rise to controversial theories, so it is hard to determine the genesis of schizophrenia and reconstruct its initial clinical picture:

1. Original written sources are scarce, not easily accessible, and often abstruse.
2. Most ancient writings refer to lists, instead of patterns of symptoms.
3. Social milieus largely determined whether a person's mental status was seen as normal or in need of medical care, as deviance to be confined or demonic or divine possession.
4. Only conspicuous symptoms were seen as components of mental disorder in antiquity.
5. Societal demands imposed on lay individuals were less stringent in pre-modern agricultural societies. Symptoms of schizophrenia now evaluated as light, soft or negative, may perhaps have existed always, remaining latent: undetectable and unrecorded.

Ancient and Medieval Societies

The existence of mental disorders was acknowledged in Pharaonic Egypt as part of the prevailing religious conception of life-cycles. Treatment consisted in propitiating benevolent supernatural forces and the departed spirit of the dead, who were invoked to grant a cure.

In India the body was deemed separate from the immortal soul, with passions (within) and darkness (outside) causing mental illness. Scholars suggest that symptoms listed are not unlike those on which our diagnostic definitions of schizophrenia and bipolar disorders are based.

Four types of insanity are found in Ayurveda and the Caraka Sa hit Sutra (6th c. BC): the first three resembling mania, depression or catatonia, and schizophrenia respectively, the fourth comprising symptoms of the previous three. A fifth type, closely resembling the third, and associated with demonic possession, was held to be incurable if chronic and inherited.

Chinese culture exhibited more naturalistic concepts with ethical dimensions regarding insanity. Loss of face was listed among causative factors, treatment, however, was the priest's prerogative, who acted as an intermediary in propitiating the spirit of the ancestor.

In cuneiform tablets we find the oldest documented testimony of the existence of insanity, with frequent references to mental disorders in Assyria. According to the persistence, advocates symptom descriptions in Babylonian records are irrefutable evidence of the existence of schizophrenia.

In the Talmud and in the old and New Testament there are frequent references to madness with symptoms similar to those in the current clinical picture of psychotic disorders. In Judaic culture their origin was not attributed solely to evil spirits but also to the individual's moral behavior; psychotic disorders were thus construed as punishment by divine decree.

In ancient Greece mental disorders were recognized early and their origin was much debated by playwrights, philosophers and physicians. Divine forces were implicated in the earlier writings. A totally naturalistic, wholly medical approach was initiated by the Hippocratic school in Kos (1). Hippocrates systematized the description of symptoms and, by adopting clinical diagnostic criteria, grouped symptoms into distinct nosological entities. At some point he explains: "by the same organ we become mad and delirious, and fears and terrors assail us some by night and some by day... All these things we endure from the brain when it is not healthy". Yet, he also regards imbalances of the four humors as differential causative factors of the mental disorders he acknowledges: mania, melancholia and phrenitis. He mentions paranoia too, as an ill-defined subcategory, though no clear-cut schizophrenia-like entity. His four humors theory was superseded: its last fervent advocate was the Cappadocian physician, Aretaeus; but two of his terms, mania and melancholia, have stood the test of time.

Galen revived partly Hippocratic taxonomy. Apart from inserting psychological insights into melancholia, Galen subsumed in it several additional symptoms that bring it closer to schizophrenia phenotypy.

Most of the available information on mental illness in the Middle Ages derives from religious sources: given the prevailing social ambience of the era, particularly in Central and Western Europe, it is loaded with bias and superstition. It was not only that church authorities saw every deviance as witchcraft and demon possession, subject to the death penalty; there were also outbreaks of the plague and extreme poverty limiting life expectancy, obscuring thus a rational and humane approach to mental disorders. There was hardly any change in the situation in the early Renaissance. Indeed, the Inquisition established by the church and guided by Malleus Maleficarum, the treatise on witchcraft, intensified the persecution of those individuals, particularly women, thought of as being inspired by the devil in their posture or behavior. (2–8)

By the 16th century most of the extant writings of the classical era were translated: as reason replaced religious fanaticism, attitudes toward the mentally ill began to change. The great figure of the time, Paracelsus maintained that mental illnesses were due to the loss of reason, with a tendency to heritability (3, 4, 7). Behavioral aberrations, at least partly fitting today's descriptions of mania and schizophrenia, were recognized as illnesses requiring care. Thus, in several parts of Europe institutions for the treatment of 'lunatics' were set up long before the Asylum period of the 18th and 19th century.

Willis, an English anatomist and physician, described the symptomatology in several cases and distinguished 'foolishness' from 'stupidity'. For some (5), his description fits the clinical picture of simple or dementia praecox schizophrenia: others disagree (9).

The Enlightenment—The Dawn of Psychiatry

The end of the enlightenment, was the beginning of the history of schizophrenia, as currently recognized. Toward the close of the 18th century an inquisitive and progressive young physician by the name of Philippe Pinel was appointed head of the Bicêtre Hospital in 1793, and head of the Salpêtrière Hospital two years later. While at Bicêtre, he was engaged in applying his reformist ideas by improving inpatients' living conditions and initiating novel, more humane approaches to the treatment of the insane, since then known as moral therapy. He secured his name in history as the man of 'one act', by unchaining mentally ill inmates, and of 'one book', the text-book "*Traité médico-philosophique; ou la manie*" published in 1801 (10). He was celebrated among his contemporaries for his book and by historians for his act (11). Until recently though, history had ignored the man who stood behind the act and sought to turn Asylums from custodial into therapeutic institutions. He was Jean-Baptiste Pussin, a tuner by profession, who was admitted at Bicêtre as a medical case and a few years later, after been declared cured, was posted as supervisor (head-nurse of sorts) at the mentally disturbed patients' section of the Hospital. He suggested and implemented, admittedly with Philippe Pinel's consent, the 'breaking of the chains' and the humane reforms at Bicêtre. A nine-page manuscript discovered by Wiener in the French State Archives, provides a detailed record of his initiatives and actions at Bicêtre and Salpêtrière— stressing particularly his belief than only if trust were established between staff and patients, was treatment feasible (12). Pinel, on the other hand, with his cross-sectional, syndromal approach to the diagnosis of insanity which he used as a criterion for the admission of patients to the Asylum, was a pioneer in the diagnosis and classification of the major psychiatric disorders. His proposed classification of mental disorders into four categories (mania, melancholia, degeneration and imbecility), expanded by Jean-Étienne Dominique Esquirol, (13) with the addition of a fifth category, partial insanity (folie partielle), laid the foundation of the French school of Psychiatry (2, 4, 7, 8, 14).

Pinel's and Esquirol's fame outshone the contribution made toward reforming Asylums into Therapeutic Institutions by several non-French alienists, including Vincenzo Chiarugi at the Bonifacio Asylum in Florence (the first to 'unchain' the insane), William Battie at St. Luke's, John Haslam at Bethlem in London, and the Tuke family in York (2, 4, 7, 8, 15).

In the diagnostic field, the 'syndromal' approach advanced by Pinel and Esquirol was widely accepted not as theoretical dogma but rather as a clinical convenience. Although heredity was often quoted in the writings of practically all alienists of the time (including the Salpêtrière group) as a possible contributing factor to madness (la folie), systematic research on etiology and pathogenetic causes was not their primary interest. In the early twenties of the 19th century a dissertation by a young physician named Antoine Bayle, a collaborator of Esquirol, caused quite a stir in Salpêtrière. Bayle provided evidence that in mental patients who also presented neurosyphilis paralytic phenomena there was an association of the clinical symptomatology with lesions in the Central Nervous System and specifically in the meninges (16). This was a landmark discovery that showed the direct relationship of a mental symptom with identified brain lesions. Still, Bayle's only reward was a reference to his thesis in Esquirol's *"Maladies Mentales"*.

Bénédict-Augustin Morel's theory of degeneration had a great impact on French Psychiatry. In *"Demence Precoce"* he distinguished the evolutionary degeneration process mainly afflicting young persons, from congenital idiocy. He took this type of degeneration to be hereditary, passed on to the offspring in subsequent generations until extinction (2, 8, 17). He might have preceded Kraepelin and Bleuler in their conceptualization of schizophrenia, had he limited his theory to a particular and distinct mental disorder rather than expanding it to cover biological degeneration in general (15).

Another eminent physician at Salpêtrière, Jean-Pierre Falret, owes his place in the history of Psychiatry to having established, with Baillarger, the clinical concept of 'circular insanity' (folie circulaire), in which depression alternates with excessive mood elevation (mania). He had thus preceded Kraepelin, who at the end of the century separated affective disorders, including Manic-Depressive Illness from 'Dementia praecox' (18).

Valentin Magnan, yet another historical figure of French Psychiatry, initially joined the Falret research team at Salpêtrière and later got the post of 'Maitre' of the Admissions Department at Sainte-Anne Asylum where he was examining thousands of patients, deciding whether Asylum admission was indicated or not. Like Falret, he was biologically orientated regarding the etiology of mental disorders. His extensive study, with Lasègue and Falret, on the classification of psychotic patients advanced the notion of subdividing delusional states into acute (bouffée délirante) and chronic (délire chronique systématique). Failing to get a university position, Magnan began lecturing at Sainte-Anne: his lectures were published in 1891. He is chiefly associated with 'chronic' systematical delusional states, an entity that was considered 'demence precoce', from Morel's reference. Kraepelin and Bleuler merged the former of Magnan's subdivisions with dementia praecox and the latter with schizophrenia, much to the chagrin of French Psychiatry, which only recently agreed that it be included in international classifications as part of schizophrenia (8, 14, 15).

Then the focus in clinical research of mental disorders shifted to German speaking countries in Central Europe, which dominated European Psychiatric thinking until the mid-20th century. This may have been due to their state-based decentralized administrative governance that fostered University Departments and Clinics combining patient care with training and research.

Among clinical investigators in the pre-Kraepelin era, we should single out Wilhelm Griesinger who established a Neuro-Psychiatric Clinic at the 'Charité' General Hospital in Berlin. Griesinger is rightly held to be the founder of Neuropsychiatry. He divided the clinic into two sections, for patients with neurological and with psychiatric illnesses. This model gave staff the opportunity to acquire clinical experience with a great range of clinical manifestations in psychotic and nonpsychotic patients, rarely seen in an Asylum, and to follow closely the course of their illness. It also provided staff and trainees with an opportunity to gain experience and establish a clinical cross-talk with other medical departments, to their mutual benefit. The Griesinger Charité Clinic implemented what is now known as consultation-liaison Psychiatry in a hospital setting (19). In his belief that all psychiatric disorders stem from the brain with a hereditary susceptibility, Griesinger was an organicist, and he espoused Heinrich Neumann's unitary concept of psychosis (einheit psychose); yet, for him symptomatology was contextual to patients' cultural milieu and experience in life. Griesinger's heritage to Psychiatry is his model for Academic Institutions of Psychiatry, widely adopted in Germany and elsewhere.

Schizophrenia's Early History

In 1863, five years before Griesinger's death at 51, the first of the two 'grandfathers' of schizophrenia arrived on the scene: Karl Kahlbaum published a book contesting Neumann's 'einheit psychose' theory, arguing that there are several distinct groups of psychosis.

He described cases in which motor symptoms prevailed, differentiating them from other psychoses (insanities). He named this distinct clinical entity Catatonia (20). Soon after, a young colleague by the name of Ewald Hecker joined him at the Clinic. Together they came to the conclusion that psychoses had to be looked at as being a composite of distinct, clinical groups not only by dint of their symptomatology, but also on account of their course and outcome. Hecker published an article amplifying Kahlbaum's prior reference to a group of adolescents that developed a progressive type of insanity, and concretized this observation by supplying a detailed clinical account of its main features, the early onset, the particular symptomatology, and the progressive course to irreversible mental deterioration. He introduced the term hebephrenia, which was later incorporated by Kraepelin as a major subgroup of his 'dementia praecox' (21). Kahlbaum and Hecker may be deemed the 'grandfathers' of schizophrenia as it is currently conceived, albeit other clinicians elsewhere, were quite active at the same period in the diagnosis and classification of schizophrenia. T. Glouston of Edinburgh University, described adolescent insanity in 1873, in terms very similar to hebephrenia and even related it to neurodevelopmental abnormalities (22).

Emil Kraepelin is generally acknowledged as the father of schizophrenia for describing it, though not naming it. His term 'dementia praecox' did not last, chiefly for being too close to Morel's old term, 'demence precoce'. He was first appointed Professor of Psychiatry in Estonia, later in Stuttgart and finally in Munich, at the Royal University Clinic, the oldest of its kind in Germany. That was when he introduced his concept of 'dementia praecox', in the 5th edition of his *"Kompendium der Psychiatrie"* by grouping together disparate groups of mental patients whose illness complied with the following criteria: early onset of psychotic symptomatology and progressive course to terminal dementia. He disregarded cause and he emphasized evolution. He was above all a bed-side clinical empiricist. His entire work was based on a meticulous study of the case histories of the Clinic's patients. It was on this clinical ground that he differentiated the affective states from dementia praecox and introduced the term 'Manic-depression' as a distinct entity. His theoretical standing among the various cause-related trends in Psychiatry was neutral and often grossly misconceived. Many Freudians still consider him the founder of a school of psychiatry that leaves the person out: that does not see patients but only cases to be labeled and classified. (23)

The truth is that Kraepelin and Freud, both born in the same year, German speaking, and living not far from one another, never crossed paths.

Biologically oriented psychiatrists, on the other hand, claim that by ignoring biological causal mechanisms, Kraepelin setback research in the field. The truth is that he did not expect to resolve the causal mystery of dementia praecox through brain pathology. Still, he did invite E. Nissle and Aloys Alzheimer to his clinic and make them his close associates, who were the most renowned Nervous System histologists of the time. Kraepelin was not unreceptive to criticism. When the irreversibility of dementia praecox, his core assumption, was challenged, he conceded that a rather small percentage of his patients did not in fact end up with dementia, though they retained some of the symptoms for life. To his three main subgroups (hebephrenia, catatonia and paranoia) he added a separate one that he called paraphrenia and, some years later, even agreed to recognize Bleuler's 'Schizophrenia simple' as a distinct entity.

With Eugen Bleuler, the god-father of schizophrenia, we come to the close of our survey of schizophrenia's historical roots (24). Bleuler was born one year after Kraepelin and Freud, and while acknowledging Kraepelin as his teacher, broke away from the latter's fundamental views on the illness. Bleuler acquired world fame (and reputation) for coining the term schizophrenia, and for his 1911 book "*Dementia Praecox oder die Gruppen der Schizophrenien*", where he contested most of the pillars on which Kraepelin had built his concept of dementia praecox. Bleuler questioned both the early onset and the progressive terminating to dementia. By proposing his primary symptoms, known as the four A's, he played down Kraepelin's symptomatology. His approach to diagnosis was syndromal, based on the patient's presented symptoms, thus avoiding the ascription to schizophrenia of disease status. He particularly emphasized the importance of thought processes and the emotional state of the patient. It is his view that patients with a given type of schizophrenia, primarily present a loosening of their association leading to the splitting (spaltung) of the mind, a misnomer that persisted for nearly a century.

Bleuler was not a formalist: indeed he attached primary significance to the content of the symptoms rather than to their descriptive attributes. As a consequence he introduced an hierarchical order in symptomatology with a weighted listing of symptoms. His views on diagnosis did not come as an epiphany, but were the result of long years of deliberation in which a Freudian influence was more than apparent. Burghölzli University Clinic, headed by Bleuler, was the first, and, at the time, the only Academic Institution that opened its doors to Freudian psychoanalysis. Freud himself admitted as much in his book on the "*History of the Psychoanalytic Movement*". The scope of Freudian influence on Bleuler's concepts about schizophrenia was evident even in his everyday professional work. In a letter to Freud he confessed that he, his wife and the clinic staff held daily sessions analyzing their dreams. In such a frame of mind perhaps, Freud's pathways of internal conflict and irrational associations may have led him to coin the term 'schizophrenia' (25).

Kraepelin's and Bleuler's impact on modern Psychiatry is enormous, particularly with regard to schizophrenia and related psychosis in both clinical practice and research. Any attempt to improve diagnostic or classification schemes revolves around these two figures and entails the adoption, rejection, or revision of their views, of which nobody can remain heedless.

Recency versus Persistency

A few remarks on the question raised in the introduction of 'recency' vs 'persistency' deem necessary.

Recency theory was advanced mainly by philosophers and historians, such as Michel Foucault, whose 1964 book, '*Histoire de la folie*', soon became the 'sacred text' against the medicalization of schizophrenia (26). He argued that schizophrenia is no illness but the ploy of rising capitalism (in tandem with industrialization and urbanization) to fill Asylums with deviants who pose a nuisance to a society greedy for profit. The massive influx into Asylums, which he calls the 'grand confinement' marked the genesis of insanity and, by extension, of schizophrenia as an illness. His views were embraced and advanced by a wide range of intellectuals and gained a hold over public opinion. They were also adopted by a few psychiatrists, such as Szasz in the US, (27) and a group led by Laing in the UK, whose impact on the clinical and research level of psychiatry was limited. Still, in the US, with the psychiatric community sharing the Analytical School's scorn of diagnosis and classification, resistance to these theories was low key, paving the way to their glorification by Hollywood in films such as "One flew over the cuckoo's nest", that spread the message that psychiatric illness is social deviance in different garb. Shorter's excellent book "*A History of Psychiatry*" (8) aptly illustrates these developments and the prevailing climate in the US and elsewhere, which fostered the Antipsychiatry Movement. Admittedly, theories of the asylogenic origin of schizophrenia, did have some beneficial effects on the professional and organizational quality of care systems for the mentally ill, fostering the deinstitutionalization movement and the establishment of community based services. Still, it is ironic that these theories would flourish just when the revolution brought about by the introduction of pharmacotherapy of schizophrenia and related psychoses, resulted in the exodus *en masse* of patients from mental institutions.

A more moderate approach, linked chronicity—rather than recency to industrialization—instead of—institutionalization—in industrialized societies (28, 29). A more medical and clinical approach advocating the recency hypothesis was Torrey's study implicating viral infection etiology of schizophrenia, linked to the rise of urbanization and population density in the 19th century (29). Hare expanded Torrey's views further (9). Their case is strengthened by the argument that, unlike depression and mania, there was no vivid written description for schizophrenia prior to the 19th century.

The hypothesis advocating the persistency of schizophrenia is based on writings that refer to persons, even in antiquity, who presented schizophrenia symptoms in their overt behavior, as well as to the existence of treatment facilities for affected persons. This view was more or less held in common by all the established authorities, Kraepelin and Bleuler included, and was defended persuasively by Jeste and Bark (5, 6). A quasi-Darwinian evolutionary biological 'speciation' theory has been proposed in recent years by Crow, arguing that schizophrenia has always existed, closely linked with epigenetic changes that led *homo sapiens* (endowed with the capacity of language) to split off from other hominids (30).

The third school is neutral toward the other two, not dismissing the likelihood of biological or environmental factors being involved in schizophrenia's origin and pathogenesis. It accepts variation of incidence of schizophrenia across cultures and over time from antiquity to our days.

No definitive conclusion can be drawn from our review on the historical roots of schizophrenia regarding the recency and persistency theories of its origin, because methodological limitations preclude reliable, evidence-based comparisons between disparate views, even should the etiology and pathogenesis of schizophrenia be established unequivocally—which is highly unlikely. Our adherence to any of the hypotheses proposed would still be based on flimsy evidence. That said, a few critical comments might be warranted.

Negativistic theories of schizophrenia's nonexistence or, at best, of its asylogenic origin, are in their majority literary essays based on meager and questionable documentation. The 'grand confinement' to Asylums in the 19th century and consequent schizophrenogenic institutionalism is hardly consistent with available statistics that indicate patients' admission rates were almost equally distributed in highly industrialized and rural regions of Europe. The viral and urbanization hypothesis may not be discarded in view of recent findings from epidemiological immunological and genetic population density interaction studies.

The 'persistence' hypothesis appears to be rather persuasive based on written descriptive data from antiquity to the 19th century. However, a case for schizophrenia as a distinct entity, as we perceive it today, cannot be made reliably by reference to schizophrenia-like symptoms, the more so when the symptoms described either lack specificity or are subsumed under other entities. Further historical documentation is needed to reduce the chronological gap.

The third hypothesis seems to be the most plausible, since, by being neutral to the other two, it espouses the notion that schizophrenia is fluctuating cross-culturally and over time (transgenerationally): that it is not unalterable from antiquity to our time, but shows variation in presenting symptoms, with social conception and tolerability affecting its detectability and recognition. Foremost among such variances, those deriving from diverse diagnostic theories and procedures are mainly accountable for observed discrepancies in rates, even if structured diagnostic tools are employed. This was best exemplified, in 1971 by the well known Joint British-American study comparing diagnostic practices between psychiatrists in both countries (31). The findings were astonishing. A great percentage of patients received disparate diagnoses. In the same patients schizophrenia was more often diagnosed in the US and Manic Depression illness in the UK. Americans held more of a Bleulerian outlook, according to DSM-II criteria, and the British more of a Kraepelinian one. Were Kraepelinian and Bleulerian criteria to be applied retrospectively to former and ancient times for reconstructing schizophrenia diagnoses, the magnitude of diagnostic discrepancies would be inconceivable.

Closing Remarks

With the introduction of the Current Diagnostic and Classification Systems, diagnostic reliability is claimed to have substantially increased mainly in Clinical Research, but validity is still lacking and utility both in research and clinical practice is still questionable. The adopted operational diagnostic criteria arranged in a multiaxial system supposedly are syndrome rather than illness oriented, atheoretical, free of etiological inferences, hierarchical axis dependent but not symptom weighted. It is rather a mixed construct, currently under revision. Issues and dilemmas for restructuring the existing DSM-IV and ICD-10 are plenty. Should schizophrenia diagnosis be categorically spectrum or distinct subgrouping oriented, symptom weighted or not, open to neuroscience inputs or strictly atheoretical, are just a few of the dilemmas. Even its name is at issue with controversial proposals in the literature for either retaining or changing it steadily increasing. It would be ironic to hold another plebiscite to decide. (32–37).

RECENT RESEARCH DEVELOPMENTS (GENETICS & IMAGING)

The rapid advances being made in the past few years in all fields of science, Neuroscience in particular, empowered Psychiatric research in Schizophrenia with new investigative tools for exploring the brain neurobiological and neurocognitive processes underlying the clinical symptomatology of the disorder. The fertile ground from which it is currently anticipated that new exciting findings in schizophrenia may spring up, is among others as Neuropsychopharmacology, Neurogenetics and Neuroimaging. The literature on both these fields is vast and thus we will confine our contribution to highlighting the latest developments in the two fields by brief comments and references of interest for further reading.

Neurogenetics

The etiology of schizophrenia remains as elusive as ever. While there are clear recognized environmental contributors to disease, it is also clear that genetic predisposition is the major determinant of who develops schizophrenia. Heritability estimates are as high as 80% (38, 39), placing schizophrenia amongst the most heritable of common diseases. Similar to other disorders with complex inheritance, it appears that at least a substantial proportion of the genetic variance results from alleles of small effect (multiple common alleles in the population contributing small-to-moderate additive or multiplicative effects). Attempts to discover such common alleles that relate directly to schizophrenia have only very recently been productive but point to very small odds ratios for individual susceptibility polymorphisms (40).

In the first years of the twenty first century several candidate susceptibility genes were identified on the basis of an initial report of linkage, and for some of these, for example dysbindin (DTNBP1) neuregulin 1 (NRG1) D-amino oxidase activator (DAOA) and Disrupted in Schizophrenia 1 (DISC1) although the evidence is not decisive, there is a substantial amount of support from follow-up studies. Intriguingly it is increasingly clear that there is considerable overlap in genetic susceptibility across the traditional binary classification of psychosis, judging from evidence that most of these genes may also influence susceptibility to bipolar disorder or clusters of mixed affective-non affective phenotypes (41).

Rapid developments in microarray technologies as well as the representation of the majority of common genetic variation in the genome by genotyping a selected set of tagging SNPs, has led to the emergence of hypothesis-free genome-wide association studies (GWAS). To date, there have been seven GWAS of schizophrenia: although not supportive for the involvement of the first generation susceptibility genes, they have either led to no obvious common variant candidates (42, 43) or pinpointed several novel susceptibility genes such as reelin (RELN) gene (44) and ZNF804A (40) that have often surpassed predetermined level of significance in multiple tested samples. While the results of these studies await further replication, it is clear that the GWAS methodology has brought unexpected reward by highlighting the involvement of copy number variants (CNV) in the aetiology of schizophrenia. CNVs are segments of DNA ranging from 1 kilobase (kb) to several megabases (Mb), and can be readily identified in GWAS, even if they occur in only one or a few subjects. The role of CNVs in schizophrenia was initially less well anticipated, since CNVs were thought to be more important in autism spectrum disorders and certain forms of mental retardation. Five genome-wide screens for large CNVs have appeared within the last few years, latest by Need et al., (43), providing unequivocal evidence for the involvement of such genomic structures in the susceptibility to schizophrenia, albeit in a small minority of cases, around 1%. It remains to be seen, which of these paradigms (common disease common-variant hypothesis vs common-disease-rare variant hypothesis) will bear more fruit in the years to come.

Despite recent advances in the genetic basis of schizophrenia the failure to identify responsible genes beyond any doubt can be attributed in part to not incorporating environmental measures of risk that may interact synergistically with susceptibility genes into the study design. This genotype- environmental interaction (G x E) approach poses a causal role not for genes or the environment in isolation but rather for their synergistic coparticipation in the cause of psychosis, where the effect of one is conditional on the other (European Network of Schizophrenia Networks for the Study of Gene-Environment Interactions) (45). G x E seems a particularly suitable approach for understanding the development of psychosis because this phenotype is known to be associated with environmentally mediated risks (high rates of schizo-phrenia in large cities, immigrant populations, traumatized individuals and canna-bis users) yet people display considerable heterogeneity in their response to those environmental exposures.(37). For the time being, the bulk of the evidence for gene-environment interactions is from epidemiological research using indirect measures of genetic risk such as positive family history or high scores of psychosis proneness measures. To date there are four replications of gene—urbanicity interaction (46) and at least two of gene-cannabis interaction (47, 48). These important early findings are now being extended to studies using direct molecular genetic measures of genetic variation in schizophrenia and psychosis proneness (49–52). The European Network of Schizophrenia Networks for the Study of Gene-Environment Interactions (45) has recently reviewed the evidence on G x E interaction in schizophrenia, and alerts to the urgent need for well documented large scale G x E studies that may provide a new promising framework for unraveling the complex etiology, severity and course of this enigmatic disorder.

Neuroimaging

Schizophrenia was one of the first targeted psychiatric disorders for imaging studies. The first report on the subject by computer tomography (CT) (53), showing enlarged brain ventricles in patients with schizophrenia compared to healthy controls was fol-lowed by hundreds of publications on the subject. The remarkable subsequent tech-nological advances in neuroimaging with the introduction of Magnetic Resonance Imaging (MRI), Functional Magnetic Resonance Imaging (fMR), fMRI spectroscopy, Diffusion Tensor Imaging (DTI), Magnetization Transfer Imaging (MTI), Single Photon Emission Computer Tomography (SPECT), Positron Emission Tomography (PET) and other innovations in hyperscanning, have offered new insights into the pathophysiol-ogy of this enigmatic disorder.

Two meta-analyses of MRI volumetric studies in schizophrenia have largely con-firmed earlier individual reports showing that patients with schizophrenia have smaller regional brain volumes in relation to age-matched healthy volunteers (54, 55). The dif-ference was more pronounced in hippocampus and amygdala. The application of voxel-based MRI (VBM) method to identify brain Gray Matter Density (GMD) has confirmed GMD decreases, which mainly occur in the temporal and frontal regions and the tha-lamus (56). According to two other meta-analyses, such GMD decreases are found not only in chronic, but also in first episode patients, and may be due to neurodevelopmental alterations or to an active, progressive neurodegenerative process (57), and similar struc-tural abnormalities, more pronounced in the hippocampus, also occur in nonaffected first-degree relatives (58).

Two very recent additional VBM studies merit particular attention due mainly to the large size of the participant subject groups. In the first one, GMD decreases in schizophrenic patients' siblings were slight, but occurred in the same brain regions as in the patients. Only the GMD decreases in the patients' group achieved statistical significance (59). The second study, a multi-site collaborative effort, has confirmed regional decreases in brain volume in superior temporal, inferior frontal, cingulated and fusiform gyri in patients with schizophrenia compared to controls, taking into account confounding factors, i.e. interactions between scanners and the effect of par-ticipating group differences (60).

Several research centers are involved in prospective volumetric studies. We will refer to three of them as being more representative and new. The Edinburgh study showed significant decline in gray matter density in the high risk group for schizophrenia, more pronounced in the temporal, the right frontal and the parietal lobes (61). Those who latter developed schizophrenia differed from those that did not in the spatial distribution of GMD pairs.

The Swiss group (62) applied even broader inclusion criteria for High Risk Schizophrenia (HRSx) in their prospective longitudinal study. All three groups, i.e. HRSx who developed Sx, HRSx who did not, and patients with a first episode of Sx displayed volumetric abnormalities, with GMD decreases compared to controls in the left insula, superior and medial temporal lobe and cingulate gyrus. Within the HRSx groups, those who developed psychosis had greater GMD decrease than those who did not. There were no differences between the HRSx groups and the first episode group. These volumetric findings were interpreted as vulnerability markers for the development of schizophrenia. The Melbourne group (63–65) have coined the term "Ultra High Risk" (UHR) in their prospective, longitudinal studies investigating neuroimaging and neuroanatomical correlates of psychosis. Their inclusion criteria for the HRSx are clinical and are the broadest compared to the two previous groups, including not only family history, but also attenuated psychotic symptomatology, brief psychotic episodes, schizotypical personality and recent functional decline, thus enriching the sample of UHR subjects. From this extensive work, they have concluded that there are few definitive markers that enable distinction of the UHR subjects who develop schizophrenia from those who do not. Neither hippocampal volume nor ventricular size were found to predict transition to the onset of the schizophrenic disorder. The decline of GM volume in prefrontal regions and anterior cingulate cortex are promising predictors, particularly if they are combined with prefrontal lobe-specific cognitive measurements, but they are not definitive. Extensive neuroanatomical changes, particularly in the medial temporal and frontal regions, were however observed during the course of the study in those UHR subjects who later developed schizophrenia. Speculatively, the group proposed genetic and/or other endogenous mechanisms, prolonged premorbid stress and other environmental mechanisms underlying the transition of UHR subjects toward schizophrenia onset.

In an attempt to discern genetic from environmental contribution to the development of schizophrenia, Lui et al., (66) investigated differences in GM by VBM between patients with schizophrenia who had and those who did not have a family history of the disease. They found that familial schizophrenia is associated with more severe GM abnormalities than sporadic schizophrenia, in several brain regions, particularly in the thalamus.

Supplementary to GM decrease, neuroimaging investigations in schizophrenia have also focused on the white matter (WM), based on the plausible assumption that disturbed connectivity may underlie schizophrenia pathology (67). The newly developed techniques of diffusion tensor imaging (DTI) and magnetic transfer imaging (MTI) provide new technical possibilities to directly investigate such connectivity abnormalities. Reviewing the available literature, Conrad and Winterer (68) concluded that there wasn't sufficient evidence yet for such WM abnormalities in schizophrenia.

Regarding functional radiotracer imaging, only Dopamine (DA) and Serotonin (5HT) receptors have thus far been adequately studied in schizophrenia with rather selective radiotracers. Due to the pronounced blocking effect of antipsychotic agents on DA receptors, it was anticipated that an increase of DA neurotransmission would be shown in schizophrenia. However, this has not been borne out. Only a few studies have found a significant increase of D2/3 dopaminergic synaptic activity in the basal ganglia of patients with schizophrenia, while most studies have reported marginal, nonsignificant changes (69).

However, two studies are worth citing in this respect. In one, caudate D2 receptor was upregulated in both affected and nonaffected monozygotic twins compared to affected and nonaffected dizygotic twins as well as to healthy twin pairs. It was thus concluded that the D2 synaptic activation in schizophrenia is under genetic control (70). Even more interesting is a very recent PET-study in which elevated radio-labeled DA uptake in the associate striatum was found, both in patients with schizophrenia and subjects with prodromal symptoms. Although in the group with prodromal symptoms the uptake was lower relative to patients, the findings suggest that DA over activity predates the onset of schizophrenia (71).

Interesting findings derived recently from a Magnetoencephalography (MEG) study. The investigators reported, using a test that, by a sophisticated computational method, assesses the dynamic synchronous mental interactions, that they were able successfully to classify individual patients, among them eleven with schizophrenia, to their respective diagnostic category (72).

As already mentioned fMRI imaging technology has gradually displaced both SPECT and PET in schizophrenia research, predominantly in the field of imaging of sensory processing and control of action.

Earlier studies with fMRI comparing patients with schizophrenia and healthy controls showed large spatial distribution of activation in both groups, involving cortical and subcortical regions with the patient's group though exhibiting significantly reduced activation of dorsolateral prefrontal cortex (DLPC) during spatial working memory paradigms (73). A later study largely confirmed the wide spatial distribution of activation in both groups, though lesser in the DLPC in the patient's group during the information maintenance testing period (74). These results were interpreted as indicating decline of prefrontal function before the onset of illness and, by extension, as representing a vulnerability marker for developing psychotic disorders (75). More recent investigations have raised the concept of "insufficiency" of DPLC in patients with schizophrenia (76), or stressed an impairment of connectivity between DPLC and other brain regions, which was present not only in medicated-chronic patients, but also in nonmedicated first episode patients and, to a lesser extent, unaffected siblings (77).

What has emerged as a rather consistent finding from these studies is that brain structural, metabolic, and hemodynamic abnormalities do exist in patients with schizophrenia and at the group level they significantly differentiate them from healthy subjects. These findings though cannot be individualized and provide a diagnostic validity factor of schizophrenia due to significant overlapping: even more so since they are lacking regional specificity. However, despite the great variance in regional distribution, the regions most frequently reported as affected are, with or without lateralization, the temporal (medial), the prefrontal (dorsomedial) lobes, the Cingulate Cortex, the hippocampus and the lateral ventricles. There is no consensus on correspondence between regional deficiencies and cognitive impairments. However, the dorsolateral prefrontal and the cingulate cortices are frequently reported as being associated with working memory and executive impairment while hippocampus reportedly is more frequently associated with verbal memory deficits.

The reported findings from neuroimaging familial studies on schizophrenia are consistent with genetic contribution being involved in the origin and possibly in the evolution of the observed abnormalities. However, whether they qualify—as some of the authors claim—as schizophrenia 'endophenotypes' according to the Gottesman and Gould criteria, (78) is at this stage unclear. It is equally uncertain whether neuroimaging findings will acquire sufficient specificity and claim clinical relevance. Even so, they provide valuable information that enriches our insight into the pathophysiology of schizophrenia and serves as an additional stepping stone to enhance further research in the field.

REFERENCES

1. Hippocrates. The Medical Works of Hippocrates. Oxford, Blackwell; 1950.
2. Alexander FG, Selesnick ST: The History of Psychiatry: An Evaluation of Psychiatric Thought and Practice from Prehistoric Times to The Present. New York, Harper & Row; 1966.
3. Evans JL. Witchcraft, demonology and renaissance psychiatry. Med J Aust 1966; 11: 34–9.
4. Mora G. Historical and Theoretical Trends in Psychiatry. Comprehensive Textbook of Psychiatry ed Freedman H, Kaplan B, Sadock B eds Vol. Sed. Ed.: Williams Wilkins, 1975.
5. Jeste DV. Did schizophrenia exist before the eighteenth century? Comprehensive Psychiatry 1985; 26: 493–503.
6. Bark NM. On the history of schizophrenia. Evidence of its existence before 1800. NYS J Med 1988; 88: 374–83.
7. Kales A, Kales J, Vela-Bueno A. Schizophrenia: Historical Perspectives In Recent Advances In Schizophrenia. Eds. By Kales A, Stefanis C, and Tablott J. Springer Verlag, 1990: 3–23.
8. Shorter E. A History of Psychiatry. Wiley; 1997.
9. Hare E. Schizophrenia as a recent disease. BJP 1988; 153: 521–31.
10. Pinel P. Traité Medico-Philosophique sur l'Aliénation Mentale, ed 2. Paris, Richard, Caille et Ravier; 1809: 252–3 (first ed. 1801).
11. Swain Gladys. Le sujet de la folie. Naissance de la psychiatrie. Privat; 1977.
12. Wiener D. Philippe Pinel et l'abolition des chaims: un document retrovive. L'information Psyc; 1980.
13. Esquirol JED: Mental Maladies. New York, Hafner Press; 1965.
14. Ey H, Bernard P et Brisset Ch. Manuel de Psychiatrie. Masson et Cia; 1960.
15. Stefanis CN. On The Concept of Schizophrenia, In Recent Advances In Schizophrenia ed by Kales A, Stefanis C and Tablott J. Springer Verlag, 1990: 24–57.
16. Bayle AL. Description of General Paralysis, Paris, Didot le Jeune; 1822.
17. Morel BA. Traité de dégénérescenses physiques, intellectuelles et morales de l'espèce humaine. Paris, Bailliere; 1857.
18. Falret JP. Memoire sur la folie circulaire. Bulletin de l' Academie de Medicine 1854; 19: 382–415.
19. Griesinger W. Mental Pathology and Therapeutics. New York, Hafner Press; 1965.
20. Kahlbaum DL. Die Katatonie Oder Das Spannungsirresein. Berlin, Hirschwald; 1874.
21. Hecker E. Die hebephrenie. Arch Pathol Ant Physiol Klin Med 1871; 52: 394–429.
22. O'Connell P, Woodruff P, Wright I et al. Developmental insanity or dementia praecox: Was the wrong concept adopted? Schiz Res 1997; 23: 97–106.
23. Kraepelin E. Psychiatrie, 8th ed. Leipzig, JA Barth; 1915.
24. Bleuler E. Dementia Praecox Oder Die Gruppe Der Schizophrenien. Leipzig, Deuticke; 1911.
25. Dalzell TG. Eugen Bleuler 150: Bleuler's reception of Freud. History of Psychiatry 2007;18: 471–82.
26. Foucault M. Histoire de la folie. Plon; 1964.
27. Szasz T. The myth of mental illness: Foundations of A Theory of Personal Conduct. New York: Harper and Row; 1974.
28. Cooper J, Sartorius N. Cultural and temporal variations in schizophrenia: a speculation on the importance of industrialization. Br J Psychiatry 1977; 130: 50–5.
29. Torrey EF, Petersen MR. The viral hypothesis of schizophrenia. Schizophr Bull 1976; 2: 136–46.
30. Crow TJ. How and why genetic linkage has not solved the problem of psychosis: review and hypothesis. Am J Psychiatry 2007; 164: 13–21.
31. Kendell RE, Cooper J, Gourley A et al. Diagnostic criteria of American and British psychiatrists. Arch Gen Psychiatry 1971; 25: 123–30.
32. Kingdon DG, Kinoshita Y, Naeem F et al. Schizophrenia can and should be renamed. BMJ 2007; 221–2.

33. Kingdon DG, Gibson A, Turkington D et al. Acceptable terminology and subgroups in schizophrenia: an exploratory study. Soc Psychiatry Psychiatr Epidemiol 2008; 43: 239–43.

34. Lieberman JA, First MB. Renaming schizophrenia. BMJ 2007; 334: 108.

35. Sugiura T, Sakamoto S, Tanaka E et al. Labeling effect of Seishin-bunretsu-byou, the Japanese translation for schizophrenia: an argument for relabeling. Int J Soc Psychiatry 2001; 47: 43–51.

36. van Os J. A Salience dysregulation syndrome. Br J Psychiatry 2009; 194: 101–3.

37. van Os J, Linscott RJ, Myin-Germeys I et al. A systematic review and meta-analysis of the psychosis continuum: Evidence for a psychosis proneness–persistence–impairment model of psychotic disorder. Psychol Med 2009; 39: 179–95.

38. Cardno AG, Gottesman II. Twin studies of schizophrenia: from bow-andarrow concordances to star wars Mx and functional genomics. Am J Med Genet 2000; 97: 12–17.

39. Sullivan PF, Kendler KS, Neale MC. Schizophrenia as a complex trait: evidence from a metaanalysis of twin studies. Arch Gen Psychiatry 2003; 60: 1187–92.

40. O'Donovan MC, Craddock N, Norton N et al. Identification of loci associated with schizophrenia by genome-wide association and follow-up. Molecular Genetics of Schizophrenia Collaboration. Nat Genet 2008; 40: 1053–5.

41. Owen MJ, Craddock N, Jablensky A. The genetic deconstruction of psychosis. Schizophr Bull 2007; 33: 905–11.

42. Sullivan PF, Lin D, Tzeng JY et al. Genomewide association for schizophrenia in the CATIE study:Results of Stage 1. Mol Psychiatry 2008; 13: 570–84.

43. Need AC, Ge D, Weale ME et al. A genome-wide investigation of SNPs and CNVs in schizophrenia. PLoS Genet 2009; 5: e1000373.

44. Shifman S, Johannesson M, Bronstein M et al. Genome-wide association identifies a common variant in the reelin gene that Increases the risk of schizophrenia only in women. PLoS Genet 2008; 4: e28.

45. The European Network of Schizophrenia Networks for the Study of Gene-Environment Interactions(EU-GEI): schizophrenia aetiology: Do gene-environment interactions hold the Key? Schiz Res 2008; 102: 21–6.

46. van Os J, Rutten BP, Poulton R. Gene-environment interactions in schizophrenia: Review of epidemiological findings and future directions. Schizophr Bull 2008; 34: 1066–82.

47. Henquet C, Krabbendam L, Spauwen J et al. Prospective cohort study of cannabis use, predisposition for psychosis, and psychotic symptoms in young people. BMJ 2005; 330: 11

48. Verdoux H, Gindre C, Sorbara F et al. Effects of cannabis and psychosis vulnerability in daily life : an experience sampling test study. Psychol Med 2003; 33: 23–32.

49. Caspi A, Moffitt TE, Cannon M et al. Moderation of the effect of adolescent-onset cannabis use on adult psychosis by a functional polymorphism in the catechol-O-methyltransferase gene: longitudinal evidence of a gene X environment interaction. Biol Psychiatry 2005; 57:1117–27.

50. Stefanis NC, Henquet C, Avramopoulos D et al. COMT Val158Met moderation of stressinduced psychosis. Psychol Med 2007; 37: 1651–6.

51. Nicodemus KK, Marenco S, Batten AJ et al. Serious obstetric complications interact with hypoxia-regulated/vascular-expression genes to influence schizophrenia risk. Mol Psychiatry 2008; 13: 873–7.

52. Stefanis NC, Trikalinos TA, Avramopoulos D et al. Associations between Neuregulin-1 and psychosis under condition of uniform acute exposure to stress—The ASPIS study (in submission).

53. Johnstone EC, Crow TJ, Frith CD et al. Celebral ventricular size and cognitive impairment in chronic schizophrenia. Lancet 1976; 2: 924–6.

54. Wright IC, Rabe-Hesketh S, Woodruff PW et al. Meta-analysis of regional brain volumes in schizophrenia. Am J Psychiatry 2000; 157: 16–25.

55. Lawrie SM, Abukmeil SS. Brain abnormality in schizophrenia: a systematic and quantitative review of volumetric magnetic resonance imaging studies. Br J Psychiatry 1998; 172:110–20.

56. Honea R, Crow T, Passingham D et al. Regional deficits in brain volume in schizophrenia: a meta-analysis of voxel-based morphometry studies. Am J Psychiatry 2005; 162: 2233–45.

57. Steen RG, Mull C, McClure R. Brain volume in first-episode schizophrenia: Systematic review and meta-analysis of magnetic resonance imaging studies. Br J Psychiatry 2006; 188: 510–8.

58. Boos H, Aleman A, Cahn W et al. Brain volumes in relatives of patients with schizophrenia. A meta-analysis. Arch Gen Psychiatry 2007; 64: 297–304.

59. Honea R, Meyer-Lindenberg A, Hobbs K et al. Is gray matter volume an intermediate phenotype for schizophrenia? A voxel-based morphometry study of patients with schizophrenia and their healthy siblings. Biol Psychiatry 2008; 63: 465–74.

60. Segall J, Turner J, Van Erp TGM et al. Voxel-based morphometric multisite collaborative study on schizophrenia. Schizophr Bull 2009; 35: 82–95.

61. Job DE, Whalley HC, Johnstone EC et al. Grey matter changes over time in high risk subjects developing schizophrenia. Neuroimage 2005; 25: 1023–30.

62. Borgwardt SJ, Riecher-Rossler A, Dazzan P et al. Regional gray matter volume abnormalities in the at rik mental state. Biol Psychiatry 2007; 61: 1148–56.

63. Pantelis C, Velakoulis D, McGorry PD et al. Neuroanatomical abnormalities before and after onset of psychosis: A cross-sectional and longitudinal MRI study. Lancet 2003; 361: 281–8.

64. Velakoulis D, Wood SJ, Wong MT et al. Hippocampal and amygdala volumes according to psychosis stage and diagnosis: a magnetic resonance imaging study of chronic schizophrenia, first-episode psychosis, and ultra-high-risk individuals. Arch Gen Psychiatry 2006; 63:139–49.

65. Wood SJ, Pantelis C, Velakoulis D et al. Progressive changes in the development toward schizophrenia: Studies in subjects at increased symptomatic risk. Schizophr Bull 2008; 34:322–9.

66. Lui S, Deng W, Huang X et al. Neuroanatomical differences between familial and sporadic schizophrenia and their parents: an optimized voxel-based morphometry study. Psych Research: Neuroimaging 2009; 171: 71–81.

67. Weinberger DR, Egan MF, Bertolino A et al Prefrontal neurons and the genetics of schizophrenia. Biol Psychiatry 2001; 50: 825–44.

68. Conrad A, Winterer G. Disturbed structural connectivity in schizophrenia-primary factor in pathology or epiphenomenon? Schizophr Bull 2008; 34: 72–92.

69. Frankle WG. Neuroreceptor imaging studies in schizophrenia. Harv Rev Psychiatry 2007; 15: 212–32.

70. Hirvonen J, van Erp TG, Huttunen J et al. Increased caudate dopamine D2 receptor availability as a genetic marker for schizophrenia. Arch Gen Psychiatry 2005; 62: 371–8.

71. Howes OD, Montgomery AJ, Asselin MC et al. Elevated striatal dopamine function linked to prodromal signs of schizophrenia. Arch Gen Psychiatry 2009; 66: 13–20.

72. Georgopoulos AP, Karageorgiou E, Leuthold AC et al: Synchronous neural interactions assessed by magnetoencephalography: A functional biomarker for brain disorders. J Neural Engl 2007; 4: 349–55.

73. Manoach DS, Gollub RL, Benson ES et al. Schizophrenic subjects show aberrant fMRI activation of dorsolateral cortex and basal ganglia during working memory performance. Biol Psychiatry 2000; 48: 99–109.

74. Cannon TD, Van Erp TG, Rosso IM et al. Fetal hypoxia and structural brain abnormalities in schizophrenic patients, their siblings and controls. Arch Gen Psychiatry 2002; 59: 35–41.

75. Morey RA, Inan S, Mitchell TV et al. Imaging frontostriatal function in ultra-high-risk, early, and chronic schizophrenia during executive processing. Arch Gen Psychiatry 2005; 62:254–62.

76. Potkin S, Turner J, Brown G. Working memory and DLPFC in schizophrenia: the FBIRN Study. Schizophr Bull 2009; 35: 19–31.

77. Woodward ND, Waldie B, Rogers B et al. Abnormal pefrontal cortical activity and connectivity during response selection in first episode psychosis, chronic schizophrenia, and unaffected siblings of individuals with schizophrenia. Schiz Res 2009; 109:182-90.

78. Gottesman II, Gould TD. The endophenotype concept in psychiatry: etymology and strategic intentions. Am J Psychiatry 2003; 160: 636–45.

2 Epidemiology and gender

Johannes Wancata, Marion Freidl, and Annemarie Unger

INTRODUCTION

Schizophrenia is a mental disorder that can result in chronic impairments and disabilities. When compared to other, more common, mental disorders such as depression or anxiety disorders, schizophrenia is relatively rare (1). Nevertheless, schizophrenia is among the most burdensome and costly illnesses worldwide (2). The "Global Burden of Disease" study showed that schizophrenia is one of the major contributors to the overall burden of disease (3).

PREVALENCE

The prevalence of a disorder is defined as the number of cases (i.e., persons suffering from an illness) present in a defined population at a given time or over a given period (4, 5). Point prevalence refers to patients who were ill (i.e., suffering from symptoms) on a defined day, and 1-year prevalence to patients who were ill at any time during the period of 1 year. Because cases that have remitted are missed by these methods, some authors suggest including all those who suffered from a defined disorder during their lifetime (i.e., lifetime prevalence). Because prevalence data provide a cross-section of the burden of disease in a population at a specific time, they can be used for planning services and resource allocation (6).

One of the most comprehensive reviews on the prevalence of schizophrenia (7) found about 130 studies on this topic. In surveys reporting point prevalence or prevalence for the period of up to 1 year, age-corrected rates showed a range from 0.09% in Tongo to 1.74% in Ireland, with a mean of 0.58%. This review reporting nearly 20-fold differences between studies included publications from all over the world since 1931. Changes in the definition of schizophrenia and differences in research methods applied (e.g., sampling, period of observation) make comparisons very difficult. A more restricted range of prevalence estimates (0.25%–0.53%) was reported by Jablensky (8) from his review of 26 epidemiological studies performed in Europe. Similarly, Eaton et al. (9) reported a median point prevalence rate of 0.32% (0.06%–0.83%) when including 25 studies where the diagnosis was given by a psychiatrist (10). A recent review (1) including 21 European studies published between 1990 and 2004 found a medium 1-year prevalence of 0.8% (0.2%–2.6%) for psychotic disorders (i.e., including not only persons with schizophrenia).

While reviews including studies with widely varying methodologies (7, 11) report markedly differing results, studies using identical methodologies across study sites, such as the International Study of Schizophrenia (12), found smaller variations of prevalence worldwide. In order to decrease the likelihood that variation of rates is an artifact of methodology, several of the more recent reviews defined their inclusion and exclusion criteria more narrowly (10, 6). This approach maximizes the comparability across studies.

Goldner et al. (6) used the following inclusion criteria for their meta-analysis: studies using ICD-9 or DSM-III and later criteria, case identification based on either standardized instruments or diagnosis by a clinician, community surveys of the

TABLE 2.1 Selected prevalence studies of schizophrenic disorders and schizophrenia (%; based on Goldner et al. (6))

			Schizophrenic disorders		Schizophrenia	
Region	Region	Sample size	1-year-prevalence	lifetime prevalence	1-year-prevalence	lifetime prevalence
Bijl et al. (13)	Netherlands	7146			0.2	0.4
Wiederlov et al. (14)	Sweden	–	0.73		0.42	
Kendler et al. (15)	United States	5877	0.5	0.7		0.15
Chen et al. (16)	Hong Kong	7229				0.12
Lethinen et al. (17)	Finland	7217		2.2		1.3
Robins& Regier (18)	United States (ECA)	19182	1.0	1.5	0.9	1.3
Oakley-Brown et al. (19)	New Zealand	1498	0.2	0.4	0.2	0.3
Hwu et al. (20)	Metropolitan Taipei of Taiwan	5005			0.28	0.3
	Small towns of Taiwan	3004			0.23	0.23
	Rural villages of Taiwan	2995			0.2	0.23
Bland et al. (21)	Canada	3258	0.4	0.6	0.3	0.6
Canino et al. (22)	Puerto Rico	1513		1.8		1.6
Best estimate (95% Confidence interval)			0.60 (0.38–0.91)	1.45 (0.8–2.37)	0.34 (0.22–0.50)	0.55 (0.37–0.80)

general population using probability sampling techniques or those that surveyed the entire population of a defined area, denominator sample sizes of at least 450 persons. Because this is one of the most sophisticated recent meta-analyses, the results are described in more detail. Table 2.1 shows some selected prevalence studies included by Goldner et al. (6) presenting their findings separately for schizophrenic disorders and schizophrenia. For schizophrenic disorders, 1-year prevalence rates ranged from 0.2% in New Zealand to 1.0% in the United States. For schizophrenia, 1-year prevalence ranged from 0.2% (Netherlands, New Zealand, rural villages in Taiwan) to 0.9% (United States, ECA study). The 1-year prevalence best-estimate rates (based on a Bayesian approach to meta-analysis) for schizophrenic disorders and for schizophrenia worldwide were 0.60% and 0.34%, respectively (Table 2.1). Lifetime prevalence of schizophrenic disorders ranged from 0.4% in New Zealand to 2.2% in Finland and in the United States. For schizophrenia, lifetime prevalence showed rates ranging from 0.12% in Hong Kong to 1.6% in Puerto Rico. The best estimates for lifetime prevalence worldwide of schizophrenic disorders and schizophrenia are 1.45% and 0.55%, respectively.

Concerning the question whether prevalence differs between countries, the results are not clear. While Goldner et al. (6) reported that lifetime prevalence is significantly

TABLE 2.2 Selected incidence studies of schizophrenia (per 100.000; based on Goldner et al. (6))

Authors	Region	Diagnostic system	1-year-incidence
Jablensky et al. (12)	World	ICD	6.9
Brewin et al. (26)	United Kingdom	ICD	4.8
Iacono & Beiser (27)	Canada	ICD	7.7
		DSM	3.6
King et al. (28)	United Kingdom	ICD	22.6
		DSM	22.0
McNaught et al. (29)	United Kingdom	DSM	21.0
Tien & Eaton (30)	United States	DSM	200
Best estimate (95%			11.1
Confidence interval)			(7.5–16.3)

lower in Asia (0.25%) than in non-Asian countries (0.88%) in their meta-analysis, other authors could not find any clear differences between countries (7). When interpreting such results, differences in health care systems and in demography must be considered that might lead to increased mortality in some countries, reducing the numbers of those that can be identified by surveys. Because many confounding factors may inflate or deflate the prevalence, comparisons of schizophrenia prevalence across countries must be interpreted with caution (5, 23).

INCIDENCE
The incidence is usually defined as the annual number of new cases within 1 year (4, 5). Incidence studies can help determine whether potential risk factors lead to the subsequent development of an illness. This information is the basis for preventive interventions and early identification of new cases (6). In principle, the estimation of incidence is based on the ability to identify the onset of disease, but, unfortunately, there is no generally accepted definition of the beginning of schizophrenia (23). The first contact with psychiatric services is often months or years after the onset of first symptoms. Prodromal and subclinical symptoms of varying duration usually precede clinical symptoms (24).

Warner and Girolamo (7) as well as Saha et al. (25) performed very comprehensive reviews and found about 50 studies on the incidence of schizophrenia worldwide. One-year incidence rates show a wide range (between 5 per 100,000 and 170 per 100,000), that is, more than 30-fold differences between studies (7). In this review, the mean age–corrected incidence for schizophrenia was 24 per 100,000 (after exclusion of very wide and very narrow diagnostic criteria). The WHO 100-country study applying identical diagnostic criteria found a more restricted range of incidence estimates (16–42 per 100,000 when using ICD-9 criteria and 2–14 per 100,000 when using CATEGO-5 criteria (23)).

Goldner et al. (6) used narrowly defined inclusion criteria for their meta-analysis (see above). Some of the 1-year incidence studies of schizophrenia selected by them are shown in Table 2.2. The incidence ranged from 3.6 per 100,000 in Canada to 200 per 100,000 in the United States. The 1-year incidence best-estimate rate for schizophrenia worldwide was 11.1 per 100,000. Studies using DSM reported rates between 3.6 and 22 per 100,000, and those using ICD reported rates between 4.8 and 22.6 per 100,000 (after excluding the U.S. ECA study, considering its extreme outlier rate).

MORTALITY

Nearly 100 years ago, Kräpelin (31) and Bleuler (32) reported that persons suffering from schizophrenia exhibit an increased mortality. Among the reasons they mentioned suicide, malnutrition, tuberculosis, and other physical diseases. The first and most comprehensive meta-analysis on mortality of schizophrenia was performed only a decade ago and reported 1.51-fold increased mortality for patients with schizophrenia as compared to the general population (33). Another systematic review (34) reported an even higher mortality for schizophrenia (2.5-fold increase). Mortality rates among schizophrenia patients were significantly increased for diseases of the cardiovascular (standardized mortality ratio [SMR] = 110), respiratory (SMR = 226), digestive (SMR = 185), and genitourinary system (SMR = 161) as well as for accidents (SMR = 216) and for suicides (SMR = 838 [33]). Smoking-related disorders were reported to be especially increased in a recent study based on data from England (35). Nearly 70% of those affected with schizophrenia (compared with about one-half in the general population) die from coronary heart disease (36). Merely neoplastic diseases do not show increased mortality rates among schizophrenia cases (35, 36). About a fifth of persons suffering from schizophrenia were reported to be victims of violence during their life time (37, 38). One study (39) found that especially men with schizophrenia exhibit an increased risk of dying by homicide, but Harris and Barraclough (40) reported from their meta-analyses that both men and women with schizophrenia show an increased risk for dying from violence.

Some authors (34, 36, 41) have speculated that the higher mortality of schizophrenia patients (as compared to the general population) has increased further during the last two decades. Some authors who found an increasing mortality among schizophrenia patients suggested that this might be due to the changing mental health care system (42). However, it should be considered that the SMRs must have increased due to the methods applied in many of these studies (irrespective of real changes of mortality).

A   In many studies, the diagnoses used for analyses are based on hospital discharge diagnoses. In the past 20 years, the definitions of schizophrenia were narrowed, frequently excluding milder forms of the disease. Because of recent changes in mental health care, it has become common that only the most severely ill or those with comorbidity are admitted to hospital. This could lead to higher SMRs.

B   Recent studies included higher proportions of persons with a shorter duration of illness, while previous studies had included more schizophrenia patients with a longer duration of illness. Because some authors found that mortality is disproportionately increased during the first years after onset of schizophrenia, we must expect higher death rates in recent studies (41).

Considering the fact that only some studies reported increasing death rates, these results must be interpreted with caution.

GENDER

For nearly 100 years (31) it has been well known that the onset of schizophrenia is earlier among men than among women. A review of more than 50 studies (43) found age differences from 1 to 10 years between women and men concerning their first admission. This difference was found regardless of which definition of onset was used (date of first hospital admission, occurrence of first symptoms of schizophrenia, or occurrence of first nonspecific signs of any mental disorder).

TABLE 2.3 Selected studies on gender-specific lifetime prevalence and annual incidence of schizophrenia (based on Goldner et al. (6))

Prevalence studies	Study site	Lifetime prevalence (%)	
		Men	Women
Bijl et al. (13)	Netherlands	0.4	0.3
Kessler et al. (47)	United States	0.6	0.8
Chen et al. (16)	Hong Kong	0.12	0.13
Lehtinen et al. (17)	Finland	1.3	1.3
Wells et al. (46)	New Zealand	0.3	0.4
Bland et al. (21)	Canada	0.5	0.6
Canino et al. (22)	Puerto Rico	1.9	1.2

Incidence studies	Study site	Annual incidence (per 100 000)	
		Men	Women
Vazquez-Barquero et al. (48)	Spain	12.7	14.4
Brewin et al. (26)	United Kingdom	10.0	5.0
Iacono & Beiser (27)	Canada	10.9	4.12

Häfner et al. (44) reported that first admission to hospital was between 4 and 6 years earlier among men than among women, depending on the definition of schizophrenia used. This finding was not attributable to differences in help seeking between men and women. Another study (45) had shown that these differences between genders are not due to sociodemographic cofounders (e.g., marriage, working status, or social class).

Despite these differences in age of onset, the overall prevalence rates are similar in most studies (7). Table 2.3 (6) shows some selected results from studies reporting gender-specific lifetime prevalence for schizophrenia. Males and females were found to have very similar rates in most studies. Despite the fact that some single studies (20) found slightly higher rates for men, these differences were not significant. Using meta-analytic techniques no significant differences could be found even when pooling the data of 57 studies (11).

The incidence rates between sexes are not as similar as those of prevalence (6, 11, 49). Among the incidence studies identified by Goldner et al. (6), two of the three studies reported male rates as being about twice as high as female rates (Table 2.3). Some authors report that incidence rates differ between sexes depending on age. Jablensky (23) reported that the age-specific incidence is significantly higher for men up to the mid-30s, but the male–female ratio becomes inverted with increasing age. In contrast, in their 10-country International Study of Schizophrenia Jablensky et al. (12) found similar cumulated incidence rates for men and women, both for broad and for narrow definitions of schizophrenia, using identical methods across study sites.

Until now, gender effects on mortality are not clear. Brown (33) reported from their meta-analysis that men as well as women show a significantly increased death rate as compared to the general population (SMR 148 and 139, respectively), but men did not differ significantly from women concerning their increased mortality. In contrast, Harris and Barraclough (40) who performed a similar meta-analysis based on a slightly different set of primary studies reported that men show a significantly higher mortality than women (SMR 156 and 141, respectively). Concerning single causes Brown (33) found a significantly higher mortality for men (SMR 956) than for women (SMR 673) only for suicide. However, he could not find significant differences for all other causes (e.g., diseases of the cardiovascular, respiratory, digestive, and genitourinary system as wells as accidents). Harris and Barraclough (40) did not identify any significant differences between genders in the causes for mortality.

MORBIDITY IN SPECIAL SAMPLES

Homelessness is a well-recognized outcome of schizophrenia, but there have been few attempts to quantify it (50). Rates vary across borders and time. A review published by Martens (51) reported prevalence rates between 1.8% and 43.0% (median 20.0) among homeless people. Unfortunately, this review did not differentiate between point prevalence, 1-year prevalence, and lifetime prevalence. The European schizophrenia cohort found that 32.8% of the British schizophrenia sample had been homeless during their lifetime with an even higher rate in metropolitan London (52).

A lot of studies have shown that severe mental disorders such as schizophrenia occur frequently among those imprisoned (53, 54). A review of 49 surveys of mental disorders among prisoners (total sample more than 19,000) reported high rates of psychotic disorders (i.e., not only schizophrenia in the narrow sense). Overall, 3.7% of male and 4.0% of female prisoners suffered from any psychotic disorder, which is a dramatically high rate compared to the general population (55).

Epidemiological studies in nonpsychiatric wards of general hospitals have shown that point prevalence of schizophrenia is similar to that reported from studies in the general population, while other mental disorders such as depression or substance abuse occur much more often (56, 57). One of the largest surveys in general hospitals reported a point prevalence of schizophrenia according to *DSM-III-R* of 0.4% among patients of internal medical wards (58).

Several authors reported that the reforms of the mental health care system in the last three decades resulted in a lower number of persons with chronic schizophrenia being admitted to psychiatric hospitals increasing the number of those living in nursing homes for the elderly (59). While a large number of studies investigated the prevalence of dementia and depression in nursing homes (60, 61), only a few studies included schizophrenia. An Austrian survey reported that 1.9% of nursing home residents are suffering from schizophrenia (62).

METHODOLOGICAL FACTORS INFLUENCING THE RESULTS OF EPIDEMIOLOGICAL STUDIES

For a long time, differences in diagnostic concepts played a critical role in the outcome of epidemiological studies of schizophrenia (23). The proportion of cases identified depends on the definition of schizophrenia used. The WHO 10-country study reported between two-fold and three-fold higher incidence rates when using broad diagnostic criteria as compared to narrow criteria for schizophrenia (12). The worldwide use of modern diagnostic systems such ICD-10 or *DSM-IV* has increased the comparability of results.

Some studies included only cases suffering from schizophrenia, while others included similar psychotic conditions (often summarized as "schizophrenic disorders").

Thus, it is not surprising that studies including other psychotic conditions beside schizophrenia reported higher prevalence estimates (see Table 2.1).

Epidemiological studies vary with regard to how and by whom schizophrenia cases are identified ("case identification"). Many of the earlier studies used psychiatric experts (i.e., psychiatrists or psychologists) having the advantage of clinical experience and knowledge about the conditions investigated (63). Using psychiatric experts increases the costs for assessment resulting in relatively small samples of several hundred persons. Considering the low prevalence and incidence of schizophrenia, larger samples would be more appropriate in order to identify a sufficient number of schizophrenia cases. This led to the introduction of highly structured research interviews using (cheaper) lay interviewers instead of psychiatric experts (23). The effects of interviewer-related variation (i.e., psychiatric experts versus lay interviewers) have been studied only in a limited way (64). In the last decade, there is an increasing concern that lay interviewers are liable to commit response errors (e.g., misinterpreting the interviewee's responses [63]).

Another critical point is the sample investigated for the identification of schizophrenia cases. Investigating only those who are in treatment in psychiatric services does not take into account all those who are not in treatment or receive medication only by primary care physicians into consideration. Community surveys based on representative samples of households (e.g., probability sample based on census lists, electoral roll, or door-to-door survey) have the advantage that all those can be included who are not in contact with psychiatric services. However, a high proportion of schizophrenia sufferers show incapacity to live independently in private households and need some kind of housing support. Community surveys based merely on household samples do not include those living in sheltered housing. Goldner et al. (6) have shown that extending the household samples by including psychiatric institutions (e.g., psychiatric homes, psychiatric hospitals) yields double or triple of the prevalence estimates. For example, lifetime prevalence of schizophrenia increased from 0.4% (pure household sample) to 1.3% when the sample was complemented by those living in psychiatric institutions (6).

FUTURE RESEARCH

While the problem of differing diagnostic criteria of schizophrenia was solved to a large extent by introducing modern diagnostic systems such as ICD and DSM, it is frequently not clear whether studies are limited to schizophrenia or included similar psychotic disorders. It might be useful to asses and to report rates for schizophrenia in the narrow sense as well as more comprehensively for schizophrenic disorders because this information might be useful for service planning and for identifying risk factors.

A variety of recent studies reported that genetic, social, and environmental factors increase the risk for schizophrenia. While this research contributed to the knowledge about the heterogeneity of risk factors for schizophrenia, our understanding of the interactions between genes and environment is rather poor.

Until now, it is unknown which biological and social differences between men and women cause the differences in morbidity. We do not know whether biological and/or social factors cause the earlier beginning among men and the lower impairment among women. Searching for the causes of these differences might result in information relevant for prevention, early recognition, and treatment.

The reasons for the dramatically increased mortality among schizophrenia sufferers are known only in part. Our knowledge on the relationship between schizophrenia and physical diseases is rather limited. Epidemiological studies focusing on the causes for increased mortality might yield information that could be used for developing preventive interventions.

Finally, the methodological problems of epidemiological research in schizophrenia mentioned above deserve more investigations of the advantages and disadvantages of different methods. It would be prudent to explore the utility of lay interviews and other assessment methods for the epidemiology of schizophrenia before starting new large-scale projects.

REFERENCES

1. Wittchen HU, Jacobi F. Size and burden of mental disorders in Europe – a critical review and appraisal of 27 studies. Eur Neuropsychopharmacol 2005; 15: 357–76.
2. Rössler W, SalizeHJ, van Os J et al. Size of burden of schizophrenia and psychotic disorders. Eur Neuropsychopharmacol 2005; 15: 399–409.
3. Murray C, Lopez A. The global Burden of Disease: A Comprehensive Assessment of Mortality and Disability from Diseases, Injuries and Risk Factors in 1990 and Projected to 2020, Cambridge: Cambridge Univ Press, 1996.
4. Rothman KJ, Greenland S. Modern Epidemiology. Philadelphia: Lippincott Williams & Wilkins, 1998.
5. Tsuang MT, Tohen M. Textbook of psychiatric epidemiology. New York: Wiley, 2002.
6. Goldner E, Hsu L, Waraich P et al. Prevalence and incidence studies of schizophrenic disorders: a systematic review of the literature. Can J Psychiatry 2002; 47: 833–43.
7. Warner R, de Girolamo G. Epidemiology of mental disorders and psychosocial problems: schizophrenia. Geneva: World Health Organisation, 1995.
8. Jablensky A. Epidemiology of schizophrenia: a European perspective. Schizophrenia Bull 1986; 12: 52–73.
9. Eaton WW, Day R, Kramer M. The use of epidemiology for risk factor research in schizophrenia: an overview and methodologic critique. In. Tsuang MT, Simpson JC eds. Handbook of schizophrenia. Vol. 3, Amsterdam: Elsevier Science, 1988: 169–204.
10. Bromet E, Dew M, Eaton W. Epidemiology of psychosis with special reference to schizophrenia. In: Tsuang MT, Tohen M eds. Textbook of psychiatric epidemiology. New York: Wiley, 2002: 365–88.
11. Saha S, Chant D, Welham J et al. A systematic review of the prevalence of schizophrenia. PLoS Medicine 2005; 2: 413–33.
12. Jablensky A, Sartorius N, Ernberg G et al. Schizophrenia: manifestations, incidence and course in different cultures: a World Health Organization ten-country study. Psychol Med – Monograph Suppl 1992; 20: 1–97.
13. Bijl R, Ravelli A, van Zessen G. Prevalence of psychiatric disorder in the general population: results of the Netherlands Mental Health Survey and Incidence Study (NEMESIS). Soc Psychiatry Psychiatr Epidemiol 1998; 33: 587–95.
14. Widerlov B, Lindstrom E, von Knorring L. One-year prevalence of long-term functional psychosis in three different areas of Uppsala. Acta Psychiatr Scand 1997; 96: 452–8.
15. Kendler KS, Gallagher TJ, Abelson JM et al. Lifetime prevalence, demographic risk factors, and diagnostic validity of nonaffective psychosis as assessed in a US community sample: The National Comorbidity Survey. Arch Gen Psychiatry 1996; 53: 1022–31.
16. Chen CN, Wong J, Lee N et al. The Shatin Community Mental Health Survey in Hong Kong. Arch Gen Psychiatry 1993; 50: 125–33.
17. Lehtinen V, Joukamaa M, Lahtela K et al. Prevalence of mental disorders among adults in Finland: basic results from the Mini Finland Health Survey. Acta Psychiatr Scand 1990; 81: 418–25.
18. Robins LN, Regier DA. Psychiatric disorders in America: The Epidemiologic Catchment Area Study. New York: The Free Press, 1991.

19. Oakley-Browne MA, Joyce PR, Wells E et al. Christchurch Psychiatric Epidemiology Study, Part II: six month and other period prevalences of specific psychiatric disorders. Aust N Z J Psychiatry 1989; 23: 327–40.
20. Hwu HG, Yeh EK, Chang LY. Prevalence of psychiatric disorders in Taiwan defined by the Chinese Diagnostic Interview Schedule. Acta Psychiatr Scand 1989; 79: 136–47.
21. Bland RC, Orn H, Newman SC. Lifetime prevalence of psychiatric disorders in Edmonton. Acta Psychiatr Scand 1988; 77 (Suppl 338): 24–32.
22. Canino GJ, Bird HR, Shrout PE et al. The prevalence of specific psychiatric disorders in Puerto Rico. Arch Gen Psychiatry 1987; 44: 727–35.
23. Jablensky A. The epidemiological horizon. In: Hirsch SR, Weinberger DR eds. Schizophrenia. Oxford: Blackwell, 2003: 203–31.
24. Häfner H, Maurer K, Löffler W et al. The influence of age and sex on the onset and early course of schizophrenia. Br J Psychiatry 1993; 162: 80–6.
25. Saha S, Welham J, Chant D et al. Incidence of schizophrenia does not vary with economic status of the country. Soc Psychiatry Psychiatr Epidemiol 2006; 41: 338–40.
26. Brewin J, Cantwell R, Dalkin T et al. Incidence of schizophrenia in Nottingham – a comparison of two cohorts: 1978-80 and 1992-94. Br J Psychiatry 1997; 171: 140–4.
27. Iacono WG, Beiser M. Are males more likely than females to develop schizophrenia? Am J Psychiatry 1992; 149: 1070–74.
28. King M, Coker E, Leavey G et al. Incidence of psychotic illness in London: comparison of ethnic groups. BMJ 1994; 309: 1115–9.
29. McNaught AS, Jeffreys SE, Harvey CA et al. The Hampstead Schizophrenia Survey 1991. II: Incidence and migration in inner London. Br J Psychiatry 1997; 170: 307–11.
30. Tien AY, Eaton WW. Psychopathologic precursors and sociodemographic risk factors for the schizophrenia syndrome. Arch Gen Psychiatry 1992,; 49P: 37–46.
31. Kräpelin E. Dementia präcox und Paraphrenia. Edinburgh: Livingstone, 1919
32. Bleuler E. Dementia präcox oder die Gruppe der Schizophrenien. Leipzig Wien: Deuticke, 1911.
33. Brown S. Excess mortality of schizophrenia: a meta-analysis. Br J Psychiatry 199; 171: 502–8.
34. Saha S, Chant D, McGrath J. A systematic review of mortality in schizophrenia. Arch Gen Psychiatry 2007; 64: 1123–31.
35. Brown S, Inskip H, Barraclough B. Causes of excess mortality in schizophrenia. Br J Psychiatry 2000; 177: 212–7.
36. Seeman M. An outcome measure in schizophrenia: mortality. Can J Psychiatry 2007; 52: 55–60.
37. Walsh E, Moran P, Scott C, et al. Prevalence of violent victimisation in severe mental illness. Br J Psychiatry 2003; 183: 233–8.
38. White MC, Chafetz L, Collins-Bride G et al. History of arrest, incarceration and victimization in community-based severely mentally ill. J Community Health 2006; 31: 123–35.
39. Hiroeh U, Appleby L, Mortensen PB et al. Death by homicide, suicide, and other unnatural causes in people with mental illness: a population-based study. Lancet 2001; 358: 2110–2.
40. Harris E, Barraclough B. Excess mortality of mental disorder. Br J Psychiatry 1998; 173: 11–53.
41. Heilä H, Haukka J, Suvisaari J et al. Mortality among patients with schizophrenia and reduced hospital care. Psychol Med 2005; 35: 725–32.
42. Ösby U, Correia N, Brandt L et al. Time trends in schizophrenia mortality in Stockholm County, Sweden: cohort study. BMJ 2000; 321: 483–4.
43. Angermayer M, Kuhn L. Gender differences in age at onset of schizophrenia. Eur Arch Psychiat Neurol Sci 1988; 237: 351–64.
44. Häfner H, Riecher A, Maurer K et al. How does gender influence age at first hospitalization for schizophrenia? A transnational case register study. Psychol Med 1989; 19: 903–18.
45. Faraone SV, Chen WJ, Goldstein JM et al. Gender differences in age at onset of schizophrenia. Br J Psychiatry 1994; 164: 625–9.

46. Wells JE, Bushnell JA, Hornblow AR et al. Christchurch Psychiatric Epidemiology Study, Part I: methodology and lifetime prevalence for specific psychiatric disorders. Aust N Z J Psychiatry 1989; 23: 315–26.

47. Kessler RC, McGonagle KA, Zhao S et al. Lifetime and 12-month prevalence of DSM-III-R psychiatric disorders in the United States. Results from the National Comorbidity Survey. Arch Gen Psychiatry 1994; 51: 8–19.

48. Vazquez-Barquero JL, Cuesta Nunez MJ, de la Varga M et al. The Cantabria first episode schizophrenia study: a summary of general findings. Acta Psychiatr Scand 1995; 91: 156–62.

49. McGrath J, Saha S, Welham J et al. A systematic review of the incidence of schizophrenia: the distribution of rates and the influence of sex, urbanicity, migrant status and methodology. BMC Med 2002; 2: 13.

50. Kooyman I, Dean K, Harvey S et al. Outcomes of public concern in schizophrenia. Br J Psychiatry 2007; 191 (Suppl 5): s29–s36.

51. Martens W. A review of physical and mental health among homeless persons. Publ Health Rev 2001; 29: 13–33.

52. Bebbington PE, Angermeyer M, Azorin J et al. The European Schizophrenia Cohort: a naturalistic prognostic and economic study. Soc Psychiatry Psychiatr Epidemiol 2005; 40: 707–17.

53. Lader D, Singleton N, Meltzer H. Psychiatric morbidity among young offenders in England and Wales. Intern Rev Psychiatry 2003; 15:144–7.

54. O'Brien M, Mortimer L, Singleton N et al. psychiatric morbidity among women prisoners in England and Wales. Intern Rev Psychiatry 2003; 15: 153–7.

55. Fazel S, Danesh J. Serious mental disorders in 23000 prisoners: a systematic review of 62 surveys. Lancet 2002; 359: 545–50.

56. Mayou R, Hawton K. Psychiatric disorder in the general hospital. Br J Psychiatry 1986; 149: 172–90.

57. Modestin J. Psychiatrische Morbidität bei intern-medizinisch hospitalisierten Patienten. Schweiz med Wschr 1977; 107: 1354–61.

58. Wancata J, Benda N, Hajji M et al. Psychiatric disorders in gynecological, surgical and medical departments of general hospitals in an urban and a rural area of Austria. Soc Psychiatry Psychiatr Epidemiol 1996; 31: 220–6.

59. Meise U, Kemmler G, Kurz M et al. Quality of the location as a principle in psychiatric health care planning. Gesundheitswesen 1996; 58 (Suppl1): 29–37.

60. Mann A, Graham N, Ashby D. Psychiatric illness in residential homes for the elderly: a survey in one London borough. Age Ageing 1984; 13: 257–65.

61. Cooper B. Home and away: the disposition of mentally ill old people in an urban population. Soc Psychiatry 1984; 19: 187–96.

62. Wancata J, Benda N, Hajji M et al. Prevalence and course of psychiatric disorders among nursing home admissions. Soc Psychiatry Psychiatr Epidemiol 1998; 33: 74–9.

63. Cooper B, Singh B. Population research and mental health policy: bridging the gap. Br J Psychiatry 2000; 176: 407–11.

64. Brugha T, Jenkins R, Taub N et al. A general population comparison of the Composite International Diagnostic Interview (CIDI) and the Schedules for Clinical Assessment in Neuropsychiatry (SCAN). Psychol Med 2001; 31: 1001–13.

3 | Interviewing the patient with schizophrenia

Florence Thibaut

Clinical interview has two main goals:

1 Making a diagnosis
2 Developing a therapeutic alliance on which treatment response depends, whatever treatment modality used.

In the first part of this chapter, we shall briefly review the history of diagnostic criteria. In the second part, we shall describe how to make a diagnosis, and then we shall try to help the interviewer to get into contact with a schizophrenic patient and to give the interviewer some safety advices.

DIAGNOSIS CRITERIA

In psychiatry, diagnosis relies only on clinical assessment, based on patient's interview. Diagnostic criteria are arbitrary and are likely to change over time as we understand more about the disease mechanisms. In medicine, physicians recognize specific symptoms (nonspecific markers of disease), syndromes (groups of symptoms that tend to co-occur), and diseases (syndromes in which the pathophysiological mechanisms are at least partially understood). In psychiatry, it is critical to remember that most of the psychiatric diagnostic categories are still at the syndromal level rather than the disease level.(1)

Kraepelin (2) approached the definition and classification of psychiatric disorders from a neurobiological perspective. He emphasized the longitudinal course of the disease in classification and dichotomized psychotic patients into manic depressive and dementia praecox. This categorization has been maintained in many nosological systems. In contrast, Bleuler (3) approached psychotic disorders from a psychological model. He focused on negative symptoms rather than on positive ones; he included mild and nonpsychotic forms in schizophrenia and emphasized cross-sectional rather than longitudinal features.

Schneider (4), like Bleuler, emphasized symptoms but considered positive symptoms as fundamental (e.g., hearing multiple voices commenting on, or conversing, about one's behavior; experiencing one's thoughts as being broadcast and heard by others; experiencing the feeling of being controlled by external forces). The symptoms were referred as first-rank symptoms of schizophrenia and were considered as almost pathognomonic of the disorder. These positive symptoms are mainly used in classifications systems.

Classifications such as the *Diagnostic and Statistical Manual of Mental Disorders* (DSM) (5) and the *International Classification of Diseases* (ICD) (6), with their operational criteria for diagnosis and their multiaxial system, have strengthened the symptom-based approach. This checkup approach followed by the use of a checklist led to the development of structured clinical interviews and questionnaires that can by used by nonpsychiatrists, especially in epidemiological studies. The decision tree for treatment is also mainly based on this approach.

HOW TO MAKE A DIAGNOSIS

Making a diagnosis is one of the two major goals of the interview, even if this goal is sometimes partially achieved.

Gauron and Dickinson (7, 8) described six types of diagnosis style:

1. The intuitive approach: A diagnosis is made very quickly during the first minutes of interview, based on a limited amount of information. The clinician remains ready for changing the diagnosis during the course of the interview if new information becomes available that invalidates the initial diagnosis. In 50% of cases, the first diagnosis was maintained up until end of the interview. Among final diagnosis, in 65% of cases, diagnoses were made after five bits of information.
2. The exclusion approach: During the interview and using an accumulation of data, different diagnoses are gradually excluded until only one remained. The diagnosis usually appears after 15 or 20 categories of information.
3. The overinclusive–indecisive approach: The clinician considers every diagnosis at the same time. For example after 26 bits of information, 6 diagnoses are still considered; after 35 bits of information, 2 diagnoses remain possible with 60% of certitude for the first one and 80% for the second one.
4. The textbook approach: All kinds of information share the same weight, and the clinician follows a strict diagnostic procedure.
5. The flexible–adaptable approach: The clinician has no preconceived idea of the diagnosis. During the interview, the diagnosis process will be guided by the informations gradually collected.

Most of the psychiatrists use a mixture of these different approaches but with various proportions. In summary, two main aspects are important: (1) the way the clinician obtains informations and the degree of organization of this latter task (structured or nonstructured), and (2) the process of thinking on the part of the interviewer (logical or not, inductive or intuitive).

Gauron and Dickinson (9) also showed, using two sequences (information given about a patient, before or after seeing a filmed interview) that, seeing the patient for about 1 minute, increased the diagnosis speed and efficiency. This means the clinician is more efficient when a quick diagnosis hypothesis is made and then can be tested during the interview.

From the 1960s, some psychiatrists have emphasized the major role of the first contact and especially of the first 5 minutes of the interview (for review, 10). It is interesting that Sandifer et al. (11) have studied the role of the first 5 minutes of the interview. In all, 60 patients were filmed during an interview at the point of admission (mean age 39 years). Psychiatrists, aged 30 to 45 years (mean duration of experience of 10 years) saw 30 interviews. After 3 minutes, there was a break (comments were written). After this break, the rest of the films were shown until the end of the interview (25 minutes). The psychiatrists wrote the time elapsed before they wrote something down. After 3 minutes of interview, 32% of psychiatrists wrote descriptive comments only, 33% wrote 2 or more diagnostic hypotheses, and 33% opted for 1 diagnostic preference. About 50% of the amount of total symptoms observed after 30 minutes were already reported after 3 minutes and 3 out of 4 symptoms reported in the first 3 minutes were considered as present after the interview session that lasted 30 minutes. Another 50% of the final diagnoses of schizophrenia (versus 56% in depressive disorders) were made during the first 3 minutes of the filmed interview. Only in 1 out of 4 times the diagnosis made during the first 3 minutes was rejected after 30 minutes. For

75% of psychiatrists who have made the diagnosis during the first three minutes the concordance for the diagnostic category with their colleagues was the same as compared with those who only wrote descriptive comments after 3 minutes.

In summary, the role of the first 5 minutes during clinical structured interview is critical in establishing a diagnosis, as 50% of the clinical symptoms are reported during this phase. But the clinician who reached early a diagnostic conclusion must be cautious about the diagnosis because there is a possibility of not paying adequate attention to further symptoms as they may appear after the first diagnosis, which in turn may lead to diagnostic errors.

HOW TO CONDUCT A FIRST INTERVIEW

Interviewing schizophrenic patients is usually a scary affair for young psychiatrists.

Several authors, such as Kurt Schneider (4), have stressed the failure of empathy and the difficulty of comprehension of a schizophrenic patient. A major difficulty in establishing contact is considered as a core element in the diagnosis of schizophrenia. Schizophrenic patients usually have trouble maintaining social distance. In addition, schizophrenic patients are often ambivalent about interviews due to past difficulties with psychiatric settings, delusions, difficulties in social relationships. Indeed it is usual that schizophrenic patients could have been put on involuntary holds and hospitalized against their will during previous hospitalizations. They could have spent hours in an emergency ward and could have been forced to take medications. This may considerably increase their apprehension during the first interview. Hence, explaining about the interview process in a manner that is reassuring can diminish the patient's anxiety.

First, the interviewer should introduce himself to the patient and mention the purpose of the interview and what he already knows about the patient. He should also tell the patient how long the interview will last and ask the patient to let him know in case he or she would find it too long to be at ease. Usually, a first interview will last almost 1 hour, but sometimes patients can only tolerate brief interviews; hence, instead of one 1-hour session, two 30-minute sessions may be a better choice. The interviewer should also make every effort to be on time or tell the patient if he is going to be late. The interviewer should try not to let the patient waiting too long at first admission before the interview.

Establishing a relationship, whenever possible, is more important than immediately trying to come to a firm diagnosis (see also 12).

Most patients do not believe they are mentally ill; therefore, starting off the interview session with a remark, "We are here to talk about your mental illness," is not recommended. In addition, some patients do not like the term *schizophrenia*. You can gain the confidence and cooperation of the patient who does not accept the existence of a psychiatric problem, or denies psychiatric symptoms, by focusing on and reducing the client's distress rather than debating over a diagnostic label, as it may not go down well with the patient, which in turn would affect the diagnostic process. By using the "what if" questions, the interviewer can identify barriers in the patient's thinking and help him or her to decrease or remove those barriers (13).

Arguing about whether the patients' experiences are true or false is not useful. The interviewer should help the patients keep their anxiety levels low so that their reality testing and abilities to cope with the interview are not compromised. Sometimes, psychotic anxiety is contagious, and the interviewer may become anxious for no discernible reason. If patients get too anxious, too angry, or too sad, you can move away from a topic to something more neutral or allow a break and come back later. The interviewer should not forget that some schizophrenic patients have difficulties with the use of metaphors, and they should pay attention to the way patients use some words with an intonation emphasis or gesture that is different from the usual one, which may help during the interview.

Making a diagnosis need not be an intrusive process. By listening to and observing a patient during the first interview, symptoms such as disorganized speech, disorganized or catatonic behavior, and affective flattening often become obvious. During the course of interview, the following items must be analyzed: reduction in facial expression, communication gestures, emotional responsiveness or interest in life events, lack of interpersonal empathy, reduction in fluidity, spontaneity of communication and flexibility of thinking, and lack of interest and initiative in social interactions.

As the interview proceeds, the patient may spontaneously refer to the voices, and the questions of the interviewer may help the patient to describe them. If there is no such spontaneous mention, the interviewer can ask, "Have you had any unusual or strange experiences such as hearing voices that no one else seems to hear?" This may be sufficient to get into a discussion of voices, and the interviewer can follow up by asking about other kinds of hallucinatory phenomena; for example, "Have you seen things that other people haven't seen or felt things when there was nothing visible?" For delusions, the interviewer can say, "Sometimes people worry more than they should that other people are spying on them or planning to get them into trouble. Has anything of that sort ever happened to you?" Similarly, questions about insertion could be asked, "Do you ever get the feeling that other people, the radio or TV are putting thoughts into your head or thought broadcasting?" Or "Do you ever get the feeling that your thoughts are being transmitted to other people or come out on the radio or TV?" Once it is apparent that the patient wants to talk about such subjects, the interviewer can ask, "When was the first time in your life that you remember hearing voices?" "When was the last time you heard the voices?" "How does it make you feel to hear the voices?" This is a point at which the patient may express some anguish at the mental affliction the voices or the delusions cause him and the interviewer can strengthen an alliance with the patient by emphasizing with the patient's distress.

From this point, the interviewer can inquire about areas of potential danger. He has to know about the patient's potential for suicide, assault, and homicide. The interviewer can ask whether the voices or the delusions ever gave the patient commands to obey, or suggestions to follow, especially ones that might involve hurting themselves or someone else. If the patient has such thoughts, it is important to know when he last had them, how close he came to acting on them, whether he is having such thoughts now and whether he wants any help with controlling his impulses. If there is current risk of dangerous behaviors the patient needs to be helped with before any other matters are addressed. Many patients who were helped to control or overcome destructive impulses before they acted on them later thanked who aided them.

SAFETY OF THE INTERVIEW
Safety for both patient and psychiatrist must be considered. Medical students starting psychiatry are often scared of patients because of patients' unpredictable behavior during sessions; in some cases, fears of verbal and physical attacks are realistic.

Therefore, we must ensure safety for both patients and interviewers before commencing the interview session. The patient who is out of control must be first subdued and brought back under control, as humanely as possible, often by putting him or her in restraints and in seclusion and/or by giving medications. A patient being in restraints and in seclusion is not necessarily a barrier to starting an interview. In fact, sitting with the patient in restraints, explaining what is being done and why, and simply being present, may be extremely important for a patient who is in fear.

Assessment of the potential for violence has to be part of an initial interview (see above, last paragraph). In addition, the interview of violent patients requires careful monitoring of subjective states of the patient and maximum safety conditions for the clinicians (e.g., presence of several people in the room and availability of other care givers if necessary) (14).

You should never forget that the interviewer is a stranger for the patient at first contact with psychiatry and the patient will have to cope with a stranger. You must be very careful in approaching the patient from the front; never approach a new/unfamiliar patient from the side or the rear. The interviewer will be tested and sometimes misperceived by the patient, especially when there are persecutory delusions. In addition, when a patient has his or her first psychotic experience, it is perceived by him or herself as a nightmare, and he may think that he has lost control of his mind and behavior or that you might be responsible for this experience.

During the interview of a new patient, you must constantly stay receptive and responsive to what the patient is doing and saying. If the patient asks whether the interviewer believes what he or she says is true (or not true), you must be very careful in your answer. If you say, "No I don't believe these delusional ideas," the risk of aggressiveness is high. You must rather explain that you are interested in the way the patient is thinking even if it is not your personal view. In some cases, you can talk about unrealistic thoughts in order to help the patient to accept care.

AT THE END OF THE INTERVIEW THE FOLLOWING ITEMS MUST BE OBTAINED

Reason for admission, physical appearance, behavior, age, gender, marital status, name of the GP, story of the current disease, symptoms of the main disease, comorbid symptoms including negative data (depressive symptoms, anxiety, suicidal ideation, addictive disorders, etc.), previous psychiatric history, family psychiatric history, previous hospitalizations or treatments, educational level, previous and current employment status, previous judiciaries, history of sexual or physical aggressions, familial or social relationships, medical history and treatments, mood and anxiety, content of thought and speech, delusions, hallucinations, emotional responsiveness or interest in others or in life events, cognitive functioning and insight, daily functioning, suggested diagnosis and differential diagnosis, risk of suicide or violence, treatment objectives (for review, 15).

The first interview is crucial for the potential therapeutic alliance especially in chronic diseases such a schizophrenia. It is important that the patient feels confident during the first interview and can trust the interviewer.

REFERENCES

1. Flaum M. The diagnosis of schizophrenia. In: Shriqui CL, HA Nasrallah HA eds. Contemporary issues in the treatment of schizophrenia. Washington, DC: American Psychiatric Press, 1995: 83–108.
2. Kraepelin E, Barclay RM, Robertson GM. Dementia praecox and paraphrenia. Edinburgh, Scotland: Livingstone E and S, 1919.
3. Bleuler E. Dementia Praecox or the group of schizophrenias (1911) Translated by Zinkin J. New York International Universities Press, 1950.

4. Schneider K. Clinical psychopathology. Translated by Hamilton MW. New York: Grune and Stratton, 1959.

5. American Psychiatric Association: Diagnostic and Statistical Manual of Mental Disorders. 4th ed. revised Washington DC American Psychiatric Association, 2000.

6. World Health Organization. The ICD-10 Classification of Mental and Behavioural Disorders: diagnostic criteria for research. Paris: Masson, 1994.

7. Gauron EF, Dickinson JK. Diagnostic decision making in psychiatry. I. Information usage. Arch Gen Psychiatry 1966; (14): 225–32.

8. Gauron EF, Dickinson JK. Diagnostic decision making in psychiatry. II. Diagnostic styles. Arch Gen Psychiatry 1966; (14): 233–37.

9. Gauron EF, Dickinson JK. The influence of seeing the patient first on diagnostic decision making in psychiatry. Am J Psychiatry 1969; (126): 199–205.

10. Bourgeois M. The first few minutes : original contact and the speed of psychiatric diagnosis. In: Pichot P, Rein W, eds. The clinical approach in psychiatry. Paris: Les empêcheurs de penser en rond, 1994: 273–86.

11. Sandifer MG, Hordern A, Green LM. The psychiatric interview: the impact of the first three minutes. Am J Psychiatry 1970; (126): 968–73.

12. Rosenbaum CP. Interviewing the patient with schizophrenia. Schizophrenia 1st edition. Ed ?? Pub ?? Ch 1. Year ?? This chapter was kindly provided by the publisher but without any references.

13. Othmer E, Othmer JP, Othmer SC. Our favourite tips for "getting in" with difficult patients. Psychiatr Clin North Am 2007; 30(2): 261–68

14. Twemlow SW. Interviewing violent patients Bull Menninger Clin 2001; 65(4): 503–21.

15. Shea SC. Psychiatric interviewing. The art of understanding 2nd ed. Saunders WR, 1998.

Evaluation of symptomatology on schizophrenia

Julio Bobes, Maria P Garcia-Portilla, Pilar A Saiz, and Manuel Bousoño

INTRODUCTION

The objective rating of mental state has long been of considerable interest in psychiatric research and more recently, with the introduction of evidence-based medicine, in daily clinical practice as well. Furthermore, with the development of new biological and psychosocial treatments, the assessment and measurement of clinical change has increased the need for instruments of evaluation suitable for this purpose.

When a psychiatric scale has demonstrated to have good psychometric properties, its use has the same strengths and limitations than the biological tests employed in other medical disciplines. Thus, clinicians must be aware that evaluation scales do not replace the clinical judgment, just as laboratory or imaging results cannot, but they complement the clinical assessment and help clinicians to make accurate diagnosis and evaluate the clinical course.

Assessment scales are useful to both clinicians and patients. They help clinicians in the identification and severity rating of clinical symptoms, impairments in daily functioning and quality of life, and side-effects, in the monitoring of clinical progress and in the evaluation of outcomes. For patients, they can be helpful in promoting adherence and enhancing the therapeutic alliance.

In this chapter, we describe what we consider the most useful scales in schizophrenia for the assessment of basic symptomatology, psychosocial functioning, and quality of life.

EVALUATION OF BASIC SYMPTOMATOLOGY

Since 1950 several scales have been developed for assessing patients with psychotic disorders. Through these 60 years, scales evolved parallel to the evolution of the psychopathological model of schizophrenia. While the oldest scales used a single-dimension approach, the newer ones used a multidimensional, for example, a two-factor model assessing positive and negative symptoms—the most popular during the 80s. In this context, Carpenter, Heinrichs, and Wagman (1) differentiate between primary negative symptoms that are present as enduring traits and may contribute to define a subtype of schizophrenia from the transitory or secondary negative ones. They employed the term "deficit syndrome" to refer to the primary negative symptoms and they developed an instrument to identify it.

In the 90s, several models with three, four or five factors were developed. The recognition of other psychopathological dimensions in schizophrenia, such as depression and cognition, stimulates the development of new specific instruments for assessing this type of symptomatology in patients with schizophrenia.

In this section we describe the most widely used instruments for assessing the classic positive and negative symptoms, as well as the deficit syndrome and depressive symptoms. Cognitive assessment is dealt in Chapter 1.5.

EVALUATION OF POSITIVE AND NEGATIVE SYMPTOMS

The Brief Psychiatric Rating Scale –BPRS; Overall and Gorham, 1962

The BPRS was developed by Overall and Gorham in 1962 (2) to provide a rapid assessment procedure to evaluate treatment change in psychiatric patients. The authors recommended its use when efficiency, speed, economy, and a comprehensive description of major symptoms were needed.

This scale derives from two larger scales, i.e., Lorr's Multidimensional Scale for Rating Psychiatric Patients (3) and Inpatient Multidimensional Psychiatric Scale (4). It is a semistructured interview that provides definitions of symptoms and some suggested direct questions in order to improve interrater reliability.

The original BPRS consisted of 16 relatively discrete symptoms, and the final version (5) included the following 18 items that assess (1) somatic concern, (2) anxiety, (3) emotional withdrawal, (4) conceptual disorganization, (5) guilt feelings, (6) tension, (7) mannerisms and posturing, (8) grandiosity, (9) depressive mood, (10) hostility, (11) suspiciousness, (12) hallucinatory behavior, (13) motor retardation, (14) uncooperativeness, (15) unusual thought content, (16) blunted affect, (17) excitement, and (18) disorientation.

Each item should be rated using a Likert severity scale ranging from 1 (*not present*) to 7 (*extremely severe*). Some items are rated on the basis of observed behavior and speech, while others depend upon the verbal report of the patient. However, raters are encouraged to seek additional sources of information about the patient's psychopathology from staff, family members, or caregivers when possible.

The instrument provides a "total pathology" score that is the sum of scores on the 18 items, and scores on the negative symptoms cluster or anergia factor, sum of scores on items 3, 13, 16, and 18, and the positive symptoms cluster, sum of scores on items 4, 11, 12, and 15.

There is an expanded BPRS version (6,7) including six new symptoms to the original BPRS that provides a more comprehensive assessment of patients with severe mental disorders. The added symptoms are: suicidality, elevated mood, bizarre behavior, self-neglect, distractibility, and motor hyperactivity. In addition, this expanded version provides specific anchor points for rating symptoms.

The Positive and Negative Syndrome Scale –PANSS; Kay, Opler, and Fiszbein, 1987

The PANSS was developed by Kay, Opler, and Fiszbein (8,9) with the aim of designing a more strictly operationalized and standardized instrument without the psychometric problems that the previous scales posed. In fact, as pointed out by Peralta et al. (10), it is this scale that is most thoroughly studied from the psychometric point of view.

This scale derives from the Brief Psychiatric Rating Scale (BPRS) (2) and the Psychopathology Rating Schedule (PRS) (11). The PANSS is a 30-item, semistructured interview categorized in 3 rationally derived scales: positive (7 items), negative (7 items), and general psychopathology (16 items),

Since its development, the structure of the PANSS has greatly evolved, although the best model of how symptoms are structured is not yet identified. To date factor-analytic studies of the PANSS have yielded different models:

– Three-factor model: delusion/hallucination, disorganization, and modified negative syndrome (12)
– Four-factor pyramidical model: hallucination–delusion (positive), excitement, negative, and depression (13)

FIVE-FACTOR MODELS

Positive, negative, excitement, cognitive, and depression/anxiety (14,15)

Positive, negative, dysphoric mood, activation, and autistic preoccupation (16)

Each item is rated using a Likert 7-point scale of severity, ranging from 1= *absent* to 7= *extreme psychopathology*. The interview provides detailed operational criteria for rating the severity of a broad range of symptoms in order to achieve a reliable and standardized method of assessment.

Rating is based upon the presence, frequency, and severity of the symptom and its influence on the patient's behavior and function. As for the items, 16 items require assessment during the interview, 12 items need both the interview and corroborative information from staff and/or family, and 2 items use only information from staff or family.

The PANSS is probably the most frequently used scale, particularly in clinical trials. Recently, Andreasen et al. (17) proposed the following operational criteria for symptomatic remission in patients with schizophrenia when using the PANSS:

Symptoms severity: a score of mild or less (≤3) simultaneously on the following 8 items: delusions (P1), unusual thought content (G9), hallucinatory behavior (P3), conceptual disorganization (P2), mannerisms/posturing (G5), blunted affect (N1), social withdrawal (N4), and lack of spontaneity (N6)

Time threshold: The symptom severity criteria must be maintained during 6 months as minimum.

Although the PANSS was originally developed for using in patients with schizophrenia, it is also used in patients with bipolar disorder.

EVALUATION OF THE DEFICIT SYNDROME

The Quality of Life Scale –QLS; Heinrichs, Hanlon, and Carpenter, 1984

The Quality of Life Scale is an instrument specifically developed by Heinrichs et al. (18) for rating the schizophrenic syndrome. It is a semistructured interview gathering information on negative symptoms and functioning.

The QLS has 21 items grouped in the following four dimensions: intrapsychic foundations (7 items), interpersonal relations (8 items), instrumental role (4 items), and common objects and activities (2 items).

Each item is rated using a Likert 7-point scale of severity ranging from 0 (*severe impairment*) to 6 (*normal functioning*). The QLS provides a global score and scores in each of the four dimensions.

The authors recommend the use of the QLS in combination with measures of other dimensions of psychopathology, in order to appreciate the significance of the QLS scores.

The Schedule for the Deficit Syndrome –SDS; Kirkpatrick et al., 1989.

The SDS is an instrument designed to categorize patients with schizophrenia into deficit and nondeficit types (19). It is based in the distinction between enduring primary negative symptoms and those negative symptoms transitory or secondary.

It is made up of 6 negative items: restricted affect, diminished emotional range, poverty of speech, curbing of interests, diminished sense of purpose, and diminished social drive.

Each item is rated by the interviewer using a Likert 5-point scale of severity ranging from 0 = *normal* to 5 = *severely impaired*. The SDS provides a global deficit/ nondeficit classification—deficit syndrome requires a score ≥2 on two of the six symptoms, and a global score (0-4) reflects the severity of the deficit syndrome.

EVALUATION OF DEPRESSIVE SYMPTOMS

The Calgary Depression Scale –CDS; Addington, Addington, and Maticka-Tyndale, 1993.

The CDS was designed for assessing depression in patients with schizophrenia at any stage of the disease and avoiding the significant overlap between extrapyramidal, negative, and depressive symptoms (20,21). It was developed by factor techniques from the Present State Examination (22) and the Hamilton Depression Rating Scale (23). Several studies have demonstrated that the CDS can satisfactorily discriminate between depression and negative symptoms in patients with schizophrenia.

It is a 9-item scale; 8 items are rated using a structured interview and the last one depends on the observation during the whole interview. The items included are depression, hopelessness, self-depreciation, guilty ideas of reference, pathological guilt, morning depression, early wakening, suicide, and observed depression.

Scores for each symptom range from 0 = *absent* to 3 = *severe*. There are descriptive anchors for every other point. The CDS provides a global score ranging from 0 to 27 points.

EVALUATION OF FUNCTIONING

Patients suffering from schizophrenia often show deterioration on their functional status, that is, social and occupational functioning, living status, and instrumental daily living activities.

Taking into account that "the ultimate clinical objective in the treatment of schizophrenia is to enable patients to lead the most productive and meaningful lives possible" (24), accurate assessment of functioning is important in evaluating the treatment needs of patients and producing successful outcomes.

The Global Assessment of Functioning –GAF- (25) and the Social and Occupational Functioning Assessment Scales –SOFAS- (25), both developed by the American Psychiatric Association, are the most used scales for the assessment of this area. However, they have been recently criticized because they incorporate psychopathological symptoms in the evaluation of functioning. Thus, a new scale, the Personal and Social Performance scale –PSP- (26) is now considered the best scale for the assessment of the functioning in patients with schizophrenia.

The Personal and Social Performance scale –PSP; Morosini et al., 2000

The PSP was developed by Morosini (26) for assessing the level of personal and social functioning in a more valid and reliable way than the SOFAS (25). Patient functioning is assessed in the following four areas: socially useful activities, including work and study; personal and social relationships; self-care; and disturbing and aggressive behaviors.

It consists of a single-item that rates global personal and social functioning using a 100-point scale divided into ten 10-point intervals. To rate this item first it is needed to rate the level of functioning in the 4 areas of functioning using a 6-point scale with operational criteria ranging from absent to very severe. Then an algorithm is applied to incorporate the degree of difficulties in the 4 areas into a single score from 0 to 100. The global score ranges described by the authors are 1 to 30: *poor functioning*, 31 to 70: *manifest disabilities*, 71 to 90: *mild difficulties*, and 91 to 100: *more than adequate functioning*.

EVALUATION OF QUALITY OF LIFE

The assessment of quality of life in patients with schizophrenia is an area of growing concern because it is considered an essential distal outcome for clinical trials and patient management (27). The assessment is based on the principle of applying medical care and interventions, bearing in mind patients' right of autonomy, which necessarily includes taking into account their opinion during diagnostic evaluation and in formulating their care plan (28).

Until recently, some doubts existed concerning whether schizophrenic patients, due to their lack of insight into their illness and cognitive deficiencies, are capable of self-assessing their quality of life. However, the results of several studies allow us to conclude that quality of life is a consistent and homogeneous concept that can be measured by self-reports even in the case of patients affected by schizophrenia.

In recent years, there has been a great effort for developing adequate quality of life instruments with conceptual framework, measurement model, and acceptable psychometric properties. For this reason, clinicians and researchers have available several psychometrically tested quality of life instruments for use with schizophrenic patients, both generic and specific. The choice of the instrument(s) will depend on the aim of the quality of life measurement, taking in account that, if possible, a generic instrument should be combined with a specific one.

In this section we describe the most widely employed generic instrument, the Short-Form Health Survey—SF 36-, and one specific instrument developed in Europe, the Lancashire Quality of Life Profile—LQoLP.

The Medical Outcome Study (MOS) 36-Item Short-Form Health Survey –SF-36; Ware and Sherbourne, 1992.

The SF-36 (29) is a well-established, widely used, generic quality of life instrument. Because it was not specifically developed for patients with schizophrenia Pukrop et al. (30) determined its validity for using in this population.

It consists of 36 items grouped into the following eight scales: physical functioning, role physical, bodily pain, general health, vitality, social functioning, role emotional, and mental health. These eight scales can be summed up into two broader dimensions: physical health and mental health.

It is a self-rated instrument; it takes approximately 15 minutes. Scores range from 0 to 100, with higher values indicating higher quality of life.

The Lancashire Quality of Life Profile –LQoLP; Oliver et al., 1996.

The LQoLP has been developed by Oliver et al. (31) from the Lehman's Quality of Life Interview (32).

This instrument combines objective and subjective measures in the following nine life domains: living situation, social relationships, work and education, legal status and safety, religion, family relations, leisure activities, finances, and health. The LQoLP also measures the following additional areas: positive and negative affect (with the Bradburn Affect-Balance Scale); self-esteem; global well-being (Cantril's Ladder and Happiness Scale); perceived quality of life; and the quality of life of the patient, independent of the patient's own opinion (with the Quality of Life Uniscale).

It is a structured self-report interview with 105 items that takes approximately 45 minutes. There is a European version, the LQoLP-EU, developed in the context of the EPSILON Study 8 (33).

CONCLUSIONS

In the last two decades, there was a great interest in the development of valid instruments for assessing schizophrenia from a multidimensional point of view. Thus, these days, clinicians have an arsenal of psychometric valid scales that allows them to take clinical decisions based on the best available information, to monitor clinical changes and to evaluate clinical outcomes, from psychopathology to quality of life.

REFERENCES

1. Carpenter WT, Heinrichs DW, Wagman AMI. Deficit and non-deficit forms of schizophrenia: the concept. Am J Psychiatr 1988; 145: 578–83.
   Overall JE, Gorham DR. The Brief Psychiatric Rating Scale. Psychological Reports 1962; 10: 799–812.
2. Lorr M, Jenkins RL, Holsopple JQ. Multidimensional Sclae for Rating Psychiatric Patients. V A Tech Bull 1953; 10: 507.
3. Lorr M, McNair DM, Klett CJ et al. A confirmation of nine postulated psychotic syndromes. Am Psychologist 1960; 15: 495.
4. Overall JE, Hollister LE. Assessment of Depression using the Brief Psychiatric Rating Scale. In: Sartorius N, Ban TA, eds. Assessment for Depression. Berlin: Springer, 1986: 159–78.
5. Lukoff D, Nuechterlein KH, Ventura J. Manual for the Expanded Brief Psychiatric Rating Scale. Schizophrenia Bull 1986; 12: 594–602.
6. Ventura J, Lukoff D, Nuechterlein KH et al. Appendix 1. Brief Psychiatric Rating Scale (BPRS). Expanded Version (4.0). Scales, anchor points, and administration manual. Int J Methods Psychiatr Res 1993; 3: 227–44.
7. Kay SR, Opler LA, Fiszbein A. Positive and Negative Syndrome Scale (PANSS). Rating manual. New York: Albert Einstein College of Medicine, 1986.
8. Kay SR, Fiszbein A, Opler LA. The Positive and Negative Syndrome Scale (PANSS) for schizophrenia. Schizophr Bull 1987; 13: 261–76.
9. Peralta V, Cuesta MJ, de Leon J. Positive and negative symptoms/síndromes in schizophrenia: reliability and validity of different diagnostic systems. Psychological Med 1995; 25: 43–50.
10. Singh MM, Kay SR. A comparative study of haloperidol and chlorpromazine in terms of clinical effects and therapeutic reversal with benztropine in schizophrenia: theoretical implications for potency differences among neuroleptics. Psychopharmacologia 1975; 43: 103–13.
11. Arndt S, Alliger RJ, Andreasen N. The distinction of positive and negative symptoms: the failure of a two-dimensional model. Br J Psychiatry 1991; 158: 317–22.
12. Kay SR, Sevy S. Pyramidical model of schizophrenia. Schizophr Bull 1990; 16: 537–45.
13. Lindenmayer JP, Bernstein-Hyman R, Grochowski S. Five-factor model of schizophrenia. Initial validation. J Nerv Ment Dis 1994; 182: 631–38.
14. Lindenmayer JP, Brown E, Baker RW et al. An excitement subscale of the positive and negative syndrome scale. Schizophr Res 2004; 68: 331–37.
15. White L, Harvey PD, Opler L, Lindenmayer JP, and the PANSS Study Group. Empirical assessment of the factorial structure of clinical symptoms in schizophrenia. A multisite, multimodel evaluation of the factorial structure of the Positive and Negative Syndrome Scale. Psychopathology 1997; 30: 263–74.
16. Andreasen NC, Carpenter WT, Kane JM et al. Remission in schizophrenia: proposed criteria and rationale for consensus. Am J Psychiatry 2005; 162: 441–49.
17. Heinrichs DW, Hanlon TE, Carpenter WT. The Quality of Life Scale: an instrument for rating the schizophrenic deficit syndrome. Schizophr Bull 1984; 10: 388–98.
18. Kirpartrick B, Buchanan RW, McKenney PD, Alphs LD, Carpenter WT Jr. The Schedule for the Deficit Syndrome: an Instrument for Research in Schizophrenia. Psychiatr Res 1989; 30: 119–23.

19. Addington D, Addington J, Schissel B. A depression rating scale for schizophrenics. Schizophr Res 1990; 3: 247–51.
20. Addington D, Addington J, Maticka-Tyndale E. Assessing depression in schizophrenia: the Calgary Depression Scale. Br J Psychiatry 1993; 163(suppl 2): 39–44.
21. Wing JK, Cooper JE, Sartorius N. The Measurement and Classification fo Psychiatric Symptoms. London: Cambridge University Press, 1974.
22. Hamilton M. A rating scale for depression. J Neurol Neurosurg Psychiat 1960; 23: 56–62.
23. Tandon R, Targum SD, Nasrallah HA, Ross R. Treatment effectiveness in schizophrenia consortium. Strategies for maximizing clinical effectiveness in the treatment of schizophrenia. J Psychiatr Practice 2006; 12: 348–63.
24. American Psychiatric Association. Diagnostic and Statistical Manual of Mental Disorders, 4th ed. Washington, DC: APA, 1994.
25. Morosini P-L, Magliano L, Brambilla L, Ugolini S, Pioli R. Development, reliability and acceptability of a new version of the DSM-IV social and Occupational Functioning 26. Assessment Scale (SOFAS) to assess routine social functioning. Acta Psychiatr Scand 2000; 101: 323–29.
27. Bobes J, García-Portilla P, Sáiz PA, Bascarán MT, Bousoño M. Quality of life measures in schizophrenia. Eur Psychiatry 2005; 20: S313–S317.
28. Bobes J. Current status of quality of life assessment in schizophrenic patients. Eur Arch Psychiatry Clin Neurosc 2001; 251(suppl 2): II/38–II/42.
29. Ware JE, Sherbourne CD. The MOS 36-Item Short-Form Health Survey (SF-36). Med Care 1992; 30 473–83.
30. Pukrop R, Schlaak V, Möller-Leimkühler AM et al. Reliability and validity of quality of life assessed by the Short-Form 36 and the Modular System for Quality of Life in patients with schizophrenia and patients with depression. Psychiatr Res 2003; 119: 63–79.
31. Oliver JPJ, Huxley PJ, Priebe S, Kaiser W. Measuring the quality of life of severly mentally ill people using the Lancashire Quality of Life Profile. Soc Psychiatry Psychiatr Epidemiol 1997; 32: 76–83.
32. Lehman AF. A Quality of Life Interview for the chronically mentally ill (QOLI). Eval Prog Planning 1988; 11: 51–62.
33. Gaite L, Vázquez-Barquero JL, Arriaga A et al. Quality of life in schizophrenia: development, reliability and internal consistency of the Lancashire Quality of Life Profile – European version. Br J Psychiatr 2000; 177(suppl 39): s49–s54.

5 Clinical characteristics of first-episode schizophrenia

Lisa P Henry, Patrick D McGorry, Meredith G Harris, and Paul Amminger

INTRODUCTION

Throughout the 20th century, numerous studies examined the clinical characteristics, illness course, and outcomes for schizophrenia cohorts (1). Until the mid-1980s, these cohorts were usually clinically heterogeneous with samples derived from predominately multiepisode, severely ill cases, and comprising individuals with varying duration of illness at different stages of the disorder (2–4). Because of this selection bias toward more chronically ill cases, the conclusions were often inevitably pessimistic, in particular regarding the long-term outcome (5). Findings from studies recruiting patients at different stages of illness may, therefore, not be representative for schizophrenia in general. More recently, the clinical and research focus has shifted from multiepisode schizophrenia cohorts to first-episode schizophrenia cohorts. First-episode cohorts have the advantage of examining both clinical characteristics at first presentation and outcomes free from the confounding issues of heterogeneous, multiepisode samples such as previous treatments, illness duration and disability, and illness-related selection. This development has contributed to the emergence of a new paradigm concerning early detection and specialized intervention programs for first-episode patients such as the Early Psychosis Prevention and Intervention Centre (EPPIC) in Melbourne, Australia (6). These programs provide early intervention strategies, specialized treatment strategies supported by clinical protocols, treatment manuals, and educational material for first episode psychosis patients and their families; the programs have been generally successful at recruiting and treating patients earlier during their first episode of psychosis (7). First-episode psychosis programs also facilitate the recruitment of patients for research purposes who are homogeneous for illness phase and have a range of psychotic disorders, thus providing a more complete picture of clinical manifestations of psychosis and the opportunity for comparison between diagnostic groups.

OUTCOME STUDIES IN FIRST-EPISODE SCHIZOPHRENIA

The past two decades have witnessed the emergence of prospective follow-up studies focusing upon first-episode psychosis (8-10) and first-episode schizophrenia cohorts (11–15). These studies provide the opportunity to examine the characteristics of psychotic disorders and to assess prognosis among a cohort, at the same phase of illness, free from the confounding effects of previous treatment interventions or secondary disability (16, 17). However, despite the obvious advantages of this approach, few large, prospective, longitudinal studies of illness course and outcome in first-episode psychosis have been conducted, reflecting the complexities and challenges of recruiting and retaining such a cohort. Studies to date have typically involved either large but heterogeneous, nonrepresentative samples (15, 18, 19) or, conversely, comparatively smaller cohorts that approximate epidemiological samples (8, 20, 21). Other limitations of first-episode follow-up studies are lack of standardized sampling methods, entry criteria and information regarding the completeness and representativeness of recruited samples. Few studies have conducted longitudinal assessments beyond 24 months; these have focused on patients with schizophrenia (13–15, 22–25). This body of work provides a resource for examining the characteristics of first-episode psychosis and schizophrenia, particularly when conducted in representative samples. However, in a recent review of the methodology, in particular the sampling procedures, of longitudinal first-episode studies published from 1996 (26), all but two studies were confidently considered representative for first-episode psychosis (8, 27). Sampling biases falling into three categories were observed: (1) the absence of data collected or reported on individuals who refused to participate, and comparisons of this group with study participants (28–38); (2) limited diagnostic range with a sampling bias toward nonaffective psychosis (schizophrenia spectrum disorder) (31–34, 36, 37); and (3) convenience samples with inevitable biases, for example, inpatients only, tertiary referrals to private hospitals, mixed first- and multiepisode samples, male predominance, and exclusion of participants without family involvement (18, 30, 34, 35, 37–40). The findings are summarized in Table 5.1. While this body of research has sought to elucidate the correlates of outcome in psychosis, the limitations of nonrepresentative first-episode psychosis studies with sampling biases, small samples, and short follow-up periods impede generalizability and validity of the results.

In summary, the consistent impression from these follow-up studies in first-episode cohorts is that individuals with schizophrenia tend to have unfavorable symptomatic and functional outcomes compared to individuals with affective psychoses (8, 30). Substance use in first-episode psychosis is associated with more persisting positive symptoms, and substance-related psychoses have in particular very poor occupational outcome (8). Negative symptoms occur in all psychotic disorders but are more frequent and prominent in schizophrenia than in affective psychoses (30). Narrower concepts of negative symptoms, conceptualized as the deficit syndrome, seem to be rather specific for schizophrenia (30). Longer duration of untreated psychosis (DUP) predicts poorer outcome independently of other variables and is not simply a proxy for other factors (27, 41). The association of DUP with treatment resistance supports the argument for early intervention as soon as possible following the onset of psychotic symptoms (28). As one of the few potentially malleable factors influencing outcome, DUP has been suggested as a target for secondary preventive efforts in first-episode schizophrenia.

Much less information is available on the clinical characteristics of first-episode schizophrenia compared to first-episode bipolar disorder with psychotic features and first-episode major depression with psychotic features upon initial presentation to a service. To our knowledge, the only epidemiological study that has been conducted is the Suffolk County Mental Health Project (40). In this study, a sample of first-admission patients was drawn from 10 inpatient and 25 outpatient facilities comparing the three groups of the most common psychotic disorders. Of the total sample, 58% of males and 29% of females had a history of substance abuse or dependence. Sex differences were reported on several background and clinical characteristics. Males were younger, less likely to have ever married, and had less years of education. Individuals with schizophrenia-related disorders were characterized by significantly more negative symptoms than were affectively ill subjects, but clinical ratings of depression were not significantly different across diagnostic groups (40). The median DUP the Suffolk County Mental Health Project was 98 days for schizophrenia, 9 days for psychotic bipolar disorder, and 22 days for psychotic depression (18).

TABLE 5.1 An overview of the sampling procedures in longitudinal first episode psychosis studies published from 1996 to 2006

Study	Diagnostic range† (% FES or FEnonAFF)	Age range‡	Male (%) area§	Catchment	Consecutive recruitment	Inpatients only	Eligible N¶	Study N#	Refusal (%)¢	Bias testing±	Study representative
Bromet et al. [40]; Craig et al. [18]		15–60	54	Yes	Not reported	Yes	Not reported	349	28	Yes	No: 3
Edwards et al. [28]	FEP (58.6%)	16–45	64	Yes	Yes	No	Not reported	347	Not reported	No	No: 1
Takei et al. [38]	FEP (44.4%)	18–44	63	Yes	Yes	Yes	Not reported	88	Not reported	No	No: 1, 3
Carbone et al. [29]	FEP (58%)	16–45	64.4	Yes	Yes	No	Not reported	347	Not reported	No	No: 1
Larsen et al. [37]	FES (81.4%)	15–55	65	Yes	Yes	Yes	Not reported	43	Not reported	No	No: 1, 2, 3
Lehtinen et al. [36]	FEnonAff (40%)	15–44	59	Yes	Yes	Not reported	165	135	18	No	No: 1, 2
Singh et al. [8]	FEP (33.7%)	16–64	59	Yes	Yes	No	167	166	0.6	N/A	Yes
Tohen et al. [39]	FEP (5.5%)	Minimum 16-years	59	No	Not reported	Yes	784	296	62	Yes	No: 3
Linszen et al. [35]	FEP (68%)	15–26	Not reported	No	Yes	Yes	Not reported	97	Not reported	No	No: 1, 3
Moeller et al. [30]	FES (49%), FESA, FEA	Not reported	Not reported	No	Yes	Yes	Not reported	374	Not reported	No	No: 1, 3
Novak-Grubic & Tavcar [34]	FES (% not reported), FESA	Not reported (mean =27years)	100	Yes at baseline	Yes	Yes	Not reported	56	Not reported	No	No: 1, 2, 3

TABLE 5.1 (Continued)

Study	Diagnostic range (% FES or FEnonAFF)†	Age range‡	Male (%) area§	Catchment	Consecutive recruitment	Inpatients only	Eligible N¶	Study N#	Refusal (%)¢	Bias testing±	Study representative
Whitehorn et al. [33]	FES (89%), FESA	Not reported	67	Not reported	Not reported	No	Not reported	103	Not reported	No	No: 1, 2
Addington et al. [31]	FES (88%)	16–50	70	Yes	Yes	No	Not reported	257	Not reported	No	No: 1, 2
Harrigan et al. [27]	FEP (57%)	16–45	71.2	Yes	Yes	No	Not reported	565	≤25	Yes	Yes: Two periods during recruitment where data collected on refusers and compared to participants.
Stirling et al. [32]	FES (83.7%),	16–50	57	Yes	Yes	No	Not reported	112	Not reported	No	No: 1, 2

† Diagnostic range: FEP= first episode psychosis, FES= first episode schizophrenia spectrum disorder, FESA= first episode schizoaffective, FEA= first episode affective psychosis, FEnonAff= first episode non-affective psychosis.
‡ Age range: Age range of study participants at recruitment.
§ Catchment area: Study conducted in a catchment area.
¶ Eligible N: Record of all eligible study subjects at recruitment.
# Study N: Participant sample size at study entry.
¢ Refusal: Those who were eligible for the study but not included because of refusal at recruitment phase.
± Bias testing: Comparison between study participants and eligible study refusals.
+ Study sample representative for FEP: Yes or No based upon sampling bias. Categories of sampling bias: 1) the absence of comparisons of study refusers with participants; 2) limited diagnostic range of FEP; and 3) convenience samples derived from specific conditions.
Re-printed with permission from Henry and colleagues

The following section presents findings on demographic and illness characteristics of individuals with first-episode schizophrenia in comparison to individuals with first-episode bipolar disorder or depressive disorder with psychotic features, from The Early Psychosis Prevention and Intervention Centre (EPPIC) long-term follow-up study of first-episode psychosis (42). The study has important strengths and is, therefore, used to demonstrate clinical characteristics of first-episode schizophrenia. First, to our knowledge it is the largest multidiagnostic, epidemiologically representative prospective long-term follow-up study, comprising a cohort of 723 individuals; second, diagnostic, functional, and clinical assessments were conducted at multiple time points, including the index presentation, using standard and reliable measures with carefully established, good or excellent interrater reliability.

METHODOLOGY

Study sample
The study sample comprised 442 first-episode patients from the EPPIC long-term follow-up study (42) who had a baseline diagnosis of schizophrenia, bipolar disorder or major depressive disorder with psychotic features.

Study design
The EPPIC long-term follow-up study was designed in an attempt to address methodological shortcomings of previous longitudinal studies in schizophrenia (42). The study provides a baseline data and a naturalistic, prospective follow-up of a large cohort of 723 consecutive patients experiencing a first episode of psychosis, a median 7.4 years after initial presentation to a specialist early psychosis service, EPPIC in Melbourne, Australia. The study was designed to describe the presenting characteristics and the long-term clinical, functional, and psychosocial outcome of 723 individuals treated at EPPIC for up to the first 2 years of illness. EPPIC (6) is a comprehensive, integrated, community-based treatment program for first-episode psychosis patients aged between 14 and 30 years, drawn from an urban-defined catchment area of approximately 850,000 in Melbourne, Australia. The catchment area is socioeconomically disadvantaged, has minimal private sector services, and those that exist typically refer first-episode psychosis cases to EPPIC. It is, therefore, estimated that the number of new cases accepted into EPPIC (approximately 240 per year) represents close to the entire treated incidence of first-episode psychosis in this age group within the catchment area (43).

The present study cohort comprises all consecutive admissions into studies conducted at EPPIC between April 1989 and January 2001. We have previously shown that the cohort is representative of the full treated incidence of first-episode psychosis treated at EPPIC in terms of epidemiological and psychopathological characteristics (1; page 56, Table 5.4). In cohort size, the EPPIC study is comparable to the early longitudinal studies of schizophrenia (4, 44, 45). The EPPIC study, however, is not limited to schizophrenia but provides detailed standardized information on the full diagnostic range of psychotic disorders.

ASSESSMENTS
The cohort underwent diagnostic, functional, and clinical assessments conducted at multiple time points using standard and reliable measures with carefully established,

good or excellent interrater reliability. The assessment instruments are reported else-where. The assessment time-points were (1) within the first few days following entry into treatment (baseline), (2) after first treatment response or stabilization (an average of 8 weeks after baseline), (3) 3 to 6 months after stabilization, (4) 12 months after sta-bilization, and (5) median 7.4 years after baseline.

For the purpose of this chapter, the standardized assessments used to assess participants' demographic characteristics, diagnosis, psychopathology, and level of functioning at baseline are presented below.

Demographics and level of functioning

Baseline demographic characteristics of participants, including gender, date of birth, age of study entry, marital status, and current work status, were assessed using the Royal Park Multidiagnostic Instrument for Psychosis (RPMIP) (46) or the Structure Clinical Interview for DSM-IV axis 1 Disorders - Patient Version (SCID I/P) (47).

Diagnosis

At baseline the RPMIP was administered to 571 subjects, while the remaining 152 subjects were administered the SCID-I/P, to ascertain Axis I diagnoses. The RPMIP was designed as a comprehensive and valid assessment and diagnostic tool for first-episode psychosis and also assessed range of psychosis illness-related variables, including duration and type of prodromal symptoms and the DUP. DUP is defined as the number of days between the onset of sustained psychotic symptoms and initia-tion of treatment. The onset of prodrome is defined as the earliest clinically significant deviation from the patient's premorbid personality. As baseline assessments were con-ducted from 1989, the RPMIP originally provided *DSM-III-R* diagnoses. Subsequently, these diagnoses were converted to *DSM-IV*.

Psychopathology

At baseline, interviewer-administered measures included the Brief Psychiatric Rating Scale-Expanded Version (BPRS-E) (48) to evaluate severity of major psychiatric symp-tom characteristics, and the Schedule for the Assessment of Negative Symptoms (SANS) (49) was used to evaluate the severity of five negative symptoms: affective blunting, alogia, avolition, anhedonia, and attention impairment.

Data Analysis

Baseline patient characteristics were compared across three baseline diagnostic groups: schizophrenia, bipolar disorder, and depressive disorder with psychotic fea-tures. One-way ANOVAs were conducted to test for differences between the diag-nostic groups for the following variables: age at first treatment, DUP, SANS total score at baseline, BPRS total, and psychotic subscale scores at baseline. Tukey hon-estly significant difference test was used for *post hoc* analyses as appropriate to test differences between individual diagnostic groups. Chi-square tests were conducted to test for differences between the diagnostic groups for the following variables: gen-der, marital status, and work status immediately prior to first treatment. The level of significance for all analyses was set at $p \leq 0.05$. All statistical analyses were carried out using SPSS (Version 14.0.2).

The following section details the baseline characteristics of the cohort in order to define the clinical characteristics of individuals with first-episode schizophrenia compared to individuals with first-episode bipolar disorder and depressive disorder with psychotic features.

RESULTS

Table 5.2 presents the *DSM-IV* psychotic diagnostic distribution of the study sample in terms of demographic, clinical, and functioning characteristics at initial presentation.

The sample comprised 261 (59.0%) individuals with schizophrenia, 94 (21.3%) individuals with bipolar disorder, and 87 (19.7%) individuals with depressive disorder with psychotic features. No age difference was found between the diagnostic groups, $F(2, 439) = 0.10$, $p = 0.90$. Chi-square test indicated significant sex differences between the diagnostic groups ($\chi^2 = 16.6$, $df = 2$, $p < 0.001$). Individuals diagnosed with schizophrenia were predominately male, while the group with bipolar disorder had an almost equal sex distribution. A t test revealed no significant difference for sex and age of onset of psychosis ($p = 0.09$). Results from a two-way between-groups ANOVA found no significant difference in the effect of age of onset of psychosis on diagnostic groups for males and females, $F(2,436) = 0.15$, $p = 0.86$.

Duration of untreated psychosis

DUP significantly differed between the diagnostic groups, $F(2, 376) = 18.80$, $p < 0.001$ (Table 5.2). Post hoc group comparisons indicated that individuals with schizophrenia had a significantly longer DUP than individuals with bipolar disorder ($p < 0.001$) and individuals with depressive disorder ($p < 0.001$).

Although DUP was longer in the depressive group than in the bipolar group, this difference was not statistically significant.

Psychopathology

The BPRS psychotic subscale mean score significantly differed between the diagnostic groups, $F(2, 351) = 6.29$, $p = 0.002$ (Table 5.2). Post hoc group comparisons indicated that individuals with schizophrenia were characterized by significantly more psychotic symptoms at initial presentation than the group with bipolar disorder ($p = 0.04$), and the group with depressive disorder ($p = 0.006$). The SANS total mean score also significantly differed between the diagnostic groups, $F(2, 321) = 52.47$, $p < 0.001$ (Table 5.2). Post hoc group comparisons revealed that the group with bipolar disorder was characterized by a significantly lower SANS total mean score compared to the group with first-episode schizophrenia ($p < 0.001$) and the group with depressive disorder ($p < 0.001$).

Psychosocial Functioning

Chi-square test revealed a significant difference between the diagnostic groups for marital status at initial presentation with the highest proportion of not married individuals in the group with first-episode schizophrenia, $\chi^2 = 14.8$, $df = 4$, $p = 0.005$. The diagnostic groups also significantly differed for work status prior to first treatment with the highest proportion of employed individuals in the group with bipolar disorder, $\chi^2 = 10.4$, $df = 4$, $p = 0.035$ (Table 5.2).

TABLE 5.2 Means (with standard deviations in parentheses) or percentages, for baseline characteristics of 442 first-episode psychosis patients grouped according to baseline psychotic diagnosis

Characteristic	Schizophrenia n = 261	Bipolar n = 94	Depressive n = 87	P value
Age at entry, years	21.9 (3.7)	22.0 (3.3)	21.8 (4.0)	NS
Gender, % Male	77.0	55.3	65.5	<0.001
Marital status, % 1				0.005
Never married	88.7	80.2	73.5	
Married/defacto	8.9	11.6	22.1	
Separated/divorced	2.4	8.1	4.4	
Work status, % 1				0.035
Employed	58.8	67.0	53.1	
Unemployed	19.2	7.7	13.6	
Student/home duties	22.1	25.3	33.3	
DUP, days § 1	364.1 (607.4)	19.1 (38.9)	102.9 (227.1)	<0.001a
Median	183.0	10.0	29.0	
SANS (total) #	29.3 (15.2)	10.9 (8.3)	27.0 (14.5)	<0.001b
BPRS (total) ¢ 1	29.5 (9.2)	27.6 (9.4)	30.1 (10.8)	NS
BPRS-PS ± 1	11.2 (3.4)	10.0 (3.8)	9.5 (4.7)	0.002a

1 Subject numbers vary between n = 324–442 for these variables
§ DUP (log transformed for analysis. Descriptive data shown here are untransformed)
# Schedule for the Assessment of Negative Symptoms at treatment entry
¢ Brief Psychiatric Rating Scale at treatment entry (18-item version)
± Psychotic subscale at treatment entry derived from the Brief Psychiatric Rating Scale (comprising suspicious-ness, hallucinations, unusual
thought content, conceptual disorganisation items) 24
a Significant post hoc differences: Schizophrenia > bipolar disorder, depressive psychotic disorder.
b Significant post hoc differences: Schizophrenia > bipolar disorder; depressive psychotic disorder > bipolar disorder.

DISCUSSION

The present cohort was younger at initial presentation compared to other studies (18, 37, 39, 50). This reflects the age range (14–30 years) accepted into the EPPIC treatment program. The observed diagnostic breakdown with about 60% individuals diagnosed with schizophrenia is similar to previous reports (see Table 5.1). In over 50 studies, males have been found to develop schizophrenia earlier in life than females (51). In the Mannheim ABC first-episode sample that used a broad definition of schizophrenia, the mean age at the emergence of the first sign of the disorder, the first negative and first positive symptom, and the maximum of positive symptoms, all differed significantly by 3 to 4 years between males and females (52). Similar observations have been reported in a pooled data analysis of WHO 10-country study (53). However, a few other studies failed to find sex differences in the age of onset of psychotic symptoms (43, 54, 55). The present study did not find a significant sex difference for age of onset of psychotic symptoms. This may be explained by the fact that the study sample included individuals during the peak onset phase of schizophrenia but not after the age of 30 years.

The higher proportion of individuals diagnosed with schizophrenia being unmarried compared to the other two groups (bipolar and depressive disorder with psychotic features) is consistent with previous reports (18, 40). We found a significant difference among the investigated diagnostic groups for work status at initial presentation with a higher proportion of employed individuals in the bipolar group compared to the other two diagnostic groups. Similar although not significant observations have been reported in a study by Singh et al. (8), which compared nonaffective and affective first-episode psychotic groups at first treatment intake. The shorter DUP in individuals with bipolar disorder may be one factor contributing to the higher employment rate in this group.

Regarding psychopathology in general, we observed no clinically relevant differences between the investigated diagnostic groups. The significant difference for negative symptoms between the bipolar disorder group and the schizophrenia group observed in the present study is consistent with a previous report by Bromet and colleagues (40). In contrast to the present study, Bromet and colleagues also found that individuals with schizophrenia were characterized by significantly more negative symptoms than individuals with major depression with psychotic features. Varying inclusion criteria and different recruitment strategies used in the studies might account for this discrepancy. The study by Bromet (40) was a multisite study with an age range of 15 to 60 years, and some participants had previously been treated for psychosis.

In the present study, DUP was substantially longer in individuals with first-episode schizophrenia compared to both individuals with first-episode bipolar disorder and individuals with a first episode of psychotic depression. This finding on DUP is consistent with the study by Craig and colleagues (18), who used similar diagnostic groupings as the present study; however, DUP was not applied as a continuous variable but categorized into four time intervals (<4 week, 4 weeks to 6 months, 6 months to 1 year, >1 year). The construct of DUP has attracted interest among clinicians and researchers, as it represents one of the few modifiable predictors of outcome in schizophrenia. There is evidence that DUP correlates moderately with short-term (29, 41, 56) and long-term (57) symptomatic and functional outcomes, independent of premorbid functioning. Attempts at modifying or targeting DUP in the form of early interventions have been generally successful at recruiting and treating patients earlier during their first episode of psychosis (7) and, therefore, reducing DUP. Reducing DUP is one of a host of objectives in the reform process in the treatment of psychotic disorders that has culminated in approximately 200 early intervention services globally that focus specifically on young people with first manifestations of psychosis (58, 59), along with guidelines specific to early psychosis included in the clinical practice guidelines for the treatment of schizophrenia (60).

LIMITATIONS

The following limitations apply to the present study: (a) We did not incorporate a leakage study, unlike previous reports that were able to identify subjects missed by an initial screening process (8, 50). However, the catchment area of EPPIC offers few alternative private sector treatment options for psychosis, and the sample includes patients treated solely as outpatients; (b) The age range of the present study was limited to 14-30 years of age. However, based upon previous incidence studies the majority (approximately 80%) of those who are likely to be affected a psychotic disorder would show relevant symptoms at the age of 30 years (61); (c) Subjects were not recruited continuously into this cohort across the full recruitment period. During periods of recruitment, however, we were able to show that the recruited subjects did not differ from those not recruited (42); (d) An important limitation is that substance abuse or dependence was not systematically recorded in the cohort.

SUMMARY OF FINDINGS

Individuals experiencing first-episode schizophrenia differed from the other investigated diagnostic groups at initial presentation to a clinical service. Based upon the findings from the current epidemiologically representative sample, the likely clinical profile at first treatment intake of individuals with first-episode schizophrenia, compared to individuals with a first-episode of psychotic bipolar disorder or depressive disorder, is predominately male, unmarried, more often unemployed, experiencing more severe positive and negative symptoms, and a lengthy DUP (>6 months).

REFERENCES

1. Hegarty JD, Baldessarini RJ, Tohen M, Waternaux C, Oepen G. One hundred years of schizophrenia: A meta-analysis of the outcome literature. American Journal of Psychiatry 1994; 151(10): 1409–16.
2. Bleuler M. The schizophrenic disorders: Long-term patient and family studies. New Haven, Conn: Yale University Press 1978.
3. Ciompi L. Catamnestic long-term study on the course of life and aging of schizophrenics. Schizophrenia Bulletin 1980; 6(4): 606–16.
4. Huber G, Gross G, Schuttler R. A long-term follow-up study of schizophrenia: Psychiatric course of illness and prognosis. Acta Psychiatrica Scandinavica 1975; 52(1): 49–57.
5. Cohen P, Cohen J. The clinician's illusion. Archives of General Psychiatry 1984; 41: 1178–82.
6. McGorry PD, Edwards J, Mihalopoulos C, Harrigan S, Jackson H. EPPIC: An evolving system of early detection and optimal management. Schizophrenia Bulletin 1996; 22(2): 305–26.
7. Melle I, Larsen TK, Haahr U et al. Reducing the duration of untreated first-episode psychosis. Archives of General Psychiatry 2004; 61: 143–50.
8. Singh SP, Croudace T, Amin S et al. Three-year outcome of first-episode psychoses in an established community psychiatric service. British Journal of Psychiatry 2000; 176: 210–6.
9. Rabiner CJ, Wegner JT, Kane JM. Outcome study of first-episode psychosis: I. Relapse rates after 1 year. American Journal of Psychiatry 1986; 143(9): 1155–8.
10. Mojtabai R, Herman D, Susser ES et al. Service use and outcomes of first-admission patients with psychotic disorders in the Suffolk County Mental Health Project. American Journal of Psychiatry 2005; 162: 1291–8.
11. Lieberman JA, Alvir JM, Woerner M et al. Prospective study of psychobiology in first-episode schizophrenia at Hillside Hospital. Schizophrenia Bulletin 1992; 18(3): 351–71.
12. Johnstone EC, MacMillan JF, Frith CD, Benn DK, Crow TJ. Further investigation of the predictors of outcome following first schizophrenic episodes. British Journal of Psychiatry 1990; 157: 182–9.
13. Mason P, Harrison G, Glazebrook C, Medley I, Dalkin T. Characteristics of outcome in schizophrenia at 13 years. British Journal of Psychiatry 1995; 167: 596–603.
14. Thara R, Henrietta M, Joseph A, Rajkumar S, Eaton W. Ten-year course of schizophrenia: The Madras longitudinal study. Acta Psychiatrica Scandinavica 1994; 90(5): 329–36.
15. Robinson DG, Woerner MG, McMeniman M, Mendelowitz A, Bilder RM. Symptomatic and functional recovery from a first episode of schizophrenia or schizoaffective disorder. American Journal of Psychiatry 2004; 161(3): 473–9.
16. Browne S, Larkin C, O'Callaghan E. Outcome studies in schizophrenia. Irish Journal of Psychological Medicine 1999; 16(4): 140–4.
17. Clarke M, O'Callaghan E. The value of first-episode studies in schizophrenia. In: Murran RM, Jones PB, eds. The Epidemiology of Schizophrenia. New York, NY: Cambridge University Press 2003: 148–66.
18. Craig TJ, Bromet EJ, Fennig S et al. Is there an association between duration of untreated psychosis and 24-month clinical outcome in a first-admission series? American Journal of Psychiatry 2000; 157(1): 606.

19. Harrison G, Hopper K, Craig T et al. Recovery from psychotic illness: A 15- and 25-year international follow-up study. British Journal of Psychiatry 2001; 178: 506–17.
20. Addington J, van Mastrigt S, Addington D. Duration of untreated psychosis: impact on 2-year outcome. Psychological Medicine 2004; 34: 277–84.
21. Craig TKJ, Garety P, Power P et al. The Lambeth Early Onset (LEO) Team: Randomised controlled trial of the effectiveness of specialised care for early psychosis. British Medical Journal 2004; 329: 1067.
22. Scully PJ, Coakley G, Kinsella A, Waddington JL. Psychopathology, executive (frontal) and general cognitive impairment in relation to duration of initially untreated versus subsequently treated psychosis in chronic schizophrenia. Psychological Medicine 1997; 27: 1303–10.
23. Group TSSR. The Scottish first episode schizophrenia study VIII. Five-year follow-up: Clinical and psychosocial findings. British Journal of Psychiatry 1992; 161: 496–500.
24. Siegel SJ, Irani F, Brensinger CM et al. Prognostic variables at intake and long-term level of function in schizophrenia. American Journal of Psychiatry 2006; 163: 433–41.
25. Bottlender R, Sato T, Jager M et al. The impact of the duration of untreated psychosis prior to first psychiatric admission on the 15-year outcome in schizophrenia. Schizophrenia Research 2003; 62: 37–44.
26. Menezes NM, Arenovich T, Zipursky RB. A systematic review of longitudinal outcome studies of first-episode psychosis. Psychological Medicine 2006; 7: 1–14.
27. Harrigan SM, McGorry PD, Krstev H. Does treatment delay in first-episode psychosis really matter? Psychological Medicine 2003; 33: 97–110.
28. Edwards J, Maude D, McGorry PD, Harrigan S, Cocks J. Prolonged recovery in first-episode psychosis. British Journal of Psychiatry 1998; 172(Supplement 33): 107–16.
29. Carbone S, Harrigan S, McGorry PD, Curry C, Elkins K. Duration of untreated psychosis and 12-month outcome in first-episode psychosis: The impact of treatment approach. Acta Psychiatrica Scandinavica 1999; 100: 96–104.
30. Moeller H-J, Bottlender R, Gross A et al. The Kraepelinian dichotomy: Preliminary results of a 15-year follow-up study on functional psychoses: Focus on negative symptoms. Schizophrenia Research 2002 Jul; 56(1-2): 87–94.
31. Addington J, Leriger E, Addington D. Symptom outcome 1 year after admission to an early psychosis program. Canadian Journal of Psychiatry 2003; 48(3): 204–7.
32. Stirling J, White C, Lewis S et al. Neurocognitive function and outcome in first-episode schizophrenia: a 10-year follow-up of an epidemiological cohort. Schizophrenia Research 2003; 65: 75–86.
33. Whitehorn D, Brown J, Richard J, Rui Q, Kopala L. Multiple dimensions of recovery in early psychosis. International Review of Psychiatry 2002; 14: 273–83.
34. Novak-Grubic V, Tavcar R. Predictors of noncompliance in males with first-episode schizophrenia, schizophreniform and schizoaffective disorder. European Psychiatry 2002; 17: 148–54.
35. Linszen D, Dingemans P, Lenior M. Early intervention and a five year follow up in young adults with a short duration of untreated psychosis: ethical implications. Schizophrenia Research 2001; 51: 55–61.
36. Lehtinen V, Aaltonen J, Koffert T, Rakkolainen V, Syvalahti E. Two-year outcome in first-episode psychosis treated according to an integrated model. Is immediate neuroleptisation always needed? European Psychiatry 2000; 15: 312–20.
37. Larsen TK, Moe LC, Vibe-Hansen L, Johannessen JO. Premorbid functioning versus duration of untreated psychosis in 1 year outcome in first-episode psychosis. Schizophrenia Research 2000; 45(1–2): 1–9.
38. Takei N, Persaud R, Woodruff P, Brockington I, Murray R M. First episodes of psychosis in Afro-Caribbean and White people. An 18-year-old follow-up population-based study. British Journal of Psychiatry 1998; 172(2): 147–53.

39. Tohen M, Strakowski SM, Zarate C Jr et al. The McLean-Harvard First-Episode Project: 6-month symptomatic and functional outcome in affective and nonaffective psychosis. Biological Psychiatry 2000; 48(6): 467–76.

40. Bromet EJ, Jandorf L, Fennig S et al. The Suffolk County Mental Health Project: demographic, pre-morbid and clinical correlates of 6-month outcome. Psychological Medicine 1996; 26: 953–62.

41. Larsen TK, McGlashan TH, Moe LC. First-episode schizophrenia: I. Early course parameters. Schizophrenia Bulletin 1996; 22(2): 241–56.

42. Henry LP, Harris MG, Amminger GP et al. Early psychosis prevention and intervention centre long-term follow-up study of first-episode psychosis: methodology and baseline characteristics. Early Intervention in Psychiatry 2007; 1(1): 49–60.

43. Amminger GP, Harris MG, Conus P et al. Treated incidence of first-episode psychosis in the catchment area of EPPIC between 1997 and 2000. Acta Psychiatrica Scandinavica 2006 114(5): 337–45.

44. Tsuang MT, Woolson RF, Fleming JA. Long-term outcome of major psychosis. Archives of General Psychiatry 1979; 36: 1295–301.

45. Ciompi L. The natural history of schizophrenia in the long term. British Journal of Psychiatry 1980; 136: 413–20.

46. McGorry PD, Singh B, Copolov DL et al. Royal Park Multidiagnostic Instrument for Psychosis: Part II. Development, reliability, and validity. Schizophrenia Bulletin. 1990; 16(3): 517–36.

47. First MB, Spitzer RL, Gibbon M, Williams JBW. Structured Clinical Interview for DSM-IV-TR Axis I Disorders, Research Version, Patient Edition. (SCID-I/P). New York: Biometrics Research, New York State Psychiatric Institute 1996.

48. Lukoff D, Liberman RP, Nuechterlein KH. Symptom monitoring in the rehabilitation of schizophrenic patients. Schizophrenia Bulletin 1986; 12: 578–93.

49. Andreasen NC. Negative symptoms in schizophrenia: definition and reliability. Archives of General Psychiatry 1982; 39: 784–8.

50. Kirkbride JB, Fearon P, Morgan C et al. Heterogeneity in incidence rates of schizophrenia and other psychotic syndromes: findings from the 3-center AeSOP study. Archives of General Psychiatry 2006 Mar; 63(3): 250–8.

51. Angermeyer MC, Kuhn L. Gender differences in age at onset of schizophrenia. Eur Arch Psychiatry Neurol Sci 1988; 237: 351–64.

52. Hafner H. Gender differences in schizophrenia. Psycho-neuroendocrinology 2003; 28 (Suppl. 2): 17–54.

53. Hambrecht M, Maurer K, Hafner H. Gender differences in schizophrenia in three cultures. Results of the WHO collaborative study on psychiatric disability. Soc Psychiatry Psychiatr Epidemiol 1992; 27: 117–21.

54. Rasanen S, Veuola J, Hakko H, Joukamaa M, Isohanni M. Gender differences in incidence and age at onset of DSM-IIIR schizophrenia. Preliminary results of the Northern Finland 1966 birth cohort study. Schizophrenia Research 1999; 37: 197–8.

55. Salokangas RK. First-contact rate for schizophrenia in community psychiatric care. Consideration of the oestrogen hypothesis. Eur Arch Psychiatry Clin Neurosci 1993; 242: 337–46.

56. McGlashan TH. Duration of untreated psychosis in first-episode schizophrenia: Marker or determinant of course? Biological Psychiatry 1999; 46(5): 899–907.

57. Harris M G, Henry LP, Harrigan S et al. The relationship between duration of untreated psychosis and outcome: An eight-year prospective study. Schizophrenia Research 2005; 79: 85–93.

58. International Early Psychosis Association Writing Group. International clinical practice guidelines for early psychosis. British Journal of Psychiatry 2005; 48(Suppl): s120–s4.

59. Bertolote J, McGorry PD. Early intervention and recovery for young people with early psychosis: consensus statement. British Journal of Psychiatry 2005; 48(Suppl): s116–s9.
60. McGorry PD, Killackey E, Lambert T, Lambert M. Roayl Australian and New Zealand College of Psychiatrists clinical practice guidelines for the treatment of schizophrenia and related disorders. Australian and New Zealand Journal of Psychiatry 2005; 39: 1–30.
61. McGrath J, Saha S, Welham J et al. A systematic review of the incidence of schizophrenia: the distribution of rates and the influence of sex, urbanicity, migrant status and methodology. BMC Med 2004; 2: 13.

Schizophrenia: Differential diagnosis and comorbidities

Carlo A Altamura, Filippo Dragogna, Sara Pozzoli, and Massimo C Mauri

INTRODUCTION

Differential diagnosis and evaluation of comorbidities, particularly for schizophrenia, represent the "core" of the psychiatrist's clinical activities. Unfortunately, there is no laboratory test for schizophrenia. Its complex spectrum of symptoms cannot be gauged with methods such as mental-status examination. Diagnosis is made by clinically examining individual family history, current symptoms, extent and quality of drug response and the presence of comorbid disorders. In particular, it may be difficult to diagnose acute (quick, severe, and brief) schizophrenia during its first episode. On the other hand, physicians must wait to establish recurrence, chronicity, and intensity, especially with regard to negative symptoms. For these reasons, psychiatrist's main goal in early diagnosis is to distinguish a schizophrenic disorder from other conditions, including other psychotic disorders, organic disorders, and drug-related conditions. Differential diagnosis for schizophrenia involves distinguishing it from bipolar disorder, schizoaffective disorder, and brief psychotic disorder. Differential diagnosis from bipolar disorders is the most problematic and important in view of therapeutic choices and maintenance programs. Schizophrenia-related changes in mood can include mania and depression; however, these changes in mood typically do not meet the criteria for full-blown mania or depression as in case of a bipolar disorder.

Psychosis as dimension is reported to be present in 50% or more of patients with bipolar disorder, usually during bipolar mania, with 48% of manic episodes accompanied by delusions, 15% by hallucinations, and 19% by a formal thought disorder. Moreover, some studies indicate similarities in psychotic symptom domains, including factors like anxiety, negative symptoms, depression, excitement, and positive symptoms in patients with bipolar mania and schizophrenia. Several authors have questioned whether schizophrenia and bipolar disorder represent separate categories of diseases or are separate dimensions of a single disorder(1, 2). Thus, it is of interest to determine whether some psychopathological dimensions in bipolar and schizophrenic patients have a different weight. Some authors reported an absence of a cognitive factor in bipolar mania, supporting the notion that bipolar patients may present fewer cognitive symptoms; the anxiety factor has a greater weight in the patients with bipolar mania, where it is the negative dimension the main factor in the studies of patients with schizophrenia (3).

However, psychosis may be even more common than is typically diagnosed and its recognition and treatment are important components in the effective treatment of bipolar patients (4, 5).

On the other hand, the recognition of comorbidities is essential for a complete therapeutic assessment, particularly in the case of medical comorbidities that can be secondary to psychiatric disorders, leading to further complication of the clinical picture.

About 40% to 80% of patients affected by schizophrenia have been found to have concurrent medical illnesses, and it was thought to aggravate the mental state in more than 40% of the patients (6).

In particular, clinicians need to be aware of the substantial rates of physical comorbidity in first episode of schizophrenic patients that may not be necessarily associated with worse longitudinal outcomes, and the findings should encourage even greater efforts at early identification and management of these conditions.

It was not until 1994 when the *Diagnostic and Statistical Manual of Mental Disorders, Fourth Edition* (DSM-IV) was published that diagnostic guidelines first permitted additional diagnoses on Axis I, such as anxiety disorder, in the presence of schizophrenia. Yet remnants of the old hierarchical diagnostic system remain, diverting attention from the pressing issue of managing what appear to be common and treatable disabling conditions, such as panic disorder and obsessive-compulsive disorder (OCD), which often occur with schizophrenia.

The proportion of subjects with an anxiety disorder (43%–45%) is reported almost identical across the three major psychoses including schizophrenia, schizoaffective disorder and bipolar disorder (7). In particular, the prevalence of social phobia (17%), panic disorder (24%–35%), and obsessive-compulsive Disorder (OCD) (13%–25%) in schizophrenia are relatively high, as are prevalences of panic disorder (15%–21%) and OCD (21%–30%) in bipolar disorder. It was also hypothesized that patients with both anxiety disorders and psychosis would have greater overall morbidity than those with psychosis alone. On the other hand, given that anxiety disorders are relatively more responsive to treatment, greater awareness of their comorbidity with psychosis should yield worthwhile clinical benefits (7).

DIFFERENTIAL DIAGNOSIS

The reliability of differentiating schizophrenia from other psychotic disorders is strengthened by the presence of several characteristic features like hallucinations, delusions, and disorganized speech, which occur in a manner consistent with the persistent course and social/occupational impairment, as outlined in the *Diagnostic and Statistical Manual of Mental Disorders* (DSM-IV) (8, 9).

Without a clear preexisting psychotic disorder, every patient experiencing an acute psychotic episode should have a wide medical workup, including medical and psychiatric histories, medication history, physical and mental status examination, laboratory evaluation, including urinalysis and toxicology screens (10, 11). When applying diagnostic criteria for schizophrenia, it is important to carefully determine modality of the onset, age of onset, quality, and course of presenting symptoms. One should also establish the presence or absence of symptoms required for the diagnosis of schizophrenia using reliable interview such as SCID or CIDI (12, 13).

It is equally important to review the presence or absence of symptoms of bipolar affective disorder and major depressive disorder because their onset usually coincides with the onset of schizophrenia.

In summary, because psychotic states are a common expression of psychiatric and medical illnesses or related to substances abuse, the evaluation of an acute psychotic episode should begin with the formulation of a broad differential diagnosis.

In any case, the *DSM-IV* (so as ICD-10) descriptive approach makes the process of differential diagnosis and evaluation of comorbidities limitative. The new dimensional approach to psychiatric disorders, scheduled in the *DSM-V* agenda, will overcome this matter by considering symptoms on a continuum from health to pathology.

At present, the following table summarizes the possible differential diagnosis of schizophrenia.

TABLE 6.1   Differential Diagnosis of Schizophrenia

Psychiatric Disorders
Schizophreniform disorder
Brief Reactive Psychosis
Mood disorders with psychotic features (Major Depressive Disorder, Bipolar Disorders)
Depression in Schizophrenia
Schizoaffective Disorder
Delusional Disorder
Hallucinatory Disorder
Psychotic Disorder Not Otherwise Specified
Paranoid, Schizotypal, Schizoid, and Borderline Personality Disorders
Mental Retardation

Psychotic Disorders Due to General Medical Conditions
Temporal-lobe epilepsy
Tumor, stroke, brain trauma
CNS infections (neurosyphilis, AIDS, herpes encephalitis)
Alzheimer's dementia
Huntington's disease
Wilson's disease
Endocrine/metabolic disorders (e.g., porphyria)
Vitamin deficiency (e.g., vitamin B_{12})
Autoimmune (e.g., systemic lupus erythematosus)

Substance-Induced Psychoses
Stimulants (amphetamine, cocaine, methampehetamine)
Hallucinogens (lysergic acid diethylamide)
Cannabinoids
Phencyclidine, ketamine
Anticholinergics (e.g., belladonna alkaloids)
Glucocorticoids
L-dopa
Histamine-H_2-blocking drugs
Alcohol withdrawal delirium
Barbiturate withdrawal delirium
Toxic (e.g., heavy metals, carbon monoxide)

PSYCHIATRIC DISORDERS

Many psychiatric disorders share symptoms with schizophrenia or have symptoms that may be confused with those of schizophrenia. The course and outcome of psychotic and other symptoms are the major factors that differentiate schizophrenia from other psychiatric disorders.

The importance of establishing not only the presence of symptoms but also their pattern and course has been recognized in current diagnostic strategies.

Schizophreniform Disorder

Schizophreniform disorder has the same characteristic symptoms of schizophrenia, but the *DSM-IV* criteria require the duration of symptoms to be at least 1 month but less than 6 months. Therefore, schizophreniform disorder is likely to be the diagnosis in patients who have an abrupt, rather than an insidious, onset.

Moreover, schizophreniform disorder patients differ from schizophrenic patients in ways such as displaying prominent emotional turmoil, intellectual confusion, or perplexity and who have a presumed greater role for psychosocial stresses (14). Also, a deterioration in social or vocational functioning is not required for schizophreniform disorder.

Be that as it may, in current diagnostic criteria, the most important distinctions between the two disorders are modality of onset and duration of episode.

Brief Reactive Psychosis

Brief reactive psychosis is a disorder characterized by sudden onset of positive psychotic symptoms (i.e., hallucinations, delusions, disorganized speech, or grossly disorganized or catatonic behavior) that last for at least 1 day but less than a month. Distinguishing a brief reactive psychosis from a schizophrenia can be harder when the patient has a preexisting personality disorder that shares some similarities to the prodrome of schizophrenia.

Another defining feature of brief reactive psychosis is the relationship with a triggering stressful event; this "stressful life event" can take many forms, including (but not limited to) the death of a loved one, professional loss, or serious adverse changes in the patient's personal life, such as the breakdown of their family through divorce, and so on.

The condition usually spontaneously resolves itself within 2 weeks, and the main goal of treatment is to prevent the patient from harming either himself or others.

Mood Disorders

To distinguish schizophrenia from bipolar mood disorder, the clinician has to evaluate first the onset of the symptoms. An abrupt onset usually identifies bipolar mood disorder with psychotic features instead of a schizophrenia, except for those cases of bipolar disorder presenting continuous, low-level psychotic symptoms.

Any psychotic symptoms associated with bipolar disorder should occur within the context of a manic or a depressive state—delusions of grandeur and hallucinations may be either wildly optimistic and grandiose, or completely disastrous and guilt-ridden. Symptoms like flight of ideas may be confused with a chronic formal thought disturbance; however, they usually they occur with other symptoms of mania, such as euphoria, decreased need for sleep, and hyperactivity. Hyperactivity and poor sleep need in patients affected by schizophrenia are usually secondary to delusions and hallucinations rather than to mood alterations.

Depression in Schizophrenia

Patients affected by schizophrenia may also experience depressive symptoms during the course of the main disorder; depressive episodes usually occur simultaneously with the typical schizophrenia symptoms. It has been reported that the prevalence of depressive symptoms during the course of schizophrenia ranges from 25% to 80%, depending on the phase of the illness, patient age, treatment setting, and the definition of depression (15).

Some authors (16) suggest that they may be related to schizophrenia when the full-blown psychosis is most evident, that is, so-called revealed depression, thus suggesting that the depression may be associated with the psychotic state itself or a subjective reaction to the experience of psychotic decompensation. Furthermore, it has classically been reported that depressive symptoms are induced by classical antipsychotics in 15%-50% of patients (pharmacogenic depression)(17). Moreover, postpsychotic depression is described as a phase of manifest depression and or social withdrawal occurring after remission of more florid psychotic symptoms with a 25%-50% frequency (18).

The clinical picture of a depressive episode in a schizophrenic patient may be confused by the classical negative symptoms of schizophrenia, as like social withdrawal, lack of interest, and psychomotor retardation. To differentiate depressive symptoms from negative symptoms, the clinician must investigate the patient's history to understand whether these symptoms occur in the context of a typical depressive illness or with other symptoms such as poor appetite, terminal insomnia, and self-reproach. The use of rating scales like Calgary for depression and SANS for negative symptoms can be helpful beside the clinical judgement and experience.

Schizoaffective Disorder

The mood symptoms in schizoaffective disorder are more prominent and last for a substantially longer time than those in schizophrenia. Schizoaffective disorder differs from schizophrenia in that both affective symptoms and the features of schizophrenia are equally prominent and occur together (14, 15). In *DSM-IV*, schizoaffective disorder is distinguished from schizophrenia by the presence of significant mood symptoms that must be present for "a substantial portion of the total duration of the disturbance" (9). The term should not be applied to patients who exhibit schizophrenic symptoms and affective symptoms only in different episodes of illness. The diagnosis of a patient with schizophrenia or mood disorder may change later to that of schizoaffective disorder, or vice versa.

Delusional Disorder

Delusional disorder (formerly paranoid disorder) can be easily confused with schizophrenia, especially the paranoid subtype of the two disorders.

Delusion in this disorder is more likely to be single, well-encapsulated and non-bizarre. The diagnosis of delusional disorder does not include hallucinations, disorganized behaviour, or negative symptoms, as in typical schizophrenia. It is possible to find further differences in the age of onset, over the age of 40 for Delusional disorder, and in social and occupational impairment that is classically more severe for schizophrenic patients.

Hallucinatory Disorder

Chronic hallucinatory psychosis is a disease that has long been considered in the French literature but is neglected by the current Anglo-Saxon classification systems, which generally classify it among the atypical forms of schizophrenia (*DSM-IV*) while in the ICD-10 classification it is included in the group of psychosis not otherwise specified.

Various authors have described the disorder, attributing it different characteristics. The first bibliographical references date back to 1911, when Gilbert Ballet first described chronic hallucinatory psychosis, which has been subsequently considered by De Clerambault, Ey, Pull, and Pichot. These Authors underlined the central nature of the hallucinatory symptoms and have suggested the nosographic autonomy of the syndrome, but each hypothesize different underlying pathogenetic mechanisms and disagreed about the prognosis. The French concept of "Psychoses Hallucinatoire Chronique" is characterized by late-onset psychosis, predominantly in females, with rich and frequent hallucinations, but almost no dissociative features or negative symptoms (19).

In any case, hallucinatory psychosis may be considered a disorder like delusional disorder characterized by hallucinations as a primary phenomenon as in the definition of Ballet with a favorable prognosis such as described by Ey.

Psychosis Not Otherwise Specified

Psychosis not otherwise specified (NOS) is a diagnostic category used when there is inadequate or contradictory informations to make a specific diagnosis or when there are psychotic symptoms that do not meet the criteria for a specific psychotic disorder. Using this category rather than forcing a choice between the more carefully defined categories may be of substantial clinical importance. It signifies that more informations need to be gathered before deciding on a specific diagnosis and making predictions concerning prognosis. Usually, especially in clinician contest, the diagnosis of psychosis NOS finds its role as a temporary category for new-onset patients until the course and nature of their symptoms help to clarify the appropriate diagnosis.

Personality Disorders

Schizoid, schizotypal, and *paranoid personality disorders* (Cluster A) have the greatest similarity to schizophrenia. These disorders may be conceptualized as having features of the schizophrenia spectrum, but to a substantially lesser degree such that they are not of sufficient magnitude in either severity or degree of social/occupational impairment to constitute schizophrenia.

Schizoid personality disorder is a condition characterized by excessive detachment from social relationships and a restricted range of expression of emotions in interpersonal settings. Occupational functioning may be impaired, particularly if interpersonal involvement is required, but individuals with this disorder may do well when they work under conditions of social isolation.

Schizotypal personality disorder is a condition characterized by acute discomfort with, and reduced capacity for, close relationships as well as by cognitive or perceptual distortions and eccentricities of behavior. It should be not diagnosed if the distrust and suspiciousness occur exclusively during the course of schizophrenia, a mood disorder with psychotic features, or another psychotic disorder. Schizotypal disorder is more common among first-degree biological relatives of those with schizophrenia showing that schizotypal personality disorder may be genetically related to schizophrenia (20).

In *paranoid personality disorder*, one might initially suspect that delusions lie behind the suspiciousness, guardedness, and hostility, but none can be found. This disorder should be not confused with schizophrenia, as no well-formed delusions, hallucinations, changes in affect, thought disorder, or other symptoms of schizophrenia are present.

Borderline personality disorder (Cluster B) is also a potential source of misdiagnosis of schizophrenia. Unlike the Cluster A patients, these patients have symptoms that may mimic the psychosis of schizophrenia, yet their illness is probably not in the schizophrenia spectrum. This personality disorder may exhibit the prodromal symptoms of schizophrenia, vague and fleeting psychotic symptoms, or display susceptibility to brief reactive psychoses. Strict application of the diagnostic criteria for schizophrenia, using reliable and narrowly defined symptoms in Criterion A of the diagnostic criteria for schizophrenia, helps to reduce these misclassifications. Additionally, the prominent affective instability and behavioral disturbances such as impulsivity and addictive and self-harm behaviors help distinguish the Cluster B personalities. In any case both Cluster A and B personality disorders can be distinguished from schizophrenia by the lack of delusions, hallucinations, and grossly disorganized behavior.

Mental Retardation

Historically, dual diagnosis of schizophrenia and mental retardation has been a source of controversy. Recent studies have shown that the symptoms and clinical features of schizophrenia in persons with mild and moderate mental retardation are similar to those of normal intelligence (21). Deficits in language ability may hamper or preclude self-reports of delusions, hallucinations, and other expressions of disordered thought that are the hallmark diagnostic criteria for schizophrenia. Nonetheless, persons with mental retardation show the full range of psychiatric disorders, including schizophrenia (10). To help clarify the diagnosis when the patient cannot give you the history you need, it is particularly important to obtain history from family informants and caregivers focusing on the presence of behaviors suggestive of psychotic symptomatology (i.e., attending and/or responding to hallucinatory experiences, suspiciousness, etc.). The development of empirically derived behavioural criteria that are less dependent upon language ability is one avenue that may provide a basis for the diagnosis of schizophrenia in persons with severe mental retardation. Because these individuals are at increased risk for tardive dyskinesia, consistent reappraisals of diagnosis and medication management in this population may be of paramount clinical importance.

PSYCHOTIC DISORDERS DUE TO GENERAL MEDICAL CONDITIONS

Many general medical and neurological conditions can present in their course psychotics symptoms that may be confused with those of schizophrenia. Clinician must keep in mind that endocrinopathies (thyroid, adrenal, pancreatic), autoimmune disorders (systemic lupus erythematosus), vitamin B_{12} deficiency, hepatic, vascular, erythropoietic, or metabolic disorders can show psychotic symptoms.

Most of these pathologies show many other symptoms and dysregulations; therefore, differential diagnosis can easily be done with a general chemistry screen, complete blood count, thyroid-function tests, urinalysis, and serological tests for evidence of an infection with syphilis or human immunodeficiency virus.

Neurological conditions are often not easy to differentiate from a first-episode psychosis. Neurological pathologies included in the schizophrenia differential diagnosis are head trauma, brain and adrenal tumors, seizures, multiple sclerosis, metachromatic leukodystrophy, Huntington's disease, and Wilson's disease. A first psychotic episode should be evaluated with diagnostic tests such as computerized tomography (CT) or magnetic resonance imaging (MRI) of the brain and electroencephalogram (EEG) may be indicated (or useful) in selected cases (22, 23). From a clinical point of view, in the case of acute psychotic disorders such as a metabolic disorder, head trauma, brain tumor, or stroke, symptoms often begin much more abruptly and may include visual hallucinations or bizarre behavior resulting from a clouded consciousness. These symptoms are usually qualitatively different from the positive symptoms that characterize schizophrenia (i.e., auditory hallucinations in the context of a clear sensorium). In more chronic disorders, such as Alzheimer's disease or Huntington's disease, symptoms that might be confused with negative symptoms are actually the result of cognitive deterioration.

The pattern of delusions and hallucinations in a temporal-lobe epilepsy (complex partial seizures) may resemble to that of a schizophrenia; nevertheless, these symptoms occur subsequent to the onset of complex partial seizures (e.g., in one case series, an average of 14 years after the onset of seizures). Specifically asking about a history of other seizure phenomena is useful in making this differential diagnosis.

SUBSTANCE-INDUCED PSYCHOTIC DISORDERS

A large number of toxic or psychoactive substances can cause psychotic reactions. Psychotic symptoms can result as adverse effects of prescribed drugs glucocorticoids, L-dopa, anticholinergics, and histamine H_2-blockers. To investigate thorough medical history, including a medication history, it is necessary to rule out potential psychotic disorders due to medication.

Finally, people may do an overdose on recreational drugs, such as cocaine or cannabinoids, or become dependent on drugs or alcohol and experience psychotic symptoms during withdrawal. While the substance induced psychosis is triggered and then sustained by intoxication or withdrawal, its effects can continue long after intoxication or withdrawal has ended.

In particular, psychotic symptoms, especially delusions and hallucinations, can result from a wide variety of substances, including alcohol, amphetamines, marijuana, cocaine, hallucinogens, inhalants, opioids, phencyclidine, and certain sedatives and anxiolytics. The diagnosis is made when symptoms begin during or less than 1 month after intoxication with or withdrawal from the implicated substance and after other psychotic disorders are ruled out. Because chronic psychoses in the context of substance abuse may begin at an earlier age than in the onset of schizophrenia in the absence of substance abuse, some authors have suggested that substance abuse precipitates the illness in the genetically predisposed subjects (67).

COMORBIDITIES

The term "comorbidity" denotes those cases in which a "distinct additional clinical entity" occurred during the clinical course of a patient who has an index disease. This term has recently become very common in psychiatry and is commonly used to indicate the simultaneous presence in an individual presenting two or more nosologically different disorders that may be either coincident or causally related. Indeed, it is used not only for those cases in which a patient receives both a psychiatric and a general medical diagnosis (e.g., major depression and hypertension) but also for those cases in which a patient receives two or more psychiatric diagnoses (e.g., major depression and panic disorder). This co-occurrence of two or more psychiatric diagnoses ("psychiatric comorbidity") has been reported to be very frequent. For instance, in the US National Comorbidity Survey, 51% of patients with a *DSM–III–R/DSM–IV* diagnosis of major depression had at least one concomitant ("comorbid") anxiety disorder and only 26% of them had no comorbid mental disorder (24). In a study based on data from the Australian National Survey of Mental Health and Well-Being 21% of people fulfilling *DSM-IV* criteria for any mental disorder met the criteria for three or more comorbid disorders (25). The co-occurrence of multiple psychiatric diagnoses is now more frequent than in the past. Certainly, this is partially a consequence of the use of standardised diagnostic interviews, which help to identify

TABLE 6.2 Comorbidities

Psychiatric comorbidities
Anxiety disorders (obsessive-compulsive disorder, panic disorder, social phobia, posttraumatic
    stress disorder)
Mental retardation
Personality disorder
Substances abuses

Medical comorbidities
Nutritional and metabolic disease (diabetes, hyperlipidaemia, obesity, osteoporosis,
    hyperprolactemia)
Malignant neoplasms
Cardiovascular diseases
Infectious disease (HIV, Hepatitis C)
Other physical illnesses

---

several clinical aspects that in the past remained unnoticed after the principal diagnosis had been made.

In schizophrenia, comorbidity includes (i) specific disorders that may have a
putative pathogenetic relationship with schizophrenia itself, and (ii) relatively common medical problems and diseases that tend to occur among schizophrenic patients
more frequently as a consequence of dysfunctional behaviours, poor self-care, or
medical neglect.

PSYCHIATRIC COMORBIDITIES
The results of the Chestnut Lodge follow-up study in the 1980s (26) showed that
schizophrenia can coexist with other forms of psychopathology and that this will
have prognostic implications for the outcome of the disorder. Comorbid conditions,
including anxiety disorders, mental retardation, personality disorders, and substances
abuses, reflect prognosis of both acute as well chronic schizophrenia.

Anxiety disorders
Comorbid anxiety disorders are common in schizophrenia, although differences in
reporting are observed across cultures. Most of the time anxiety is considered secondary to the psychotic condition and is expected to improve in parallel with the psychotic
symptoms (27). The existence of a comorbid anxiety disorder is related to positive
symptoms, suggesting that anxiety is related to the acute exacerbation of schizophrenia. Available studies point to the fact that the presence of a comorbid anxiety disorder
has a deleterious effect on the prognosis of schizophrenia (7).

Obsessive-compulsive disorder (OCD)
OCD is the best documented comorbidity condition. The presence of obsessive-
compulsive (OC) symptoms in schizophrenic patients has been long recognized. In
the last 20 years, several studies have estimated the prevalence of OCD comorbidity in schizophrenic patients ranging from 0% to 55%; this great variability is probably related to differences of sample (chronicity, recruiting methods, etc.) and the use
of different diagnostic instruments (28). OC symptoms could be a predictor of poor

outcome in schizophrenia: Patients with OC are more likely to be unemployed, to be hospitalized, and to have worse functioning levels at follow-up.

Panic disorder

Epidemiological data found panic attacks to be frequent (45%) in patients with schizophrenia (29). Schizophrenic patients with panic attacks had elevated rates of coexisting mental disorders, psychotic symptoms, and health service utilization. Panic attacks are associated with an increased risk for comorbid alcohol or substance use disorder. Some authors found a concurrence in 43% with a higher rate in paranoid schizophrenics, and schizophrenic patients with panic attacks showed more depressive symptoms, greater hostility, and a lower level of functioning (30, 31).

Social phobia

Social phobia may have a high frequency in schizophrenic patients, ranging from 8.2% to 36.6%. In comparison with other schizophrenics, those with social phobia are reported to have more suicide attempts of a greater lethality and a lower social adjustment (32). Furthermore, the presence of comorbid social phobia is a significant predictor of worse quality of life in several domains.

Posttraumatic stress disorder (PTSD)

Studies dedicated to the presence of PTSD in schizophrenia illustrate the complexity of anxiety comorbidity in schizophrenia and the variable outcomes that can result from different analytic approaches (17). The *DSM-IV* does not consider psychotic-related symptoms as stressors; however, studies that were able to show that psychotic symptoms and hospitalization were a relevant contribution to the traumatization of the subjects, with estimated frequencies as high as 51% among schizophrenic patients (33).

Mental retardation

As many schizophrenics regress cognitively to the point of mental deficiency, the distinction between true developmental and functional retardation in the adult poses a recurrent diagnostic problem (15).

Kraepelin estimated that about 7% of all cases of dementia praecox arose in individuals with premorbid cognitive impairment. Few studies in the past 25 years have attempted to take a holistic approach to the biological origins of schizophrenia in subjects with learning disability. Prevalence estimates of schizophrenia in persons with mental retardation have varied from 2% to 14% (34). Accurate determination of prevalence rates of schizophrenia in people with mental retardation is complicated by many diagnostic problems. These problems include distinguishing true hallucinations from developmentally appropriate behaviours such as self-talk and talking to imaginary friends. Recent studies have found higher incidences of schizophrenia in those with mild or moderate intellectual disabilities compared with those with more severe intellectual disabilities (35). However, it remains unclear whether these findings reflect true prevalence rates or whether they merely reflect the problems in the detection of schizophrenia and psychosis in people with more severe intellectual disabilities.

Much of the emphasis on the diagnosing of schizophrenia in subjects with mental retardation is in developing methods to improve the ability to diagnose this disorder.

Recently some studies investigated neuropathology in terms of prefrontal lobe cortical folding in a cohort of individuals comorbid for schizophrenia and mental retardation and people with schizophrenia alone, and it was not possible to make any distinction (36). It seems, therefore, that the brain structure of people with intellectual disabilities and schizophrenia resembles that of people with schizophrenia more closely than that of those with intellectual disabilities alone.

These findings support the hypothesis that these comorbid individuals should, therefore, be conceptualized as suffering from severe, early onset schizophrenia that caused their low IQ, rather than intellectual disabilities complicated by psychosis.

Personality disorders

It has long been thought that the presence of comorbid Axis II disorders contribute to a poorer short-term as well as long-term outcome in psychiatric disorders. In most patients, personality pathology precedes current psychopathology, suggesting that personality factors may contribute to the occurrence of psychiatric disorders (37). However, this does not exclude the possibility that personality pathology originates from or deteriorates through serious or recurrent psychopathology (38).

A relevant issue is that some Axis I and Axis II disorders bear a strong interfamilial relationship. For instance, the most powerful of these is probably the genetic, physiological, and pharmacological evidence supporting the hypothesis that schizotypal personality disorder and schizophrenia have a strong genetic interrelationship (39, 40).

About gender differences, there is evidence to show that schizophrenia is more common in males than females, and past research provides an empirical support for the higher prevalence of personality disorders in males than in females. It is reasonable also to suggest that the higher prevalence of personality disorder in men is a contributor to the poor outcome.

Substance abuses

A number of studies suggest a high level of comorbidity between substance abuse and schizophrenia, and approximately half of the patients suffering from schizophrenia have also been substance abusers at some point during their illness (41).

Literature data on outpatients report that 35% of schizophrenics are currently diagnosed with alcoholic abuse. Other abused substances were cocaine (20%), heroin (3%), and marijuana (60%) (42).

The comorbidity of schizophrenia and substance abuse is associated with more frequent relapses, more positive symptoms and depression, cognitive impairment, and a poorer outcome and treatment response. Several hypotheses have been put forward to explain the relationship between schizophrenia and substance abuse: It has been hypothesized that substance abuse may increase the risk of schizophrenia, at least in vulnerable individuals; the self-medication hypothesis suggests that patients abuse drugs to alleviate the symptoms of psychosis or the debilitating side effects caused by antipsychotic medications, such as extrapyramidal symptoms; finally, it could be a merely coincidental association of two psychiatric disorders that have similar age peaks in the distribution of onset and prevalence but without any causal interrelation.

A high incidence of substance abuse is also observed in first-episode patients, among whom the rates of substance abuse have been found to range from 20% to 30% (43, 44).

Among patients with substance abuse or dependence, the onset of substance abuse precedes the onset of psychosis by several years in most cases and only in a minority of cases begins at the time of a first episode or later.

Literature data reveal that 60% of first-admission schizophrenic patients had started substance abuse before their first hospitalization and that the onset of cannabis abuse preceded the onset of psychotic symptoms by at least 1 year in 69% of cases and that most of the patients had started substance abuse several years before the onset of psychosis (44). Several authors observed that alcohol and cannabis were the main substances for most first-episode patients (44). Substance abuse also involves stimulants, anxiolytics, hallucinogens, antiparkinsonian drugs, as well as caffeine and tobacco.

In the WHO 10-country study, a history of alcohol use in the year preceding the first contact was elicited in 57% of the male patients, and in three of the study areas drug abuse, mainly cannabis and cocaine, was reported by 24-41% of the patients (45).

MEDICAL COMORBIDITY IN SCHIZOPHRENIA

Schizophrenia has been described as a "life-shortening disease". Without considering suicide (68, 69), which accounts for less than a third of premature deaths, people diagnosed with schizophrenia can expect to live 9–12 years fewer, on average, than those in the general population. High mortality and morbidity in schizophrenia may be attributed to an environment in which unhealthy and high-risk behaviours such as smoking, substance abuse, lack of exercise, and poor diet are prevalent (21, 46).

Smoking-related fatalities are significantly higher in people with schizophrenia than in the general population. Smoking is a good example of how behavior and treatment interact to increase morbidity at a number of levels. It is a risk factor for respiratory and ischaemic heart disease and stroke, and, by reducing available plasma levels of antipsychotics, it may influence the patient's behavior and the treatment outcome.

With respect to diet, the cognitive and social deficit symptoms of schizophrenia may make patients prone to choosing easily obtainable "fast" foods as their major source of nutrition. The same deficits, especially those to do with motivation, often leave the patient without any desire to keep physically active to counter the effects of their poor diet and maintain general fitness. This is further complicated by psychotropic side effects, particularly Parkinsonism, sedation and neuroleptic-induced cognitive deficits, which can compound these problems. Together, these lifestyle factors increase the risk or severity of medical conditions, particularly the development of metabolic syndrome characterized by obesity, insulin resistance, dyslipidaemia, impaired glucose tolerance, and hypertension.

Physical disease is common among patients with schizophrenia but is rarely diagnosed. Concurrent medical illnesses have been found among inpatients (46%-80%) and among outpatients with schizophrenia (20%-43%). In 46% of the patients, a physical illness was thought to aggravate the mental state, and in 7%, it was life threatening (47). Schizophrenic patients have a dramatically increased risk of poisoning with psychotropic drugs (50 fold for men and 20 fold for women).

In addition to a generally increased susceptibility to infections prior to hospitalization, schizophrenic patients have higher-than-expected rates of diabetes, arteriosclerotic disease, and myocardial infarction, and middle-ear disease, irritable bowel syndrome, and some rare genetic or idiopathic disorders such as acute intermittent porphyria. HIV infection has a 5%-7% estimated prevalence in patients with schizophrenia in the United States (48).

This heavy burden of medical morbidity remains largely underrecognized because schizophrenic patients with comorbid conditions are usually excluded from research studies.

NUTRITIONAL AND METABOLIC DISEASE

Diabetes
In people with schizophrenia has been found increased risk of developing glucose-regulation abnormalities, insulin resistance, and type 2 diabetes mellitus (49). Lifestyle factors (poor diet, sedentary behavior) could exacerbate the problem; however, antipsychotic agents, particularly clozapine and olanzapine, also increase the propensity to develop diabetes.

Hyperlipidaemia
Fat levels are more high in people with schizophrenia than general population. Antipsychotic mediations have been associated with the development of hyperlipidemia (both related to, and independent of, weight gain) (50). Phenothiazines (e.g., chlorpromazine) tend to raise triglyceride levels and reduce levels of high-density lipoproteins, such as atypical antipsychotics, particularly clozapine and olanzapine, are associated with increased levels of fasting glucose and lipids (51).

Obesity
The obesity problem is one of the most serious comorbidities due to the fatal long-term cardiovascular consequences (52). About 40%–62% of people with schizophrenia are obese or overweight (53). Both typical and atypical antipsychotics can induce weight gain, particularly atypicals, clozapine, and olanzapine, and cause rapid weight increase. Other more plausible reasons for the increase of obesity are lifestyle factors like self-neglect, smoking, negative symptoms, lack of exercise, poor diet, and poor ability to modify incorrect behavior.

Osteoporosis
People with schizophrenia have been found to have accelerated rates of osteoporosis (54) that are attributed to antipsychotic-driven decreases in oestrogen and testosterone, reduced calcium due to smoking and alcoholism, and polydipsia.

Hyperprolactinemia
High doses of typical antipsychotics and the atypical antipsychotics risperidone and amisulpride raise prolactin levels, causing galactorrhoea, amenorrhoea, oligomenorrhoea, sexual dysfunction, and reduced bone mineral density, and contributing to cardiovascular disease (55).

Malignant neoplasms
The hypothesis that people with schizophrenia have a decreased risk of cancer was formulated for the first time in 1909 (Commission of Lunacy for England and Wales).

Most of the population-based incidence studies carried out in Denmark, Japan, Hawaii, Australia, Finland, Israel, the United States, and the United Kingdom revealed a decreased cancer risk in persons with schizophrenia (56). Considering specific cancer sites, the results are also contradictory (57, 58). For example, some studies showed decreased risks of lung cancer in schizophrenia, while others showed increased risks. A possible exception is prostate cancer, which was consistently found to be rarer in schizophrenic patients compared to the general population (59).

Cardiovascular disease (hypertension, cardiac arrhythmias)
Mortality studies have shown consistently that people with schizophrenia die more frequently from cardiovascular diseases (ischaemic heart disease, cardiac arrhythmias, and myocardial infarction) and experience sudden death than control populations (60). The increased risk of cardiac problem can be due by metabolic syndrome (hypertension, hyperlipidaemia, hyperglycaemia, insulin resistance, and obesity) and lifestyle factors (smoking, alcoholism, poor diet, lack of exercise).

Infectious disease
The prevalence of HIV positivity in people with schizophrenia, estimated to be 4%–23%, is generally higher than in the general population (0.6% in the general population of America according to a WHO statistic) (61). Also Hepatitis C has increased prevalence in people with schizophrenia compared with the general population. A number of reasons account for the high HIV prevalence among people with mental disorders. One is the high frequency of substance abuse in these populations. Other factors may be sexual risk behaviours (e.g., lack of condom use, trading sex for money and drugs, and a reduced knowledge about HIV-related issues).

Other physical illnesses
Incidence of irritable bowel syndrome in people with schizophrenia is 19% (versus 2.5% in the general population). Prevalence of Helicobacter pylori infection is significantly higher in people with schizophrenia (odds ratio, 3.0) (62).

There are a number of relatively large studies that showed sexual dysfunction to be more frequent in people with schizophrenia compared to normal controls (63).

Increased prevalence of incontinence in people with schizophrenia have also been reported (64).

CONCLUSIONS
At present, in *DSM-IV* diagnostic criteria such as ICD-10, schizophrenia is defined as a discrete category rather than in terms of different dimensions leading to heterogeneous clinical patterns. Moreover current diagnostic criteria for schizophrenia do not include neurobiological signs or symptoms.

In the future, it is likely descriptive approaches will be complemented by the inclusion of putative, etiological, or pathophysiological indications.

All of this could be useful for a clear and definitive diagnostic process and a resolution of differential diagnosis problems, at least theoretically.

On the other hand, in the case of patients with symptoms of multiple disorders, a reliance on discrete categories may lead to artificial boundary conditions and/or increased rates of comorbidity (65).

One approach is to identify psychopathological dimensions and groups of symptoms that occur together by chance alone and more often than would be expected, using exploratory factor analysis.

Certainly dimensional models of psychopathology have pragmatic limitations as well. The question of whether a dimensional model describes more accurately than a categorical model the biological nature of schizophrenia remains open.

In any case, dimensions are not diagnosis specific, yet current categorical diagnosis requires dimensional specificity; for instance, affective and dimension has been identified in people affected by different psychoses, on the other hand in major mood syndromes, psychotic dimension has been found.

In conclusion, current evidences support the complementary use of both categorical and dimensional representations of psychoses, including schizophrenia.

Diagnostic models using both categorical diagnoses and dimensions have better predictive validity than either model independently. Moreover, flexible scoring of dimensions across all psychotic patients can be more informative also in terms of pharmacological response (66).

Furthermore, the concept of endophenotypes should be taken into account. Endophenotypes are present in quantifiable traits, often not easy to ascertain, and are thought to reflect an intermediate place in the pathway between genes and the disorder. Endophenotype abnormalities in domains such as neurophysiology or neurocognition occur in schizophrenic patients as well as their clinically "unaffected" relatives. Endophenotype reflects polymorphisms in the DNA of schizophrenia spectrum subjects, creating vulnerability to develop schizophrenia.

Combining dimensional approach and endophenotypes, analysis will surely lead, in the next years, to a more accurate and precise diagnosis, restricting further the diagnostic "conceptual" frame for schizophrenia and possibly enlarging that of related disorders included in the "psychotic spectrum."

REFERENCES

1. Smith MJ, Barch DM, Csernansky. Bridging the gap between schizophrenia and psychotic mood disorders: Relating neurocognitive deficits to psychopathology. JG.Schizophr Res 2009 Jan; 107(1): 69–75.
2. Bora E, Yucel M, Fornito A et al. Major psychoses with mixed psychotic and mood symptoms: are mixed psychoses associated with different neurobiological markers? Acta Psychiatr Scand 2008 Sep; 118(3): 172–87.
3. Lindenmayer JP, Bossie CA, Kujawa M et al. Dimensions of psychosis in patients with bipolar mania as measured by the positive and negative syndrome scale. Psychopathology 2008; 41: 264–70.
4. Altamura AC. Drug-resistance phenomena in major psychoses: their discrimination and causal mechanisms. Clin Neuropharmacol 1990; 13 (S1): 1–15.
5. Altamura AC, Bassetti R, Cattaneo E et al.Some biological correlates of drug resistance in schizophrenia: a multidimensional approach. World J Biol Psychiatry 2005; 6 Suppl 2: 23–30.
6. Bora E, Yucel M, Fornito A et al.. Major psychoses with mixed psychotic and mood symptoms: are mixed psychoses associated with different neurobiological markers? Acta Psychiatr Scand 2008 Sep118(3)172–87.
7. Braga RJ, Petrides G, Figueira I. Anxiety disorders in schizophrenia. Compr Psychiatry 2004 Nov-Dec; 45(6)460–8.
8. Flaum M, Schultz SK. Core symptoms of schizophrenia. Ann Med 1996; 28(6): 525–31.
9. American Psychiatric Association. Diagnostic and Statistical Manual of Mental Disorders. 4th ed. Washington, DC: American Psychiatric Press, 1994: 290–315.

10. Carpenter WT, Buchanan RW. Schizophrenia. N Engl J Med 1994; 330: 681–90.
11. The expert consensus guideline series Treatment of schizophrenia 1999. J Clin Psychiatry 1999; 60(suppl 11): 3–80.
12. Spitzer RL, Williams JB, Gibbon M et al. The Structured Clinical Interview for DSM-III-R (SCID). I: History, rationale, and description; Arch Gen Psychiatry 1992; 49(8): 624–9.
13. Tacchini G, Coppola MT, Musazzi A et al. Multinational validation of the Composite International Diagnostic Interview (CIDI). Minerva Psichiatr 1994; 35(2): 63–80.
14. Tsuang MT, Loyd DW. Other psychotic disorders. In: Michels R, ed. Psychiatry. Philadelphia: JP Lippincott 1985; 1(70): 1–17.
15. Tsuang MT, Demsey M, Rauscher F. A study of "atypical schizophrenia": a comparison with schizophrenia and affective disorder by sex, age of admission, precipitant, outcome, and family history. Arch Gen Psychiatry 1976; 33: 1157–60.
16. Knights A, Hirsch SR. "Revealed" Depression and drug treatment for schizophrenia Arch Gen Psychiatry 1981 Jul; 38(7): 806–11.
17. Buckley PF, Miller BJ, Lehrer DS et al. Psychiatric Comorbidities and Schizophrenia. Schizophr Bull 2008 Nov 14; vol: page span.
18. Kendler KS, Tsuang MT. Nosology of paranoid, schizophrenic, and other paranoid psychoses. Schizophr Bull 1981; 7: 594–610.
19. Mauri MC, Gaietta M, Dragogna F et al. Hallucinatory disorder, an original clinical picture? Clinical and imaging data. Prog Neuropsychopharmacol Biol Psychiatry 2008; 32(2): 523–30.
20. Faraone SV, Kremen WS, Lyons MJ et al. Diagnostic accuracy and linkage analysis: how useful are schizophrenia spectrum phenotypes? Am J Psychiatry 1995; 152(9): 1286–90.
21. Wright EC. The presentation of mental illness in mentally retarded adults. Br J Psychiatry 1982; 141: 496–502.
22. Lishman WA. Organic Psychiatry: The Psychological Consequences of Cerebral Disorder. Oxford: Blackwell Scientific, 1978.
23. Slater E, Beard AW. The schizophrenia-like psychoses of epilepsy. I. Psychiatric aspects. Br J Psychiatry 1963; 109: 95–150.
24. Kendler KS, Gallagher TJ, Abelson JM et al. Lifetime prevalence, demographic risk factors, and diagnostic validity of nonaffective psychosis as assessed in a US community sample. The National Comorbidity Survey. Arch Gen Psychiatry 1996 Nov; 53(11): 1022–31.
25. Australian Bureau of Statistics. Mental Health and Wellbeing: Profile of Adults, Australia. Australia, Catalogue no., 4326.0. Canberra: Australian Bureau of Statistics, 1997.
26. McGlashan TH. A selective review of recent North American long-term follow up studies of schizophrenia. Schizophr Bull 1988; 14(4): 515–42.
27. Hall CW. Psychiatric Presentations of Medical Illness: Somatopsychic Disorders. New York: SP Medical and Scientific Books, 1980.
28. Byerly M, Goodman W, Acholonu W et al. Obsessive compulsive symptoms in schizophrenia: frequency and clinical features. Schizophr Res 2005 Jul 15; 76(2-3): 309–16.
29. Goodwin R, Lyons JS, McNally RJ. Panic attacks in schizophrenia. Schizophr Res 2002; 58: 213–20.
30. Chen CY, Liu CY, Yang YY. Correlation of panic attacks and hostility in chronic schizophrenia. Psychiatry Clin Neurosci 2001; 55: 383–7.
31. Ciapparelli A, Paggini R, Marazziti D et al. Comorbidity with axis I anxiety disorders in remitted psychotic patients 1 year after hospitalization. CNS Spectr 2007; 12: 913–19.
32. Pallanti S, Quercioli L, Hollander E. Social anxiety in outpatients with schizophrenia: a relevant cause of disability. Am J Psychiatry 2004 Jan; 161(1): 53–8.
33. Priebe S, Bro¨ker M, Gunkel S. Involuntary admission and posttraumatic stress disorder symptoms in schizophrenia patients. Compr Psychiatry 1998; 39: 220–24.
34. Hemmings CP. Schizophrenia spectrum disorders in people with intellectual disabilities. Curr Opin Psychiatry 2006 Sep; 19(5): 470–4.
35. Reichenberg A, Weiser M, Rapp MA et al. Elaboration on premorbid intellectual performance in schizophrenia: premorbid intellectual decline and risk for schizophrenia. Arch Gen Psychiatry 2005 Dec; 62(12): 1297–304.

36. Bonnici HM, William T, Moorhead J et al. Pre-frontal lobe gyrification index in schizophrenia, mental retardation and comorbid groups: an automated study. Neuroimage 2007 Apr 1; 35(2): 648–54.
37. Newton-Howes G, Tyrer P, North B, et al.. The prevalence of personality disorder in schizophrenia and psychotic disorders: systematic review of rates and explanatory modelling. Psychol Med. 2008 Aug; 38(8): 1075-82
38. Widiger TA, Trull TJ Personality and psychopathology: an application of the five-factor model. J Pers 1992 Jun; 60(2): 363–93.
39. Fanous AH, Kendler KS The genetic relationship of personality to major depression and schizophrenia. Neurotox Res 2004; 6(1): 43–50.
40. Schürhoff F, Szöke A, Chevalier F et al. Schizotypal dimensions: an intermediate phenotype associated with the COMT high activity allele. Am J Med Genet B Neuropsychiatr Genet 2007 Jan 5; 144B(1): 64–8.
41. Green AI, Drake RE, Brunette MF et al. Schizophrenia and co-occurring substance use disorder. Am J Psychiatry 2007 Mar; 164(3): 402–8.
42. Buckley PF. Substance abuse in schizophrenia: a review. J Clin Psychiatry 1998; 59 Suppl 3: 26–30.
43. Archie S, Rush BR, Akhtar-Danesh N et al. Substance use and abuse in first-episode psychosis: prevalence before and after early intervention. Schizophr Bull 2007 Nov; 33(6): 1354–63.
44. Larsen TK, Melle I, Auestad B et al. Substance abuse in first-episode non-affective psychosis. Schizophr Res 2006 Dec; 88(1-3): 55–62.
45. Victor M, Hope JM. The phenomenon of auditory hallucinations in chronic alcoholism: a critical evaluation of the status of alcoholic hallucinosis. J Nerv Ment Dis 1958; 126: 451–81.
46. Tsuang MT, Simpson JC, Kronfol Z. Subtypes of drug abuse with psychosis: demographic characteristics, clinical features, and family history. Arch Gen Psychiatry 1982; 39: 141–7.
47. Muck-Jørgensen P, Mors O, Mortensen PB, Ewald H. The schizophrenic patient in the somatic hospital Acta Psychiatr Scand Suppl 2000; (407): 96–9.
48. Leucht S, Burkard T, Henderson J et al. Physical illness and schizophrenia: a review of the literature. Acta Psychiatr Scand 2007 Nov; 116(5): 317–33.
49. McCreadie RG. Scottish Schizophrenia Lifestyle Group. Diet, smoking and cardiovascular risk in people with schizophrenia: descriptive study. Br J Psychiatry 2003 Dec; 183: 534–9.
50. McEvoy JP, Meyer JM, Goff DC et al. Prevalence of the metabolic syndrome in patients with schizophrenia: baseline results from the Clinical Antipsychotic Trials of Intervention Effectiveness (CATIE) schizophrenia trial and comparison with national estimates from NHANES III. Schizophr Res 2005 Dec 1; 80(1): 19–32.
51. Saari K, Jokelainen J, Veijola J et al. Serum lipids in schizophrenia and other functional psychoses: a general population northern Finland 1966 birth cohort survey. Acta Psychiatr Scand 2004 Oct; 110(4): 279–85.
52. Wetterling T, Pest S, Müssigbrodt H et al. Bodyweight in inpatients with schizophrenia. Psychiatr Prax 2004 Jul; 31(5): 250–4.
53. Allison DB, Mentore JL, Heo M et al.Antipsychotic-induced weight gain: a comprehensive research synthesis. Am J Psychiatry 1999 Nov; 156(11): 1686–96.
54. Halbreich U, Palter S. Accelerated osteoporosis in psychiatric patients: possible pathophysiological processes. Schizophr Bull 1996; 22(3): 447–54.
55. Peveler RC, Branford D, Citrome L et al. Antipsychotics and hyperprolactinaemia: clinical recommendations. J Psychopharmacol 2008 Mar; 22(2 Suppl): 98–103.
56. Barak Y, Achiron A, Mandel M et al. Reduced cancer incidence among patients with schizophrenia. Cancer 2005 Dec 15; 104(12): 2817–21.
57. Mortensen PB. The incidence of cancer in schizophrenic patients. J Epidemiol Community Health 1989 Mar; 43(1): 43–7.
58. Lichtermann D, Ekelund J, Pukkala E et al. Incidence of cancer among persons with schizophrenia and their relatives. Arch Gen Psychiatry. 2001 Jun; 58(6): 573–8.

59. Mortensen PB. Neuroleptic medication and reduced risk of prostate cancer in schizophrenic patients. Acta Psychiatr Scand 1992 May; 85(5): 390–3.
60. Brown S, Inskip H, Barraclough B. Causes of the excess mortality of schizophrenia. Br J Psychiatry 2000 Sep; 177: 212–7.
61. Cournos F, McKinnon K, Sullivan G Schizophrenia and comorbid human immunodeficiency virus or hepatitis C virus. J Clin Psychiatry 2005; 66 (Suppl 6): 27–33.
62. De Hert M, Hautekeete M, De Wilde D et al. High prevalence of Helicobacter pylori in institutionalized schizophrenic patients. Schizophr Res 1997 Aug 29; 26(2–3):243–4.
63. Macdonald S, Halliday J, MacEwan T et al. Nithsdale Schizophrenia Surveys 24: sexual dysfunction. Case-control study. Br J Psychiatry 2003 Jan; 182: 50–6.
64. Bonney WW, Gupta S, Hunter DR et al. Bladder dysfunction in schizophrenia. Schizophr Res 1997 Jun 20; 25(3): 243–9.
65. Aukes MF, Alizadeh BZ, Sitskoorn MM, et al. Genetic overlap among intelligence and other candidate endophenotypes for schizophrenia. Biol Psychiatry 2009 Mar 15; 65(6): 527–34.
66. Altamura AC, Bobo WV, Meltzer HY. Factors affecting outcome in schizophrenia and their relevance for psychopharmacological treatment. Int Clin Psychopharmacol 2007; 22(5): 249–67.
67. Degenhardt L, Hall W, Lynskey M. Testing hypotheses about the relationship between cannabis use and psychosis. Drug Alcohol Depend. 2003 Jul 20; 71(1): 37–48.
68. Altamura AC, Mundo E, Bassetti R, et al. Transcultural differences in suicide attempters: analysis on a high-risk population of patients with schizophrenia or schizoaffective disorder. Schizophr Res. 2007 Jan; 89(1-3): 140–6.
69. Altamura AC, Bassetti R, Bignotti S, et al. Clinical variables related to suicide attempts in schizophrenic patients: a retrospective study. Schizophr Res. 2003 Mar 1; 60(1): 47–55.

7 | Neurocognition and schizophrenia

Gabriele Sachs

INTRODUCTION

Cognitive deficits represent a core feature in schizophrenia (1, 2) and have substantial influence on the course of the illness, on noncompliance, and on psychosocial functioning. These cognitive deficits were described initially by Kraepelin (3).

Since the development of antipsychotics, however, the main focus was put on treating positive and negative symptoms rather than cognitive functions. Only in the recent past, the interest in cognitive functions has reawakened. This is partially due to the increasing knowledge of the relationship between cognitive and psychosocial functional deficits (4).

Cognitive deficits have a considerable influence on everyday life and also help predict the development of the patient's psychosocial functioning and social integration. In addition, cognitive deficits are relevant to compliance as they reduce the motivation to go through therapy and the commitment to work in the therapeutic alliance.

NEUROCOGNITIVE DYSFUNCTIONS

In patients with schizophrenia, various domains of cognitive functions are impaired, including attention, memory, learning, executive functions, motor functions, and speech.

Cognitive deficits become apparent in more than 85% of the schizophrenic patients. In the study by Bilder et al. 2000 (5), first-episode patients with schizophrenia or schizoaffective disorder evidenced a generalized deficit, i.e., their results in most cognitive tests showed a standard deviation of 1.5 below the performance of the healthy controls, which indicates a severe deficit.

These cognitive impairments in patients with schizophrenia are stable suggesting the existence of "trait markers": They occur before the onset of the illness and are present at the beginning and during remission phases. Recent studies indicate that cognitive deficits play a significant role in early diagnosis and prevention. Deficits in information processing are of high value for predicting the beginning of psychotic symptoms (6, 7). They cannot primarily be seen as a medication effect, as deficits also occur without medication (8).

ATTENTION

Attention dysfunctions are one of the most important domains of cognitive deficits in patients with schizophrenia. The impairments include different components of attentional functioning such as the ability to detect relevant stimuli, to focus attention on certain relevant stimuli, and suppress or ignore irrelevant stimuli at the same time (selective attention), as well as to sustain attention on a stimulus until it is processed (sustained attention or vigilance). The deficits of the information processing capacity can be found in patients with schizophrenia during high demand (9). Patients process irrelevant information consciously which leads to an overstraining of the patient's processing capacity (10).

MEMORY AND LEARNING

In patients with schizophrenia, various memory functions are impaired. A meta-analysis (11) of more than 204 studies showed that verbal memory was disturbed more than any other area. Compared to healthy controls, patients with schizophrenia are less able to recognize numbers, words, and faces they have seen before; these specific deficits are present in both visual and verbal memory. In addition, patients with schizophrenia have difficulty in retaining and consolidating factual information as in the semantic memory (12). Saykin et al. (13) found that encoding, storage, reproduction as well as recognition can be impaired. Also, the ability to associate between pieces of information can be diminished. In addition, deficits in short-term memory and working memory have been found. Two components of working memory are the brief storage system and the executive system. According to the Baddeley model (14), working memory refers to the temporary storage of information that is being processed in any cognitive task. Such tasks require an increased usage of encoding strategies that represent a particular problem for patients with schizophrenia.

EXECUTIVE FUNCTIONS

Executive functioning includes the ability to solve problems, to formulate strategies, and to evaluate their usefulness (15), which is important for everyday life and social activities and for performing tasks. Studies also show considerable deficits in the areas of planning, executing, and controlling actions (16). Patients with schizophrenia perform tasks with a high executive component with a standard deviation of 1.4 below the performance of healthy controls (17). This planning deficit is a lack in the ability to combine and process information from varying sources. The degree of impairment differs in various phases of the illness.

COGNITION, BRAIN STRUCTURE, AND NEURAL NETWORK DEFICITS

Using neurocognitive tests and structural/functional brain imaging, correlations between cognitive deficits, brain anomalies, and neuronal dysfunctional brain areas have been detected.

In a meta-analysis (18), the volume of the whole brain was described to be associated with neuropsychological functioning. The prefrontal cortex seems to be correlated with attention and working memory, thalamic anomalies with executive functions and the hippocampal volume has been associated with verbal memory. Enlargement of ventricles in patients is associated with deficits in attention and executive functioning.

To investigate specific brain activation patterns of the illness, cognitive paradigms are applied. In brain imaging studies, differences were found between patients and healthy controls in the activation of their corticolimbic and frontoparietal brain areas as well as in the anterior cingulum when performing selective attention tests (distractibility by irrelevant stimuli) (19). Hypofrontality has been one of the most prominent and consistent findings in schizophrenic disorders. Frequently, the Continuous Performance Test (CPT) was used to investigate the performance of a patient's attention and working memory. Studies in which the CPT was applied showed that in comparison to healthy controls activation of the dorsolateral prefrontal cortex and the cingulum was reduced in schizophrenic patients (20, 21). Schneider et al. (22) demonstrated in first-episode patients with schizophrenia a hypoactivation of the parietal lobe (precuneus) and at the same time a hyperactivation of the inferior frontal areas. From these data, the conclusion was drawn that there is no general, detectable hypoactivation in the inferior frontal areas.

TABLE 7.1   Neurocognition and structural/functional brain-imaging

Cognitive domains	Functional deficits	Structural deficits (18)
Attention, Working memory	Lateral prefrontal cortex Anterior cingulate (20, 21, 22)	Anterior cingulate, Ventral frontal, parietal occipital, left frontal lobe
Verbal and spatial memory	Inferior prefrontal cortex Superior temporal cortex Hippocampus (24, 25)	Hippocampus, Parahippocampus Cerebellum
Verbal fluency	Lateral temporal cortex	Superior temporal gyrus
Executive function	Lateral prefrontal cortex (26)	Thalamus, Anterior cingulate, Ventral frontal lobe, Parahippocampus

In regard to memory functions, deficits were primarily found in the episodic as well as in the semantic memory. Functional impairments were mostly noted during encoding and memory retrieval (23, 24). Both hypoactivation in the left inferior prefrontal cortex and hyperactivation in the left superior temporal gyrus were detected with male schizophrenic patients during semantic processing (25). Discrepant findings were reported in relation to hippocampus, areas of the medial temporal cortex, and dorsolateral prefrontal cortex (26). However, studies about the connectivity of frontal brain areas also stress the complex networking between dorsolateral cortex, subcortical structures, and also the cerebellum (27).

NEUROCOGNITIVE DYSFUNCTIONS AND ENDOPHENOTYPES

Neuropsychological deficits in patients with schizophrenia can also be seen as endophenotypes that could be associated with possible disposition genes (28). Studies suggest that working memory and associated structural and functional abnormalities in prefrontal cortex "are reflective of an inherited diathesis to schizophrenia" (29). Working memory, attention, reaction time to visual targets, and verbal memory retrieval deficits make contributions to the prediction of genetic loading. Weinberger et al. (30) reported the influence of the catechol-O-methyltransferase gene (COMT) on chromosome 22 with valine allele associated with prefrontal hypofunction. Egan et al. 2001 (31) investigated the effect of the COMT Val/Met genotype in the frontal lobe function and the risk for schizophrenia. COMT Val allele has an impact on prefrontal cognition. Furthermore, the G-protein signaling the subtype 4 (RGS4) gene, the disrupted-in-schizophrenia-1 (DISC1) gene on chromosome 1, showed evidence of association with decreased prefrontal cognitive function (32). These findings implicate genetic factors as playing a role in the abnormalities of prefrontal cortex and working memory in schizophrenia. Among the genes that may contribute to disturbances in structure and functioning of the temporal cortex and hippocampus, dysbindin, neuregulin, and G72 are candidates in relation to verbal learning and memory deficits (33, 34).

DIAGNOSTIC METHODS AND TREATMENT STRATEGIES

To remedy the lack of an accepted standard for measuring cognitive change in schizophrenia and improve the diagnostics of cognitive deficits the American National Institutes of Health (NIMH) has initiated the MATRICS program (Measurement and Treatment Research to Improve Cognition in Schizophrenia) (35).

The aim is to develop a consensus with regard to a cognitive battery for clinical trials of cognition-enhancing treatments for schizophrenia. In addition, the American Food and Drug Administration (FDA) demands that medication does not only improve cognitive deficits but also improves social functioning and working performance (36).

TABLE 7.2 Domains of Cognitive Deficits in Schizophrenia (35, 36) Neuropsychological Tests MCCB- MATRICS Consensus Cognitive Battery

Domains	Test
Information processing	Symbol Coding (BACS)
	Fluency: Animal Naming (Fluency) (BVMT-R)
	Trail Making Test – connect numbers (TMT)
Attention/Vigilance	Continuous Performance Test–Identical Pairs (CPT-IP)
Working memory (nonverbal)	Wechsler Memory Scale (WMS-II)
Working memory (verbal)	Letter-Number Span (LNS)
Verbal learning	Hopkins Verbal Learning Test–Revised (HVLT-R)
Visual learning	Brief Visuospatial Memory Test–Revised (BVMT-R)
Logical thinking and problem solving	Neuropsychological Assessment Battery (NAB): Mazes
Social cognition	Mayer-Salovey-Caruso Emotional Intelligence Test (MSCEIT): Managing Emotions

As a first step, tools were developed that identify essential target criteria to measure cognitive functions. The MATRICS Committee was employed to select a final battery of 10 tests, the consensus cognitive battery (MCCB) (37), to establish an accepted way to evaluate cognition-enhancing agents. The next step will be to develop specific neuropharmacological therapies that will then be tested in multicenter studies. For this, several research centers have teamed up in the NIMH-TURNS project (Treatment Units for Research on Neurocognition and Schizophrenia) (38). In the following, the most promising targets of the neurotransmitter systems are listed, which, according to current knowledge, play an important role in the pathogenesis of cognitive deficits in schizophrenia: D1 dopamin receptor in the prefrontal cortex, serotonin receptor in prefrontal and anterior cingular cortex, excitatory and gluamatergic synapses, the nicotinic acetyl receptor in the hippocampus, the muscarinic acetyl receptor, and GABAergic systems (39). First examples of the respective medication with an effect on these specific target structures are currently being tested for approval by the FDA as so called cognitive enhancing agents.

THE NEUROPHARMACOLOGY OF COGNITION

The introduction of atypical antipsychotics leads to a certain positive effect on negative and cognitive symptoms. They were also better tolerated and had fewer side effects on motor and affective functions. The particular advantages of atypical antipsychotics are mainly their positive influence on cognitive symptoms and their possible influence on the long-term course of illness. Due to current debates about healthcare economics, there were discussions in the recent past whether atypical antipsychotics improve cognitive deficits more than typical antipsychotics. Previous data showed that atypical antipsychotics are more effective than the older typical ones. In the study by Bilder et al. (40), olanzapine and risperidone were superior to haloperidol. Positive effects became apparent, specifically, in the domains of learning and information processing (41). However, one important limitation of these results is that, in contrast to atypical antipsychotics, the typical antipsychotics (haloperidol in most cases) were administered in very high dosages. Even when typical antipsychotics were given in a lower dosage, no significant differences were found compared to atypical antipsychotics (42). Interestingly, in the CATIE study (Clinical Antipsychotic Trials of Intervention Effectiveness) that compares the atypical antipsychotics—olanzapine, quetiapine und risperidone (later ziprasidone)—to the typical perphenazine, only low effects were found with regard to

TABLE 7.3 The effect of antipsychotics on cognitive deficits in patients with schizophrenia

Author	N (study design)	Medication effects – mean doses (mg/d)
Bilder et al. (40)	101, chronic double blind, 14-weeks	Olanzapine (20.2mg), Risperidone (8.3mg) > Clozapine (452mg), Haloperidol (19.6mg) Olanzapine attention, Risperidone memory
Green et al. (42)	62, stable double blind, 2-year	Haloperidol (5mg) = Risperidone (6mg) global score
Keefe et al. (45)	400, first episode double-blind, 52-weeks	Olanzapine (11.7mg) = Quetiapine (506mg) = Risperidone (2.4mg)
Harvey et al. (46)	289, first episode double blind, 8-weeks	Quetiapine (200–800mg) = Risperidone (2–8mg) neurocognition and social competence
Harvey et al. (47)	130, resistant double blind	Ziprasidone > Clozapine Composite score
Meltzer et al. (48)	40, resistant double blind, 6-month	High-dose Olanzapine (34mg) = Clozapine (564mg)
Harvey et al. (50)	133, acute symptoms double blind, 6-month	Ziprasidone (114.17mg) = Olanzapine (12.27mg)
Kern et al. (51)	169, stable open label, 8 and 26 weeks	Aripiprazole (30mg) > Olanzapine (15mg) verbal learning at week 8

cognitive deficits. After a period of 18 months, perphenazine was even superior to olanzapine and risperidone, but there was a very high drop-out rate (approximately 268 of almost 1,500 patients) (43). However, the meta-analysis by Woodward et al. (44) shows that, in general, atypical antipsychotics can achieve better effects than typical antipsychotics. In studies in which atypical antipsychotics were compared exclusively to each other, there were improvements to be observed in the cognitive domains. In the study by Keefe et al. (45) that investigated 400 first-episode patients, no significant differences were detected between olanzapine, quetiapine und risperidone after 52 weeks, with low effects in the cognitive domains. A significant correlation was, however, detected between the improvement in cognition and the functional outcome (46).

Comparing various atypical antipsychotics in a meta-analysis, Woodward et al. (44) found that some of them differ in specific cognitive domains. Significant differences were discovered in the areas of attention and verbal fluency.

In a comparison between clozapine and ziprasidone (47), the latter had a better effect on therapy-resistant patients. Olanzapine, at higher doses, demonstrated a similar efficacy to clozapine in treatment-resistant schizophrenia (48). Further, cognitive performance was similarly improved by ziprasidone and olanzapine when administered over a 6-month period (49). In the open, comparative clinical trial of aripiprazole and olanzapine, improvements in the secondary verbal memory were significantly more perceivable with aripiprazole (50).

It should be noted, however, that there are still some limitations in the results of the currently existing studies. First, the impact of antipsychotics on cognitive deficits should also be compared to the performance of healthy controls in order to exclude any possible practice effect (51). Second, new antipsychotics do not only improve positive symptoms but also negative symptoms and cognitive deficits, although there have been only low effects. Nevertheless, more comprehensive double-blind studies are needed to further verify their impact.

The advantages of using atypical antipsychotics to treat cognitive deficits of patients with schizophrenia are the low side effects and the better tolerability in the long-term course of the disease. In choosing the appropriate atypical antipsychotic for a patient, it is, however, essential to carefully consider for each individual the medication's efficacy on cognitive deficits, as this can significantly influence the patient's psychosocial functioning.

COGNITIVE TRAINING AND REMEDIATION

In addition to treatment with psychopharmacological agents, neuropsychological rehabilitation programs can further improve cognitive functioning and psychosocial problem solving (52). Cognitive remediation programs have been found to enhance attention and vigilance, memory, and executive function (53, 54). A recent meta-analysis by McGurk et al. (55), which includes 26 studies, established that cognitive remediation in combination with psychiatric rehabilitation is more effective than cognitive remediation alone.

SUMMARY AND FUTURE DEVELOPMENTS

Cognitive deficits and functional impairments are important target criteria in the treatment of patients with schizophrenia. They are related to neuronal dysfunctional activation patterns. Integrative treatment strategies combining the use of atypical antipsychotics and cognitive remediation are more likely to have a positive impact on the long-term course of the illness as well as on the psychosocial integration.

In the future, one can expect an increasing number of treatment studies about neurobiological aspects of cognitive deficits. They may reveal in which way dysfunctional activation patterns can be influenced in certain brain areas. Currently, a number of new substances are tested that can possibly be used as cognitive enhancers in addition to existing therapy options so that cognitive deficits and the psychosocial functioning of a patient with schizophrenia can be improved.

REFERENCES

1. Heinrichs RW, Zakzanis KK. Neurocognitive deficit in schizophrenia: a quantitative review of the evidence. Neuropsychology 1998; 12: 426–45.
2. Sachs G, Steger-Wuchse D, Kryspin-Exner I et al. Facial recognition deficits and cognition in schizophrenia. Schizophr Res 2004; 68(1): 27–35.
3. Kraepelin E. Dementia Praecox and Paraphrenia. Edinburgh: Livingstone, 1919.
4. Green MF, Kern RS, Braff DL et al. Neurocognitive deficits and functional outcome in schizophrenia: are we measuring the "right stuff"? Schizophr Bull 2000; 26, 119–36.
5. Bilder RM, Goldman RS, Robinson D et al. Neuropsychology of first-episode schizophrenia: initial characterization and clinical correlates. Am J Psychiatry 2000; 157(4): 549–59.
6. Lencz T, Smith CW, McLaughlin D et al. Generalized and specific neurocognitive deficits in prodromal schizophrenia. Biol Psychiatry 2006; 59: 863–71.
7. Rund BR, Melle I, Friis S et al. The course of neurocognitive functioning in first-episode psychosis and its relation to premorbid adjustment, duration of untreated psychosis, and relapse. Schizophr Res 2007; 91: 132–40.
8. Saykin AJ, Gur RC, Gur RE. Neuropsychological function in schizophrenia: selective impairment in memory and learning. Arch Gen Psychiatry 1991; 48: 618–24.
9. Nuechterlein KH, Dawson ME. Information processing and attentional functioning in the developmental course of schizophrenic disorders. Schizophr Bull 1984; 10(2): 160–203.
10. Nuechterlein KH, Dawson ME, Green MF. Information-processing abnormalities as neuropsychological vulnerability indicators for schizophrenia. Acta Psych Scan 1994; 90: 71–9.
11. Aleman A, Ron Hijman MA, de Haan EHF et al. Memory impairment in schizophenia: a meta-analysis. Am J Psychiatry 1999; 156(9): 1358–66.
12. Rosell SL, David AS. Are semantic deficits in schizphrenia due to problems with access or storage? Schizophr Res 2006; 82(2–3): 121–34.

13. Saykin AJ, Gur RC, Gur RE. Neuropsychological function in schizophrenia: selective impairment in memory and learning. Arch Gen Psychiatry 1991; 48: 618–24.
14. Baddeley A. Working memory: the interface between memory and cognition. J of Cognitive Neuroscience 1992; 4: 281–8.
15. Hutton SB, Puri BK, Duncan LJ. Executive function in first-episode schizophrenia. Psychol Med 1998; 28: 463–73.
16. Kurtz MM. Symptoms versus neurocognitive skills as correlates of everyday functioning in severe mental illness. Expert Rev Neurother 2006; 6(1): 47–56.
17. Gur RE, Calkins ME, Gur RC et al. The Consortium on the Genetics of schizophrenia: neurocognitive endophenotypes. Schizophr Bull 2007; 33: 49–68.
18. Crespo-Facorro B, Barbadillo L, Pelayo-Teran JM et al. Neuropsychological functioning and brain structure in schizophrenia. Int Rev Psychiatry 2007; 19(4): 325–36.
19. Liddle PF, Laurens KR, Kiehl KA et al. Abnormal function of the brain system supporting motivated attention in medicated patients with schizophrenia: an fMRI study. Psychol Med 2006; 36(8): 1097–108.
20. Tan HY, Sust S, Buckholtz JW et al. Dysfunctional prefrontal regional specialization and compensation in schizophrenia. Am J Psychiatry 2006; 163 (11): 1996–77.
21. Harrison BJ, Yücel M, Fornito A et al. Characterizing anterior cingulate activation in chronic schizophrenia: a group and single-subject fMRI study. Acta Psychiatr Scand 2007; 116(4): 271–9.
22. Schneider F, habel U, Reske M et al. Neural correlates of working memory dysfunction in first-episode schizophrenia patients: an fMRI multi-center study. Schizophr Res 2007; 89(1–3): 198–210.
23. Eyler LT, Jeste DV, Brown GG. Brain response abnormalities during verbal learning among patients with schizophrenia. Psychiatry Res 2008; 162(1): 11–24.
24. Ragland JD, Moelter ST, Bhati MT et al. Effect of retrieval effort and switching demand on fMRI activation during semantic word generation in schizophrenia. Schizophr Res 2008; 99(1–3): 312–23.
25. Achim AM, Lepage M. Episodic memory-related activation in schizophrenia: meta-analysis. Br J Psychiatry 2005; 187: 500–9.
26. Meyer – Lindenberg A, Poline JB, Kohn PD et al. Evidence for abnormal cortical functional connectivity during working memory in schizophrenia. Am J Psychiatry 2001; 158(11): 1809–17.
27. Andreasen NC, O`Leary DS, Cizadlo T. Schizophrenia and cognitive dysmetria: a positron-emission tomography study of dysfunctional prefrontal-thalamic-cerebellar circuitry. Proc Natl Acad Sci 1996; 93(18): 9985–90.
28. Meyer – Lindenberg A, Nichols T, Callicott JH et al. Impact of complex genetic variation in COMT on human brain function. Mol Psychiatry 2006; 11(9): 867–77.
29. Cannon TD, Keller MC. Endophenotypes in the genetic analyses of mental disorders. Annu Rev Clin Psychol 2006; 2: 267–90.
30. Weinberger DR, Egan MF, Bertolino A. Prefrontal neurons and the genetics of schizophrenia. Biol Psychiatry 2001; 50(11): 825–44.
31. Egan MF, Goldberg TE, Kolachana BS et al. Effect of COMT Val108/158 Met genotype on frontal lobe function and risk for schizophrenia. Proc Natl Acad Sci 2001; 98(12): 6917–22.
32. Cannon TD, Hennah W, van Erp TG et al. Association of DISC1/TRAX haplotypes with schizophrenia, reduced prefrontal gray matter, and impaired short- and long-term memory. Arch Gen Psychiatry 2005; 62(11): 1205–13.
33. Talbot K, Eidem WL, Tinsley CL et al. Dysbindin-1 is reduced in intrinsic, glutamatergic terminals of the hippocampal formation in schizophrenia. J Clin Invest 2004; 113(9): 1353–63.
34. Numakawa T, Yagasaki Y, Ishimoto T et al. Evidence of novel neuronal functions of dysbindin, a susceptibility gene for schizophrenia. Hum Mol Genet 2004; 13(21): 2699–708.
35. Marder SR, Fenton WS. Measurement and treatment research to improve conition in schizophrenia: NIMH MATRICS initiative to support the development of agents for improving cognition in schizophrenia. Schizophr Res 2004; 72: 5–10.

36. Green MF, Nuechterlein KH, Gold JM et al. Approaching a consensus cognitive battery for clinical trials in schizophrenia: the NIMH-MATRICS conference to select cognitive domains and test criteria. Biol Psychiatry 2004; 56: 301–7.
37. Green MF, Nuechterlein KH, Kern RS et al. Functional Co-Primary Measures for Clinical Trials in Schizophrenia: Results from the MATRICS Psychometric and standardization study. Am J Psychiatry 2008; 165: 221–8.
38. Buchanan RW, Davis M, Goff D et al. A summery of the FDA-NIMH-MATRICS workshop on clinical trial design for neurocognitive drugs for schizophrenia. Schizophr Bull 2005; 31: 5–19.
39. Tamminga CA. The neurobiology of cognition in schizophrenia. J Clin Psychiatry 2006; 67 Suppl: 9–13.
40. Bilder RM, Goldman RS, Volavka J et al. Neurocognitive effects of Clozapine, Olanzapine, Risperidone, and Haloperidol in patients with chronic schizophrenia or schizoaffective disorder. Am J Psychiatry 2002; 159: 1018–28.
41. Keefe RS, Young CA, Rock SL et al. One-year double-blind study of the neurocognitive efficacy of olanzapine, risperidone, and haloperidol in schizophrenia. Schizophr Res 2006; 81: 1–15.
42. Green MF, Marder SR, Glynn SM et al. The neurocognitive effects of low-dose Haloperidol: A two-year comparison with Risperidon. Biol Psychiatry 2002; 51: 972–8.
43. Keefe RS, Bilder RM, Davis S et al. Neurocognitive effects of antipsychotic medications in patients with chronic schizophrenia in the CATIE trial. Arch Gen Psychiatry 2007; 64: 633–47.
44. Woodward ND, Purdon SE, Meltzer HY et al. A meta-analysis of neuropsychological change to Clozapine, Olanzapine, Quetiapine, and Risperidone in schizophrenia. Int J Neuropsychopharmacol 2005; 8: 457–72.
45. Keefe RS, Sweeney JA, Gu H et al. Effects of Olanzapine, Quetiapine, and Risperidone on neurocognitive function in early psychosis: A randomized, double-blind 52-week comparison. Am J Psychiatry 2007; 164: 1061–71.
46. Harvey PD, Patterson TL, Potter LS et al. Improvement in social competence with short-term atypical antipsychotic treatment: A randomized, double-blind comparison of Quetiapine versus Risperidone for social competence, social cognition, and neuropsychological functioning. Am J Psychiatry 2006; 163: 1918–25.
47. Harvey PD, Sacchetti E, Galluzzo A et al. A randomized double-blind comparison of Ziprasidone vs. Clozapine for cognition in patients with schizophrenia selected for resistance or intolerance to previous treatment. Schizophr Res 2007, epub ahead of print
48. Meltzer HY, Bobo WV, Roy A et al. A randomized, double-blind comparison of Clozapine and high-dose Olanzapine in treatment-resistant patients with schizophrenia. J Clin Psychiary 2008; 69(2): 274–85.
49. Harvey PD, Bowie CR, Loebel A. Neuropsychological normalization with long-term atypical antipsychotic treatment: results of a six-month randomized, double-blind comparison of Ziprasidone vs. Olanzapine. J Neuropsychiatry Clin Neurosci 2006; 18: 54–63.
50. Kern RS, Green MF, Cornblatt BA et al. The neurocognitive effects of Aripiprazole: an open-label comparison with Olanzapine. Psychopharmacology 2006; 187(3): 312–20.
51. Goldberg RE, Goldman RS, Burdick KE et al. Cognitive improvement after treatment with second-generation antipsychotic medications in first-episode schizophrenia. Arch Gen Psychiatry 2007; 64(10): 1115–22.
52. Medalia A, Richardson R. What predicts a good response to cognitive remediation interventions? Schizophr Bull 2005; 31(4): 942–53.
53. Sartory G, Zorn C, Groetzinger G et al. Computerized cognitive remediation improves verbal learning and processing speed in schizophrenia. Schizophrenia Research 2005; 75: 219–23.
54. Velligan DI, Kern RS, Gold JM et al. Cognitive rehabilitation for schizophrenia and the putative role of motivation and expectancies. Schizophr Bull 2006; 32(3): 474–85.
55. McGurk SR, Twamley EW, Sitzer DI et al. A meta-analysis of cognitive remediation in schizophrenia. Am J Psychiatry 2007; 164: 1791–802.

8   Genetic and epigenetic factors in schizophrenia

Alexandra Schosser and Peter McGuffin

INTRODUCTION

An inherited component to schizophrenia has been long established and even noted by Emil Kraepelin in his classical textbook on psychiatry (1). Since Kraepelin´s observations, extensive family, twin, and adoption studies have provided compelling evidence that schizophrenia not only tends to run in families but that this is largely due to genes. However, the mode of inheritance is clearly non-Mendelian, nor can it be, as was once thought, explained by a single gene with incomplete penetrance (i.e., where individuals who carry the gene do not necessarily express the illness). Rather, schizophrenia is best explained by a polygenic multifactorial model where many genes, each of small effect, combine with environmental factors and that the disorder results once a critical threshold of liability is exceeded. This "common disease-common alleles with multiple genes of small effect" model is the basis for large-scale genetic association and genome-wide association studies.

FAMILY STUDIES

The lifetime expectancy for schizophrenia in the general population worldwide is around 1%, but much higher figures have been consistently found in relatives of people with schizophrenia (2). The risk increases as the degree of genetic affinity with the affected family member increases. An approximately nine-fold increase in risk of schizophrenia in first-degree relatives has been found, and the risk rises as high as 46% among offspring of parents both of whom suffer from schizophrenia (2). The largest study of recurrence risks in relatives to date, based on a Swedish population cohort of more than 7 million individuals, was carried out by Lichtenstein et al. (3), finding a sibling relative risk (λs) of 8.55.

TWIN STUDIES

Twin studies of schizophrenia (reviewed in Cardno and Gottesman) (4) have consistently found higher concordance rates for monozygotic (MZ) twins than dizygotic (DZ) twins. This can be taken as evidence of a genetic contribution to the disorder, as MZ twins have exactly the same genes, whereas DZ twins share, on average, only half their genes, and it is a reasonable assumption that both types of twins share the environment to roughly the same extent. The probandwise concordance rate for schizophrenia in MZ twin pairs is 48% compared with 17% for DZ twin pairs (see Figure 8.1). This corresponds to heritability estimates of about 80%–85% (5). Despite the strong and consistent evidence for genetic influence provided by twin studies, the discordance rate for MZ twins indicates the importance of nongenetic factors.

Adoption studies permit to differentiate genetic factors from environmental factors that could potentially cause familiality. Similarities between individuals adopted away at birth and their biological relatives are likely to be due to shared genes, whereas

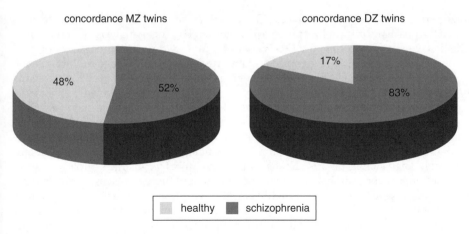

concordance MZ twins   concordance DZ twins

FIGURE 8.1 The higher concordance rate in monozygotic (Mz) twin pairs (48%) compared to dizygotic (Dz) twin pairs (17%) can be taken as evidence of a genetic contribution to schizophrenia. However, the concordance rate in Mz twins (who have 100% of genes in common) indicates the importance of non-genetic factors in schizophrenia aetiology.

similarities between adoptees and the adoptive family are likely to be due to shared environment. The risk of schizophrenia is consistently found to be associated with the presence of the illness in biological parents but not in the adoptive parents who share the same environment as probands (6, 7, 8). This implies that growing up in a family with schizophrenics does not increase the risk for schizophrenia beyond the risk due to genes. A large adoption study carried out in Finland (9) showed that about 10% of adoptees who had a schizophrenic biological parent showed some form of psychosis, whereas 1% of control adoptees had similar disorders, but it also found evidence of an interaction between genes and early social environment in that the risk of psychosis was greatest in those offspring of schizophrenic mothers adopted into poorly functioning families.

MOLECULAR GENETIC STUDIES
Current research focuses mainly on detecting common polymorphisms associated with disease susceptibility ('common disease – common variant' model), although there has been recent debate about the occurrence of highly penetrant, rare mutations of large effect ('common disease – rare variant') in at least some cases, as well as epigenetic variation (see below).

LINKAGE STUDIES
In genetic linkage studies, large families with multiply affected members or affected sibling pairs are studied to try and find a genetic marker that cosegregates with the disease. The first wave of systematic genetic linkage studies were performed in the 1980s and early 1990s. Some early claims were made for linkage with classical markers (e.g., HLA), but these could not be replicated (10). The first was a claim for linkage with a DNA marker on chromosome 5q for Icelandic and British families (11); however, this linkage could not be confirmed combining data from five other studies in other countries (12). To date, more than 30 genome-wide linkage scans have been performed in

schizophrenia and two meta-analyses (13, 14) both identified the chromosomal regions 8p and 22q as harboring schizophrenia-risk genes. The meta-analysis of 20 genome-wide linkage scans performed by Lewis et al. (14) indicated greater consistency of linkage results than previously recognized and reported significant linkage to chromosome 2q. Linkage was suggested for ten other regions, including 6p and 8p. However, it is unlikely that all of these linkage findings are true, as the regions suggested by the Lewis et al. (14) meta-analysis implicated more than 3,000 genes (18% of all known genes). In short, the results of genome-wide linkage studies do not appear to converge, and no genomic region was identified by more than a few studies and an improbably large fraction of the genome (about half) was implicated by at least one study. It has been difficult to detect linkage signals because linkage analysis requires very large samples to detect the small effects contributing to schizophrenia susceptibility, whereas in single-gene disorders this approach had been highly effective for identifying genes of large effect. Interestingly, linkage data from genome scans of schizophrenia and bipolar disorder indicated putative linkages to both disorders in the same regions of the genome, for example, 13q and 22q (15), indicating an overlap in genetic susceptibility.

ASSOCIATION STUDIES

Genetic association studies, which evaluate the relationship between specific gene variants and the risk of developing schizophrenia, are potentially more powerful than linkage studies for detecting susceptibility genes of small effect size. However, the weakness of these studies is that an association can only be detected if a DNA marker is itself the functional gene or very close to it (i.e., in linkage disequilibrium). Thus, while linkage approaches can systematically scan the genome with just a few hundred DNA markers, far more DNA markers are required to systematically scan the genome for allelic association. As a consequence, until recently association studies were not systematic and were restricted to candidate genes. However, the Wellcome Trust Case Control Consortium (WTCCC) study (16) investigating seven common diseases, including bipolar disorder, convincingly demonstrated the benefits of genome-wide association studies (GWAS) in genetic research on common disorders. At least seven GWAS of schizophrenia have been either published recently or are currently on going (see below).

Positional and functional candidate genes

Candidate genes are genes that might be involved in a particular disease. Positional candidate genes are genes that map within a chromosomal region that is implicated by linkage, and functional (or biological) candidate genes might be involved in the neurotransmitter system that is implicated by the psychoactive drugs used to treat a disorder. At least 649 candidate genes have been investigated in schizophrenia (www.schizophreniaforum.org/res/sczgene/dbindex.asp); however, the candidate gene approach has not yielded replicable associations with schizophrenia that meet a high standard of proof. Interestingly, several schizophrenia candidate genes are probably not specific, and there is evidence of substantial overlap with other psychotic disorders, including bipolar disorder.

Neuregulin 1 (NRG1)

Following the linkage evidence to 8p, fine mapping in Icelandic families identified two risk haplotypes within the gene for Neuregulin 1 (NRG1) (17). This initial finding has been replicated in multiple schizophrenic samples, but not in all (for meta-analysis see 18). Due to its multifaceted role in the development of the nervous system, NRG1 is a plausible candidate gene for schizophrenia (19). Recent studies have associated NRG1 with bipolar disorder, suggesting that it is one of the genes accounting for the overlap between schizophrenia and bipolar disorder (20).

Dysbindin (DTNBP1)
Fine mapping of the linkage region on chromosome 6p pointed to DTNBP1 as a candidate gene for schizophrenia (21). In addition, DTNBP1 is an important functional candidate gene, as it is found exclusively in neurones and has a role in synaptic structure and signalling. A meta-analysis (22) found only a weak association with schizophrenia that was not significant after multiple testing. The DTNBP1 gene is located in a region that has also received genome-wide significant linkage support in bipolar disorder, and DTNBP1 has been associated with both disorders (23, 24).

Disrupted-in-Schizophrenia 1 (DISC1)
The disrupted-in-schizophrenia 1 (DISC1) gene was initially identified at the breakpoint of a balanced translocation (1, 11) (q42.1; q14.3), which segregated with major mental illness (schizophrenia, schizoaffective disorder, bipolar affective disorder, unipolar affective disorder, and adolescent conduct disorder) in a large Scottish family (25). A number of key central nervous system proteins, thought to be highly relevant to the development of mental illness, have also been identified as interacting partners (for review see 26), and several DISC1 interactors have been defined as independent genetic susceptibility factors for major mental illness. DISC1 is plausible functionally and structurally, as it is expressed in neurones and has a role in brain development, neuronal migration, and differentiation (27), thus supporting the neurodevelopmental hypothesis of schizophrenia. DISC1 has been associated with schizophrenia, schizoaffective disorder, bipolar disorder, and depression (28, 29, 30).

Catechol-O-Methyl Transferase (COMT)
COMT is located on chromosome 22q and maps to the velocardiofacial syndrome (VCFS) microdeletion region. Patients suffering from VCFS have a high risk of developing schizophrenia, thus making COMT a positional candidate gene (31). In addition, COMT is a catabolic enzyme involved in the degradation of dopamine, especially in the frontal cortex. A widely studied valine-to-methionine (Val/Met) polymorphism results, respectively, in high- and low-activity forms of the enzymes (32). However, an association of COMT with schizophrenia (33) could not be replicated (34, 35).

D-amino acid oxidase activator (DAOA)
Chumakov et al. (36) examined markers in the 13q14–q32 linkage region, identifying two genes, G72 (now called D-amino acid oxidase activator, DAOA) and G30. DAOA functionally interacts with D-amino acid oxidase (DAO), affecting serum D-serine levels. Many subsequent studies have attempted to replicate the association, but the results have been mixed. A recent meta-analysis (37) found weak evidence of association between the G72/G30 genes and schizophrenia.

Dopminergic genes
Dopamine dysfunction is well recognized in schizophrenia and the theory of elevated dopamine neurotransmission has led to investigation of dopaminergic genes (e.g., dopamine D2 and dopamine D3 receptors) as functional candidates. However, there is still insufficient evidence to suggest a link between functional dopaminergic genes and schizophrenia (38).

GENOME-WIDE ASSOCIATION

Genome-wide association studies (GWAS) using large samples (sample sizes usually exceed 1,000 cases and 1,000 controls) have recently become possible, and these studies routinely genotype each individual for 400,000–900,000 genetic markers. The first adequately designed and powered GWAS, from the WTCCC study (16), investigated 14,000 patients and 3,000 shared population controls and 7 diseases, including bipolar disorder (2,000 cases).

The first large case-controlled genome-wide association studies in schizophrenia have been published recently (39, 40, 41), and GWAS data for approximately 12,000 subjects with schizophrenia and approximately 14,000 controls will shortly be available for meta-analysis. Nearly all investigators performing GWAS of schizophrenia have agreed to participate in the Psychiatric GWAS Consortium (http://pgc.unc.edu), which will conduct high-quality meta-analyses of schizophrenia, attention-deficit hyperactivity disorder, autism, bipolar disorder, and major depressive disorder (42). This type of collaborative work is likely to form the basis of future research in schizophrenia genetics.

GENETIC RELATIONSHIP BETWEEN SCHIZOPHRENIA AND AFFECTIVE DISORDERS

Traditionally, psychiatric genetic research has proceeded under the assumption that schizophrenia and bipolar disorder are separate disease entities with separate underlying etiologies (the "Kraepelinian dichotomy"). However, the clinical reality is that many individuals have features that fall between these two entities and have both prominent mood and psychotic features, thus raising the possibility that there is not a neat biological distinction between schizophrenia and bipolar disorder. Indeed, there is evidence of the genetic relationship between schizophrenia and affective disorders, mainly bipolar disorder. Results from family studies show that there are families with multiple cases of schizophrenia, bipolar disorder, and cases with psychosis and mood disorder. Relatives of schizophrenic patients have an increased rate of bipolar disorder; schizoaffective disorder occurs at increased rate in families of both schizophrenia and bipolar disorder; and both schizophrenia and bipolar disorder occur at increased rate in families with schizoaffective disorder. Other studies reported a link of both schizophrenia and bipolar disorder to unipolar depression (43, 44). An analysis of the Maudsley twin series (45) demonstrated that the overlap of familial vulnerabilities is due to genetic factors shared between schizophrenia and mania. Linkage and association studies subsequently revealed that a substantial proportion of schizophrenia susceptibility genes are apparently also involved in the etiology of bipolar disorder (e.g., DISC1, NRG1, DTNBP1, DAOA, COMT).

COPY NUMBER VARIATIONS (CNVs)

CNVs are segments of DNA, for which copy-number differences (e.g., duplications or insertions, deletions) have been revealed by comparison of two or more genomes. There is accumulating evidence that multiple rare de novo (and some inherited) CNVs contribute to the genetic component of vulnerability to schizophrenia (46). For example, the 22q11.2 deletion syndrome (VCFS) is associated with a 3-Mb microdeletion, and approximately 25% of patients have psychiatric manifestations, including schizophrenia, attention-deficit hyperactivity disorder (ADHD), or autism spectrum disorders. A large genome-wide survey of rare CNVs (47) found deletions within the region critical for VCFS as expected and further identified large deletions on chromosomes 1q21.1 and 15q13.3. Another study found significant association of schizophrenia and related psychoses with three deletions (including 1q21.1 and 15q13.3) in two samples (48). These first results provide strong support that effects of multiple rare structural variants contribute to schizophrenia pathogenesis.

EPIGENETICS
Epigenetics refers to the regulation of various genomic functions, including gene expression, which are not based on DNA sequence but rather controlled by heritable and potentially reversible chemical modifications of DNA and/or the chromatin structure (e.g., DNA methylation, chromatin modification)(49). DNA methylation is a relatively stable epigenetic mark; that is, DNA methylation patterns are transmitted from maternal chromatids to daughter chromatids during mitosis (epigenetic inheritance system). However, the degree of mitotic fidelity of epigenetic patterns is approximately three orders of magnitudes lower in comparison to DNA sequences (epigenetic metastability), thus significant epigenetic differences may accumulate over time across the cells. Although it was generally believed that epigenetic patterns are erased in the early stages of germline cell development, there is increasing evidence that some epigenetic modifications can also be transmitted transgenerationally via germline cells (50).

EPIGENETICS AND SCHIZOPHRENIA
Traditionally, it has been thought that schizophrenia results from the interaction of predisposing genes and hazardous environmental factors; however, partial epigenetic stability (metastability) of gene regulation is consistent with various nonmendelian irregularities of schizophrenia (e.g., clinically indistinguishable sporadic and familial cases, discordance of monozygotic twins, late disease onset, fluctuating course of psychotic symptoms, sexual dimorphism, parental origin effect, and coincidence with major hormonal changes in the organism) (51). Although there have been speculations about the role of epigenetic phenomena in schizophrenia since the early 1990 (52), it is only more recently that techniques have become available to put such notions to the test. A recent study found a number of loci to be epigenetically altered in the brain of schizophrenia and bipolar disorder patients relative to unaffected controls (53). It is of particular interest that environmental factors in schizophrenia may induce epigenetic changes resulting from promoter DNA methylation affecting gene expression in neural systems relevant for the disease (54). Such changes may be especially problematic in individuals with genetic susceptibility to the disease.

EPIGENETIC THEORY OF SCHIZOPHRENIA VERSUS HAZARDOUS ENVIRONMENT
Phenotypic discordance in MZ twin pairs (see above) has traditionally been interpreted as evidence of the role of hazardous environment; however, thus far no specific exogenous factor that would unequivocally increase the risk for schizophrenia has been identified (51). Besides, if a child born to an affected parent is raised in a healthy family, the disease risk does not decrease, and similar rates for schizophrenia have been found among the offspring of MZ cotwins who were discordant for the disease (2). It has been hypothesized that MZ twins might exhibit many random epigenetic differences, and possibly only one of the cotwins might reach the critical mass

of epigenetic misregulation resulting in some specific phenotype (55, 56), for example, schizophrenia. Thus, the epigenetic model of schizophrenia can be thought of as a result of a chain of deviant epigenetic events, beginning with an epigenetic change during gametogenesis or embryogenesis that increases the risk for schizophrenia, but is not sufficient to cause the disease. The degree of epigenetic misregulation is further increased or decreased by external environmental factors, stochastic events, and hormones, and only a fraction of the predisposed individuals may reach the threshold resulting in clinical symptoms of disease (50).

SUMMARY

The results from family, twin, and adoption studies suggest that schizophrenia is familial and that genetic effects are the predominant model of its familiarity. Until recently, candidate gene association studies and genome-wide linkage studies were performed to localize genetic variation for schizophrenia. Genome-wide association studies (GWAS) now allow hypothesis-free systematic screens of the whole genome and thus supersede the need for the selection of arbitrary candidate genes, which was often based on uncertain theories about the aetiology of the disorder.

REFERENCES

1. Kraepelin E. Psychiatrie, 6th edn. Barth, Leipzig, 1899.
2. Gottesman II. Schizophrenia Genesis: The Origins of Madness. New York: Freeman, 1991.
3. Lichtenstein P, Björk C, Hultman CM. Recurrence risks for schizophrenia in a Swedish national cohort. Psychol Med 2006; 36: 1417–25.
4. Cardno AG, Gottesman II. Twin studies of schizophrenia: from bow-and-arrow concordances to Star Wars MX and functional genomics. Am J Med Genet 2000; 97: 12–17.
5. Sullivan PF, Kendler KS, Neale MC. Schizophrenia as a complex trait: evidence from a meta-analysis of twin studies. Arch Gen Psychiatry 2003; 60(12): 1187–92.
6. Heston LL, Denney D. Interactions between early life experience and biological factors in schizophrenia. In D. Rosenthal & S. Kety, eds. The Transmission of Schizophrenia. Oxford, UK: Pergamon Press, 1968: 363–76.
7. Rosenthal D, Wender PH, Kety SS et al. The adopted-away offspring of schizophrenics. Am J Psychiatry 1971; 128: 307–11.
8. Kety SS, Rosenthal D, Wender PH et al. Mental illness in the biological and adoptive families of adopted individuals who have become schizophrenic: a preliminary report based on psychiatric interviews. Proc Annu Meet Am Psychopathol Assoc 1975; vol: 147–65.
9. Tienari P, Wynne LC, Sorri A et al. Genotype-environment interaction in schizophrenia-spectrum disorder. Long-term follow-up study of Finnish adoptees. Br J Psychiatry 2004; 184: 216–22.
10. McGuffin P, Sturt E. Genetic markers in schizophrenia. Hum Hered 1986; 36(2): 65.
11. Sherrington R, Brynjolfsson J, Petursson H et al. Localization of a susceptibility locus for schizophrenia on chromosome 5. Nature 1988; 336: 164–7.
12. McGuffin P, Sargeant M, Hetti G et al. Exclusion of a schizophrenia susceptibility gene from the chromosome 5q11–q13 region: new data and a reanalysis of previous reports. Am J Hum Genet 1990; 47(3): 524–35.
13. Badner JA, Gershon ES. Meta-analysis of whole-genome linkage scans of bipolar disorder and schizophrenia. Mol Psychiatry 2002; 7: 405–11.
14. Lewis CM, Levinson DF, Wise LH et al. Genome scan meta-analysis of schizophrenia and bipolar disorder, part II: schizophrenia. Am J Hum Genet 2003; 73: 34–48.
15. Berrettini WH. Susceptibility loci for bipolar disorder: overlap with inherited vulnerability to schizophrenia. Biol Psychiatry 2000; 47: 245–51.

16. The Wellcome Trust Case Control Consortium. Genome-wide association study of 14,000 cases of seven common diseases and 3,000 shared controls. Nature 2007; 447: 661–78.
17. Stefansson H, Sigurdsson E, Steinthorsdottir V et al. Neuregulin 1 and susceptibility to schizophrenia. Am J Hum Genet 2002; 71: 877–92.
18. Dawei L, Collier DA, He L. Meta-analysis shows strong positive association of the neuregulin 1 (NRG1) gene with schizophrenia. Hum Mol Genet 2006; 15(12): 1995–2002.
19. Harrison PJ, Law AJ. Neuregulin 1 and schizophrenia: genetics, gene expression, and neurobiology. Biol Psychiatry 2006; 60(2): 132–40.
20. Serretti A, Mandelli L. The genetics of bipolar disorder: genome 'hot regions', genes, new potential candidates and future directions. Mol Psychiatry 2008; 13(8): 742–71.
21. Straub RE, Jiang Y, MacLean CJ et al. Genetic variation in the 6p22.3 gene DTNBP1, the human ortholog of the mouse dysbindin gene, is associated with schizophrenia. Am J Hum Genet 2002; 71(2): 337–48.
22. Li D, He L. Association study between the dystrobrevin binding protein 1 gene (DTNBP1) and schizophrenia: a meta-analysis. Schizophr Res 2007a; 96: 112–8.
23. Fallin MD, Lasseter VK, Avramopoulos D et al. Bipolar I disorder and schizophrenia: a 440-single-nucleotide polymporphism screen of 64 candidate genes among Ashkenazi Jewish case-parent trios. Am J Hum Genet 2005; 77(6): 918–36.
24. Gaysina D, Cohen-Woods S, Chow PC et al. Association of the dystrobrevin binding protein 1 gene (DTNBP1) in a bipolar case-control study (BACCS). Am J Med Genet B Neuropsychiatr Genet 2008, in press.
25. Millar JK, Wilson-Annan JC, Anderson S et al. Disruption of two novel genes by a translocation co-segregating with schizophrenia. Hum Mol Genet 2000; 9(9): 1415–23.
26. Chubb JE, Bradshaw NJ, Soares DC et al. The DISC locus in psychiatric illness. Mol Psychiatry 2008; 13: 36–64.
27. Matsuzaki S, Tohyama M. Molecular mechanism of schizophrenia with reference to disrupted-in-schizophrenia 1 (DISC1). Neurochem Int 2007; 51: 165–72.
28. Hodgkinson CA, Goldman D, Jaeger J et al. Disrupted in schizophrenia 1 (DISC1): association with schizophrenia, schizoaffective disorder, and bipolar disorder. Am J Hum Genet 2004; 75(5): 862–72.
29. Schosser A, Gaysina D, Cohen-Woods S et al. Association of DISC1 and TSNAX genes and affective disorders in the Depression Case-Control (DeCC) and Bipolar Affective Case-Control (BACC) studies. Mol Psychiatry 2009, in press.
30. Hashimoto R, Numakawa T, Ohnishi T et al. Impact of the DISC1 Ser704Cys polymorphism on risk for major depression, brain morpology and ERK signaling. Hum Mol Genet 2006; 15(20): 3024–33.
31. Gothelf D, Feinstein C, Thompson T et al. Risk factors for the emergence of psychotic disorders in adolescents with 22q11.2 deletion syndrome. Am J Psychiatry 2007; 164: 663–9.
32. Williams HJ, Owen MJ, O'Donovan MC. Is COMT a susceptibility gene for schizophrenia? Schizophr Bull 2007; 33: 635–41.
33. Egan MF, Goldberg TE, Kolachana BS et al. Effect of COMT Val108/158 Met genotype on frontal lobe function and risk for schizophrenia. Proc Natl Acad Sci USA 2001; 98(12): 6917–22.
34. Sanders AR, Duan J, Levinson DF et al. No significant association of 14 candidate genes with schizophrenia in a large European ancestry sample: implications for psychiatric genetics. Am J Psychiatry 2008; 165: 497–506.
35. Munafo MR, Bowes L, Clark TG et al. Lack of association of the COMT (Val158/108Met) gene and schizophrenia: a meta-analysis of case-control studies. Mol Psychiatry 2005; 10: 765–70.
36. Chumakov I, Blumenfeld M, Guerassimenko O et al. Genetic and physiological data implicating the new human gene G72 and the gene for D-amino acid oxidase in schizophrenia. Proc Natl Acad Sci USA 2002; 99: 13675–80.

37. Li D, He L. G72/G30 genes and schizophrenia: a systematic meta-analysis of association studies. Genetics 2007b; 175(2): 917–22.

38. Talkowski ME, Bamne M, Mansour H et al. Dopamine genes and schizophrenia: case closed or evidence pending? Schizophr Bull 2007; 33: 1071–81.

39. Lencz T, Morgan TV, Athanasiou M et al. Converging evidence for a pseudoautosomal cytokine receptor gene locus in schizophrenia. Mol Psychiatry 2007; 12: 572–80.

40. Shifman S, Johannesson M, Bronstein M et al. Genome-wide association identifies a common variant in the reelin gene that increases the risk of schizophrenia only in women. PLOS Genetics 2008; 4: e28.

41. Sullivan PF, Lin D, Tzeng JY et al. Genomewide association for schizophrenia in the CATIE study: results of stage 1. Mol Psychiatry 2008a; 13: 570–84.

42. Sullivan PF. Schizophrenia genetics: the search for a hard lead. Curr Opin Psychiatry 2008b; 21: 157–60.

43. Craddock N, O'Donovan MC, Owen MJ. The genetics of schizophrenia and bipolar disorder: dissecting psychosis. J Med Genet 2005; 42: 193–204.

44. Maier W, Höfgen B, Zobel A et al. Genetic models of schizophrenia and bipolar disorder: overlapping inheritance or discrete gentotypes? Eur Arch Psychiatry Clin Neurosci 2005; 255(3): 159–66.

45. Cardno AG, Rijsdijk FV, Sham PC et al. A twin study of genetic relationships between psychotic symptoms. Am J Psychiatry 2002; 159: 539–45.

46. Cook EH, Scherer W. Copy-number variations associated with neuropsychiatric conditions. Nature 2008; 455: 919–23.

47. The International Schizophrenia Consortium. Rare chromosomal deletions and duplications increase risk of schizophrenia. Nature 2008; 455: 237–41.

48. Stefansson H, Rujescu D, Cichon S et al. Large recurrent microdeletions associated with schizophrenia. Nature 2008; 455: 232–6.

49. Henikoff S, Matzke MA. Exploring and explaining epigenetic effects. Trends Genet 1997; 13: 293–5.

50. Oh G, Petronis A. Environmental studies of schizophrenia through the prism of epigenetics. Schizphr Bull 2008; 34: 1122–9.

51. Petronis A. The origin of schizophrenia: genetic thesis, epigenetic antithesis, and resolving synthesis. Biol Psychiatry 2004; 55: 965–70.

52. McGuffin P, Asherson P, Owen M et al. The strength of the genetic effect. Is there room for an environmental influence in the aetiology of schizophrenia? Br J Psychiatry 1994; 164: 593–9.

53. Mill J, Tang T, Kaminsky Z et al. Epigenomic profiling reveals DNA-methylation changes associated with major psychosis. Am J Hum Genet 2008; 82(3): 696–711.

54. European Network of Schizophrenia Networks for the Study of Gene-Environment Interaction. Schizophrenia aetiology: do gene-environment interactions hold the key? Schizophr Res 2008; 102: 21–6.

55. Weksberg R, Shuman C, Caluseriu O et al. Discordant KCNQ10T1 imprinting in sets of monozygotic twins discordant for Beckwith-Wiedemann syndrome. Hum Mol Genet 2002; 11: 1317–25.

56. Petronis A, Gottesman II, Kan PX et al. Monozygotic twins exhibit numerous epigenetic differences: clues to twin discordance? Schizophr Bull 2003; 29: 169–78.

9 Brain abnormalities in schizophrenia

Bernhard Bogerts, Johann Steiner, and Hans-Gert Bernstein

INTRODUCTION

The search for structural changes in the brains of schizophrenics initially began about 100 years ago when Emil Kraepelin told two of his assistants, Alois Alzheimer and Franz Nissl, to look for the neuropathology of "dementia precox." Both of them, and, some decades later, Vogt and colleagues described various cytopathological changes in neocortical and thalamic regions of schizophrenics, which later were discussed controversially. At the first international conference of neuropathology 1952 in Rome, the opinion prevailed that no structural changes exist in brains of schizophrenics; in the same year, the first neuroleptics were introduced and the focus of interest shifted to neurochemical and psychodynamic theories (1). However, several early pneumencephalographic studies already gave evidence for ventricular and cortical sulcal enlargement especially in chronic patients (2) that later were fully confirmed by CT and MRI studies. Several meta-analytical reviews on structural imaging findings in schizophrenia (see chapter on neuroimaging) give convincing evidence that there is a subtle statistical decrease of whole brain volume (by about 3%), enlargement of the lateral ventricles by about 30%, and of cortical sulci as well as bilateral reduction of temporal lobes (by ca. 6%) and hippocampus (by 10%). Such changes can be recognized by clinical routine assessment of CT or MRI scans in about one third of the patients. The majority of brains appear to be structurally normal, and the changes, if present, vary from patient to patient. This argues for considerable inhomogenity of brain abnormalities in schizophrenia.

The major problem in looking for brain abnormalities in schizophrenia is the considerable heterogeneity not only in the structural findings but also in the clinical symptoms and course of the disease. This is not surprising, since the term "schizophrenia" remains until today an diagnostic construct that was defined decades ago by leading authorities in the field (Kraepelin, Schneider, Bleuler) and is now defined by committees setting up operationalized criteria for the clinical diagnosis. Thus, it becomes more and more likely that schizophrenia comprises a quite inhomogeneous group of different neuropathologies and pathophysiologies resulting in similar clinical symptoms (comparable, for example, to "dementia," "fever," or "rheumatism"). This might explain the enormous variance of all neurobiological finding in schizophrenic patients that is also characteristic for neuropathological studies, that are summarized in this chapter.

Despite the enormous advances that have been achieved by the introduction of structural and functional imaging methods to clarify the neurobiology of schizophrenia, only postmortem investigations applying modern microscopic, biochemical, and molecular biological techniques may help to clarify the cellular basis of schizophrenia, and the cellular and molecular pathologic mechanisms behind these disturbances. During the past two decades, a plethora of studies has been published pointing not only to alterations in mean volumes, neuron and glial cell densities in different brain areas in schizophrenia, but also to characteristic changes in neurotransmitter/receptor systems, growth factors, hormones, regulatory proteins, and brain energy metabolism.

Though one can hardly find a brain area that has not been suspected of being involved in the neuropathology of schizophrenia, recent research has mainly concentrated on a few regions that appear to be most affected. Robust evidence from several, replicated studies shows that the limbic system (especially the medial temporal lobe including the hippocampal formation, parahippocampal gyrus, entorhinal cortex, and amygdala), the heteromodal association cortex (prefrontal, cingulate, parietal, and temporal cortex) and the thalamus show the most prominent structural alterations in schizophrenia. Besides, the caudate nucleus, the nucleus accumbens, the cerebellum, the hypothalamus, the septal area, and certain brain stem nuclei show subtle structural changes.

LIMBIC SYSTEM
More than 30 years ago, Stevens (3) and Torrey and Peterson (4) had postulated that schizophrenia may be linked to dysfunction of limbic structures. Subsequent microscopic inspection of brains of schizophrenics revealed that major temporo-limbic structures—hippocampal formation, parahippocampal gyrus, and amygdala, as well as the internal pallidum—are significantly smaller in schizophrenia (5–7). This key observation has been confirmed in many, but not all, subsequent studies (for review, see Woodruff et al. (8); Harrison (9); Chance et al. (10)). Further MRI and postmortem work reported reduced gray matter volumes of the cingulate cortex in schizophrenia (reviewed by Heckers (11); Wang et al. (12)), while conflicting data exist on other limbic structures with regard to altered volumes: entorhinal cortex (13, 14), amygdala (5, 15–17), and mammillary bodies (18). The size of some smaller limbic structures such as the septal region (19) and the habenula (20) appears to be normal.

HIPPOCAMPUS
Cytoarchitectural changes in the hippocampal formation have been prominent among the various neuropathological abnormalities reported in schizophrenia. Numerous studies report a reduction of neuronal size, neuronal density and/or a disorganization of hippocampal or parahippocampal neurons in schizophrenia, with the most pronounced changes being found in left hippocampal subfields CA4 and the subiculum (9, 21). In addition, reduced adult hippocampal neurogenesis seems to be a characteristic feature of schizophrenia (22). These findings, in the absence of neurodegenerative changes, as indicated by the lack of gliosis and other typical signs of brain atrophy, suggest that there may be alterations in the neural connections (i.e., axons, dendrites, and synapses) in schizophrenia. These may represent the anatomical correlate of the aberrant functional connectivity described in neuroimaging studies (summarized by Burns et al. (23); Harrison (9); Talamini et al. (24)). There is converging evidence that a fundamental pathology of schizophrenia involves dysfunction of synaptic transmission and neural connectivity, including synaptic and dendritic markers (25). Among the synaptic marker proteins shown to be altered in the hippocampus of schizophrenics are synaptophysin, complexin-II, and the neuregulin-1 receptor ErbB4 (25, 26). Although the identity of the affected hippocampal circuits remains unclear, there is evidence for glutamatergic, GABAergic, cholinergic, and dopaminergic involvement (25, 27–29). Analysis of micro (mi)RNA expression in postmortem temporolimbic areas revealed significant upregulation of miRNA 181b expression in schizophrenia (30). This is a significant finding, as this particular miRNA controls the expression of, among other proteins, AMPA receptors and the calcium sensor protein VILIP-1,

which both of which have been found to be dysregulated in hippocampi of schizophrenics (31). It had been suggested that hippocampal pathology in schizophrenia is likely to be associated with the positive symptoms of the disease (32). However, more recent data support the idea that structural hippocampal involvement may be more connected with neuropsychological impairments (9, 24). Recent findings suggest that hippocampal volume changes in schizophrenia might be under partial control of the neuregulin-1 gene (33).

AMYGDALA
Due to the pivotal role of the amygdala in neuropsychiatric disorders, much effort has been made to reveal structural changes of this limbic region in schizophrenia. The results are controversial, however. Several clinical neuroimaging and postmortem studies found significant reductions in the mean volume of the amygdala in schizophrenic patients compared with controls (5, 15–17). In contrast, Heckers et al. (34) and Chance et al. (10) did not observe volume reductions of the amygdala in postmortem brains of patients with schizophrenia. Reductions of the neuronal density of individual amygdaloid nuclei were reported by Berretta et al. (35) and Kreczmanski et al. (17).

ENTORHINAL CORTEX
Prominent alterations in cell architecture have been found in another important limbic structure, the entorhinal cortex. An influential paper of Jakob and Beckmann (36) reported cytoarchitectonic abnormalities in the rostral part of the region as well as displacement of special nerve cell groups (heterotopic pre-α cell clusters). Because these findings were interpreted as a sign of disturbance of neuronal migration during cortical development (thereby giving considerable impetus to the neurodevelopmental hypothesis of schizophrenia), much work has been invested since then to learn more about entorhinal neuronal disarray in schizophrenia. Findings supporting (37–39) and questioning (13, 40, 41) the value of the original data have been published thereafter.

CINGULATE CORTEX
Early work from Braitenberg et al. (42) and Benes and Bird (43) demonstrated histological changes in the anterior cingulate cortex (reviewed in Heckers (11)). These findings that have later on been confirmed and considerably extended, comprise: decrease in laminar thickness (44), significantly reduced density of nonpyramidal neurons and/or deficit in GABAergic interneurons (45–48), reduced somal size of neurons (49, 50), increased number of parvalbumin-expressing interneurons in cortical layers V and VI (51), reduced synaptic density (52), overall glial cell loss but increase of S100B immunolabeled glial cells in paranoid schizophrenics (53, 54), and changes in the expression of myelin-related gene transcripts (55). Others could not confirm alterations in neuronal density and/or somal size in schizophrenia (56). Interestingly, no changes in the density of calbindin-expressing interneurons were found in the posterior cingulate cortex of schizophrenics (57).

With regard to some smaller limbic structures, it can be stated that they are affected differently by schizophrenia: No cell alterations were reported for the septum (19) and the habenula (20), whereas a considerable reduction was observed in the mammillary bodies, which was mainly attributable to fewer parvalbumin-containing neurons projecting to the anterior thalamus (18). Table 9.1.

TABLE 9.1

Neuropathological findings in schizophrenia

A) *Limbic structures*
   Hippocampus
   • reduced volumes (1, 5, 7, 9, 16)
   • smaller neurons (9, 21)
   • alterations in synaptic and dendritic markers (25, 26, 31)
   • changes in glutamate, GABA and neuregulin receptors (26–28, 13)
   Amygdala
   • Smaller or unchanged volumes (16, 17, 10, 34)
   • decreased neuronal density (17, 35)
   Entorhinal cortex, parahippocampal gyrus
   • reduced volume (7, 9)
   • cellular disarray (36-39) or unchanged architecture (13, 40, 41)
   Cingulate cortex
   • decreased neuronal density (11, 42, 43)
   • reduced size of neurons (49,50)
   • deficit in GABAergic interneurons (45–48)
   • increase in parvalbumin-expressing interneurons in deeper layers (51)

B) *Cortical areas*
   Dorsolateral prefrontal cortex
   • elevation of neuronal density, reduction of "neuropil" (68, 69)
   • left-right anomalies in cell densities (70)
   • loss of parvalbumin-expressing interneurons (61, 62)
   • reduced GAD expression (63–65)
   • altered neuronal expression of neuregulin-1 isoforms (26, 72, 73)

C) *Thalamus*
   • reduced volume or no change of the mediodorsal (MD) nucleus (84, 85, 89–91)
   • reduced or unchanged density of MD neurons (86–88, 89–91)
   • reduced volume and cell density of the pulvinar (88, 94, 95)
   • reduced volume of the posterior nucleus (96)
   • loss of parvalbumin-expressing neurons in the anteroventral nucleus (91)

D) *Basal ganglia*
   • smaller globus pallidus internus in catatonic patients (7, 17, 106)
   • volume increases in both the striatum and globus pallidus in neuroleptic treated patients (34, 107).
   • loss of nitrergic and cholinergic interneurons (110, 111)

DORSOLATERAL PREFRONTAL CORTEX

The dorsolateral prefrontal cortex (DLPF) is regarded to play a major role the pathophysiology of schizophrenia. Hence, much attention has been paid to structural changes in this brain area. Decreased gray matter volumes have been reported by structural imaging and postmortem studies (8, 58–60). While consensus exists as to reduced gray matter volumes, inconsistent findings have been published about possible cellular pathology. After morphometric analyses of prefrontal neurons in schizophrenia, Reynold et al. (61) and Cotter et al. (62) revealed a selective loss of parvalbumin-immunoreactive GABAergic interneurons. It is not yet completely clear whether these interneurons are really lost or whether there is a disease-related reduction of the GABA synthesizing enzyme, GAD, in surviving neurons (63-65). No changes in the number of calcium-binding proteins were observed by Tooney and Stahl (66), whereas the neuronal expression of certain calcium-sensor proteins was altered (67). A significant elevation in the neuronal density of layers II, III, IV, and VI neurons was observed in Brodman area 9 by Selemon et al. (68, 69), while cytoarchitectonic abnormalities were absent in another part of the DLPF, the Brodman area 44 (68). Since increased densities could be explained by a shrinkage of cortical thickness without a loss of neurons, the "reduced neuropil hypothesis" was created, meaning that the connecting elements between neurons are affected. Anomalies of asymmetry of pyramidal cell density between the left and right hemispheres, but no change in neuronal shape or density was described by Cullen et al. (70). Recently, an increase in neuregulin-1 expression in the DLPF has been reported in schizophrenia (71). Interestingly, neuregulin-1β immunoreactive DLPF neurons were found to be increased (72), whereas another neuregulin isoform, neuregulin-1α, was found to be decreased in DLPF neurons (73). This is of interest, as polymorphisms of the neuregulin-1 gene have repeatedly been shown to be linked with schizophrenia (for review, see Harrison and Law (26)). However, the upregulation of neuregulin-1β isoforms, which may be linked with disease-related NMDA hypofunction (74), might be, in part, the result of long-term treatment of the patients with neuroleptics.

Concerning non-neuronal cells, a subtle astroglial pathology has been reported by Rajkowska et al. (2002), but questioned by others (75).

In schizophrenic brains, characteristic changes have also been observed in interstitial white matter neurons positioned below DLPF gray matter: increased density (76–78), and reduced reelin (78) and neuregulin-1α (73) expression. These alterations may be taken as morphological evidence of an early developmental component to schizophrenia (78). Recently, a prominent deficit of gray matter (perineuronal) oligodendrocytes was found in the prefrontal cortex of schizophrenia, which might have an influence on the reduced somal size of neurons (79). White matter oligodendroglial cells in the frontal lobe have been reported to be reduced in density by several groups (for recent considerations on the functional relevance, see Segal et al. (80)). Pathology of oligodendroglial cells may underlie deficit myelination of axons and thus may contribute to intracerebral misconnectivity in schizophrenics.

THALAMUS

The thalamus is a complex brain structure, which is composed of numerous nuclei with different functions, and is a key information processing center in facilitating sensory discrimination and cognitive processes, which are obviously disturbed in schizophrenia. There is growing evidence showing structural and functional thalamic abnormalities in this disease. Contradictory data exist for a smaller total volume of the thalamus and an altered shape of this brain region (for recent review, see Harms et al. (81)). An initial report on thalamic structural pathology showed reduced thickness of the periventricular gray matter in postmortem brains of schizophrenics (82). Subsequent morphologic work has mainly concentrated on the mediodorsal (MD) thalamic nucleus, a brain structure that is linked to other brain areas known to show alterations in schizophrenia: the prefrontal, medial temporal cortex, and basal forebrain (83). Remarkable reductions in volume and total cell number of MD nucleus have been observed by Pakkenberg and Gundersen (84, 85). The presence of smaller and fewer neurons in the MD nucleus has been confirmed by others (86–88), while Cullen et al. (89), Dorph-Petersen et al. (90), and Danos et al. (91) failed to replicate these findings. Other thalamic nuclei with reported structural deficits in schizophrenia involve the anteroventral nucleus (92, 93), pulvinar (88, 94, 95), and ventral lateral posterior nucleus (96), whereas no changes have been seen in the posterior medial nucleus (86) and some limbic thalamic nuclei (97). The absence of the adhesion interthalamica has been regarded as a structural marker of developmental neuropathology in schizophrenia (98). Taking into account the key role of thalamic nuclei in information processing and pronounced structural abnormalities of the thalamus in schizophrenia, Andreasen presented the hypothesis that a defect in circuitry connecting thalamus, frontal cortex, and cerebellum may be central to patients with schizophrenia (termed "cognitive dysmetria") (99). With regard to thalamic neurotransmission, it has been shown that markers for glutamatergic (92, 100, 101) and dopaminergic (102) mechanisms may be altered in schizophrenia, while GABAergic interneurons appear unaffected (103). Finally, DISC-1, a gene linked to schizophrenia, was found to be abnormally expressed in thalamic neurons of schizophrenics (104).

BASAL GANGLIA
The basal ganglia consist of the caudate nucleus, putamen, neostriatum, and accumbens nucleus. This complex brain structure came into the focus of schizophrenia research, as they are involved in sensory, motor, and cognitive processes known to be disturbed in schizophrenia, and as they play important roles in the dopamine hypothesis of schizophrenia (105). Initial postmortem studies of basal ganglia did not show abnormalities, except for a smaller globus pallidus internum in catatonic patients (7, 106). However, subsequent postmortem investigations demonstrated volume increases in both the striatum and globus pallidus (34, 107). Because MRI studies with drug-naïve schizophrenics found basal ganglia to be normal, the suggestion was made that the hypertrophic effect, which manifests itself in volume increases, might be the result of long-term medication (for review, see Lang et al. (108)). This assumption found support by antipsychotic treatment experiments with animals (109). However, there are also reports of slightly reduced basal ganglia volumes in schizophrenia (for overview, see Kreczmanski et al. (17)). Reported basal ganglia cell loss and/or malformation mainly points to nitric oxide synthase immunoreactive and cholininergic interneurons (110, 111).

HYPOTHALAMUS
Endocrine and neuroendocrine abnormalities in schizophrenia have been extensively described (reviewed by Brown (112)). Hence, structural abnormalities of hypothalamic nuclei may exist in schizophrenia. Recent neuroimaging studies yielded conflicting results in that both increased (113) and decreased (114) hypothalamic volumes have been measured in schizophrenics. At the cellular level, changes have been described in the number of neurophysin-containing (115), nitric oxide synthase (NOS) immunoreactive (116), β-endorphin-expressing (29), parvalbumin-immunoreactive (18), and beacon-like-immunoreactive hypothalamic (117) neurons, while the number of vasopressin-expressing supraoptic neurons was unchanged in schizophrenia (118).

CEREBELLUM
Due to the suggested involvement of the cerebellum in disturbed cortico-thalamo-cerebellar circuits in schizophrenia (99), increasing emphasis is given to disease-related structural changes of this brain region. Several postmortem investigations have shown that there is cerebellar atrophy in schizophrenia, whereby the vermis is most affected

TABLE 9.2

Pathology of glia cells

- deficit in olgodendrocytes (80, 81)
- microglia activation (?) (166-172)
- no increased glia cell densities, no gliosis (1, 62)
- loss of astroglia cells (?) (75, 76)

TABLE 9.3

Neuroanatomical indicators of a neurodevelopmental disorder

- abnormal or unchanged cytoarchitecture in hippocampus, entorhinal and frontal cortex (36–41)
- absence of gliosis (129)
- reduced structural cerebral asymmetry (130, 131)
- absence of interthalamic adhesion (98)
- altered cortical gyral patterns (131)

TABLE 9.4

Support for the neuroinflammatory/autoimmune hypothesis of schizophrenia

- similarity of long-term course with autoimmune diseases (e.g. rheumatoid arthritis, psoriasis, multiple sclerosis)
- association with specific haplotypes of the human leucocyte antigen HLA (135)
- increased prevalence of antibodies for cytomegalovirus, herpes and toxoplasma gondii (136–139)
- higher rates of influenza infection during pregnancy (138–140)
- increased autoantibody production against cerebral muscarinic receptors (152, 153)
- association of polymorphisms for IL-1ß and IL-1RA with ventricular enlargement (158, 159)

(119–122). Reduced vermal Purkinje cell size but no gliosis were found in cerebellum of schizophrenics (123, 124). Histochemically, a decrease in reelin and GAD67 expression (125) and an increase in NOS (126, 127), CREB, and Elk-1 expressions (128) have been observed. Table 9.2–9.4.

NEURODEVELOPMENTAL OR NEURODEGENERATIVE CHANGES?

The findings of cellular disarray in the entorhinal cortex and hippocampus (36, 37) gave rise to the concept that the brain pathology in schizophrenia has a neuro-developmental origin: meaning that the changes are acquired before birth or very early in life. The first reports of such cytoarchitectural changes later have been questioned (40, 41) and remained a matter of controversy; however, the failure to demonstrate gliosis in postmortem brains of schizophrenics (129) and MRI findings of altered cortical sulcal and gyral patterns, as well as absence or reduction of cerebral asymmetry (130, 131), which is acquired before birth, again supported the view that the disease has an essential neurodevelopmenal component. On the other hand, in a minority of patients, the long-term course of schizophrenia shows a progressive worsening of clinical symptoms, and several more recent follow-up MRI studies showed progressive structural changes in the first years after the onset of the psychosis (for a review, see De Haan L, Bakker JM (132)). Therefore, a primary neurodevelopmental factor predating the beginning of obvious psychotic symptoms may later be accompanied by a secondary atrophic process, or alternatively, some patients might have a predominant neurodevelopmental, while others might have a more progressive brain pathology.

THE IMMUNE HYPOTHESIS OF SCHIZOPHRENIA

Historical indications of a possible significance of neuroinflammatory processes (infectious or autoimmune) in schizophrenia were provided by the positive effects of fever therapy (with attenuated strains of salmonella typhii, plasmodium malariae, or mycobacterium tuberculosis) and a lower incidence of rheumatoid arthritis in schizophrenia (133, 134). The onset of schizophrenia in early adulthood, with progressive as well as benign courses, exacerbations, and remissions, shows similarities to autoimmune disorders (e.g., multiple sclerosis, psoriasis) and may lead to the speculation of similar pathogenetic components. Various autoimmune diseases show a statistically significant correlation with specific haplotypes of human leukocyte antigen (HLA). Such correlations were also found in schizophrenia (135).

The neuroinflammatory hypothesis is further supported by an association of schizophrenia with cytomegalovirus and herpes viruses (136). A recent meta-analysis, which summarized seven studies including only patients with first-episode schizophrenia and 16 studies including patients in all clinical phases, resulted in an increased prevalence of antibodies to toxoplasma gondii in individuals with schizophrenia (136). According to the current state of knowledge, a toxoplasma gondii infection can lead to an activation of astrocytes with increased synthesis of kynurenic acid, a physiological NMDA- and nACh-receptor antagonist (137). In recent years, it is just these two transmitter systems that have increasingly become the focus of scientific investigations on schizophrenia (in addition to the previously favored dopamine hypothesis). Influenza infections during pregnancy are also associated with an increased risk of psychosis in the child (138, 139). This may be caused by persistent changes in GABA-ergic transmission in the offspring (140).

In 1962, Kamp and colleagues reported on morphologically atypical lymphocytes in schizophrenia (141). These cells were characterized by a strong basophilic cytoplasm with vacuoles, a large nucleus-to-cytoplasm ratio, and an often irregularly shaped nucleus with euchromatin structure. Atypical lymphocytes were also termed the P-lymphocyte (142) or the blast-type atypical lymphocyte (BTAL) (143). However, other workgroups were unable to confirm these observations (144–146). Rudolf et al. concluded that positive findings might be explained by performing studies not under blinded conditions, and by artifacts due to venepuncture and staining procedures (146). Interaction of dopamine with D2 and D3 dopamine receptors is known to activate the adhesion of T-cells via β1-integrin, promoting the extravasation of blast-like T cells into the central nervous system (147). This mechanism can be suppressed by neuroleptic drugs (148).

However, T-cell activity or function may not only be altered by neuroleptic drugs, but also by schizophrenia-related pathophysiological mechanisms. Riedel et al. observed a reduced Type-IV delayed skin hypersensitivity reaction after intracutaneous application of antigens (Tetanus, Diphtheria, Streptococcus, Tuberculin, Candida albicans, Trichophyton-mentagrophytes, Proteus-mirabilis) in drug-free schizophrenic patients (149). Furthermore, Craddock et al. showed lower proliferative responses in T cells from both unmedicated and minimally medicated schizophrenia patients, compared to well-matched controls (150). As reviewed by Schuld et al., some *in vitro* lymphocyte stimulation studies revealed a decreased secretion of Type 1 cytokines, such as interferon-γ (IFN-γ) and interleukin-2 (IL-2) (151). These findings were interpreted as indication for a suppression of the Th1 subset of T helper cells with decreased cellular immunity as well as a coexisting dominance of the Th2 system and activation of the humoral immunity in schizophrenia. Publications on an increased autoantibody production, for example, against cholinergic muscarinic receptors in cerebrospinal fluid and serum of individuals with schizophrenia, are pointing to the same direction (152, 153). According to Elenkov et al., this scenario is characteristic of the influence of catecholamines on the immune system, perhaps due to schizophrenia-related changes in neurotransmission or in terms of a nonspecific stress reaction (154). Functional consequences of a Th2 activation in schizophrenia are an inhibition of astro-/microglial indoleamine 2, 3 dioxygenase (IDO) and an activation of astroglial tryptophan 2, 3-dioxygenase (TDO) (155). Both mechanisms contribute to an increased degradation of tryptophan to kynurenic acid, a naturally occurring NMDA receptor antagonist (see above). In a clinical study, the COX-2-inhibitor celecoxib, which seems to rebalance the Th1/Th2 shift, was a successful add-on, especially to cognitive functioning in schizophrenic patients (156). However, the Th2 shift hypothesis is currently under debate, as a recent meta-analysis of 62 studies on cytokine levels in schizophrenia does not support this theoretical construct (157). Autoimmune diseases like rheumatoid arthritis, Type I diabetes and multiple sclerosis do not fit well into the Th1/Th2 paradigm. Recent work indicates that two other T-cell subsets might play a role in these cases, namely, IL-17-producing T cells (Th17) that induce autoimmunity and Foxp3+ regulatory T cells (Treg) that inhibit autoimmune tissue injury (157).

In a genetic association study of several candidate cytokine genes, namely, IL-1β, IL-1 receptor antagonist (IL-1RA), IL-10, and an additionally performed metaanalysis, IL-1β was suggested to play a role in predisposition to schizophrenia in 819 Caucasians but not in the Asian population (158). Polymorphisms of IL-1β and IL-1RA showed an association with a significant enlargement of both ventricles in schizophrenic patients (159). Moreover, polymorphisms of IL-2, IL-4, and a gene locus near the CSF2Rα (colony stimulating factor, cytokine receptor 2 alpha) were identified to be significantly associated with schizophrenia (160, 161).

To date, altered immunological parameters have been investigated mainly in the peripheral blood and cerebrospinal fluid of individuals with schizophrenia. For instance, a comprehensive neuropathological investigation of toxoplasma gondii in the brain tissue of schizophrenic patients is lacking until now. However, some studies investigated the numerical distribution of microglial cells in schizophrenia. Microglia are a type of glial cell that acts as the first and main form of active immune defense in the central nervous system. Several microglial markers have been investigated in the brain tissue of schizophrenic patients, including MHC-II, CD40, CD68, and the peripheral-type benzodiazepine receptor. Some postmortem studies have suggested microglial activation in this context (162, 163), whereas others provided evidence against this notion (164-169).

These findings may indicate a role of inflammatory processes in schizophrenia. However, data have to be carefully interpreted due to interference of stress and the effect of weight gain (adipokines) on immunological parameters. It must be pointed out that, even in studies showing immunological alterations, most of the subjects with schizophrenia showed no clinical evidence of immunologic dysfunction. This suggests that, if immunologic processes do play a role in schizophrenia, this is likely to be the case in only a relatively small subgroup.

SUMMARY AND CONCLUSIONS

The major problem in exploring brain abnormalities in schizophrenia is the considerable variability of clinical symptoms and long-term course of the illness that is paralleled by an enormous heterogeneity of nearly all neurobiological findings in this disease including the neuropathological anomalies summarized in this chapter. This is not surprising since *schizophrenia* is rather a diagnostic construct than a nosological entity. Hence, it is an important future task to look for neurobiological correlates of more narrowly defined psychotic syndromes such as delusions, hallucinations, paranoid ideas, thought disorder, cognitive impairment, or other so-called endophenotypes independent of the respective diagnostic construct. Nevertheless, taking all types of patients presenting with schizophrenia together, there are well-replicated statistical differences on the macroscopic level, which usually have a broad overlap with the normal control range, including subtle volume reductions of frontal, temporal, and parietal cortex, hippocampus and thalamus paralleled by ventricular and cortical sulcal enlargement in many cases. In contrast to most well-known neurological and degenerative brain diseases, the subtle brain tissue loss in schizophrenia is not accompanied by a significant loss of nerve cells or by reactive gliosis. The focus of pathology in brains of schizophrenics are the connecting elements between the nerve cell bodies (synaptic components, axons, dendrites), glial cells, and interneurons. This kind of neuropathology seems be especially pronounced in limbic regions, of which the hippocampus is the best investigated structure, and in neocortical association areas and thalamus. Cellular disarray in limbic and frontal cortex, abnormal gyrification and reduced structural asymmetry are strong arguments for a neurodevelopmental origin of schizophrenia, which might be accompanied by a later occurring progressive pathogenetic factor. It is unclear what causes the additional atrophic changes; there is, however, increasing evidence that inflammatory or autoimmune mechanisms contribute to the inhomogeneous etiology of the illness.

It remains totally unknown which neurobiological factors are responsible for the first appearance of the fully developed psychotic symptoms, which usually do not occur before puberty, and for the typical long-term course of schizophrenia characterized by exacerbations and remissions. Biochemical and neurohormonal alterations might be more promising candidates to answer this important question than static structural anomalies.

REFERENCES

1. Bogerts B, Liebermann J. Neuropathology in the study of psychiatric disease. In: Costa e Silva A, Nadelson CC, eds. In International Review of Psychiatry. Washington DC: American Psychiatric Press, 1993: 515–55.
2. Huber G. Chronische Schizophrenie, Synopsis klinischer und neuroradiologischer Untersuchungen. Heidelberg: Hütig-Verlag, 1961.
3. Stevens JR. An anatomy of schizophrenia? Arch Gen Psychiatry 1973; 29: 177–89.
4. Torrey EF, Peterson MR. Schizophrenia and the limbic system. Lancet 1974; 2: 942–6.
5. Bogerts B. Zur Neuropathologie der Schizophrenien. Fortschr Neurol Psychiatr 1984; 52: 428–37.
6. Bogerts B. Schizophrenien als Erkrankungen des limbischen Systems. In: Huber G, ed. Basisstadien endogener Psychosen und das Borderline-Problem. Stuttgart: Schattauer, 1985: 163–79.
7. Bogerts B, Meertz E, Schonfeldt-Bausch R. Basal ganglia and limbic system pathology in schizophrenia. A morphometric study of brain volume and shrinkage. Arch Gen Psychiatry 1985; 42: 784–91.

8. Woodruff PW, Wright IC, Shuriquie N et al. Structural brain abnormalities in male schizophrenics reflect fronto-temporal dissociation. Psychol Med 1997; 27: 1257–66.

9. Harrison PJ. The hippocampus in schizophrenia: a review of the neuropathological evidence and its pathophysiological implications. Psychopharmacology (Berl) 2004; 174: 151–62.

10. Chance SA, Esiri MM, Crow TJ. Amygdala volume in schizophrenia: post-mortem study and review of magnetic resonance imaging findings. Br J Psychiatry 2002; 180: 331–8.

11. Heckers S. Neuropathology of schizophrenia: cortex, thalamus, basal ganglia, and neurotransmitter-specific projection systems. Schizophr Bull 1997; 23: 403–21.

12. Wang L, Hosakere M, Trein JC et al. Abnormalities of cingulate gyrus neuroanatomy in schizophrenia. Schizophr Res 2007; 93: 66–78.

13. Krimer LS, Herman MM, Saunders RC et al. A qualitative and quantitative analysis of the entorhinal cortex in schizophrenia. Cereb Cortex 1997; 7: 732–9.

14. Kalus P, Slotboom J, Gallinat J et al. New evidence for involvement of the entorhinal region in schizophrenia: a combined MRI volumetric and DTI study. Neuroimage 2005; 24: 1122–9.

15. Lawrie SM, Abukmeil SS. Brain abnormality in schizophrenia. A systematic and quantitative review of volumetric magnetic resonance imaging studies. Br J Psychiatry 1998; 172: 110–20.

16. Wright IC, Rabe-Hesketh S, Woodruff PW et al. Meta-analysis of regional brain volumes in schizophrenia. Am J Psychiatry 2000; 157: 16–25.

17. Kreczmanski P, Heinsen H, Mantua V et al. Volume, neuron density and total neuron number in five subcortical regions in schizophrenia. Brain 2007; 130: 678–92.

18. Bernstein HG, Krause S, Krell D et al. Strongly reduced number of parvalbumin-immunoreactive projection neurons in the mammillary bodies in schizophrenia: further evidence for limbic neuropathology. Ann N Y Acad Sci 2007; 1096: 120–7.

19. Brisch R, Bernstein HG, Krell D et al. Volumetric analysis of septal region in schizophrenia and affective disorder. Eur Arch Psychiatry Clin Neurosci 2007; 257: 140–8.

20. Ranft K, Krell D, Danos P et al. Reduced volumes of the habenular complex in depression. World J Biol Psychiatry 2002; 3: 27.

21. Dwork AJ. Postmortem studies of the hippocampal formation in schizophrenia. Schizophr Bull 1997; 23: 385–402.

22. Reif A, Fritzen S, Finger M et al. Neural stem cell proliferation is decreased in schizophrenia, but not in depression. Mol Psychiatry 2006; 11: 514–22.

23. Burns J, Job D, Bastin ME et al. Structural disconnectivity in schizophrenia: a diffusion tensor magnetic resonance imaging study. Br J Psychiatry 2003; 182: 439–43.

24. Talamini LM, Meeter M, Elvevag B et al. Reduced parahippocampal connectivity produces schizophrenia-like memory deficits in simulated neural circuits with reduced parahippocampal connectivity. Arch Gen Psychiatry 2005; 62: 485–93.

25. Sawada K, Barr AM, Nakamura M et al. Hippocampal complexin proteins and cognitive dysfunction in schizophrenia. Arch Gen Psychiatry 2005; 62: 263–72.

26. Harrison PJ, Law AJ. Neuregulin 1 and schizophrenia: genetics, gene expression, and neurobiology. Biol Psychiatry 2006; 60: 132–40.

27. Heckers S, Stone D, Walsh J et al. Differential hippocampal expression of glutamic acid decarboxylase 65 and 67 messenger RNA in bipolar disorder and schizophrenia. Arch Gen Psychiatry 2002; 59: 521–9

28. Woodruff-Pak DS, Gould TJ. Neuronal nicotinic acetylcholine receptors: involvement in Alzheimer's disease and schizophrenia. Behav Cogn Neurosci Rev 2002; 1: 5–20.

29. Bernstein HG, Krell D, Emrich HM et al. Fewer beta-endorphin expressing arcuate nucleus neurons and reduced beta-endorphinergic innervation of paraventricular neurons in schizophrenics and patients with depression. Cell Mol Biol (Noisy-le-grand) 2002; 48 Online Pub: OL259–65.

30. Beveridge NJ, Tooney PA, Carroll AP et al. Dysregulation of miRNA 181b in the temporal cortex in schizophrenia. Hum Mol Genet 2008; 17(8): 1156–68.

31. Bernstein HG, Braunewell KH, Spilker C et al. Hippocampal expression of the calcium sensor protein visinin-like protein-1 in schizophrenia. Neuroreport 2002; 13: 393–6.
32. Bogerts B. The temporolimbic system theory of positive schizophrenic symptoms. Schizophr Bull 1997; 23: 423–35.
33. Gruber O, Falkai P, Schneider-Axmann T et al. Neuregulin-1 haplotype HAP(ICE) is associated with lower hippocampal volumes in schizophrenic patients and in non-affected family members. J Psychiatr Res 2008; 43(1): 1–6.
34. Heckers S, Heinsen H, Heinsen Y et al. Cortex, white matter, and basal ganglia in schizophrenia: a volumetric postmortem study. Biol Psychiatry 1991; 29: 556–66.
35. Berretta S, Pantazopoulos H, Lange N. Neuron numbers and volume of the amygdala in subjects diagnosed with bipolar disorder or schizophrenia. Biol Psychiatry 2007; 62: 884–93.
36. Jakob H, Beckmann H. Prenatal developmental disturbances in the limbic allocortex in schizophrenics. J Neural Transm 1986; 65: 303–26.
37. Arnold SE, Hyman BT, Van Hoesen GW et al. Some cytoarchitectural abnormalities of the entorhinal cortex in schizophrenia. Arch Gen Psychiatry 1991; 48: 625–32.
38. Falkai P, Schneider-Axmann T, Honer WG. Entorhinal cortex pre-alpha cell clusters in schizophrenia: quantitative evidence of a developmental abnormality. Biol Psychiatry 2000; 47: 937–43.
39. Kovalenko S, Bergmann A, Schneider-Axmann T et al. Regio entorhinalis in schizophrenia: more evidence for migrational disturbances and suggestions for a new biological hypothesis. Pharmacopsychiatry 2003; 36 Suppl 3: S158–61.
40. Heinsen H, Gossmann E, Rub U et al. Variability in the human entorhinal region may confound neuropsychiatric diagnoses. Acta Anat (Basel) 1996; 157: 226–37.
41. Bernstein HG, Krell D, Baumann B et al. Morphometric studies of the entorhinal cortex in neuropsychiatric patients and controls: clusters of heterotopically displaced lamina II neurons are not indicative of schizophrenia. Schizophr Res 1998; 33: 125–32.
42. Braitenberg V. Ricerche istopatologiche sulla corteccia frontale di schizofrenici. Proceedings of the First International Congress of Neuropathology. Turin: Rosenberg & Sellier, 1952: 621–6.
43. Benes FM, Bird ED. An analysis of the arrangement of neurons in the cingulate cortex of schizophrenic patients. Arch Gen Psychiatry 1987; 44: 608–16.
44. Bouras C, Kovari E, Hof PR et al. Anterior cingulate cortex pathology in schizophrenia and bipolar disorder. Acta Neuropathol 2001; 102: 373–9.
45. Benes FM, Vincent SL, Todtenkopf M. The density of pyramidal and nonpyramidal neurons in anterior cingulate cortex of schizophrenic and bipolar subjects. Biol Psychiatry 2001; 50: 395–406.
46. Cotter D, Landau S, Beasley C et al. The density and spatial distribution of GABAergic neurons, labelled using calcium binding proteins, in the anterior cingulate cortex in major depressive disorder, bipolar disorder, and schizophrenia. Biol Psychiatry 2002; 51: 377–86.
47. Todtenkopf MS, Vincent SL, Benes FM. A cross-study meta-analysis and three-dimensional comparison of cell counting in the anterior cingulate cortex of schizophrenic and bipolar brain. Schizophr Res 2005; 73: 79–89.
48. Woo TU, Walsh JP, Benes FM. Density of glutamic acid decarboxylase 67 messenger RNA-containing neurons that express the N-methyl-D-aspartate receptor subunit NR2A in the anterior cingulate cortex in schizophrenia and bipolar disorder. Arch Gen Psychiatry 2004; 61: 649–57.
49. Chana G, Landau S, Beasley C et al. Two-dimensional assessment of cytoarchitecture in the anterior cingulate cortex in major depressive disorder, bipolar disorder, and schizophrenia: evidence for decreased neuronal somal size and increased neuronal density. Biol Psychiatry 2003; 53: 1086–98.
50. Gittins R, Harrison PJ. Neuronal density, size and shape in the human anterior cingulate cortex: a comparison of Nissl and NeuN staining. Brain Res Bull 2004; 63: 155–60.

51. Kalus P, Senitz D, Beckmann H. Altered distribution of parvalbumin-immunoreactive local circuit neurons in the anterior cingulate cortex of schizophrenic patients. Psychiatry Res 1997; 75: 49–59.
52. Aganova EA, Uranova NA. Morphometric analysis of synaptic contacts in the anterior limbic cortex in the endogenous psychoses. Neurosci Behav Physiol 1992; 22: 59–65.
53. Stark AK, Uylings HB, Sanz-Arigita E et al. Glial cell loss in the anterior cingulate cortex, a subregion of the prefrontal cortex, in subjects with schizophrenia. Am J Psychiatry 2004; 161: 882–8.
54. Steiner J, Bernstein HG, Bielau H et al. S100B-immunopositive glia is elevated in paranoid as compared to residual schizophrenia: A morphometric study. J Psychiatr Res 2007; 42(10): 868–76.
55. McCullumsmith RE, Gupta D, Beneyto M et al. Expression of transcripts for myelination-related genes in the anterior cingulate cortex in schizophrenia. Schizophr Res 2007; 90: 15–27.
56. Law AJ, Harrison PJ. The distribution and morphology of prefrontal cortex pyramidal neurons identified using anti-neurofilament antibodies SMI32, N200 and FNP7. Normative data and a comparison in subjects with schizophrenia, bipolar disorder or major depression. J Psychiatr Res 2003; 37: 487–99.
57. Wheeler DG, Dixon G, Harper CG. No differences in calcium-binding protein immunoreactivity in the posterior cingulate and visual cortex: schizophrenia and controls. Prog Neuropsychopharmacol Biol Psychiatry 2006; 30: 630–9.
58. Schlaepfer TE, Harris GJ, Tien AY et al. Decreased regional cortical gray matter volume in schizophrenia. Am J Psychiatry 1994; 151: 842–8.
59. Gur RE, Cowell PE, Latshaw A et al. Reduced dorsal and orbital prefrontal gray matter volumes in schizophrenia. Arch Gen Psychiatry 2000; 57: 761–68.
60. Galderisi S, Quarantelli M, Volpe U et al. Patterns of structural MRI abnormalities in deficit and nondeficit schizophrenia. Schizophr Bull 2008; 34: 393–401.
61. Reynolds GP, Beasley CL, Zhang ZJ. Understanding the neurotransmitter pathology of schizophrenia: selective deficits of subtypes of cortical GABAergic neurons. J Neural Transm 2002; 109: 881–9.
62. Cotter D, Mackay D, Chana G et al. Reduced neuronal size and glial cell density in area 9 of the dorsolateral prefrontal cortex in subjects with major depressive disorder. Cereb Cortex 2002; 12: 386–94.
63. Akbarian S, Kim JJ, Potkin SG et al. Gene expression for glutamic acid decarboxylase is reduced without loss of neurons in prefrontal cortex of schizophrenics. Arch Gen Psychiatry 1995; 52: 258–66.
64. Lewis DA, Levitt P. Schizophrenia as a disorder of neurodevelopment. Annu Rev Neurosci 2002; 25: 409–32.
65. Hashimoto T, Bazmi HH, Mirnics K et al. Conserved Regional Patterns of GABA-Related Transcript Expression in the Neocortex of Subjects With Schizophrenia. Am J Psychiatry 2008; 165(4): 479–89
66. Tooney PA, Chahl LA. Neurons expressing calcium-binding proteins in the prefrontal cortex in schizophrenia. Prog Neuropsychopharmacol Biol Psychiatry 2004; 28: 273–8.
67. Bernstein HG, Sahin J, Smalla KH et al. A reduced number of cortical neurons show increased Caldendrin protein levels in chronic schizophrenia. Schizophr Res 2007; 96: 246–56.
68. Selemon LD, Mrzljak J, Kleinman JE et al. Regional specificity in the neuropathologic substrates of schizophrenia: a morphometric analysis of Broca's area 44 and area 9. Arch Gen Psychiatry 2003; 60: 69–77.
69. Selemon LD, Rajkowska G, Goldman-Rakic PS. Elevated neuronal density in prefrontal area 46 in brains from schizophrenic patients: application of a three-dimensional, stereologic counting method. J Comp Neurol 1998; 392: 402–12.
70. Cullen TJ, Walker MA, Eastwood SL et al. Anomalies of asymmetry of pyramidal cell density and structure in dorsolateral prefrontal cortex in schizophrenia. Br J Psychiatry 2006; 188: 26–31.

71. Hashimoto R, Straub RE, Weickert CS et al. Expression analysis of neuregulin-1 in the dorsolateral prefrontal cortex in schizophrenia. Mol Psychiatry 2004; 9: 299–307.

72. Chong VZ, Thompson M, Beltaifa S et al. Elevated neuregulin-1 and ErbB4 protein in the prefrontal cortex of schizophrenic patients. Schizophr Res 2008; 100: 270–80.

73. Bertram I, Bernstein HG, Lendeckel U et al. Immunohistochemical evidence for impaired neuregulin-1 signaling in the prefrontal cortex in schizophrenia and in unipolar depression. Ann N Y Acad Sci 2007; 1096: 147–56.

74. Hahn CG, Wang HY, Cho DS et al. Altered neuregulin 1-erbB4 signaling contributes to NMDA receptor hypofunction in schizophrenia. Nat Med 2006; 12: 824–8.

75. Weis S, Llenos IC. GFAP-immunopositive astrocytes in schizophrenia. Schizophr Res 2004; 67: 293–95.

76. Kirkpatrick B, Conley RC, Kakoyannis A et al. Interstitial cells of the white matter in the inferior parietal cortex in schizophrenia: An unbiased cell-counting study. Synapse 1999; 34, 95–102.

77. Kirkpatrick B, Messias NC, Conley RR et al. Interstitial cells of the white matter in the dorsolateral prefrontal cortex in deficit and nondeficit schizophrenia. J Nerv Ment Dis 2003; 191: 563–7.

78. Eastwood SL, Harrison PJ. Interstitial white matter neuron density in the dorsolateral prefrontal cortex and parahippocampal gyrus in schizophrenia. Schizophr Res 2005; 79: 181–8

79. Vostrikov VM, Uranova NA, Orlovskaya DD. Deficit of perineuronal oligodendrocytes in the prefrontal cortex in schizophrenia and mood disorders. Schizophr Res 2007; 94: 273–80.

80. Segal D, Koschnick JR, Slegers LH et al. Oligodendrocyte pathophysiology: a new view of schizophrenia. Int J Neuropsychopharmacol 2007; 10: 503–11.

81. Harms MP, Wang L, Mamah D et al. Thalamic shape abnormalities in individuals with schizophrenia and their nonpsychotic siblings. J Neurosci 2007; 27: 13835–42.

82. Lesch A, Bogerts B. The diencephalon in schizophrenia: evidence for reduced thickness of the periventricular grey matter. Eur Arch Psychiatry Neurol Sci 1984; 234: 212–9.

83. Jones EG. Cortical development and thalamic pathology in schizophrenia. Schizophr Bull 1997; 23: 483–501.

84. Pakkenberg B. The volume of the mediodorsal thalamic nucleus in treated and untreated schizophrenics. Schizophr Res 1992; 7: 95–100.

85. Pakkenberg B, Gundersen HJ. New stereological method for obtaining unbiased and efficient estimates of total nerve cell number in human brain areas. Exemplified by the mediodorsal thalamic nucleus in schizophrenics. Apmis 1989; 97: 677–81.

86. Popken GJ, Bunney WE Jr, Potkin SG et al. Subnucleus-specific loss of neurons in medial thalamus of schizophrenics. Proc Natl Acad Sci U S A 2000; 97: 9276–80.

87. Young KA, Manaye KF, Liang C et al. Reduced number of mediodorsal and anterior thalamic neurons in schizophrenia. Biol Psychiatry 2000; 47: 944–53.

88. Byne W, Buchsbaum MS, Mattiace LA et al. Postmortem assessment of thalamic nuclear volumes in subjects with schizophrenia. Am J Psychiatry 2002; 159: 59–65.

89. Cullen TJ, Walker MA, Parkinson N et al. A postmortem study of the mediodorsal nucleus of the thalamus in schizophrenia. Schizophr Res 2003; 60: 157–66.

90. Dorph-Petersen KA, Pierri JN, Sun Z et al. Stereological analysis of the mediodorsal thalamic nucleus in schizophrenia: volume, neuron number, and cell types. J Comp Neurol 2004; 472: 449–62.

91. Danos P, Schmidt A, Baumann B et al. Volume and neuron number of the mediodorsal thalamic nucleus in schizophrenia: a replication study. Psychiatry Res 2005; 140: 281–9.

92. Danos P, Baumann B, Bernstein HG et al. Schizophrenia and anteroventral thalamic nucleus: selective decrease of parvalbumin-immunoreactive thalamocortical projection neurons. Psychiatry Res 1998; 82: 1–10.

93. Byne W, Kidkardnee S, Tatusov A et al. Schizophrenia-associated reduction of neuronal and oligodendrocyte numbers in the anterior principal thalamic nucleus. Schizophr Res 2006; 85: 245–53.

94. Byne W, Fernandes J, Haroutunian V et al. Reduction of right medial pulvinar volume and neuron number in schizophrenia. Schizophr Res 2007; 90: 71–5.

95. Danos P, Baumann B, Kramer A et al. Volumes of association thalamic nuclei in schizophrenia: a postmortem study. Schizophr Res 2003; 60: 141–55.

96. Danos P, Baumann B, Bernstein HG et al. The ventral lateral posterior nucleus of the thalamus in schizophrenia: a post-mortem study. Psychiatry Res 2002; 114: 1–9.

97. Young KA, Holcomb LA, Yazdani U et al. Elevated neuron number in the limbic thalamus in major depression. Am J Psychiatry 2004; 161: 1270–7.

98. Snyder PJ, Bogerts B, Wu H et al. Absence of the adhesio interthalamica as a marker of early developmental neuropathology in schizophrenia: an MRI and postmortem histologic study. J Neuroimaging 1998; 8: 159–63.

99. Andreasen NC. The role of the thalamus in schizophrenia. Can J Psychiatry 1997; 42: 27–33.

100. Kristiansen LV, Meador-Woodruff JH. Abnormal striatal expression of transcripts encoding NMDA interacting PSD proteins in schizophrenia, bipolar disorder and major depression. Schizophr Res 2005; 78: 87–93.

101. Watis L, Chen SH, Chua HC et al. Glutamatergic abnormalities of the thalamus in schizophrenia: a systematic review. J Neural Transm 2008; 115: 493–511.

102. Clinton SM, Ibrahim HM, Frey KA et al. Dopaminergic abnormalities in select thalamic nuclei in schizophrenia: involvement of the intracellular signal integrating proteins calcyon and spinophilin. Am J Psychiatry 2005; 162: 1859–71.

103. Dixon G, Harper CG. No evidence for selective GABAergic interneuron deficits in the anterior thalamic complex of patients with schizophrenia. Prog Neuropsychopharmacol Biol Psychiatry 2004; 28: 1045–51.

104. Roberts RC. Schizophrenia in translation: disrupted in schizophrenia (DISC1): integrating clinical and basic findings. Schizophr Bull 2007; 33: 11–15.

105. Toda M, Abi-Dargham A. Dopamine hypothesis of schizophrenia: making sense of it all. Curr Psychiatry Rep 2007; 9: 329–36.

106. Bogerts B, Falkai P, Haupts M et al. Post-mortem volume measurements of limbic system and basal ganglia structures in chronic schizophrenics. Initial results from a new brain collection. Schizophr Res 1990; 3: 295–301.

107. Lauer M, Beckmann H. The human striatum in schizophrenia. I. Increase in overall relative striatal volume in schizophrenics. Psychiatry Res 1997; 68: 87–98.

108. Lang DJ, Kopala LC, Vandorpe RA et al. An MRI study of basal ganglia volumes in first-episode schizophrenia patients treated with risperidone. Am J Psychiatry 2001; 158: 625–31.

109. Anderson SM, Bari AA, Pierce RC. Administration of the D1-like dopamine receptor antagonist SCH-23390 into the medial nucleus accumbens shell attenuates cocaine priming-induced reinstatement of drug-seeking behavior in rats. Psychopharmacology (Berl) 2003; 168: 132–8.

110. Lauer M, Johannes S, Fritzen S et al. Morphological abnormalities in nitric-oxide-synthase-positive striatal interneurons of schizophrenic patients. Neuropsychobiology 2005; 52: 111–7.

111. Holt DJ, Bachus SE, Hyde TM et al. Reduced density of cholinergic interneurons in the ventral striatum in schizophrenia: an in situ hybridization study. Biol Psychiatry 2005; 58: 408–16.

112. Brown JS Jr. Effects of Bisphenol-A and Other Endocrine Disruptors Compared With Abnormalities of Schizophrenia: An Endocrine-Disruption Theory of Schizophrenia. Schizophr Bull 2008; 35(1): 256–78.

113. Goldstein JM, Seidman LJ, Makris N et al. Hypothalamic abnormalities in schizophrenia: sex effects and genetic vulnerability. Biol Psychiatry 2007; 61: 935–45.

114. Koolschijn PC, van Haren NE, Hulshoff Pol HE et al. Hypothalamus volume in twin pairs discordant for schizophrenia. Eur Neuropsychopharmacol 2008; 18: 312–5.

115. Mai JK, Berger K, Sofroniew MW. Morphometric evaluation of neurophysin-immunoreactivity in the human brain: pronounced interindividual variability and evidence for altered staining patterns in schizophrenia. J Hirnforsch 1993; 34: 133–54.

116. Bernstein HG, Stanarius A, Baumann B et al. Nitric oxide synthase-containing neurons in the human hypothalamus: reduced number of immunoreactive cells in the paraventricular nucleus of depressive patients and schizophrenics. Neuroscience 1998; 83: 867–75.

117. Bernstein HG, Lendeckel U, Dobrowolny H et al. Beacon-like/ubiquitin-5-like immuno-reactivity is highly expressed in human hypothalamus and increased in haloperidol-treated schizophrenics and a rat model of schizophrenia. Psychoneuroendocrinology 2008; 33: 340–51.

118. Malidelis YI, Panayotacopoulou MT, van Heerikhuize JJ et al. Absence of a difference in the neurosecretory activity of supraoptic nucleus vasopressin neurons of neuroleptic-treated schizophrenic patients. Neuroendocrinology 2005; 82: 63–9.

119. Weinberger DR, Kleinman JE, Luchins DJ et al. Cerebellar pathology in schizophrenia: a controlled postmortem study. Am J Psychiatry 1980; 137: 359–61.

120. Luchins DJ, Morihisa JM, Weinberger DR et al. Cerebral asymmetry and cerebellar atrophy in schizophrenia: a controlled postmortem study. Am J Psychiatry 1981; 138: 1501–3.

121. Martin P, Albers M. Cerebellum and schizophrenia: a selective review. Schizophr Bull 1995; 21: 241–50.

122. Supprian T, Ulmar G, Bauer M et al. Cerebellar vermis area in schizophrenic patients – a post-mortem study. Schizophr Res 2000; 42: 19–28.

123. Tran KD, Smutzer GS, Doty RL et al. Reduced Purkinje cell size in the cerebellar vermis of elderly patients with schizophrenia. Am J Psychiatry 1998; 155: 1288–90.

124. Fatemi SH, Laurence JA, Araghi-Niknam M et al. Glial fibrillary acidic protein is reduced in cerebellum of subjects with major depression, but not schizophrenia. Schizophr Res 2004; 69: 317–23.

125. Guidotti A, Auta J, Davis JM et al. Decrease in reelin and glutamic acid decarboxylase67 (GAD67) expression in schizophrenia and bipolar disorder: a postmortem brain study. Arch Gen Psychiatry 2000; 57: 1061–9.

126. Bernstein HG, Krell D, Braunewell KH et al. Increased number of nitric oxide synthase immunoreactive Purkinje cells and dentate nucleus neurons in schizophrenia. J Neurocytol 2001; 30: 661–70.

127. Karson CN, Griffin WS, Mrak RE et al. Nitric oxide synthase (NOS) in schizophrenia: increases in cerebellar vermis. Mol Chem Neuropathol 1996; 27: 275–84.

128. Kyosseva SV, Elbein AD, Hutton TL et al. Increased levels of transcription factors Elk-1, cyclic adenosine monophosphate response element-binding protein, and activating transcription factor 2 in the cerebellar vermis of schizophrenic patients. Arch Gen Psychiatry 2000; 57: 685–91.

129. Falkai P, Honer WG, David S et al. No evidence for astrogliosis in brains of schizophrenic patients. A post-mortem study. Neuropathol Appl Neurobiol 1999; 25: 48–53.

130. Falkai P, Schneider T, Greve B et al. Reduced frontal and occipital lobe asymmetry on the CT-scans of schizophrenic patients. Its specificity and clinical significance. J Neural Transm 1995; 99: 63–77.

131. Vogeley K, Schneider-Axmann T, Pfeiffer U et al. Disturbed gyrification of the prefrontal region in male schizophrenic patients: A morphometric postmortem study. Am J Psychiatry 2000; 157: 34–9.

132. de Haan L, Bakker JM, de Haan P et al. Overview of neuropathological theories of schizophrenia: from degeneration to progressive developmental disorder. Effect of ischemic pretreatment on heat shock protein 72, neurologic outcome, and histopathologic outcome in a rabbit model of spinal cord ischemia. Psychopathology 2004; 37: 1–7.

133. Gorwood P, Pouchot J, Vinceneux P et al. Rheumatoid arthritis and schizophrenia: a negative association at a dimensional level. Schizophr Res 2004; 66: 21–9.

134. Wagner-Jauregg J. Über die Einwirkung fieberhafter Erkrankungen auf Psychosen. Allgemeine Zeitschrift für Psychiatrie 1887; 27: 93–131.

135. Nunes SO, Borelli SD, Matsuo T et al. The association of the HLA in patients with schizophrenia, schizoaffective disorder, and in their biological relatives. Schizophr Res 2005; 76: 195–8.

136. Torrey EF, Bartko JJ, Lun ZR et al. Antibodies to Toxoplasma gondii in patients with schizophrenia: a meta-analysis. Schizophr Bull 2007; 33: 729–36.
137. Schwarcz R, Hunter CA. Toxoplasma gondii and schizophrenia: linkage through astrocyte-derived kynurenic acid? Schizophr Bull 2007; 33: 652–3.
138. Babulas V, Factor-Litvak P, Goetz R et al. Prenatal exposure to maternal genital and reproductive infections and adult schizophrenia. Am J Psychiatry 2006; 163: 927–9.
139. Brown AS. The risk for schizophrenia from childhood and adult infections. Am J Psychiatry 2008; 165: 7–10.
140. Nyffeler M, Meyer U, Yee BK et al. Maternal immune activation during pregnancy increases limbic GABAA receptor immunoreactivity in the adult offspring: implications for schizophrenia. Neuroscience 2006; 143: 51–62.
141. Kamp HV. Nuclear changes in the white blood cells of patients with schizophrenic reaction: a preliminary report. J Neuropsychiatry 1962; 4: 1–3.
142. Hirata-Hibi M, Higashi S, Tachibana T et al. Stimulated lymphocytes in schizophrenia. Arch Gen Psychiatry 1982; 39: 82–7.
143. Kokai M, Morita Y, Fukuda H et al. Immunophenotypic studies on atypical lymphocytes in psychiatric patients. Psychiatry Res 1998; 77: 105–12.
144. DeLisi LE, Goodman S, Neckers LM et al. An analysis of lymphocyte subpopulations in schizophrenic patients. Biol Psychiatry 1982; 17: 1003–9.
145. Fieve RR, Blumenthal B, Little B. The relationship of atypical lymphocytes, phenothiazines, and schizophrenia. Arch Gen Psychiatry 1966; 15: 529–34.
146. Rudolf S, Schlenke P, Broocks A et al. Search for atypical lymphocytes in schizophrenia. World J Biol Psychiatry 2004; 5: 33–7.
147. Watanabe Y, Nakayama T, Nagakubo D et al. Dopamine selectively induces migration and homing of naive CD8+ T cells via dopamine receptor D3. J Immunol 2006; 176: 848–56.
148. Levite M, Chowers Y, Ganor Y et al. Dopamine interacts directly with its D3 and D2 receptors on normal human T cells, and activates beta1 integrin function. Eur J Immunol 2001; 31: 3504–12.
149. Riedel M, Spellmann I, Schwarz MJ et al. Decreased T cellular immune response in schizophrenic patients. J Psychiatr Res 2007; 41: 3–7.
150. Craddock RM, Lockstone HE, Rider DA et al. Altered T-cell function in schizophrenia: a cellular model to investigate molecular disease mechanisms. PLoS ONE 2007; 2: e692.
151. Schuld A, Hinze-Selch D, Pollmaecher T. Cytokine network in patients with schizophrenia and its significance for the pathophysiology of the illness. Nervenarzt 2004; 75: 215–26.
152. Borda T, Perez Rivera R, Joensen L et al. Antibodies against cerebral M1 cholinergic muscarinic receptor from schizophrenic patients: molecular interaction. J Immunol 2002; 168: 3667–74.
153. Tanaka S, Matsunaga H, Kimura M et al. Autoantibodies against four kinds of neurotransmitter receptors in psychiatric disorders. J Neuroimmunol 2003; 14: 155–64.
154. Elenkov IJ, Wilder RL, Chrousos GP et al. The sympathetic nerve - an integrative interface between two supersystems: the brain and the immune system. Pharmacol Rev 2000; 52: 595–638.
155. Müller N, Schwarz M. Schizophrenia as an inflammation-mediated dysbalance of glutamatergic neurotransmission. Neurotox Res 2006; 10: 131–48.
156. Akhondzadeh S, Tabatabaee M, Amini H et al. Celecoxib as adjunctive therapy in schizophrenia: a double-blind, randomized and placebo-controlled trial. Schizophr Res 2007; 90: 179–85.
157. Potvin S, Stip E, Sepehry AA et al. Inflammatory Cytokine Alterations in Schizophrenia: A Systematic Quantitative Review. Biol Psychiatry 2007, [doi:10.1016/j.biopsych.2007.1009.1024].
158. Shirts BH, Wood J, Yolken RH et al. Association study of IL10, IL1beta, and IL1RN and schizophrenia using tag SNPs from a comprehensive database: suggestive association with rs16944 at IL1beta. Schizophr Res 2006; 88: 235–44.

159. Papiol S, Molina V, Desco M et al. Ventricular enlargement in schizophrenia is associated with a genetic polymorphism at the interleukin-1 receptor antagonist gene. Neuroimage 2005; 27: 1002–6.

160. Schwarz MJ, Kronig H, Riedel M et al. IL-2 and IL-4 polymorphisms as candidate genes in schizophrenia. Eur Arch Psychiatry Clin Neurosci 2006; 256: 72–6.

161. Lencz T, Morgan TV, Athanasiou M et al. Converging evidence for a pseudoautosomal cytokine receptor gene locus in schizophrenia. Mol Psychiatry 2007; 12: 572–80.

162. Bayer TA, Buslei R, Havas L, et al. Evidence for activation of microglia in patients with psychiatric illnesses. Neurosci Lett 1999, 271, 126-128

163. Radewicz K, Garey LJ, Gentleman SM, et al. Increase in HLA-DR immunoreactive microglia in frontal and temporal cortex of chronic schizophrenics. J Neuropathol Exp Neurol 2000, 59, 137-150

164. Arnold SE, Trojanowski JQ, Gur RE, et al. Absence of neurodegeneration and neural injury in the cerebral cortex in a sample of elderly patients with schizophrenia. Arch Gen Psychiatry 1998, 55, 225-232

165. Falke E, Han LY, Arnold SE. Absence of neurodegeneration in the thalamus and caudate of elderly patients with schizophrenia. Psychiatry Res 2000, 93, 103-110

166. Kurumaji A, Wakai T, Toru M. Decreases in peripheral-type benzodiazepine receptors in postmortem brains of chronic schizophrenics. J Neural Transm 1997, 104, 1361-1370

167. Steiner J, Mawrin C, Ziegeler A, et al. Distribution of HLA-DR-positive microglia in schizophrenia reflects impaired cerebral lateralization. Acta Neuropathol 2006, 112, 305-316

168. Togo T, Akiyama H, Kondo H, et al. Expression of CD40 in the brain of Alzheimer's disease and other neurological diseases. Brain Res 2000, 885, 117-121

169. Steiner J, Bielau H, Brisch R, et al. Immunological aspects in the neurobiology of suicide: Elevated microglial density in schizophrenia and depression is associated with suicide. J Psychiatr Res 2008, 42, 151-157

170. Arnold SE, Trojanowski JQ, Gur RE et al. Absence of neurodegeneration and neural injury in the cerebral cortex in a sample of elderly patients with schizophrenia. Arch Gen Psychiatry 1998; 55: 225–32.

171. Falke E, Han LY, Arnold SE. Absence of neurodegeneration in the thalamus and caudate of elderly patients with schizophrenia. Psychiatry Res 2000; 93: 103–10.

172. Kurumaji A, Wakai T, Toru M. Decreases in peripheral-type benzodiazepine receptors in postmortem brains of chronic schizophrenics. J Neural Transm 1997; 104: 1361–70.

173. Steiner J, Mawrin C, Ziegeler A et al. Distribution of HLA-DR-positive microglia in schizophrenia reflects impaired cerebral lateralization. Acta Neuropathol 2006; 112: 305–16.

174. Togo T, Akiyama H, Kondo H et al. Expression of CD40 in the brain of Alzheimer's disease and other neurological diseases. Brain Res 2000; 885: 117–21.

175. Steiner J, Bielau H, Brisch R et al. Immunological aspects in the neurobiology of suicide: Elevated microglial density in schizophrenia and depression is associated with suicide. J Psychiatr Res 2008; 42: 151–7.

10 Imaging in schizophrenia

Wiepke Cahn, Neeltje EM van Haren, and Rene S Kahn

INTRODUCTION

In the past, evidence was lacking to show that schizophrenia is a brain disease. This notion was mainly based on finding no or little abnormalities in postmortem brains of patients with schizophrenia. (1) This resulted in searching for other supposed causes like failing family interactions. In the 60s and 70s, clinical investigators concluded that faulty interactions between the family members, particularly between mother and child, could cause or worsen schizophrenia. (2) For years, parents had to carry the burden of guilt, as they were to blame for their children's illness. Through new *in vivo* neuroimaging techniques, such as computer tomography (CT), enlarged ventricles were found to be present in schizophrenia. (3) This finding consequently offered a new impulse to further explore the neurobiological causes of schizophrenia. Over the years and through technical progress, it was possible to study the brain more extensively *in vivo*. The use of magnetic resonance imaging (MRI) allowed for the quantification of gray and white matter and for measurement of discrete, cortical and subcortical structures (Figure 10.1). In a meta-analysis of Wright et al., (4) it was convincingly shown that brain-volume abnormalities are present in schizophrenia. The volume of the body of the lateral ventricle was found to be increased (16%) while cerebral volume was reduced (2%). The latter was primarily attributed to a decrease in gray matter volume (2%). Nevertheless, a small but significant reduction was found in white matter (1%) (see also Table 10.1). The improved quality of the MRI scans made it also possible to manually delineate brain areas of interest. Regional pathology indicates larger reductions in temporal and frontal lobe (5) and more specifically in medial temporal structures (hippocampus and amygdale) (6, 7).

That schizophrenia is a brain disease is substantiated with the extensive abnormalities found in cognitive function. Studies examining the brain function, as opposed to brain structure, found that the prefrontal cortex and those areas, especially temporal and parietal cortices, cerebellum, striatum, and thalamus that are anatomically connected to the prefrontal cortex, seem to be affected in schizophrenia (8) .

TABLE 10.1 (adapted from Wright et al. 2000)

Structure	percentage of volume change
Gray matter	−2%
White matter	−1%
Superior temporal gyrus	−7%
Amygdala/hippocampus	−6%
Parahippocampal gyrus	−6%
Thalamus	−4%
Frontal lobes	−2%
globus pallidus	+24%
putamen	+6%
caudate	+4%

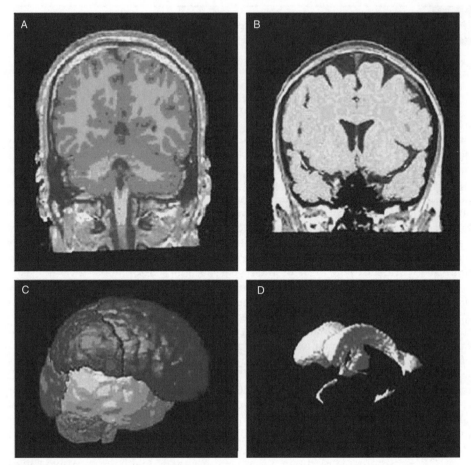

FIGURE 10.1

Many attempts have been made to unravel the etiology of schizophrenia. Through epidemiological studies in families, including those in twins, it has been shown schizophrenia must be genetic and environmental of origin, (9) with an estimated heritability of 80%. (10) Evidence is growing that these genetic and environmental influences are reflected on the brain structure (and function); thus brain imaging could also be useful while studying the etiology of schizophrenia. This chapter will focus on structural MRI studies performed in schizophrenia and will give an overview about the relationship between structural brain abnormalities, genetic and environmental influences, and clinical characteristics.

SCHIZOPHRENIA, A PROGRESSIVE BRAIN DISEASE
Based on the neurodevelopmental theory of schizophrenia, there was a notion that much of the brain abnormalities are present at illness onset and that these structural abnormalities remain stable over time. Indeed, results of early longitudinal pneumoencephalography and CT studies supported this notion. Nevertheless, the debate of

brain abnormalities being static or progressive over time became relevant again in schizophrenia research based on observations of deteriorating cognitive and daily life functioning, (11) suggesting schizophrenia to be a progressive illness. In one of the largest cross-sectional MRI studies across the adult age range smaller gray matter volume was found to be more pronounced with increasing age in patients with schizophrenia compared to healthy individuals. This suggests progressive loss of cerebral gray matter in schizophrenia patients. (12) Using a voxel-based morphometry approach distinct focal areas in the brains of schizophrenia showed decreases of the gray-matter density in the frontal and temporal cortices, left hippocampus, the insula, and left amygdala. Interestingly, the left amygdale-density decrease was more pronounced in the older than in the younger patients. (13) Moreover, in patients significant decreases in white-matter density were found in the corpus callosum, right internal capsule, and right anterior commissure (14), which may suggest aberrant interhemispheric connectivity in schizophrenia.

In the past decade, many studies have focused on investigating the effects of a prodromal phase and/or first psychotic episode on the brain. (7) Studying the early phase of the illness is useful because the confounding effects of chronicity and long-term medication can be excluded. Moreover, one is able to prospectively examine the brains of patients with schizophrenia. MRI studies in subjects with increased symptomatic risks found few definitive markers that distinguish those who go on to develop the illness from those who do not. The two most consistently abnormal brain regions in schizophrenia research, the hippocampi and the lateral ventricles, were not significantly different from healthy controls prior to psychosis onset. However, cortical thickness in the anterior cingulate was found reduced (15). Also MRI studies in antipsychotic naïve patients showed a relative paucity of brain abnormalities that stands in marked contrast with findings in more chronic patients with schizophrenia (16). Several explanations can be contemplated to elucidate the discrepancy in brain abnormalities between those patients who are chronically ill and those who are in the early phase of the illness. Medication might increase brain abnormalities and could contribute to these brain-volume changes. Finding few brain abnormalities in the prodromal phase and in antipsychotic naïve patients with schizophrenia could also be the result of a selection bias favoring the inclusion of patients who have a less severe form of schizophrenia, and last but not least, progression of the illness may lead to an increase of brain abnormalities.

There is a growing body of evidence that brain abnormalities become greater in schizophrenia over the course of the illness (see also Figure 10.2). Various reviews of (longitudinal) MRI studies in patients with (first episode) schizophrenia conclude that there is accelerated loss of gray matter, particularly in the frontotemporal cortical areas, as well as sulcal and ventricular expansion over time. (17, 7, 18) In schizophrenia a 3% gray-matter decrease is found with a 0.5% decrease per year, which is consistent with the result of postmortem studies in schizophrenia. (18) Although changes in brain-volume over time are reported in both first-episode patients and chronic patients with schizophrenia, the magnitude in first-episode patients (e.g., −1.2% in 1 year for whole brain volume) (19) suggests that these brain-volume reductions are particularly prominent during the first years of illness (20). Furthermore, the findings imply that the brain-volume changes are nonlinear over time. This notion has been supported by imaging studies both in adolescence and adults with schizophrenia. In subjects with childhood-onset schizophrenia, a differential nonlinear progression of brain volumes was found during adolescence, with the total cerebrum and hippocampus decreasing and lateral ventricles increasing in the childhood-onset schizophrenia subjects

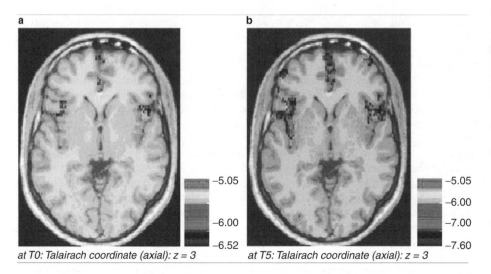

at T0: Talairach coordinate (axial): z = 3   at T5: Talairach coordinate (axial): z = 3

FIGURE 10.2

compared to healthy children. (21) Also, the trajectory of volume change over time differed between adult patients with schizophrenia and healthy individuals. Instead of a curved trajectory that was found for cerebral (gray) matter volume change in healthy subjects across the adult age range, patients showed a linear decrease over time (22).

BRAIN MORPHOLOGY AND GENETIC FACTORS IN SCHIZOPHRENIA
As mentioned previously, the vulnerability for developing schizophrenia is highly genetic. Examining brain volumes in nonpsychotic first-degree relatives of schizophrenic patients might clarify some of the causes of the brain abnormalities observed in probands. In recent years, several studies have measured brain volumes in unaffected relatives of patients with schizophrenia compared with those of healthy subjects. Most of these imaging studies showed smaller total brain volumes, larger ventricular volume, and smaller medial temporal lobe structures (24). Interestingly, a study on discordant monozygotic twins also reported smaller intracranial volumes in monozygotic patients with schizophrenia and their cotwins as compared to healthy monozygotic twins and suggested that increased genetic risk to develop schizophrenia might be related to reduced brain growth early in life (23).

A recent meta-analysis, which integrated the results of 25 MRI studies, compared brain volumes of 1,065 nonpsychotic first-degree relatives of patients with schizophrenia with those of 1,100 healthy control subjects to determine the magnitude and extent of brain-volume differences in first-degree relatives of patients with schizophrenia (24). It was found that brain volumes in relatives of patients with schizophrenia differ from those of healthy control subjects, with effect sizes in the small-to-moderate range. The largest effect was found in hippocampal volume, with relatives of patients having smaller volumes than healthy control subjects. In addition, total gray matter volume and third-ventricle volume are smaller in relatives compared with healthy control subjects. Although total brain and white matter volume did not differ significantly in relatives compared with healthy controls, both structures showed a trend toward significance. When patients with schizophrenia were compared to first-degree relatives, significantly smaller hippocampal volumes were found in patients.

Thus, through this meta-analysis, it was confirmed that brain abnormalities are (partly) related to the risk of developing schizophrenia. It further implies that brain volume reductions could well predate the clinical onset of schizophrenia and argues against the notion that the brain abnormalities in schizophrenia are solely caused by antipsychotics. These conclusions were strengthened by the finding that the brain structures affected in relatives are the same as those reported to be abnormal in patients. Interestingly, the similarity between brain abnormalities in patients and their nonpsychotic relatives was further enforced by a longitudinal study, finding progressive brain abnormalities in the nonaffected cotwins of patients with schizophrenia (25).

Recent studies have focused on testing specific genetic markers in a known candidate gene for association with endophenotypes. Structural brain parameters have been shown to be useful endophenotypes for studies in psychiatric illnesses. Recently, the available studies that reported on the influence of genotype on brain volume in schizophrenia were reviewed, and it was concluded that there is sufficient evidence to use of structural neuroimaging as an endophenotype to investigate a complex phenotype such as schizophrenia. However, so far, no single causal pathway emerges from these studies. (26)

BRAIN MORPHOLOGY AND ENVIRONMENTAL FACTORS IN SCHIZOPHRENIA

Although it is well established that environmental factors contribute to the development of schizophrenia, very few studies have been conducted to examine environmental factors in relation to brain morphology. Reduction of hippocampal volume in schizophrenia has been associated with severe pregnancy and birth complications (27). Furthermore, an interaction between genetic vulnerability and environmental factors in schizophrenia has been found, as fetal hypoxia was associated with greater structural brain abnormalities not only in patients with schizophrenia but also in their healthy siblings. Gray matter (most strongly in the temporal lobe) and hippocampal volumes were reduced, and CSF was increased in patients and healthy siblings as compared to healthy comparison subjects (28, 29).

Cannabis use is highly prevalent in schizophrenia and might increase the risk of developing schizophrenia (30). To examine the effect of cannabis on brain morphology, a cross-sectional study was designed in which patients with recent-onset schizophrenia and an additional *DSM-IV* lifetime diagnosis of cannabis abuse or dependence were compared to patients who were cannabis naïve. No differences were found in global brain and caudate nucleus volumes. (31) However, the effects of cannabis on the brain morphology became apparent in a 5-year longitudinal MRI study, as the progressive gray matter decrease was more pronounced in patients who continued using cannabis after illness onset as compared to patients and healthy subjects who did not use cannabis during the follow-up period. (32) Furthermore, patients who continued to use cannabis showed a less pronounced improvement in positive and negative symptoms as compared to nonusing patients. Although further studies need to be conducted to confirm whether the brain-volume loss is a direct or an indirect effect of cannabis in schizophrenia, this study suggests that some of the harmful effects of cannabis on the course of illness may be explained by its effect on the progression of brain changes in schizophrenia.

Until now, there is only indirect evidence that life events might affect brain volumes in schizophrenia, as lower gray and white matter volumes in schizophrenia are associated with a dysregulated, dopaminergic, and noradrenergic-mediated stress response.

(33) Some preliminary results show that through exercise (cycling versus table tennis) hippocampal atrophy in patients with schizophrenia could be reversed. (34)

Thus, it appears that (some) environmental factors do affect brain volumes in schizophrenia, but the extent of their contribution is unclear. Furthermore, there are various environmental factors, such as alcohol and drug abuse other than cannabis, nutritional state, social isolation,(7) and immigrant status (35) that could very well influence brain volumes, but these have not been examined at all.

BRAIN MORPHOLOGY AND ANTIPSYCHOTIC MEDICATION

It has long been argued that the brain-volume changes found in schizophrenia are (partly) caused by the antipsychotic medication. Indeed, in the early stages of schizophrenia, progressive decreases in gray matter (19) and frontal lobe volume (36, 37) have been found associated with the amount of antipsychotic medication taken. Those patients who were prescribed the highest doses of antipsychotic medication also had the greatest progressive decreases in brain volumes. Nevertheless, this brain volume decrease might not be a direct effect of the medication as those who are prescribed the highest doses of antipsychotic medication are generally the most severely ill patients. Increases and decreases in brain volumes depend on the type of antipsychotic medication. Basal ganglia volumes decrease by administering typical antipsychotic medication and increase (or normalize) by administering atypical medication or clozapine. (38, 39) Recent longitudinal MRI studies have shown that olanzapine and clozapine actually attenuates brain tissue loss in schizophrenia, whereas typical antipsychotic medication do not. (40, 41, 42)

BRAIN MORPHOLOGY AND ITS CLINICAL CORRELATES IN SCHIZOPHRENIA

Brain-volume reductions are present in schizophrenia, (4, 17, 18) but these reductions are only relevant if they are associated to the clinical characteristics and outcome in schizophrenia. The most consistent finding of longitudinal MRI studies in first-episode and chronic schizophrenia is the relationship between reduced brain volume (gray matter decrements and ventricular increments) and poor outcome (18, 42). Psychotic symptoms have also been examined in relation to brain-volume loss over time. A recent MRI study investigated the relationship between psychosis and brain-volume change in first-episode patients with schizophrenia (43) over the first 5 years of illness. Associations between gray matter volume loss, lateral- and third-ventricle volume increase, and longer duration of psychosis were found. Total duration of psychotic symptoms was further associated with greater decreases in total brain and cerebellar volume. Other MRI studies that examined smaller brain structures found reduced volumes of the medial temporal lobe, superior temporal gyrus, and hippocampal volumes in patients with psychotic symptoms. (44, 45) These findings suggest that brain-volume loss over time could be attributable to the "toxic" effects of the psychotic state. (11, 46, 47)

Both Kraepelin and Bleuler proposed that cognitive disturbances in schizophrenia are expressions of brain abnormalities. A selective review on the relationship between brain structure and neurocognition in schizophrenia concluded that whole brain volume appears to correlate with the measures of general intelligence as well as with a range of specific cognitive functions in normal controls and female schizophrenia patients, but this relationship is disrupted in male patients. Other brain structures have also been examined in relation to cognitive function, but it remains unclear which brain abnormalities in relation to cognition are disease specific. Furthermore, methodological issues do limit the interpretation and the implication of these findings. (48)

Although research has provided a wealth of information about brain structure (and function) in schizophrenia, there has been very little influence on clinical practice. One study examined global brain volumes as a predictor of outcome in schizophrenia, but found no associations between the brain-volume measurements at the onset of the illness and clinical and functional outcome after 2 years. (49) The use of two MRI measurements, however, appears to be more informative. Early dynamic brain-volume changes predicted longer-term outcome as patients with the greatest decrease in gray matter in the first year also had the highest negative symptom scores and were less likely to live independently 5 years after the first evaluation (50). Nevertheless, serial scanning might be a problem due to limited imaging facilities/capacity.

FUTURE DIRECTIONS IN IMAGING RESEARCH

Neuroimaging research has taught us that patients with schizophrenia have reduced brain volumes and has provided us with information about the genetic and environmental effects on the brain and about the neurobiology of symptoms in schizophrenia. Neuroimaging findings further suggest anomalies in neurodevelopmental trajectory with different regions of the brain being affected at the various stages of the illness. Longitudinal MRI studies are needed with subjects who carry a high risk for schizophrenia and (life) long follow-up periods. Genes need to be studied that are relevant to brain maturation and, because it is not clear which brain abnormalities are specific for schizophrenia, comparative research (i.e., schizophrenia versus other psychiatric disorders) needs to be conducted. Last but not least, we need to examine the underlying active pathophysiological processes with new imaging techniques such as DTI, MTR, fMRI, and ultra high-field imaging, explaining the progressive brain-volume changes found in schizophrenia.

REFERENCES

1. Harrison PJ. The neuropathology of schizophrenia. A critical review of the data and their interpretation. Brain 1999 Apr; 122 (Pt 4): 593–624.
2. Liem JH. Family studies of schizophrenia: an update and commentary. Schizophr Bull 1980; 6(3): 429–55.
3. Johnstone EC, Crow TJ, Frith CD et al. Cerebral ventricular size and cognitive impairment in chronic schizophrenia. Lancet 1976 Oct; 2 (7992): 924–6.
4. Wright IC, Rabe-Hesketh S, Woodruff PW et al. Meta-analysis of regional brain volumes in schizophrenia. Am J Psychiatry 2000 Jan; 157(1): 16–25.
5. Gur RE, Keshavan MS, Lawrie SM. Deconstructing psychosis with human brain imaging. Schizophr Bull 2007 Jul; 33(4): 921–31. Epub 2007 Jun 4. Review. PMID: 17548845 (PubMed – indexed for MEDLINE).
6. Nelson MD, Saykin AJ, Flashman LA et al. Hippocampal volume reduction in schizophrenia as assessed by magnetic resonance imaging: a meta-analytic study (see comments). Arch Gen Psychiatry 1998 May; 55(5): 433–40.
7. Steen RG, Mull C, McClure R et al. Brain volume in first-episode schizophrenia: systematic review and meta-analysis of magnetic resonance imaging studies. Br J Psychiatry 2006 Jun; 188; 510–8.
8. Weinberger DR, Egan MF, Bertolino A et al. Prefrontal neurons and the genetics of schizophrenia. Biol Psychiatry 2001 Dec; 50(11): 825–44.

9. Gottesman II, Erlenmeyer-Kimling L. Family and twin strategies as a head start in defining prodromes and endophenotypes for hypothetical early-interventions in schizophrenia. Schizophr Res 2001 Aug; 51(1): 93–102.

10. Cardno AG, Marshall EJ, Coid B et al. Heritability estimates for psychotic disorders: the Maudsley twin psychosis series. Arch Gen Psychiatry 1999 Feb; 56 (2): 162–8.

11. Lieberman JA. Is schizophrenia a neurodegenerative disorder? A clinical and neurobiological perspective. Biol Psychiatry 1999 Sep; 46(6): 729–39.

12. Hulshoff Pol HE, Schnack HG, Bertens MG et al. Volume changes in gray matter in patients with schizophrenia. Am J Psychiatry 2002 Feb; 159(2): 244–50.

13. Hulshoff Pol HE, Schnack HG, Mandl RC et al. Focal gray matter density changes in schizophrenia. Arch Gen Psychiatry 2001 Dec; 58(12): 1118–25.

14. Hulshoff Pol HE, Schnack HG, Mandl RC et al. Focal white matter density changes in schizophrenia: reduced inter-hemispheric connectivity. Neuroimage 2004 Jan; 21(1): 27–35.

15. Wood SJ, Pantelis C, Velakoulis D et al. Progressive changes in the development toward schizophrenia: studies in subjects at increased symptomatic risk. Schizophr Bull 2008 Mar; 34(2): 322–9.

16. Cahn W, Hulshoff Pol HE, Bongers M et al. Brain morphology in antipsychotic-naive schizophrenia: a study of multiple brain structures. Br J Psychiatry Suppl 2002 Sep; 43: s66–s72.

17. Pantelis C, Yucel M, Wood SJ et al. Structural brain imaging evidence for multiple pathological processes at different stages of brain development in schizophrenia. Schizophr Bull 2005 Jul; 31(3): 672–96.

18. Hulshoff Pol HE, Kahn RS. What happens after the first episode? A review of progressive brain changes in chronically ill patients with schizophrenia. Schizophr Bull 2008 Mar; 34(2): 354–66.

19. Cahn W, Hulshoff Pol HE, Lems EB et al. Brain volume changes in first-episode schizophrenia: a 1-year follow-up study. Arch Gen Psychiatry 2002 Nov; 59(11): 1002–10.

20. Kasai K, Shenton ME, Salisbury DF et al. Progressive decrease of left Heschl gyrus and planum temporale gray matter volume in first-episode schizophrenia: a longitudinal magnetic resonance imaging study. Arch Gen Psychiatry 2003 Aug; 60(8): 766–75.

21. Giedd JN, Blumenthal J, Jeffries NO et al. Brain development during childhood and adolescence: a longitudinal MRI study. Nat Neurosci 1999 Oct; 2(10): 861–3.

22. van Haren NE, Hulshoff Pol HE, Schnack HG et al. Progressive brain volume decrease across the course of the illness in schizophrenia: a 5-year follow-up MRI study. Biol Psychiatry 2008 Jan; 63(1): 106–13.

23. Baare WF, van Oel CJ, Hulshoff Pol HE et al. Volumes of brain structures in twins discordant for schizophrenia. Arch Gen Psychiatry 2001 Jan; 58(1): 33–40.

24. Boos HB, Aleman A, Cahn W et al. Brain volumes in relatives of patients with schizophrenia: a meta-analysis. Arch Gen Psychiatry 2007 Mar; 64(3): 297–304.

25. Brans RG, van Haren NE; Baal CM et al. Heritability of brain volume changes over time in twin pairs discordant for schizophrenia. Arch Gen Psychiatry, In press.

26. van Haren NE, Bakker SC, Kahn RS. Genes and structural brain imaging in schizophrenia. Curr Opin Psychiatry 2008 Mar; 21(2): 161–7.

27. Stefanis N, Frangou S, Yakeley J et al. Hippocampal volume reduction in schizophrenia: effects of genetic risk and pregnancy and birth complications. Biol Psychiatry 1999 Sep; 46 (5): 697–702.

28. van Erp TG, Saleh PA, Rosso IM et al. Contributions of genetic risk and fetal hypoxia to hippocampal volume in patients with schizophrenia or schizoaffective disorder, their unaffected siblings, and healthy unrelated volunteers. Am J Psychiatry 2002 Sep; 159(9): 1514–20.

29. Cannon TD, van Erp TG, Rosso IM et al. Fetal hypoxia and structural brain abnormalities in schizophrenic patients, their siblings, and controls. Arch Gen Psychiatry 2002 Jan; 59(1): 35–41.

30. Zammit S, Allebeck P, Andreasson S et al. Self reported cannabis use as a risk factor for schizophrenia in Swedish conscripts of 1969: historical cohort study. BMJ 2002 Nov; 325 (7374): 1199.
31. Cahn W, Hulshoff Pol HE, Caspers E et al. Cannabis and Brain Morphology in Recent-onset Schizophrenia. Schizophr Res 2004; 67: 305–7.
32. Rais M, Cahn W, van Haren NE et al. Excessive brain volume loss over time in cannabis-using first-episode schizophrenia patients. Am J Psychiatry 2008 Apr; 165(4): 490–6.
33. Marcelis M, Cavalier E, Gielen J et al. Abnormal response to metabolic stress in schizophrenia: marker of vulnerability or acquired sensitization? Psychol Med 2004 Aug; 34(6): 1103–11.
34. Pajonk F, Wobrock T, Gruber O et al. Hippocampal plasticity in response to exercise in schizophrenia. Arch Gen Psychiatry, in press.
35. Selten JP, Veen N, Feller W et al. Incidence of psychotic disorders in immigrant groups to The Netherlands. Br J Psychiatry 2001 Sep; 178: 367–72.
36. Gur RE, Cowell PE, Turetsky BI et al. A follow-up magnetic resonance imaging study of schizophrenia. Relationship of neuroanatomical changes to clinical and neurobehavioral measures. Arch Gen Psychiatry 1998 Feb; 55(2):145–52.
37. Madsen AL, Karle A, Rubin P et al. Progressive atrophy of the frontal lobes in first-episode schizophrenia: interaction with clinical course and neuroleptic treatment. Acta Psychiatr Scand 1999 Nov; 100(5): 367–74.
38. Chakos MH, Lieberman JA, Bilder RM et al. Increase in caudate nuclei volumes of first-episode schizophrenic patients taking antipsychotic drugs. Am J Psychiatry 1994 Oct; 151 (10): 1430–6.
39. Scheepers FE, de Wied CC, Hulshoff Pol HE et al. The effect of clozapine on caudate nucleus volume in schizophrenic patients previously treated with typical antipsychotics. Neuropsychopharmacology 2001 Jan; 24(1): 47–54.
40. Lieberman JA, Tollefson GD, Charles C et al. Antipsychotic drug effects on brain morphology in first-episode psychosis. Arch Gen Psychiatry 2005 Apr; 62(4): 361–70.
41. van Haren NE, Hulshoff Pol HE, Schnack HG et al. Focal gray matter changes in schizophrenia across the course of the illness: a 5-year follow-up study. Neuropsychopharmacology 2008 Apr; 18 (4): 312–5.
42. DeLisi LE. The concept of progressive brain change in schizophrenia: implications forunderstanding schizophrenia. Schizophr Bull 2008 Mar; 34(2): 312–21.
43. Cahn W, Rais M, Stigter FP et al. Psychosis and brain volume changes during the first five years of schizophrenia. European Neurpsychoparmacology, in press.
44. Gur RE, Cowell PE, Latshaw A et al. Reduced dorsal and orbital prefrontal gray matter volumes in schizophrenia. Arch Gen Psychiatry 2000 Aug; 57(8): 761–8.
45. Kurachi M. Pathogenesis of schizophrenia: Part I. Symptomathology, cognitive characteristics and brain morphology. Psychiatry and Clin Neurosci 2003 Feb; 57(1): 3–8.
46. McGlashan TH. Is active psychosis neurotoxic? Schizophr. Bull 2006 Oct; 32(4): 609–13.
47. Seok Jeong B, Kwon JS, Yoon Kim S et al. Functional imaging evidence of the relationship between recurrent psychotic episodes and neurodegenerative course in schizophrenia. Psychiatry Res 2005 Aug; 139(3): 219–28.
48. Antonova E, Sharma T, Morris R et al. The relationship between brain structure and neurocognition in schizophrenia: a selective review. Schizophr Res Review 2004 Oct; 70(2–3): 117–45.
49. van Haren NE, Cahn W, Hulshoff Pol HE et al. Brain volumes as predictor of outcome in recent-onset schizophrenia: a multi-center MRI study. Schizophr Res 2003 Nov; 64(1): 41–52.
50. Cahn W, van Haren NE, Hulshoff Pol HE et al. Brain volume changes in the first year of illness and 5-year outcome of schizophrenia.Br J Psychiatry 2006 Oct; 189: 381–2.

11 | Biochemical alterations in schizophrenia

Birte Yding Glenthoj, Lars V Kristiansen, Hans Rasmussen, and Bob Oranje

BIOCHEMICAL ALTERATIONS IN SCHIZOPHRENIA

Most candidate genes for schizophrenia are either directly or indirectly related to neural plasticity, synaptogenesis, or transmitter function within brain circuits that are involved in information processing (for review, see 1, 2). In accordance, multiple neurotransmitters have been implicated in the disturbances in early information processing and higher cognitive functions that are believed to constitute core features in schizophrenia. These disturbances are primarily genetically determined and considered to be important markers for the disease (see Chapter 2.6). They are also believed to predispose for development of positive and/or negative schizophrenic symptoms (3–6) and are, therefore, central for most (neurochemical) hypotheses for schizophrenia. Given the heterogenic character of the disease, different transmitter systems within different brain loops are likely to be involved in different patients. In addition, it is important to keep in mind that the disturbances observed in the patients might be secondary adaptive changes to primary dysfunctions. Nevertheless, an abundant literature has demonstrated transmitter disturbances in patients with schizophrenia, and pharmacological treatment is the cornerstone for all other interventions in this disease. In the following, we will describe the systems that most constantly have been found altered in schizophrenia (Table 11.1).

TABLE 11.1 Transmitter systems in schizophrenia

| Transmitter | Receptors in CNS | | Examples of proven or potential mechanisms for treatment of schizophrenia |
	Receptors	Mechanism	
Dopamine	D1, D5 "*D1-like*"	GPCR	D2 antagonism (typical and atypical neuroleptics), D3 enhancement (PFC).
	D2, D3, D4 "*D2-like*"	GPCR	
Serotonin	5-HT$_{1, 2, 4, 5, 6, 7}$	GPCR	5-HT$_{2A}$ modulation by most atypica neuroleptics, combined 5-HT$_{1A}$/D2 modulation.
Noradrenaline	α_1, α_2 and β		Several atypical neuroleptics interact with NE system (α_1 and $\alpha2$ antagonism).
Glutamate	NMDA	Ionotropic	D-serine, glycine, mGluR2-3 agonist
	AMPA	Ionotropic	(LY2140023),
	Kainate	onotropic	Ampakines, mGluR5 agonists,
	MGluR1-8	GPCR	
GABA	GABA$_A$	Ionotropic	GABA$_{\alpha2}$ receptor subunit agonist (MK-0777)
	GABA$_B$	GPCR	

DOPAMINE

The brain dopaminergic system has been in focus in schizophrenia research for nearly half a century. Dopamine (DA) receptors are divided into a D_1-like family (D_1 and D_5 receptors) and a D_2-like family (D_2, D_3, and D_4 receptors) (7–10). They are G-protein-linked receptors, meaning that they do not, like fast responding receptors, directly gate ion channels. Instead, stimulation of the receptor induces a cascade of intracellular events whereby DA modulates the neuron's response to other transmitter systems or induces long-term changes in synaptic plasticity. The latter might be of importance for development of dopaminergic sensitization (see later). Especially DA D_2 receptors have been implicated in the pathophysiology of schizophrenia. All presently used antipsychotic drugs are D_2 antagonists. These receptors are found in high concentrations in the basal ganglia and in much lower concentrations in extrastriatal areas such as the thalamus, the temporolimbic region, and the frontal cortex. In addition to the postsynaptic D_2 receptors, there are also presynaptic D_2 autoreceptors. In this way, D_2 receptors regulate both DA release and DA-activated neuronal activity. The literature further supports involvement of D_1 receptors in aspects of schizophrenic symptomathology. These receptors are likewise found in high concentrations in the striatum. In addition, D_1 receptors are distributed in cortical areas, including the prefrontal cortex (PFC). In addition, data suggest a possible involvement of D_3 and D_4 receptors in schizophrenia. However, these findings are more conflicting and will not be discussed further here.

Dopamine pathways

The dopaminergic projections in the brain were originally divided into the nigrostriatal, the mesolimbic, the mesocortical, and the tuberoinfundibular pathways (11). In addition, a more complex dopaminergic thalamic pathway also exists. Especially the mesolimbic and the mesocortical systems, and also the thalamic dopaminergic system (12) have been implicated in the pathophysiology of schizophrenia. The mesolimbic pathway projects from dopaminergic cell bodies in the ventral tegmental area (VTA) to limbic structures, such as the nucleus accumbens in the ventral striatum, amygdala, and hippocampus, whereas the mesocortical system projects from cell bodies in the VTA to cortical regions, including PFC. The mesolimbic system is associated with motivation and reward mechanisms and has also been linked to development of positive symptoms (13, 14). The mesocortical system has primarily been related to cognitive and negative symptoms.

Dopamine hypotheses of schizophrenia

The classical DA hypothesis for schizophrenia suggested that schizophrenia was the result of increased DA activity in the brain (15, 16). This hypothesis was supported by numerous studies demonstrating a relationship between affinity for striatal DA D_2 receptors and antipsychotic effect (17, 18) and by the psychotogenic effect of DA-enhancing compounds (19, 20). Postmortem measurements of DA receptor densities have generally reported increases in DA receptors in the basal ganglia in patients with schizophrenia, but these changes are most likely a consequence of an adaptive upregulation of receptors following previous treatment with DA blockers. Most imaging studies (PET or SPECT) of unmedicated or antipsychotic-naïve patients have not reported significant elevations of D_2 receptors in the striatum. Laruelle (21) did, however, in a meta-analysis observe a small but significant increase in D2 density. However, upregulation of D_2 receptors does not necessarily indicate basal dopaminergic hyperactivity but, as suggested by Grace, is consistent with decreased tonic DA release in the striatum combined with episodic or phasic increased DA release (22). A basal subcortical hypoactivity combined with an episodic increase is also in agreement with sensitization of the subcortical dopaminergic system in schizophrenia as proposed previously (for review, see 4, 5, 23, 24). In addition, we have previously provided pre-clinical evidence for such a hypothesis, (25, 26) and one of the most robust findings in more recent clinical *in vivo* studies has been increased amphetamine-induced DA release in the striatum in patients compared to healthy controls (27).

Corticostriatal–thalamocortical macrocircuits

Disturbances in information processing are core features of the disease. Thus, neu-rochemical, structural, and functional disturbances have been found in numerous studies in the corticostriatal thalamocortical macrocircuits originally described by Alexander and collaborators (28, 29). These feed-back loops basically involve projec-tions from cortex to striatum (glutamatergic) to the globus pallidum (GABAergic), or SN pars reticulata, to the thalamus (GABAergic), and back to the cortex (glutamater-gic). They have been functionally divided into parallel prefrontal, limbic, occulomotor, and motor loops that connect specific areas of cortex with specific regions in stria-tum and thalamus (28). These functional loops are further modulated by input from hippocampus and amygdala, dopaminergic cells in the VTA and striatum, cortical modulation of VTA, and by other cortical regions (30–32). Dysfunction in the flow of information in any of these loops or their connections can theoretically lead to devel-opment of schizophrenic symptoms. Carlsson was the first to propose a revised DA hypothesis for schizophrenia based on transmitter disturbances in these corticostriatal–thalamocortical macrocircuits (33). Carlsson suggested that either cortical glutamater-gic hypoactivity or subcortical dopaminergic hyperactivity could result in an overload of information, thus limiting the ability to gate this information. The latter would then lead to positive psychotic symptoms. This hypothesis was later extended to include other transmitter systems, including the dopaminergic, glutamatergic and GABAergic systems such as the cholinergic, noradrenergic, and serotonergic systems (3) and has furthermore subsequently been adapted and modified. As an example, we have, pro-posed a modified filter hypothesis for progressive dopaminergic sensitization based on primary a (glutamatergic) dysfunction in these circuits (4, 25, 26). Because increased DA release in relation to psychotic episodes or environmental stress, including expo-sure to many simultaneous stimuli, most likely will add to a progressive endogenous sensitization, this hypothesis emphasizes the importance of early intervention and protecting patients from environmental stressors.

Frontal microcircuits

Countless studies have confirmed significant interaction between cortical and sub-cortical DA activity and also pointed to a key role of DA activity in frontal microcir-cuits for schizophrenic symptomatology (see 34). In addition to the above described macrocircuits, which gate the flow of information to the cortex, microcircuits within the frontal cortex are believed to regulate the representation of information within the frontal networks. Seamans and Yang have proposed a so-called *two-state dynamic model of DA function in PFC9 (35)*. According to this model, predominant D_1 receptor activity results in increased inhibition of incoming stimuli, that is, closure of the gate and stabilization of selected goal-related activity associated with working memory. In this way D_1 activation enhances the robustness of the working memory. The authors call this dynamic State 2. Increased D_1 activity in PFC will, on the other hand, result in a narrowing of incoming stimuli. Accordingly, the network will be locked into encoding a single input, possibly leading to stereotyped thoughts and behavior. The authors suggest that such a deadlocked State 2 will initiate social isolation and lead to development of negative symptoms. Low D_1 activity, on the other hand, will have the opposite effect, that is, destabilization of State 2 causing premature termination of information in working memory prior to the completion of thoughts or actions. The model is in accordance with many preclinical and some clinical studies emphasizing the importance of frontal D_1 activity for working memory (36, 37).

Seamans and Yang (35) call the functional state with an open gate for State 1. In this state, D_2 activity predominates. The open gate allows multiple inputs to be represented in the network at the same time. State 1 is essential in order for the organism to receive sufficient stimuli, whereas a switch to State 2 is necessary to avoid contamination of information processing. Hence, Seamans and Yang propose that increased prefrontal D_2 receptor activity result in random, tangential, or intrusive thoughts and development of positive psychotic symptoms. We have recently provided the first clinical support for this model by demonstrating a significant correlation between frontal D_2 receptor binding in antipsychotic-naïve, first-episode schizophrenia patients (males) and positive psychotic symptoms (38). In addition, we observed a hemispheric imbalance in thalamic D_2 receptors. In addition, four other groups (39–42) have recently published similar data on extrastriatal D_2 receptors in antipsychotic-naïve, first-episode schizophrenia patients. Three of these studies similarly implicated changes in thalamic dopaminergic activity.

CONCLUSION DOPAMINE
One of the most robust findings in schizophrenia research has been a correlation between increased striatal DA release and psychosis. The literature further supports involvement of frontal D_1 and D_2 receptors in the development of positive and negative symptoms and cognitive disturbances. An increased disposition to episodic subcortical DA release is suggested to be the result of a (secondary) sensitization of the subcortical dopaminergic system. Cortical and subcortical DA systems interact with each other and with other transmitter systems, and subcortical changes in DA activity might be the result of glutamatergic and/or dopaminergic disturbances in cortical microcircuits as well as corticostriatal–thalamocortical macrocircuits.

SEROTONIN
During the 1950s, it was discovered that another monoamine neurotransmitter, serotonin (5-hydroxtryptamine, 5-HT), clinically had similar effects as lysergic acid diethylamide (LSD), a drug known to cause psychotic symptoms (43). This observation led to a hyper serotonin hypothesis of schizophrenia, which has mainly focused on the $5\text{-}HT_{2A}$ receptor subtype. The $5\text{-}HT_{2A}$ receptor has a wide distribution in the brain with a high density in cortical areas, lower density in the midbrain and thalamic areas, and very low expression in the cerebellum (44). Numerous studies have, either directly or via interactions with the dopaminergic system, implicated the $5\text{-}HT_{2A}$ receptor in the pathophysiology of schizophrenia (see4, 5, 45). According to the serotonin DA hypothesis, the unique feature of an atypical antipsychotic drug is its higher affinity for the $5\text{-}HT_{2A}$ receptor than to the D_2 receptor. This high $5\text{-}HT_{2A}$ affinity may account for the improved treatment effects of negative and cognitive symptoms as well as the

minimal extrapyramidal side effects. Neuroimaging studies show that during optimal dosing of atypical antipsychotic drugs, the occupancy of 5-HT$_{2A}$ receptors in the cortex far exceeds D$_2$ occupancy in the striatum (46, 47). These data are furthermore bolstered by a significant relationship between genetic variation in the 5-HT$_{2A}$ receptor gene and clinical response to clozapine (48, 49). Postmortem studies of brain tissue from schizophrenic patients suggest cortical serotonergic dysfunction. Eleven out of 15 postmortem studies report decreased 5-HT$_{2A/C}$ receptor expression in cortical areas, in particular in the frontal cortex (for references, see 50). However, these studies are, just like other postmortem studies, limited by confounders, for example, previous treatment with antipsychotic drugs, which likely decreases 5-HT$_{2A}$ receptor expression. Impairment in working memory is one of the central cognitive markers or endophenotypes of schizophrenia (51). Therefore, it is noteworthy that prefrontal 5-HT$_{2A}$ receptors also seem to be involved in working memory (52).

With the introduction of selective 5-HT$_{2A}$ receptor PET ligands, it is now possible to examine 5-HT$_{2A}$ receptor density in the living human brain and study how antipsychotic medication blocks these receptors. In antipsychotic-naïve schizophrenic patients, only a few PET studies of the 5-HT$_{2A}$ receptor have been carried out and the results are conflicting. Three PET studies found no difference in 5-HT$_{2A}$ binding between schizophrenic patients and healthy controls (53–55). One study on the other hand found decreased binding in the left lateral frontal cortex in schizophrenia (56). These studies are limited by small samples. Moreover, the ligands, [18F]setoperone and [11C]N-methylspiperone, which were used in these studies, have a relatively poor 5-HT$_{2A}$ receptor selectivity making them unsuitable for measuring subcortical 5-HT$_{2A}$ binding. The largest and most recent PET study, which used the highly selective ligand, [18F]altanserin analyzed both cortical and subcortical 5-HT$_{2A}$ binding in 15 drug-naïve schizophrenic patients (50) and found increased 5-HT$_{2A}$ receptor binding in the caudate nucleus. This finding indicates a direct or indirect role for striatal 5-HT$_{2A}$ receptors in the pathophysiology of schizophrenia. However, more research is warranted to clarify the role of 5-HT$_{2A}$ receptor activity with respect to psychopathology, information processing, and other neurobiological measures in large samples of antipsychotic-naive schizophrenic patients.

NORADRENALINE

Norepinephrine (noradrenaline) (NE) is synthesized from DA. In 1971, Stein and Wise (57) were the first to propose that this monoamine neurotransmitter was also involved in the pathophysiology of schizophrenia. Evidence for involvement of the noradrenergic system in schizophrenia has increased over the years (58–64). The initial noradrenergic hypothesis of schizophrenia proposed an increased noradrenergic transmission in schizophrenia, but recently a revision was proposed by Yamamoto and Hornykiewicz (65), which, similar to the revised DA hypothesis of schizophrenia, proposed that hyperactivity in the central noradrenergic system gives rise to the positive symptoms of schizophrenia, while hypoactivity leads to negative symptoms.

There are seven noradrenergic cell clusters in the central nervous system (CNS): In the brainstem, these are the lateral tegmental neurons and the locus coeruleus (LC). The LC, although consisting of only a small number of neurons, is the most widely projecting CNS nucleus known and is responsible for approximately 90% of the noradrenergic innervation in the forebrain and 70 % of the total NE in the brain (66). Currently, two superfamilies of adrenergic receptors have been identified (α and β), with three subfamilies: $α_1$, $α_2$ and β, with each consisting three receptor subtypes ($α_{1a}$, $α_{1b}$, $α_{1d}$; $α_{2a}$, $α_{2b}$, $α_{2c}$; $β_1$, $β_2$, $β_3$) (67). Whereas the $α_1$ and $α_2$ receptor families seem to be predominantly involved in cognition, the β_1 and β_2 receptors seem to be involved in regulation of emotional memory, while the β_3 receptors are not believed to be present in the CNS. The projections from the LC to PFC seem to be the most important for noradrenergic regulation of cognition: Moderate levels of NE seem to enhance PFC control of behavior, and hence increase cognition, whereas higher levels, caused by intense stress, seem to switch off PFC all together, and hence disrupt cognition (68). Based on this notion, Arnsten et al (69, 70) proposed a model in which the balance between α_1 and α_2 receptor activity of PFC plays an important role: Moderate NE levels activate α_2 receptors, which enhance PFC function, while higher levels of NE increasingly activate α_1 receptors, which impair PFC function. In this model, α_2 receptors are thought to be more sensitive to simulation with NE than α_1 receptors. Presumably, is the postsynaptic α_2 activity that is thought to improve PFC function and thus cognition, either directly (61, 71) or by stimulating DA (presumably D_1) output to PFC (72). PFC is involved in a large number of the previously mentioned information processing or cognitive markers for schizophrenia, for example, in executive functioning, working memory, attention, and sensory gating, and there is a vast amount of human and other primate literature providing evidence for noradrenergic modulation in all of these processes (73–78). It is, however, important to keep in mind that also the two previously described monoamine systems—not to say the glutamatergic system—likewise have a significant impact on these functions and that all the four systems interact with each other and with other transmitter systems, both in PFC and in the corticostriatal–thalamocortical circuits (3).

Many antipsychotics show affinity for noradrenergic receptors, but this is usually coincidental, and in one direction only: They block noradrenergic α_1 and/or α_2 receptors (72, 79). However, several researchers suggest that not only 5-HT_{2A} but also α_1– and/or α_2 receptors affinity is important for an antipsychotic compounds' "atypicality," that is, superior efficacy to treat both symptomatology and cognitive deficits in schizophrenia (72, 79, 80). According to the model of Arnsten et al (69, 70), reduction of α_1 activity deals with only one part of the problem, the stress-related hyperactivity of NA in CNS, which might partially restore cognition. Once the stress has been overcome, blockage of α_2 receptors in PFC due to antipsychotic treatment would still largely impair the PFC, and thus still impair cognition (61, 71). Indeed, in three studies in which schizophrenia patients were treated with a combination of antipsychotics and α_2 agonists, they improved with regards to both cognition and symptomatology (81–83).

GLUTAMATE

The importance of glutamate-mediated excitatory neurotransmission for normal brain function is illustrated by the ubiquitous expression of receptors for this neurotransmitter in the brain (84, 85). Several lines of evidence have implicated changes in glutamate signaling in the pathophysiology of schizophrenia. Clinical studies have found that administration of phencyclidine (PCP) or ketamine, both potent noncompetitive antagonists of the N-methyl-D-aspargine (NMDA) glutamate receptor, in normal individuals, induce behavioral changes that mimic positive, negative, and cognitive symptoms of schizophrenia. Consistent with these observations, and further indicating a central role for altered glutamate function in this illness, NMDA receptor antagonism was also found to worsen psychotic symptoms in patients with schizophrenia (86). Based on these clinical studies, a hypothesis for decreased glutamate-mediated signaling in schizophrenia has been formulated (87). The relation of disturbances in information processing to dysfunctional neurotransmission in PFC and in the corticostriatal–thalamocortical loops, hippocampus, and amygdala has previously been discussed. Due to the central importance of excitatory signaling by glutamatergic pyramidal neurons for flow of information in these circuits, it is obvious that dysfunctional glutamate signaling will have major implications for early information processing as well as higher cognitive functions, and hereby, for development of schizophrenic symptoms.

Besides NMDA receptors, glutamate function in the CNS is mediated by the ionotropic alpha-amino-3-hydroxy-5-methyl-4-isoxazolepropionic acid (AMPA) and kainate receptors as well as a group of G-protein-coupled metabotropic glutamate receptors (mGluRs) (88). At the ultrastructural level, synaptic transmission is controlled by expression of glutamate receptors in pre- and post-synaptic compartments as well as in glia cells, which collaborate to control synaptic functions such as presynaptic glutamate storage and release; mechanisms for glutamate reuptake, and integrated postsynaptic signaling (89). In the postsynaptic compartment, a complex structural network of receptor-associated proteins, termed the *postsynaptic density* (PSD), is centrally involved in regulating activity in the postsynaptic neuron. Furthermore, recent studies indicate that the PSD additionally could play an essential role in coordinating glutamate function with that of other neurotransmitters, including DA (90, 91).

Results from genetic and postmortem studies in patients with schizophrenia emphasize the complex nature of glutamate-related changes in schizophrenia (92–94). Studies in animal models have provided further insight into molecular aspects of positive, negative, and cognitive symptoms related to schizophrenia (95–97). Hence, recent studies indicate that NMDA receptors assembled from either of the two major subunits in PFC neurons, NR2A, or NR2B might functionally affect cellular signaling in opposing ways (98, 99). This, in turn, might help explain these receptor's differential roles in synaptic plasticity, which is the molecular correlate of learning and memory at the cellular level and which is severely compromised in schizophrenia (100). In particular, the NR2B-containing receptor, which in recent studies have been selectively associated with brain-derived neurotrophic factor (BDNF) signaling through the TrkB receptor as well as the NR2B-NMDA receptor's selective interaction with the Ca2+ calmodulin kinase II (CaMKII) in the postsynaptic neuron, might perform a central function as regulator of these cognitive processes (101, 102). Further studies are, however, needed to determine the role subunit-specific molecular interactions play in the pathophysiology of specific symptoms of schizophrenia.

Founded on the glutamate hypofunction hypothesis of schizophrenia, modulation of glutamate signaling by pharmaceutical targeting of glutamate receptors in the CNS has been proposed as a potent alternative strategy for treatment (103). Several attempts to enhance glutamate signaling in patients have involved administration of novel compounds with direct or indirect modulatory effects on AMPA and NMDA receptor function. These include ampakines (AMPA receptor interacting compounds) and different NMDA receptor coagonists and modulatory compounds (104–106). Although somewhat effective, these clinical trials unfortunately have not entirely had the expected therapeutic efficacy. However, in a recent clinical study, the compound LY2140023, which is an agonist of presynaptic mGluR2/3 receptors that regulate synaptic glutamate release, proved as effective as olanzapine in treating positive and negative symptoms in patients with schizophrenia (107). This proof-of-concept study, which was based on studies using animals to model different symptoms of schizophrenia, indicates an important clinical potential of targeting glutamate function in schizophrenia. Novel strategies based on subtype-specific receptor modulation, such as of the NR2B-NMDA receptor subunit, might help target symptoms that are currently not well treated, including negative and cognitive symptoms.

GABA

As the principal mediator of inhibitory signaling in the brain, the-aminobutyric acid (GABA) neurotransmitter plays an important role in control of neuronal activity in the CNS, in particular, as the primary modulator of cortical excitatory signaling(108). In inhibitory neurons, GABA is synthesized from glutamate by the L-Glutamic Acid Decaboxylase (GAD) enzyme, which exists as two major isoforms termed GAD67 and GAD65 (109). In inhibitory neurons, the GAD67 and GAD65 proteins, associated with distinct intracellular compartments, might have different functional regulation and contribute differentially to GABA synthesis (110, 111). Several studies have implicated altered GABA biosynthesis as a central component of the pathophysiology of schizophrenia (112). Hence, genetic linkage studies have found several GAD-associated loci linked to schizophrenia, and observations in postmortem brain have found decreased expression of GAD67 in schizophrenia (113). Decreased expression of GAD67 has furthermore been replicated in a ketamine-based animal model for schizophrenia, indicating that this biochemical change in GABA synthesis might be associated with altered glutamate signaling in PFC (114).

GABA neurotransmission is mediated by the ionotropic $GABA_A$ and $GABA_C$ receptors as well as the G-protein-coupled $GABA_B$ metabotropic receptor (115, 116). Whereas $GABA_C$ receptors are principally expressed in the retina, the $GABA_A$ and $GABA_B$ receptors are widely expressed throughout the CNS (117). The ligand-gated $GABA_A$ receptor is the target of several CNS-active compounds, including benzodiazepines. $GABA_A$ receptors are widely expressed in presynaptic nerve terminals, extrasynaptic areas, and axon-initial segments, where, through subunit-dependent and complex cellular regulatory mechanisms, mediate fast hyperpolarization of the postsynaptic neuron through its selective permeability to chloride ions (118, 119). The inhibitory $GABA_B$ receptor, which is expressed and function as a G-protein-coupled heterodimer assembled from the $GABA_{B1}$ and $GABA_{B2}$ receptor isoforms, is expressed in both pre- and post-synaptic neurons where it mediates slow synaptic inhibition (120, 121).

Altered inhibitory GABA function has been proposed to play a central role in the pathophysiology of schizophrenia (122). In particular, dysfunctional inhibition of excitatory neurons in PFC and hippocampus has been implicated as a mechanism that might be involved in dysfunction of cortical activity in schizophrenic patients (122, 123). Most postmortem studies have focused on changes in $GABA_A$ receptor expression. Hence, transcript expression for the different $GABA_A$ receptor subunits has been reported increased, decreased, or unaltered in cortex (124, 125), while muscimol binding and quantitative immunohistochemical analyses generally have indicated increased $GABA_A$ receptor expression in cortex (126–128). Such an increase likely could be secondary to decreased GABA synthesis.

In the cortical neuronal architecture, GABA neurons differ in their morphological, biochemical, and functional characteristics. Hence, based on biochemical and anatomical parameters, GABA neurons in cortex can be classified into three main groups that functionally exert different inhibitory control of cortical pyramidal neurons or other GABA neurons. At the molecular level, these functionally distinct classes of inhibitory neurons are differentiated by their selective expression of the Ca2+-binding proteins: parvalbumin (PV), calbindin, and calretinin (129). These biochemical differences in subclasses of inhibitory neurons have helped identify differential changes associated with select cortical inhibitory neurons in schizophrenia (130). Hence, expression of GAD67 was found to be selectively reduced in PV-positive GABA neurons, while expression of this enzyme in other neuronal inhibitory subtypes was not significantly altered (131). Due to the selective expression of PV in fast-spiking chandelier cells that preferentially provide inhibitory input to the axon-initial segments of pyramidal neurons, which regulate cortical gamma band activation, these data indicate an important role for altered inhibitory synchronization of integrated cortical activity in schizophrenia (132). Fine tuning of neuronal activity in PFC pyramidal cells is central for several types of cognition that are dysfunctional in schizophrenia (133). Furthermore, altered inhibitory function in corticolimbic circuits might additionally be involved in psychosis (134). Convergence of several neurotransmitter systems such as GABA, glutamate, and DA in regulation of cortical neuronal activity, therefore, indicate the importance of regulated PFC activity in higher brain functions with relevance to several symptoms of schizophrenia including cognition (134).

Recent genetic and biochemical studies have implicated altered signaling by the brain-derived growth factor (BDNF) in changes related to GAD67 expression in inhibitory PV-positive neurons and regulation of activity in PFC pyramidal neurons (135). In particular, altered expression of the BDNF receptor, TrkB, was found to be directly correlated with changes in GAD67 expression in PFC PV-GABA neurons in postmortem brain (136). This study indicates that this growth factor plays an essential role in cortical changes related to inhibitory signaling. As altered BDNF signaling might also underlie changes to excitatory cortical neurotransmission in schizophrenia, BDNF signaling appears as a key player in molecular changes that are associated with symptoms of higher cortical function (137, 138). Future molecular studies will help define such changes at the molecular level, and hopefully these studies can be translated into novel treatment strategies.

NCAM

The neural cell adhesion molecule NCAM is a differentially spliced transmembrane neural protein that is expressed in the CNS as three main isoforms of 120, 140, and 180 kDaltons (139). NCAM performs key functions during neurogenesis and is furthermore involved in the molecular synaptic events that modulate the synaptic changes that mediate learning and memory (140). Besides alternative splicing, posttranslational modification by polysialic acid (PSA) drastically influences normal NCAM functions, which involve specific protein–protein interactions and regulation of several downstream signaling pathways (141).

Due to its role in normal brain development and neural plasticity, altered NCAM function has been proposed to play a role in the pathophysiology of schizophrenia (142). Allelic variation of the NCAM gene and altered expression of different NCAM isoforms in the CNS has been reported in schizophrenia (143–146). NCAM function, in part, involves activation of the fibroblastic growth factor receptor (FGFR) (141, 147). This interaction is highly dependent on PSA modification of NCAM, which changes its conformation to allow direct binding of FGFR (148). Several studies have linked NMDA receptor activity with PSA-NCAM-induced plasticity (149–152). Interestingly, PSA-NCAM has also been proposed as an important regulator of cognitive functions that are altered in schizophrenia (153). Hence, in a recent study, the PSA-dependent interaction with FGFR in hippocampal slices was shown to exclusively involve a particular subtype of the NMDA receptor that is involved in specific functions related to cognition (154). In addition, altered NCAM functional expression and modification by PSD during development has been proposed to mediate lasting functional changes in PV-positive GABA inhibitory neurons that regulate cortical function (113, 155). The cause of altered PSA modification of NCAM in schizophrenia is not known; however, based on genetic evidence, it might involve genetic variation in the gene that encode the enzyme sialyltransterase, which is responsible for PSA transfer to NCAM (156, 157). Combined, these studies, therefore, indicate a possible involvement of NCAM in specific molecular events that regulate synaptic function in neurons of the prefrontal cortex (PFC) (142, 158). Combined, these studies provide evidence linking development of the nervous system at the molecular level with synaptic plasticity, excitatory, and inhibitory cortical function and, therefore, important clues in understanding the biochemical changes associated with schizophrenia.

CONCLUSION

Several brain transmitter systems are central for our understanding of the pathophysiological processes in schizophrenia. We have described several hypotheses that in our opinion are the most promising and/or best validated, but have, due to limited space, had to leave out other likewise relevant biochemical hypotheses involving, among others, the cholinergic system; cannabinoid receptors; histamine; peptide neurotransmitters such as neurokinin, neurotensin, and cholecystokinin; and nitric oxide—not to say potential disturbances in a vast number of tropic factors and intracellular processes. The latter we have only very briefly touched upon, but they will, no doubt, increased attention in the future. Also, we would like to mention the alpha-7-nicotine cholinergic receptor has been related to genetic transmission of one of the functional markers for schizophrenia; that is, deficits in sensory gating (P50 suppression) (159, 160) and nicotinic (161) as well as other cholinergic compounds are currently being tested in patients with schizophrenia.

REFERENCES

1. Harrison PJ, Weinberger DR. Schizophrenia genes within cortical neural circuits. Molecular Psychiatry 2005; 10(4): 420.
2. Harrison PJ, Weinberger DR. Schizophrenia genes, gene expression, and neuropathology: on the matter of their convergence. Mol Psychiatry 2005; 10(1): 40–68; image 5.
3. Carlsson A. The neurochemical circuitry of schizophrenia. Pharmacopsychiatry 2006; 39: 4.
4. Glenthoj BY, Hemmingsen R. Transmitter dysfunction during the process of schizophrenia. Acta Psychiatr Scand Suppl 1999; 395: 105–12.
5. Glenthoj BY, Hemmingsen R. Dopaminergic sensitization: implications for the pathogenesis of schizophrenia. Prog Neuropsychopharmacol Biol Psychiatry 1997; 21(1): 23–46.
6. Geyer MA, Krebs-Thomson K, Braff DL, Swerdlow NR. Pharmacological studies of prepulse inhibition models of sensorimotor gating deficits in schizophrenia: a decade in review. Psychopharmacology (Berl) 2001; 156(2–3): 117–54.
7. Sokoloff P, Giros B, Martres MP, Bouthenet ML, Schwartz JC. Molecular cloning and characterization of a novel dopamine receptor (D3) as a target for neuroleptics. Nature 1990; 347(6289): 146–51.
8. Sunahara RK, Guan HC, O'Dowd BF et al. Cloning of the gene for a human dopamine D5 receptor with higher affinity for dopamine than D1. Nature 1991; 350(6319): 614–9.
9. Tiberi M, Jarvie KR, Silvia C et al. Cloning, molecular characterization, and chromosomal assignment of a gene encoding a second D1 dopamine receptor subtype: differential expression pattern in rat brain compared with the D1A receptor. Proc Natl Acad Sci U S A 1991; 88(17): 7491–5.
10. Van Tol HH, Bunzow JR, Guan HC et al. Cloning of the gene for a human dopamine D4 receptor with high affinity for the antipsychotic clozapine. Nature 1991; 350(6319): 610–4.
11. Lindvall O, Bjorklund A, Skagerberg G. Dopamine-containing neurons in the spinal cord: anatomy and some functional aspects. Ann Neurol 1983; 14(3): 255–60.

12. Takahashi H, Higuchi M, Suhara T. The role of extrastriatal dopamine D2 receptors in schizophrenia. Biol Psychiatry 2006; 59(10): 919–28.
13. Kapur S, Mizrahi R, Li M. From dopamine to salience to psychosis–linking biology, pharmacology and phenomenology of psychosis. Schizophr Res 2005; 79(1): 59–68.
14. Kapur S, Mamo D. Half a century of antipsychotics and still a central role for dopamine D2 receptors. Prog Neuropsychopharmacol Biol Psychiatry 2003; 27(7): 1081–90.
15. Carlsson A. Antipsychotic drugs and catecholamine synapses. J Psychiatr Res 1974; 11: 57–64.
16. Carlsson A, Lindqvist M. Effect of Chlorpromazine or Haloperidol on Formation of 3methoxytyramine and Normetanephrine in Mouse Brain. Acta pharmacologica et toxicologica 1963; 20: 140–4.
17. Seeman P, Lee T, Chau-Wong M, Wong K. Antipsychotic drug doses and neuroleptic/dopamine receptors. Nature 1976; 261(5562): 717–9.
18. Farde L, Wiesel FA, Halldin C, Sedvall G. Central D2-dopamine receptor occupancy in schizophrenic patients treated with antipsychotic drugs. Arch Gen Psychiatry 1988; 45(1): 71–6.
19. Randrup A, Munkvad I. Pharmacology and physiology of stereotyped behavior. J Psychiatr Res 1974; 11: 1–10.
20. Lieberman JA, Kinon BJ, Loebel AD. Dopaminergic mechanisms in idiopathic and drug-induced psychoses. Schizophr Bull 1990; 16(1): 97–110.
21. Laruelle M. Imaging dopamine transmission in schizophrenia. A review and meta-analysis. Q J Nucl Med 1998; 42(3): 211–21.
22. Grace AA. Phasic versus tonic dopamine release and the modulation of dopamine system responsivity: a hypothesis for the etiology of schizophrenia. Neuroscience 1991; 41(1): 1–24.
23. Glenthoj BY. The brain dopaminergic system. Pharmacological, behavioural and electrophysiological studies. Dan Med Bull 1995; 42(1): 1–21.
24. Laruelle M, Abi-Dargham A. Dopamine as the wind of the psychotic fire: new evidence from brain imaging studies. J Psychopharmacol 1999; 13(4): 358–71.
25. Glenthoj B, Mogensen J, Laursen H, Holm S, Hemmingsen R. Electrical sensitization of the meso-limbic dopaminergic system in rats: a pathogenetic model for schizophrenia. Brain Res 1993; 619(1–2): 39–54.
26. Glenthoj BY, Mogensen J, Laursen H, Hemmingsen R. Dopaminergic sensitization of rats with and without early prefrontal lesions: implications for the pathogenesis of schizophrenia. Int J Neuropsychopharmcol 1999; 2(4): 271–81.
27. Laruelle M. The role of endogenous sensitization in the pathophysiology of schizophrenia: implications from recent brain imaging studies. Brain Res Brain Res Rev 2000; 31(2-3): 371–84.
28. Alexander GE, Crutcher MD, DeLong MR. Basal ganglia-thalamocortical circuits: parallel substrates for motor, oculomotor, "prefrontal" and "limbic" functions. Prog Brain Res 1990; 85: 119–46.
29. Alexander GE, DeLong MR, Strick PL. Parallel organization of functionally segregated circuits linking basal ganglia and cortex. Annu Rev Neurosci 1986; 9: 357–81.
30. Grace AA. Gating of information flow within the limbic system and the pathophysiology of schizophrenia. Brain Res Brain Res Rev 2000; 31(2–3): 330–41.
31. Grace AA, Moore H, O'Donnell P. The modulation of corticoaccumbens transmission by limbic afferents and dopamine: a model for the pathophysiology of schizophrenia. Adv Pharmacol 1998; 42: 721–4.
32. Rosenkranz JA, Grace AA. Cellular mechanisms of infralimbic and prelimbic prefrontal cortical inhibition and dopaminergic modulation of basolateral amygdala neurons in vivo. J Neurosci 2002; 22(1): 324–37.
33. Carlsson A. The current status of the dopamine hypothesis of schizophrenia. Neuropsychopharmacology 1988; 1(3): 179–86.

34. Winterer G, Weinberger DR. Genes, dopamine and cortical signal-to-noise ratio in schizophrenia. Trends Neurosci 2004; 27(11): 683–90.
35. Seamans JK, Yang CR. The principal features and mechanisms of dopamine modulation in the prefrontal cortex. Prog Neurobiol 2004; 74(1): 1–58.
36. Abi-Dargham A, Mawlawi O, Lombardo I et al. Prefrontal dopamine D1 receptors and working memory in schizophrenia. J Neurosci 2002; 22(9): 3708–19.
37. Goldman-Rakic PS, Castner SA, Svensson TH, Siever LJ, Williams GV. Targeting the dopamine D1 receptor in schizophrenia: insights for cognitive dysfunction. Psychopharmacology (Berl) 2004; 174(1): 3–16.
38. Glenthoj BY, Mackeprang T, Svarer C et al. Frontal dopamine D(2/3) receptor binding in drug-naive first-episode schizophrenic patients correlates with positive psychotic symptoms and gender. Biol Psychiatry 2006; 60(6): 9.
39. Yasuno F, Suhara T, Okubo Y et al. Low dopamine d(2) receptor binding in subregions of the thalamus in schizophrenia. Am J Psychiatry 2004; 161(6): 1016–22.
40. Talvik M, Nordstrom AL, Olsson H, Halldin C, Farde L. Decreased thalamic D2/D3 receptor binding in drug-naive patients with schizophrenia: a PET study with [11C]FLB 457.Int J Neuropsychopharmacol 2003; 6(4): 361–70.
41. Buchsbaum MS, Christian BT, Lehrer DS et al. D2/D3 dopamine receptor binding with [F-18]fallypride in thalamus and cortex of patients with schizophrenia. Schizophr Res 2006; 85(1–3): 232–44.
42. Tuppurainen H, Kuikka J, Viinamaki H et al. Extrastriatal dopamine D 2/3 receptor density and distribution in drug-naive schizophrenic patients. Mol Psychiatry 2003; 8(4): 453–5.
43. Gaddum JH, Hameed KA. Drugs which antagonize 5-hydroxytryptamine. British journal of pharmacology and chemotherapy 1954; 9(2): 240–8.
44. Adams KH, Pinborg LH, Svarer C et al. A database of [(18)F]-altanserin binding to 5-HT(2A) receptors in normal volunteers: normative data and relationship to physiological and demographic variables. Neuroimage 2004; 21(3): 1105–13.
45. Meltzer HY, Li Z, Kaneda Y, Ichikawa J. Serotonin receptors: their key role in drugs to treat schizophrenia. Prog Neuropsychopharmacol Biol Psychiatry 2003; 27(7): 1159–72.
46. Farde L, Nyberg S, Oxenstierna G et al. Positron emission tomography studies on D2 and 5-HT2 receptor binding in risperidone-treated schizophrenic patients. J Clin Psychopharmacol 1995; 15(1 Suppl 1): 19S–23S.
47. Kapur S, Zipursky RB, Remington G et al. 5-HT2 and D2 receptor occupancy of olanzapine in schizophrenia: a PET investigation. Am J Psychiatry 1998; 155(7): 921–8.
48. Arranz MJ, Munro J, Sham P, et al. Meta-analysis of studies on genetic variation in 5-HT2A receptors and clozapine response. Schizophr Res 1998; 32(2): 93–9.
49. Arranz MJ, Munro J, Owen MJ et al. Evidence for association between polymorphisms in the promoter and coding regions of the 5-HT2A receptor gene and response to clozapine. Mol Psychiatry 1998; 3(1): 61–6.
50. Erritzoe D, Rasmussen H, Kristiansen KT et al. Cortical and Subcortical 5-HT(2A) Receptor Binding in Neuroleptic-Naive First-Episode Schizophrenic Patients. Neuropsychopharmacology 2008.
51. Conklin HM, Curtis CE, Calkins ME, Iacono WG. Working memory functioning in schizophrenia patients and their first-degree relatives: cognitive functioning shedding light on etiology. Neuropsychologia 2005; 43(6): 930–42.
52. Williams GV, Rao SG, Goldman-Rakic PS. The physiological role of 5-HT2A receptors in working memory. J Neurosci 2002; 22(7): 2843–54.
53. Lewis R, Kapur S, Jones C et al. Serotonin 5-HT2 receptors in schizophrenia: a PET study using [18F]setoperone in neuroleptic-naive patients and normal subjects. Am J Psychiatry 1999; 156(1): 72–8.
54. Okubo Y, Suhara T, Suzuki K et al. Serotonin 5-HT2 receptors in schizophrenic patients studied by positron emission tomography. Life Sci 2000; 66(25): 2455–64.

55. Trichard C, Paillere-Martinot ML, Attar-Levy D et al. No serotonin 5-HT2A receptor density abnormality in the cortex of schizophrenic patients studied with PET. Schizophr Res 1998; 31(1): 13–7.

56. Ngan ET, Yatham LN, Ruth TJ, Liddle PF. Decreased serotonin 2A receptor densities in neuroleptic-naive patients with schizophrenia: A PET study using [(18)F]setoperone. Am J Psychiatry 2000; 157(6): 1016–8.

57. Stein L, Wise CD. Possible etiology of schizophrenia: progressive damage to the noradrenergic reward system by 6-hydroxydopamine. Science 1971; 171(975): 1032–6.

58. Farley IJ, Price KS, McCullough E et al. Norepinephrine in chronic paranoid schizophrenia: above-normal levels in limbic forebrain. Science 1978; 200(4340): 456–8.

59. Friedman JI, Temporini H, Davis KL. Pharmacologic strategies for augmenting cognitive performance in schizophrenia. Biol Psychiatry 1999; 45(1): 1–16.

60. Kaneko M, Honda K, Kanno T et al. Plasma free 3-methoxy-4-hydroxyphenylglycol in acute schizophrenics before and after treatment. Neuropsychobiology 1992; 25(3): 126–9.

61. Arnsten AF. Adrenergic targets for the treatment of cognitive deficits in schizophrenia. Psychopharmacology (Berl) 2004; 174(1): 25–31.

62. Lake CR, Kleinman JE, Kafka MS et al. Norepinephrine metabolism in schizophrenia. In: Henn FA, deLisi LE, eds. Neurochemistry and Neuropharamcology of Schizophrenia. New York Elsevier Science Publishing; 1987: 227.

63. Yamamoto K, Ozawa N, Shinba T, Hoshino T, Yoshii M. Possible noradrenergic dysfunction in schizophrenia. Brain Res Bull 1994; 35(5–6): 529–43.

64. Dajas F, Barbeito L, Martinez-Pesquera G et al. Plasma noradrenaline and clinical psychopathology in schizophrenia. A correlation analysis. Neuropsychobiology 1983; 10(2–3): 70–4.

65. Yamamoto K, Hornykiewicz O. Proposal for a noradrenaline hypothesis of schizophrenia. Prog Neuropsychopharmacol Biol Psychiatry 2004; 28(5): 913–22.

66. Szabo ST, Gould TD, Manji HK. Neurotransmitters, receptors, signal transduction, and second messengers in psychiatric doisorders. In: Schatzberg AF, Nemeroff CB, eds. Textbook of Psychopharmacology. 3 ed. Arlington: American Psychiatric publishing; 2004.

67. Hein L. [The alpha 2-adrenergic receptors: molecular structure and in vivo function]. Zeitschrift fur Kardiologie 2001; 90(9): 607–12.

68. Chamberlain SR, Muller U, Blackwell AD, Robbins TW, Sahakian BJ. Noradrenergic modulation of working memory and emotional memory in humans. Psychopharmacology (Berl) 2006; 188(4): 397–407.

69. Arnsten AF, Mathew R, Ubriani R, Taylor JR, Li BM. Alpha-1 noradrenergic receptor stimulation impairs prefrontal cortical cognitive function. Biol Psychiatry 1999; 45(1): 26–31.

70. Ramos BP, Arnsten AF. Adrenergic pharmacology and cognition: focus on the prefrontal cortex. Pharmacol Ther 2007; 113(3): 523–36.

71. Arnsten AF, Steere JC, Hunt RD. The contribution of alpha 2-noradrenergic mechanisms of prefrontal cortical cognitive function. Potential significance for attention-deficit hyperactivity disorder. Arch Gen Psychiatry 1996; 53(5): 448–55.

72. Svensson TH. Alpha-adrenoceptor modulation hypothesis of antipsychotic atypicality. Prog Neuropsychopharmacol Biol Psychiatry 2003; 27(7): 1145–58.

73. Li BM, Mao ZM, Wang M, Mei ZT. Alpha-2 adrenergic modulation of prefrontal cortical neuronal activity related to spatial working memory in monkeys. Neuropsychopharmacology 1999; 21(5): 601–10.

74. Coull JT, Nobre AC, Frith CD. The noradrenergic alpha2 agonist clonidine modulates behavioural and neuroanatomical correlates of human attentional orienting and alerting. Cereb Cortex 2001; 11(1): 73–84.

75. Jakala P, Sirvio J, Riekkinen M et al. Guanfacine and clonidine, alpha 2-agonists, improve paired associates learning, but not delayed matching to sample, in humans. Neuropsychopharmacology 1999; 20(2): 119–30.

76. Coull JT, Middleton HC, Robbins TW, Sahakian BJ. Contrasting effects of clonidine and diazepam on tests of working memory and planning. Psychopharmacology (Berl) 1995; 120(3): 311–21.
77. Jakala P, Riekkinen M, Sirvio J et al. Guanfacine, but not clonidine, improves planning and working memory performance in humans. Neuropsychopharmacology 1999; 20(5): 460–70.
78. Ma CL, Arnsten AF, Li BM. Locomotor hyperactivity induced by blockade of prefrontal cortical alpha2-adrenoceptors in monkeys. Biol Psychiatry 2005; 57(2): 192–5.
79. Friedman JI, Adler DN, Davis KL. The role of norepinephrine in the pathophysiology of cognitive disorders: potential applications to the treatment of cognitive dysfunction in schizophrenia and Alzheimer's disease. Biol Psychiatry 1999; 46(9): 1243–52.
80. Litman RE, Pickar D. Noradrenergic systems: A target for augmenting pharmacotherapy. In: Breier A, ed. The New Pharmacotherapy of Schizophrenia. Washington: American Psychiatric Pres; 1996: 133–52.
81. Maas JW, Miller AL, Tekell JL et al. Clonidine plus haloperidol in the treatment of schizophrenia/psychosis. J Clin Psychopharmacol 1995; 15(5): 361–4.
82. Friedman JI, Adler DN, Temporini HD et al. Guanfacine treatment of cognitive impairment in schizophrenia. Neuropsychopharmacology 2001; 25(3): 402–9.
83. van Kammen DP, Peters JL, van Kammen WB et al. Clonidine treatment of schizophrenia: can we predict treatment response? Psychiatry Res 1989; 27(3): 297–311.
84. Brose N, Gasic GP, Vetter DE, Sullivan JM, Heinemann SF. Protein chemical characterization and immunocytochemical localization of the NMDA receptor subunit NMDA R1. J Biol Chem 1993; 268(30): 22663–71.
85. Breese CR, Leonard SS. Glutamate receptor subtype expression in human postmortem brain. J Mol Neurosci 1993; 4(4): 263–75.
86. Lahti AC, Weiler MA, Tamara Michaelidis BA, Parwani A, Tamminga CA. Effects of ketamine in normal and schizophrenic volunteers. Neuropsychopharmacology 2001; 25(4): 455–67.
87. Coyle JT. The glutamatergic dysfunction hypothesis for schizophrenia. Harv Rev Psychiatry 1996; 3(5): 241–53.
88. Kew JN, Kemp JA. Ionotropic and metabotropic glutamate receptor structure and pharmacology. Psychopharmacology (Berl) 2005; 179(1): 4–29.
89. Takumi Y, Matsubara A, Rinvik E, Ottersen OP. The arrangement of glutamate receptors in excitatory synapses. Ann N Y Acad Sci 1999; 868: 474–82.
90. Hashimoto R, Tankou S, Takeda M, Sawa A. Postsynaptic density: a key convergent site for schizophrenia susceptibility factors and possible target for drug development. Drugs Today (Barc) 2007; 43(9): 645–54.
91. Gu WH, Yang S, Shi WX, Jin GZ, Zhen XC. Requirement of PSD-95 for dopamine D1 receptor modulating glutamate NR1a/NR2B receptor function. Acta Pharmacol Sin 2007; 28(6): 756–62.
92. Shibata H, Aramaki T, Sakai M et al. Association study of polymorphisms in the GluR7, KA1 and KA2 kainate receptor genes (GRIK3, GRIK4, GRIK5) with schizophrenia. Psychiatry Res 2006; 141(1): 39–51.
93. Collier DA, Li T. The genetics of schizophrenia: glutamate not dopamine? Eur J Pharmacol 2003; 480(1–3): 177–84.
94. Beneyto M, Kristiansen LV, McCullumsmith RE, Meador-Woodruff J. Glutamatergic mechanisms in schizophrenia. current psychosis and therapeutic reports 2006; 4: 27–33.
95. Rujescu D, Bender A, Keck M et al. A pharmacological model for psychosis based on N-methyl-D-aspartate receptor hypofunction: molecular, cellular, functional and behavioral abnormalities. Biol Psychiatry 2006; 59(8): 721–9.
96. Mouri A, Noda Y, Enomoto T, Nabeshima T. Phencyclidine animal models of schizophrenia: approaches from abnormality of glutamatergic neurotransmission and neurodevelopment. Neurochem Int 2007; 51(2–4): 173–84.

97. Pratt JA, Winchester C, Egerton A, Cochran SM, Morris BJ. Modellilng prefrontal cortex deficits in schizophrenia: implications for treatment. Br J Pharmacol 2008; 153(Suppl 1): 5.
98. Bartlett TE, Bannister NJ, Collett VJ et al. Differential roles of NR2A and NR2B-containing NMDA receptors in LTP and LTD in the CA1 region of two-week old rat hippocampus. Neuropharmacology 2007; 52(1): 60–70.
99. Chen Q, He S, Hu XL et al. Differential roles of NR2A- and NR2B-containing NMDA receptors in activity-dependent brain-derived neurotrophic factor gene regulation and limbic epileptogenesis. J Neurosci 2007; 27(3): 542–52.
100. Stephan KE, Baldeweg T, Friston KJ. Synaptic plasticity and dysconnection in schizophrenia. Biol Psychiatry 2006; 59(10): 929–39.
101. Zhou Y, Takahashi E, Li W et al. Interactions between the NR2B receptor and CaMKII modulate synaptic plasticity and spatial learning. J Neurosci 2007; 27(50): 13843–53.
102. Pillai A. Brain-derived neurotropic factor/TrkB signaling in the pathogenesis and novel pharmacotherapy of schizophrenia. Neurosignals 2008; 16(2–3): 183–93.
103. Tuominen HJ, Tiihonen J, Wahlbeck K. Glutamatergic drugs for schizophrenia: a systematic review and meta-analysis. Schizophr Res 2005; 72(2–3): 225–34.
104. Goff DC, Leahy L, Berman I et al. A placebo-controlled pilot study of the ampakine CX516 added to clozapine in schizophrenia. J Clin Psychopharmacol 2001; 21(5): 484–7.
105. Olsen CK, Kreilgaard M, Didriksen M. Positive modulation of glutamatergic receptors potentiates the suppressive effects of antipsychotics on conditioned avoidance responding in rats. Pharmacol Biochem Behav 2006; 84(2): 259–65.
106. Tsai GE, Yang P, Chang YC, Chong MY. D-alanine added to antipsychotics for the treatment of schizophrenia. Biol Psychiatry 2006; 59(3): 230–4.
107. Patil ST, Zhang L, Martenyi F et al. Activation of mGlu2/3 receptors as a new approach to treat schizophrenia: a randomized Phase 2 clinical trial. Nat Med 2007; 13(9): 1102–7.
108. Petroff OAC. GABA and glutamate in the human brain. The Neuroscientist 2002; 8(6): 11.
109. Pinal CS, Tobin AJ. Uniqueness and redundancy in GABA production. Perspect Dev Neurobiol 1998; 5(2–3): 109–18.
110. Martin DL, Rimvall K. Regulation of gamma-aminobutyric acid synthesis in the brain. J Neurochem 1993; 60(2): 395–407.
111. Martin DL, Barke KE. Are GAD65 and GAD67 associated with specific pools of GABA in brain? Perspect Dev Neurobiol 1998; 5(2–3): 119–29.
112. Blum BP, Mann JJ. The GABAergic system in schizophrenia. Int J Neuropsychopharmacol 2002; 5(2): 159–79.
113. Akbarian S, Huang HS. Molecular and cellular mechanisms of altered GAD1/GAD67 expression in schizophrenia and related disorders. Brain Res Rev 2006; 52(2): 293–304.
114. Zhang Y, Behrens M, Lisman JE. Prolonged Exposure to NMDAR Antagonist Suppresses Inhibitory Synaptic Transmission in Prefrontal Cortex. J Neurophysiol 2008.
115. Watanabe M, Maemura K, Kanbara K, Tamayama T, Hayasaki H. GABA and GABA receptors in the central nervous system and other organs. Int Rev Cytol 2002; 213: 1–47.
116. Enz R, Cutting GR. Molecular composition of GABAC receptors. Vision Res 1998; 38(10): 1431–41.
117. Mohler H, Knoflach F, Paysan J et al. Heterogeneity of GABAA-receptors: cell-specific expression, pharmacology, and regulation. Neurochem Res 1995; 20(5): 631–6.
118. Kullmann DM, Ruiz A, Rusakov DM et al. Presynaptic, extrasynaptic and axonal GABAA receptors in the CNS: where and why? Prog Biophys Mol Biol 2005; 87(1): 33–46.
119. Michels G, Moss SJ. GABAA receptors: properties and trafficking. Crit Rev Biochem Mol Biol 2007; 42(1): 3–14.
120. Huang ZJ. GABAB receptor isoforms caught in action at the scene. Neuron 2006; 50(4): 521–4.
121. Jones KA, Tamm JA, Craig DA Ph D, Yao W, Panico R. Signal transduction by GABA(B) receptor heterodimers. Neuropsychopharmacology 2000; 23(4 Suppl): S41–9.

122. Benes FM, Berretta S. GABAergic interneurons: implications for understanding schizophrenia and bipolar disorder. Neuropsychopharmacology 2001; 25(1): 1–27.
123. Braun I, Genius J, Grunze H et al. Alterations of hippocampal and prefrontal GABAergic interneurons in an animal model of psychosis induced by NMDA receptor antagonism. Schizophr Res 2007; 97(1–3): 254–63.
124. Ohnuma T, Augood SJ, Arai H, McKenna PJ, Emson PC. Measurement of GABAergic parameters in the prefrontal cortex in schizophrenia: focus on GABA content, GABA(A) receptor alpha-1 subunit messenger RNA and human GABA transporter-1 (HGAT-1) messenger RNA expression. Neuroscience 1999; 93(2): 441–8.
125. Akbarian S, Huntsman MM, Kim JJ et al. GABAA receptor subunit gene expression in human prefrontal cortex: comparison of schizophrenics and controls. Cereb Cortex 1995; 5(6): 550–60.
126. Deng C, Huang XF. Increased density of GABAA receptors in the superior temporal gyrus in schizophrenia. Exp Brain Res 2006; 168(4): 587–90. Epub 2005 Dec 16.
127. Dean B, Hussain T, Hayes W et al. Changes in serotonin2A and GABA(A) receptors in schizophrenia: studies on the human dorsolateral prefrontal cortex. J Neurochem 1999; 72(4): 1593–9.
128. Ishikawa M, Mizukami K, Iwakiri M, Hidaka S, Asada T. Immunohistochemical and immunoblot study of GABA(A) alpha1 and beta2/3 subunits in the prefrontal cortex of subjects with schizophrenia and bipolar disorder. Neurosci Res 2004; 50(1): 77–84.
129. Kawaguchi Y, Kubota Y. GABAergic cell subtypes and their synaptic connections in rat frontal cortex. Cereb Cortex 1997; 7(6): 476–86.
130. Conde F, Lund JS, Jacobowitz DM, Baimbridge KG, Lewis DA. Local circuit neurons immunoreactive for calretinin, calbindin D-28k or parvalbumin in monkey prefrontal cortex: distribution and morphology. J Comp Neurol 1994; 341(1): 95–116.
131. Volk DW, Austin MC, Pierri JN, Sampson AR, Lewis DA. Decreased glutamic acid decarboxylase67 messenger RNA expression in a subset of prefrontal cortical gamma-aminobutyric acid neurons in subjects with schizophrenia. Arch Gen Psychiatry 2000; 57(3): 237–45.
132. Lewis DA, Hashimoto T, Volk DW. Cortical inhibitory neurons and schizophrenia. Nat Rev Neurosci 2005; 6(4): 312–24.
133. Lewis DA, Hashimoto T. Deciphering the disease process of schizophrenia: the contribution of cortical gaba neurons. Int Rev Neurobiol 2007; 78: 109–31.
134. Daskalakis ZJ, Fitzgerald PB, Christensen BK. The role of cortical inhibition in the pathophysiology and treatment of schizophrenia. Brain Res Rev 2007; 56: 15.
135. Hashimoto T, Lewis DA. BDNF Val66Met polymorphism and GAD67 mRNA expression in the prefrontal cortex of subjects with schizophrenia. Am J Psychiatry 2006; 163(3): 534–7.
136. Hashimoto T, Bergen SE, Nguyen QL et al. Relationship of brain-derived neurotrophic factor and its receptor TrkB to altered inhibitory prefrontal circuitry in schizophrenia. J Neurosci 2005; 25(2): 372–83.
137. Lang UE, Puls I, Muller DJ, Strutz-Seebohm N, Gallinat J. Molecular mechanisms of schizophrenia. Cell Physiol Biochem 2007; 20(6): 687–702.
138. Crozier RA, Black IB, Plummer MR. Blockade of NR2B-containing NMDA receptors prevents BDNF enhancement of glutamatergic transmission in hippocampal neurons. Learn Mem 1999; 6(3): 257–66.
139. Reyes AA, Schulte SV, Small S, Akeson R. Distinct NCAM splicing events are differentially regulated during rat brain development. Brain Res Mol Brain Res 1993; 17(3–4): 201–11.
140. Panicker AK, Buhusi M, Thelen K, Maness PF. Cellular signalling mechanisms of neural cell adhesion molecules. Front Biosci 2003; 8: d900–11.
141. Hinsby AM, Berezin V, Bock E. Molecular mechanisms of NCAM function. Front Biosci 2004; 9: 2227–44.
142. Brennaman LH, Maness PF. NCAM in Neuropsychiatric and Neurodegenerative Disorders. Neurochem Res 2008.

143. Atz ME, Rollins B, Vawter MP. NCAM1 association study of bipolar disorder and schizophrenia: polymorphisms and alternatively spliced isoforms lead to similarities and differences. Psychiatr Genet 2007; 17(2): 55–67.

144. Barbeau D, Liang JJ, Robitalille Y, Quirion R, Srivastava LK. Decreased expression of the embryonic form of the neural cell adhesion molecule in schizophrenic brains. Proc Natl Acad Sci U S A 1995; 92(7): 2785–9.

145. Vawter MP. Dysregulation of the neural cell adhesion molecule and neuropsychiatric disorders. Eur J Pharmacol 2000; 405(1–3): 385–95.

146. Vawter MP, Frye MA, Hemperly JJ et al. Elevated concentration of N-CAM VASE isoforms in schizophrenia. J Psychiatr Res 2000; 34(1): 25–34.

147. Francavilla C, Loeffler S, Piccini D et al. Neural cell adhesion molecule regulates the cellular response to fibroblast growth factor. J Cell Sci 2007; 120(Pt24): 6.

148. Kiselyov VV, Soroka V, Berezin V, Bock E. Structural biology of NCAM homophillic binding and activation of FGFR. J Neurochem 2005; 94(5): 10.

149. sytnyk V, Leshchynska I, Nikonenko AG, Schachner M. NCAM promotes assembly and activity-dependent remodeling of the postsynaptic signaling complex. J Cell Biol 2006; 174(7): 1071–85.

150. Singh J, Kaur G. Neuroprotection mediated by subtoxic dose of NMDA in SH-SY5Y neuroblastoma cultures: activity-dependent regulation of PSA-NCAM expression. Brain Res Mol Brain Res 2005; 137(1–2): 223–34.

151. Dityatev A, Dityateva G, Sytnyk V et al. Polysialylated neural cell adhesion molecule promotes remodeling and formation of hippocampal synapses. J Neurosci 2004; 24(42): 9372–82.

152. Butler AK, Uryu K, Rougon G, Chesselet MF. N-methyl-D-aspartate receptor blockade affects polysialylated neural cell adhesion molecule expression and synaptic density during striatal development. Neuroscience 1999; 89(9): 1169–81.

153. Vicente AM, Macciardi F, Verga M et al. NCAM and schizophrenia: genetic studies. Mol Psychiatry 1997; 2(1): 65–9.

154. Hammond MS, Sims C, Parameshwaren K et al. Neural cell adhesion molecule-associated polysialic acid inhibits NR2B-Containing N-methyl-D-aspartate receptors and prevents glutamate-induced cell death. J Biol Chem 2006; 281(46): 34859–69.

155. Brennaman LH, Maness PF. Developmental regulation of GABAergic interneuron branching and synaptic development in the prefrontal cortex by soluble neural cell adhesion molecule. Mol Cell Neurosci 2008; 37(4): 781–93.

156. Arai M, Yamada K, Toyota T et al. Association between polymorphisms in the promoter region of the sialyltransferase 8B (SIAT8B) gene and schizophrenia. Biol Psychiatry 2006; 59(7): 652–9.

157. Muhlenhoff M, Eckhardt M, Bethe A, Frosch M, Gerardy-Schahn R. Polysialylation of NCAM by a single enzyme. Curr Biol 1996; 6(9): 1188–91.

158. Sullivan PF, Keefe RS, Lange LA et al. NCAM1 and neurocognition in schizophrenia. Biol Psychiatry 2007; 61(7): 902–10.

159. Olincy A, Harris JG, Johnson LL et al. Proof-of-concept trial of an alpha7 nicotinic agonist in schizophrenia. Arch Gen Psychiatry 2006; 63(6): 630–8.

160. Freedman R, Coon H, Myles-Worsley M et al. Linkage of a neurophysiological deficit in schizophrenia to a chromosome 15 locus. Proc Natl Acad Sci U S A 1997; 94(2): 587–92.

161. Freedman R, Olincy A, Buchanan RW et al. Initial Phase 2 Trial of a Nicotinic Agonist in Schizophrenia. Am J Psychiatry 2008.

Dopamine dysregulation in the brain network of decision-making: Can this explain the psychopathology of schizophrenia?

Seyed M Assadi, Murat Yücel, and Christos Pantelis

INTRODUCTION

Individuals need to continuously decide between two or more options in their everyday lives. Recent animal and human studies suggest that the dorsal anterior cingulate cortex (dACC) and its related subcortical structures are at the center of a brain network that makes such decisions (1–5). Decision making is a complex process and involves various elements such as analyzing different costs and benefits and their probabilities, taking account of previous outcomes, mobilizing resources, and processing different motor variables for pursuing the preferred option. Taken as a whole, however, it can be considered as a cycle of two general processes of evaluation and execution (Figure 12.1). Evaluation refers to all events that lead to a new decision. The process starts with exposure to a new set of options and ends in an overall preference. This includes cost-benefit analysis and outcome appraisal. Execution refers to all events that attempt to actualize the preference. Execution starts with an overall preference and ends with the attainment of the preferred option. This requires motivation to action and action sequencing. Recent studies have shown that the dACC and its related subcortical structures are involved in both evaluation and execution of decisions (4–8). Moreover, it seems that the dopamine system modulates this network at multiple levels to optimize both processes (5, 9). The present chapter reviews the abnormality of the decision-making network in schizophrenia to suggest that this disorder is associated with pervasive abnormalities in this network and its dopamine regulation. The review focuses on the dACC, basal ganglia, and thalamus. We then introduce a model that considers how the abnormal decision-making network can contribute to the psychopathology of schizophrenia.

ABNORMAL DECISION-MAKING NETWORK IN SCHIZOPHRENIA

DORSAL ANTERIOR CINGULATE

Gross Anomalies

Structural neuroimaging studies have shown that schizophrenia is associated with a reduction in dACC gray matter volume or thickness (10–18). The neuropathological studies have confirmed this reduction (19, 20). Some neuroimaging studies have suggested that these gray matter changes may be related to psychosis onset (21, 22), may progress over time (23–27), and extend from the upper tier of the dACC (28) toward the lower tier (18). However, some studies have not found these changes (29), and more longitudinal studies are warranted to investigate the precise changes in this region over the course of schizophrenia.

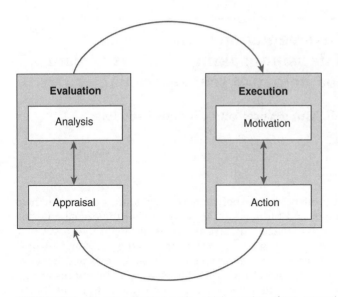

FIGURE 12.1 Decision-making cycle, which consists of two general processes. The first process is evaluation, which is comprised of analysis of cost and benefit and appraisal of pervious outcomes. Evaluation ends in an overall preference for one option over other competing options. The second process is execution of the preference and consists of motivation and action. Motivation refers to mobilization of resources and action to planning a sequence of movements to attain the chosen option. Execution ends in attaining the preferred option.

Functional Abnormality

Several functional neuroimaging studies have found abnormal activity of the dACC in individuals with schizophrenia during working-memory tasks (12, 30) as well as the tasks that are closely related to decision making. Further, dysmorphology of the dACC has been associated with abnormal performance on such tasks (31, 32). As suggested recently, the diverse roles attributed to the dACC might point toward the different elements of decision making; hence, some of the neuropsychological tests probably assess some aspects of this decision making (9). They include abnormal performance in the multisource interference task (33), stroop tasks (34–38), priming tasks (39), verbal fluency tasks (40), auditory oddball tasks (41), choice anticipation tasks (42), continuous performance tasks (43), and the random number generation task (44). Consistent with the findings above, an electrophysiological study found abnormal information processing in the dACC during an auditory choice reaction task (45). Almost all of the above-mentioned tasks are related to response selection, error monitoring, or executive control. Therefore, these studies provide some evidence that the activity of the dACC is abnormal in patients with schizophrenia during the evaluation or execution processes of decision making. However, further studies are required directly to assess decision making in patients with schizophrenia.

Abnormal Circuitry

Previous studies have provided evidence that the anterior cingulate cortex (ACC) is abnormal in schizophrenia both in intrinsic circuits (microcircuitry) and in its connections with other brain regions (macrocircuitry). At the microcircuit level, there is a significant neuronal reduction in the ACC. Magnetic resonance spectroscopy studies have suggested neuronal loss in the ACC (46), which appears more prominent in the dACC (47). Neuropathological studies have reported a reduction in the density of pyramidal neurons in layer IV (48, 49) and of interneurons in layer II (50, 51), with a compensatory increase in $GABA_A$ receptor binding activity in layers II and III (52). However, the changes related to the GABAergic interneurons are not specific to schizophrenia, and are also found in affective psychosis (53). At the macrocircuit level, studies have found increased glutamatergic fibers in layer II, which are believed to be afferent fibers originating from other brain regions (54). This is accompanied with an increase in NMDA and AMPA receptor binding in the same layer (55). These abnormally dense innervations have been proposed to selectively originate from either the basolateral amygdala (54) or the thalamus (56). These suggestions, however, should be directly tested. Diffusion tensor imaging studies have suggested a general disturbance in the white matter connectivity of the ACC with other brain regions (56–60). PET studies have also suggested such disconnections (61, 62).

Collectively, there is evidence that the connectivity between the ACC and other cortical and subcortical regions is disturbed in patients with schizophrenia. In addition, schizophrenia is accompanied by a nonspecific decrease in GABAergic interneurons and a specific increase in glutamatergic inputs in layer II. Further studies are required to replicate these findings in the dorsal portion of the ACC.

Dopamine Dysregulation

It has been suggested that dysfunction of the dACC in schizophrenia is linked to dopamine dysregulation because abnormal activation of the dACC in patients with schizophrenia during cognitive tasks can be improved by manipulation of dopaminergic transmission (40). Several studies have reported abnormal dopamine neurotransmission in the ACC of patients with schizophrenia. Most recent PET studies have found a significant decrease in D2 receptor binding in the ACC of drug-naïve patients (62–64). One study, however, failed to show this change (65). Decrease in D1 receptor binding has also been reported in the ACC (66, 67), though some studies failed to detect this change (68, 69). The reason for this discrepancy might be the difference in method or sample characteristics (69).

Abnormality in the dopamine system has been found at the neuronal level. The neuropathological studies have shown a "miswiring" of dopaminergic projections to the ACC. In cortical layer II, the density of tyrosine hydroxylase–immunoreactive varicosities in contact with nonpyramidal cells was three times higher than that of pyramidal neurons (53, 54). This suggests a shift of dopamine projections away from pyramidal neurons to interneurons. Further studies are warranted to confirm that the abnormality occurs throughout the ACC including the dACC.

It has been recently proposed that the dopamine system modulates the pattern of activity in the prefrontal network via a complex interplay with a variety of ionic and synaptic currents, especially GABA and NMDA currents (70–72) (Figure 12.2). The model has shown that a predominantly D2 receptor activation leads to a net reduction in network inhibition. As a result, multiple inputs can gain access to the prefrontal network. This allows multiple representations to be processed in the prefrontal network simultaneously. On the other hand, a predominantly D1 receptor activation leads to a net increase in network inhibition so that only strong inputs can persist in

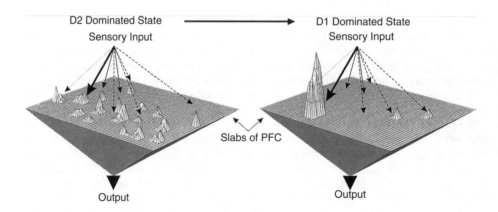

FIGURE 12.2 Effect of D1 vs. D2 receptor activation on the prefrontal network. The blue arrow shows the normal course of network activation in decision-making, which begins with a D2-dominant evaluation state and progress to a D1-dominant execution state. In schizophrenia, progression to D1-dominant state is defective. This leads to stagnation in the evaluation phase, characterized by roving among different associations and inability to choose and pursue an appropriate array of ideas. Reproduced with permission from Seamans et al (71).

the prefrontal network. We have recently suggested that these two states fit well with the evaluation and execution phases of decision making (9). First, the transient D2 state allows multiple representations to exist simultaneously, which is required for cost-benefit analysis and the comparison of different options. Subsequently, the long-lasting D1 state stabilizes the selected representation and shuts off the influence of other representations, thereby maintaining the animal's focus on the selected option. In this model, it is proposed that dopamine dysregulation in the prefrontal network would shift the network toward a persistent D2 state (73), which may lead to stagnation in the decision-making cycle.

Although this model provides a good framework for explaining how dopamine dysregulation disturbs decision-making processes in the dACC, further studies are required specifically to tailor the model to the dACC of patients with schizophrenia. The model was originally developed to examine the effect of the dopamine system on the dorsolateral prefrontal cortex (71). Two of the neuropathological abnormalities mentioned above are unique to the ACC and have not been observed in the dorsolateral prefrontal cortex. These include increased glutamatergic inputs and dopaminergic miswiring in layer II (54). Therefore, further clarification of the effect of these unique regional variations on the brain network of decision making will prove informative.

RELATED SUBCORTICAL STRUCTURES

The dACC is connected with several cortical and subcortical structures. The basal ganglia and the thalamus make a cortical–subcortical loop with the dACC (74). Specifically, the dACC is connected with the ventromedial and dorsolateral portions of the striatum (75, 76) and the mediodorsal and anteroventral nuclei of the thalamus (77–80). The loop is intensely innervated by amygdala, hippocampal, and dopamine projections (81–85). In patients with schizophrenia, there is ample evidence for abnormality in these subcortical structures, for dysregulation in their dopamine innervations, and for disturbance in their connectivity with the dACC. In the following, we briefly review the findings related to the basal ganglia and thalamus. However, it is noteworthy that these subcortical regions are not exclusively connected with the ACC, but are also linked with other medial prefrontal/orbitofrontal regions (75).

Basal Ganglia

There is considerable evidence that the dACC closely interacts with the striatum during decision making (1–3). The lower tier of the ACC is linked to the ventromedial striatum (i.e., the NAc and ventral putamen) while the upper tier is linked to the dorsolateral striatum (i.e., the dorsal caudate and the putamen)(75).

Structural abnormalities: The available evidence suggests that antipsychotic medications change striatal volume over time (86–89). Studies on drug-naïve patients, however, have also shown changes in striatal volume, with several studies reporting an absolute or relative volume reduction of the caudate in patients with drug-naïve schizophrenia and related disorders (87, 89–96). Some studies, however, have failed to find this volume reduction (97–100). Findings regarding putamen volume in drug-naïve patients are inconclusive, with evidence for significant enlargement (96) or volume reduction (87, 101), while other studies do not report any significant change (89, 94, 98, 99). Few studies have assessed NAc volume separately in patients with drug-naïve schizophrenia, with one study reporting subtle volume reduction (87) while another did not find any change (98).

Postmortem studies, as expected from the numerous confounding factors and diverse methodologies, are controversial. In these studies, changes in striatal volume, neuron density, or neuron number range from significant increases to significant decreases (see for example 102).

Functional abnormality: Functional imaging studies have suggested a significant reduction in resting striatal metabolism in drug-naïve patients (89, 103, 104), and a few recent studies identified abnormal activation of the striatum during decision-making tasks. One recent study reported reduced activation of the ventral striatum in drug-free patients during the presentation of cues that indicated reward (105), while an fMRI study found hypoactivity of the caudate along with the ACC during priming tasks (39). In another study, reduced activation of the ACC and basal ganglia has been found in schizophrenic patients during the forced-choice visual oddball task (106). Finally, two studies found that a procedural learning task, which normally activates the dACC and caudate, failed to adequately activate these regions in patients with schizophrenia (107, 108). Although the task did not directly assess decision making, participants were required to determine the location of asterisks appearing on a screen either sequentially or randomly. The task, therefore, included some features of error detection and response selection.

Dopamine dysregulation: Dopamine dysregulation in the striatum of patients with schizophrenia has been inferred from the correlation between the antipsychotic effect and striatal D2 receptor occupancy (109). It has been shown that striatal D2 blockade significantly predicts antipsychotic response (110, 111). Dopamine dysregulation has been studied more directly by assessment of the dopamine binding in patients with schizophrenia. Several studies have suggested an increased baseline D2 receptor occupancy by dopamine in the striatum of drug-free and drug-naïve patients (112–115), though one study failed to find a significant change in striatal D2 binding in drug-naïve patients (116). Finally, a twin study found that increased caudate D2 dop-amine was associated with poor performance on neuropsychological tasks in a sample of patients with schizophrenia and their unaffected cotwins. This study concluded that the striatal dopamine dysregulation might be a trait related to psychosis vulner-ability (117). Studies have not found any significant change in striatal D1 binding in drug-naïve patients (67–69).

Thalamus

The ACC is connected with the mediodorsal (MD) (77, 80, 118) and anteroventral nuclei (AV) (78, 79) of the thalamus. Recent studies have shown that there are two complementary circuits between the ACC and the AV nucleus. Parvalbumin-positive thalamic neurons project to the middle cortical layers in an area-specific manner, while calbindin-positive thalamic neurons project to the superficial cortical layers over widespread areas. The former projections are proposed to be a "driver" pathway that transmits data, while the latter projections seem to be a "modulator" pathway that modifies data (79).

Structural abnormalities: Like the basal ganglia, there is evidence that antipsychotic medications change the volume of the thalamus. However, studies on drug-naïve, first-episode patients have shown that the overall volume of the thalamus is probably reduced in schizophrenia (see for review 119). Moreover, a few studies have reported a decrease in the volume of the MD nucleus in drug-naïve patients (96, 120–122), and a recent study reported reduced thalamic volume in twin pairs concordant for schizo-phrenia compared with control twins, suggesting a genetic contribution to the thalamic volume reduction (123).

There is evidence for abnormal neural connectivity between the ACC and the thalamus in patients with schizophrenia (124, 125). A recent diffusion tensor imaging study found significantly elevated mean diffusivity measures within the ACC and the MD nucleus of the thalamus in schizophrenic patients; this might suggest an altered connectivity between these regions (59). This is also supported in another study show-ing that there was a lack of correlation between the volumes of the ACC and thala-mus in patients with schizophrenia compared with control subjects (126). Further, a neuropathological study has found that the density of parvalbumin-positive thalamic axon terminals in the middle layers of the prefrontal cortex was significantly lower in patients with schizophrenia, compared with patients with major depressive disorder and haloperidol-treated monkeys (127). This finding indicates that data transmission from the thalamus to the cortex is abnormal in schizophrenia.

Functional abnormality: Studies in drug-naïve patients have shown decreased baseline metabolism in the whole thalamus (128) and in the MD nucleus (129). Several studies demonstrated abnormal activation of the thalamus during different neuropsy-chological tasks (see for review 119).

More important, there is evidence for abnormal metabolic connectivity between the dACC and the MD nucleus during decision-making tasks. Two studies showed that the dACC and thalamus were hypoactive in schizophrenia patients during oddball tasks, which assess response selection and cognitive control (130, 131). In another study, the thalamus and the dACC showed decreased blood flow during recall tasks in which patients were required to distinguish between target and nontarget stimuli (132, but see 133). Yet another study found that patients with schizophrenia exhibited relatively lower metabolic rates in the MD nucleus and the dACC during a spatial attention task, which required selection of a target stimulus from competing surrounding stimuli (134). In a more recent study, metabolic disconnection was reported between the MD nucleus and the upper tier of the dACC during a serial verbal learning task. Although this task was not designed to assess decision making, patients with schizophrenia exhibited more perseveration and intrusion errors during the task, suggesting abnormal executive control (135). However, none of the above-mentioned tasks directly assessed the core elements of decision making, and further studies are warranted in which options with different costs and benefits are simultaneously presented for selection.

Dopamine dysregulation: Three recent PET studies have confirmed a decrease in D2 binding in the thalamus of drug-naïve patients with schizophrenia, especially in the MD nucleus (63, 65, 136). Thalamic D1 binding, however, was not significantly changed (68).

HYPOTHESIS
There is evidence that the dACC and its related subcortical regions are at the center of a brain network responsible for choosing between different options and pursuing the selected one. The dopamine system seems to be crucial in the normal function of this decision-making network by modulating the network in different regions. Dopamine has a bimodal effect (73), which first allows the network to compare different representations during an evaluation phase, and then focuses the network on the preferred representation during the execution phase (9). Our review of previous studies indicates that this decision-making network is abnormal in schizophrenia at both microcircuit and macrocircuit levels. There is also significant dopamine dysregulation throughout this network. However, inconsistencies do exist and future studies are warranted to assess the concept of decision making in patients with schizophrenia.

Below, we propose that an abnormality of the decision-making network in schizophrenia is relevant to its psychopathology. We discuss the possible impact of an abnormal decision-making network on the three dimensions of psychotic symptoms separately. These dimensions include positive symptoms, negative symptoms, and disorganization (137, 138). We then consider whether the model is relevant to understanding the effect of antipsychotic and behavioral treatments on patients with schizophrenia. We suggest that the model could provide a general framework to help generate new testable hypotheses about schizophrenia and related psychotic disorders.

Disorganization
Several years ago, Liddle and colleagues showed that the disorganization dimension was associated with increased blood flow to the dACC (139). This has been replicated by some (140–142), though not all subsequent studies (143). One of these studies found an inverse correlation between the severity of formal thought disorder and dACC blood flow (140). This study also reported a positive correlation of formal thought disorders and striatal blood flow.

We suggest that abnormality in the decision-making network could satisfactorily explain the disorganization symptoms of schizophrenia. As explained above, there is evidence that the decision-making network is responsible for selecting certain options and pursuing those options. This response selection could be as concrete as chasing a chosen prey out of a herd or as abstract as pursuing a given array of mental representations from a number of competing representations. Formal thought disorder is generally characterized by the inability of patients to pursue a series of ideas appropriately. Patients shift prematurely between different arrays of mental representations so that they continuously rove between different associations (as seen in loosening of associations) or different arrays of ideas (as seen in flight of ideas).

These phenomena could be explained by a strong D2 state in the two-state model (Figure 12.2). Although this model has been used to explain abnormal working memory relevant to the dorsolateral prefrontal cortex of schizophrenia patients (71, 144), we propose that this model can also explain the effect of abnormal decision making relevant to the psychopathology of schizophrenia. Dopamine dysregulation would cause an abnormally persistent D2 state (73), characterized by simultaneous existence of overflowing representations in the dACC network. This, in the extreme case, results in numerous selections, which are chosen inappropriately and are terminated prematurely. The condition is clearly inefficient and causes intense network activation, which is reflected in high metabolic consumption as observed in most of the PET studies mentioned earlier. The current model has similarities and differences with the previous hypotheses. Seamans and Yang (73) have proposed that disorganization results from a persistent D2 state in the working memory network. The current model suggests that it may occur due to an abnormality in the decision-making network. Winterer and Weinberger (144) have proposed that a persistent D2 state in the prefrontal network causes positive symptoms such as hallucinations and delusions, while the current model argues that dopamine dysregulation is not directly involved in the generation of hallucinations and delusions (see below).

Positive symptoms

There is accumulating evidence that positive symptoms (e.g., hallucinations and delusions) are associated with abnormality in the dACC, striatum, and thalamus and in the dopamine projections to these regions. Structural studies have shown a negative correlation between positive symptoms and the grey matter volumes of the ACC (10, 145) and the NAc (146). Several functional neuroimaging studies have found an association between positive symptoms and ACC activity in resting states. However, inconsistencies exist as some studies report a negative correlation (142, 147) and others a positive correlation (141, 148), while other studies do not find any association with Schneiderian symptoms (149). Two of these studies also found a negative correlation between positive symptoms and activity of the striatum and thalamus (142, 147).

Increased activity of the ACC and its dorsal part has been found by almost all the studies that assessed patients while they were experiencing positive symptoms. One study found hyperactivity in the ACC after the provocation of psychotic symptoms by ketamine administration (150). Another study showed the ACC hyperactivity during free selection movements in schizophrenia patients experiencing delusions of control (151). Several studies reported hyperactivity of the dACC during auditory hallucinations (152–154). The latter also found hyperactivity in the striatum and the thalamus. Finally, it has been found that dopamine D2 binding in the ACC of patients with schizophrenia is negatively related to the severity of positive symptoms (64).

However, dACC dysfunction is unlikely to be involved in the generation of positive symptoms. Animal studies have shown that the dACC-NAc circuit is not involved in perception (5, 9, 155). In other words, it is unlikely that the circuit is involved in the initial processing of abnormal sensory experiences or mental representations. The role of this circuit probably starts off when these representations are present simultaneously with others in the prefrontal network and are ready for analysis. Indeed, studies suggest that other brain regions are involved in the development of abnormal representations (150, 156, 157). We propose that the decision-making network is involved in the next step, that is, when the individual should decide on whether psychotic representations are significant enough to be pursued instead of other representations. In line with this argument, studies on the time course of hallucinations have shown that the dACC is activated when the hallucination is fully developed and becomes conscious (153), showing that the dACC is not involved in the early stages of the development of hallucinations. In this model, psychotic representations (including percepts, thoughts, and behaviors) are seen as options competing with other representations for dominance in the dACC network. Psychotic representations enchant patients. They are unusual, often acute experiences; they are voices that warn patients about an imminent danger or ideas that gratify them as being unique and genius. These experiences, however, are too costly to be pursued. They are not in harmony with other mental representations, demanding an extensive reconstruction of the internal world and a dramatic change in social relationships. On the other hand, socially acceptable ideas and behaviors are less acute or attention grabbing; they are normal routines and ordinary experiences. However, they are less costly and are facilitated by social norms and routines.

We propose that the normal decision-making circuit tends not to pursue psychotic representations. As proposed by Phillips and colleagues (158), the maximum response cost that the animal would afford for a given benefit follows a hyperbolic curve (Figure 12.3). Therefore, however salient a representation may be, if it is too costly, the subject will not choose to pursue it (e.g., Point A in Figure 12.1). Dopamine dysregulation and "miswiring," however, might lead to failure to take account of the costs and might bias the subject toward choosing "enchanting" psychotic representations. This is depicted in Figure 12.1 as an upward shift in the cost-benefit curve, which consequently would include the salient but costly psychotic representations (i.e. Point A in Figure 12.1). Overall, we propose that the decision-making network is not involved in the generation of positive symptoms but is important in the way that the individual responds to the preexisting symptoms. The abnormality of this network causes the individual to "pursue" such symptoms even to the point of psychosocial dysfunction.

Indeed, such an abnormal shift in decision making, rather than psychotic symptoms per se, can be considered the hallmark of psychotic disorders. This is reflected in psychiatric classifications where psychotic symptoms are regarded as disorders if, and only if, they make the individual dysfunctional. In other words, psychotic symptoms make the individual ill, if they force the individual away from socially acceptable ideas and behaviors. This argument is well supported by studies showing that psychotic symptoms such as hallucinations and delusions are considerably more prevalent than psychotic disorders. Hallucinations are experienced in 33% of adolescents and delusions in 24% (159), showing that these phenomena are 20 to 30 times more common than psychotic disorders in the age range during which schizophrenia usually begins. The main reason that they are not considered as psychiatric disorders is that they do not significantly distract individuals from socially acceptable behaviors. Consistent with the above argument, recent studies have shown that patients are more preoccupied and convinced about delusional ideas than non-patients (160, 161), showing that patients differ from nonpatients in their "pursuit" of the delusions. This is also in line with a recent study showing that the gray matter abnormality in the dACC coincides with the beginning of schizophrenia (21–23, 28), with evidence for progressive grey matter loss in the ACC during transition to active psychosis (25, 29). However, these findings need to be confirmed by further longitudinal studies.

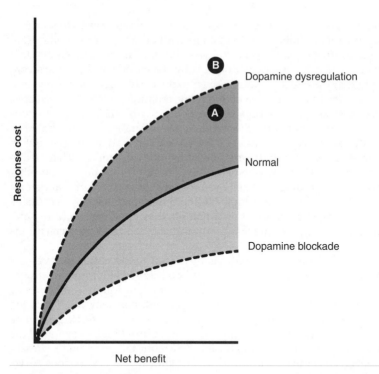

FIGURE 12.3   The proposed effect of dopamine on the maximum affordable cost (modified from Phillips et al (158). The maximum response cost as a function of reward magnitude follows a hyperbolic curve. Dysregulation or blockade of the dopamine system shifts the curve upwards or downwards, respectively. Dopamine dysregulation refers to the "mis-wiring" observed in the ACC of patients with schizophrenia. This is substituted for dopamine enhancement in the original model. The rationale has been discussed elsewhere (6).

Negative symptoms

The results of anterior cingulotomy provide clues about a possible relationship between the abnormality in the decision-making network and negative symptoms. Anterior cingulotomy usually destroys the dACC region (162). The lesion is reported to cause difficulty both in initiating and sustaining behavioral responses (163, 164). This is clearly in line with the model that the dACC and related subcortical regions are involved in choosing and pursuing an action. Cingulotomy patients are also described by their family as undergoing subtle personality and behavioral changes; they are unable to focus, get frustrated easily and become passive, laissez-faire, and emotionally blunted (165). Therefore, it seems plausible that intensive atrophy or pervasive hypoactivity of the dACC and related subcortical structures result in indecisiveness, avolition in initiating, and impersistence in pursuing goal-directed behaviors.

The neuroimaging studies partly support this argument. Magnetic resonance spectroscopy studies have found reduced levels of NAA in the ACC, which has been associated with the severity of blunted affect (47, 166), suggesting that neuronal loss and dysfunction of this area is relevant to negative symptoms of schizophrenia. In a more recent study, thinner ACC in prepsychotic "ultra-high-risk" individuals was also associated with greater negative symptoms (22). Functional neuroimaging studies have also reported decreased blood flow or metabolism of the ACC (167, 168), the striatum (105, 147, 168), or the thalamus (147, 167, 168), including the MD nucleus (129) in patients with negative symptoms. However, not all studies are consistent, with at least one functional neuroimaging study failing to find an association between the ACC activity and negative symptoms (169). That study, however, assessed medicated patients after a 5-day washout period. Association between decreased dopamine D1 binding in the ACC and negative symptoms is controversial, with one study reporting an association (67) while another was negative (69).

Token economy—a reward-based intervention

Token economy is a type of behavioral therapy introduced in the 1950s and 1960s for long-stay hospital patients. Despite its success, the method has fallen out of favor in the deinstitutionalization era, partly because the method required highly controlled environments (170). In this therapeutic discipline, tokens were awarded for socially acceptable behaviors and could be used to buy ward privileges. For example, if the patient met criteria for appropriate grooming and social interactions, they would have been offered certain tokens that could be used to acquire or purchase certain privileges, such as buying cigarettes, snacks, personal radios, or to have leave from hospital. The method was successful in promoting socially desirable conduct and to minimize inappropriate or other psychotically driven behaviors (171).

Token economy is a good example of decision making in which patient choice is constrained and patients must choose between psychotic behaviors and socially acceptable conduct in a well-controlled environment. Although patients do not choose the socially acceptable options ordinarily, they are more likely to choose them by increasing the benefit derived from these options with tokens. Token economy, therefore, does not change the abnormal cost–benefit curve per se, rather it manipulates the cost and benefits of behavioral options. This can be depicted by a rightward shift of Point B in Figure 12.1 so that the point comes under the cost–benefit curve. In other words, token economy increases the benefit of the socially acceptable behaviors and makes it more cost-effective than psychotic behaviors.

Antipsychotics

There is evidence that antipsychotic medications act via dopamine blockade. Their clinical effect is linked with striatal D2 receptor occupancy (111). This continuous D2 inhibition is reflected in D2 receptor upregulation (172–174) and D1 receptor downregulation (175, 176) in subjects treated with antipsychotics. Therefore, it seems that antipsychotic medications, through blocking D2 receptors, force the dACC network away from a predominantly D2 state and act to stabilize the network (73). This would dampen disorganization symptoms in schizophrenia. In line with this argument, studies have shown that antipsychotics normalize dACC activity, potentially resulting in a more efficient and stable network (150, 177, 178). Moreover, the superiority of clozapine over other antipsychotics has been attributed to a clozapine-induced change in dACC activity (179–181).

In addition, antipsychotics help patients to ignore positive symptoms. Well-replicated animal studies have shown that the dopamine blockade causes a dramatic decrease in the maximum response cost that subjects would afford for a given option. In other words, antipsychotic medications cause a downward shift in the cost–benefit curve (Figure 12.1), thereby reducing the probability that patients would continue to pursue "lavish" positive symptoms. This can be depicted as a downward shift in the dopamine dysregulation curve in Figure 12.1, so that the curve no longer covers Point A. This is in line with the studies showing that antipsychotics may not necessarily eradicate positive symptoms but prevent them from disturbing or engaging patients (182). The finding shows that antipsychotics merely dampen choosing and pursuing psychotic representations.

CONCLUSION AND FUTURE DIRECTION

The present chapter uses concepts developed in the basic neurosciences to explain the clinical syndrome of schizophrenia. A review of animal and human studies indicates that a brain network consisting of the dACC, striatum, and thalamus is important in several elements of decision making. All those elements, however, deal either with the evaluation or execution phase of decision making. Further, the evidence suggests that the dopamine system modulates this network at multiple levels to facilitate an optimal cost–benefit decision. In the present chapter, we reviewed the findings regarding an abnormality of the decision-making network in schizophrenia. We demonstrated that there is considerable evidence for a pervasive abnormality of this network and its dopamine regulation, though further studies are warranted to assess unexplored aspects and to resolve the inconsistencies.

In this chapter, we also proposed a model about how the abnormal decision-making network could contribute to the psychopathology of schizophrenia. We proposed that (i) stagnation in the activity of the decision-making network would lead to disorganization symptoms such as loosening of associations and frequent derailments; (ii) the network is not directly involved in the experience of positive symptoms; instead, we proposed that dopamine-related disturbances in the cost–benefit analysis force patients to pursue their delusions and hallucinations to a point of psychosocial dysfunction; (iii) negative symptoms such as indecisiveness, avolition, and impersistence might result from an intense hypofunction of this network; and (iv) behavioral and pharmacological treatments may act to modify decision making to help patients work through their symptoms.

In conclusion, the concept of abnormal decision making may explain some aspects of the psychopathology of schizophrenia as well as the effect of behavioral and pharmacological treatments on abnormal symptoms. However, these hypotheses require examination in future studies. One important step for future work would be to develop a human decision-making test that specifically assesses the type of decision-making that the dACC network is involved in, that is, short-term, exploiting, effort-related decision making. The test should incorporate both evaluation and execution phases and should be versatile enough to be conducted with neuroimaging techniques. The test can consist of two options with different amounts of reward that require different levels of effort but should control for the time that subjects spend on each option to rule out time-related costs. Such a test can be used in patients with schizophrenia to assess which aspects of their decision making are abnormal, to examine whether these abnormalities are associated with the structural and functional problems in the dACC network, and finally to evaluate whether these abnormalities are related to the clinical symptoms of schizophrenia.

REFERENCES

1. Hampton AN, O'Doherty JP. Decoding the neural substrates of reward-related decision making with functional MRI. Proc Natl Acad Sci USA 2007; 104(4): 1377–82.
2. Ernst M, Nelson EE, McClure EB et al. Choice selection and reward anticipation: an fMRI study. Neuropsychologia 2004; 42(12): 1585–97.

3. Eshel N, Nelson EE, Blair RJ, Pine DS, Ernst M. Neural substrates of choice selection in adults and adolescents: development of the ventrolateral prefrontal and anterior cingulate cortices. Neuropsychologia 2007; 45(6): 1270–9.

4. Rushworth MF, Walton ME, Kennerley SW, Bannerman DM. Action sets and decisions in the medial frontal cortex. Trends Cogn Sci 2004; 8(9): 410–7.

5. Salamone JD, Correa M, Farrar A, Mingote SM. Effort-related functions of nucleus accumbens dopamine and associated forebrain circuits. Psychopharmacology (Berl) 2007; 191(3): 461–82.

6. Kennerley SW, Walton ME, Behrens TE, Buckley MJ, Rushworth MF. Optimal decision making and the anterior cingulate cortex. Nat Neurosci 2006; 9(7): 940–7.

7. Critchley HD. Neural mechanisms of autonomic, affective, and cognitive integration. J Comp Neurol 2005; 493(1): 154–66.

8. Dosenbach NU, Visscher KM, Palmer ED et al. A core system for the implementation of task sets. Neuron 2006; 50(5): 799–812.

9. Assadi S, Yücel M, Pantelis C. Dopamine modulates neural networks involved in effort-based decision making. Neurosci Biobehav Rev 2009; 33: 383-393.

10. Choi JS, Kang DH, Kim JJ et al. Decreased caudal anterior cingulate gyrus volume and positive symptoms in schizophrenia. Psychiatry Res 2005; 139(3): 239–47.

11. Davatzikos C, Shen D, Gur RC et al. Whole-brain morphometric study of schizophrenia revealing a spatially complex set of focal abnormalities. Arch Gen Psychiatry 2005; 62(11): 1218–27.

12. Haznedar MM, Buchsbaum MS, Hazlett EA et al. Cingulate gyrus volume and metabolism in the schizophrenia spectrum. Schizophr Res 2004; 71(2–3): 249–62.

13. Job DE, Whalley HC, McConnell S et al. Structural gray matter differences between first-episode schizophrenics and normal controls using voxel-based morphometry. Neuroimage 2002; 17(2): 880–9.

14. Kawasaki Y, Suzuki M, Nohara S et al. Structural brain differences in patients with schizophrenia and schizotypal disorder demonstrated by voxel-based morphometry. Eur Arch Psychiatry Clin Neurosci 2004; 254(6): 406–14.

15. Kuperberg GR, Broome MR, McGuire PK et al. Regionally localized thinning of the cerebral cortex in schizophrenia. Arch Gen Psychiatry 2003; 60(9): 878–88.

16. Mitelman SA, Shihabuddin L, Brickman AM, Hazlett EA, Buchsbaum MS. Volume of the cingulate and outcome in schizophrenia. Schizophr Res 2005; 72(2–3): 91–108.

17. Narr KL, Toga AW, Szeszko P et al. Cortical thinning in cingulate and occipital cortices in first episode schizophrenia. Biol Psychiatry 2005; 58(1): 32–40.

18. Vidal CN, Rapoport JL, Hayashi KM et al. Dynamically spreading frontal and cingulate deficits mapped in adolescents with schizophrenia. Arch Gen Psychiatry 2006; 63(1): 25–34.

19. Bouras C, Kovari E, Hof PR, Riederer BM, Giannakopoulos P. Anterior cingulate cortex pathology in schizophrenia and bipolar disorder. Acta Neuropathol 2001; 102(4): 373–9.

20. Kreczmanski P, Schmidt-Kastner R, Heinsen H et al. Stereological studies of capillary length density in the frontal cortex of schizophrenics. Acta Neuropathol 2005; 109(5): 510–8.

21. Wood SJ, Pantelis C, Velakoulis D et al. Progressive changes in the development toward schizophrenia: studies in subjects at increased symptomatic risk. Schizophr Bull 2008; 34(2): 322–9.

22. Fornito A, Yung AR, Wood SJ et al. Anatomic abnormalities of the anterior cingulate cortex before psychosis onset: an MRI study of ultra-high-risk individuals. Biol Psychiatry 2008; 64(9): 758–65.

23. Borgwardt SJ, Riecher-Rossler A, Dazzan P et al. Regional gray matter volume abnormalities in the at risk mental state. Biol Psychiatry 2007; 61(10): 1148–56.

24. Farrow TF, Whitford TJ, Williams LM, Gomes L, Harris AW. Diagnosis-related regional gray matter loss over two years in first episode schizophrenia and bipolar disorder. Biol Psychiatry 2005; 58(9): 713–23.

25. Pantelis C, Velakoulis D, McGorry PD et al. Neuroanatomical abnormalities before and after onset of psychosis: a cross-sectional and longitudinal MRI comparison. Lancet 2003; 361(9354): 281–8.

26. Pantelis C, Velakoulis D, Wood SJ et al. Neuroimaging and emerging psychotic disorders: the Melbourne ultra-high risk studies. Int Rev Psychiatry 2007; 19(4): 371–81.

27. Pantelis C, Yücel M, Wood SJ et al. Structural brain imaging evidence for multiple pathological processes at different stages of brain development in schizophrenia. Schizophr Bull 2005; 31(3): 672–96.

28. Fornito A, Yücel M, Wood SJ et al. Surface-based morphometry of the anterior cingulate cortex in first episode schizophrenia. Hum Brain Mapp 2008; 29(4): 478–89.

29. Job DE, Whalley HC, Johnstone EC, Lawrie SM. Grey matter changes over time in high risk subjects developing schizophrenia. Neuroimage 2005; 25(4): 1023–30.

30. Meyer-Lindenberg A, Poline JB, Kohn PD et al. Evidence for abnormal cortical functional connectivity during working memory in schizophrenia. Am J Psychiatry 2001; 158(11): 1809–17.

31. Fornito A, Yücel M, Wood S et al. Individual differences in anterior cingulate/paracingulate morphology are related to executive functions in healthy males. Cereb Cortex 2004; 14(4): 424–31.

32. Fornito A, Yücel M, Wood SJ et al. Morphology of the paracingulate sulcus and executive cognition in schizophrenia. Schizophr Res 2006; 88(1–3): 192–7.

33. Heckers S, Weiss AP, Deckersbach T et al. Anterior cingulate cortex activation during cognitive interference in schizophrenia. Am J Psychiatry 2004; 161(4): 707–15.

34. Carter CS, Mintun M, Nichols T, Cohen JD. Anterior cingulate gyrus dysfunction and selective attention deficits in schizophrenia: [15O]H2O PET study during single-trial Stroop task performance. Am J Psychiatry 1997; 154(12): 1670–5.

35. Kerns JG, Cohen JD, MacDonald AW 3rd et al. Decreased conflict- and error-related activity in the anterior cingulate cortex in subjects with schizophrenia. Am J Psychiatry 2005; 162(10): 1833–9.

36. Weiss EM, Siedentopf C, Golaszewski S et al. Brain activation patterns during a selective attention test–a functional MRI study in healthy volunteers and unmedicated patients during an acute episode of schizophrenia. Psychiatry Res 2007; 154(1): 31–40.

37. Yücel M, Brewer WJ, Harrison BJ et al. Anterior cingulate activation in antipsychotic-naive first-episode schizophrenia. Acta Psychiatr Scand 2007; 115(2): 155–8.

38. Yücel M, Pantelis C, Stuart GW et al. Anterior cingulate activation during Stroop task performance: a PET to MRI coregistration study of individual patients with schizophrenia. Am J Psychiatry 2002; 159(2): 251–4.

39. Dehaene S, Artiges E, Naccache L et al. Conscious and subliminal conflicts in normal subjects and patients with schizophrenia: the role of the anterior cingulate. Proc Natl Acad Sci U S A 2003; 100(23): 13722–7.

40. Dolan RJ, Fletcher P, Frith CD et al. Dopaminergic modulation of impaired cognitive activation in the anterior cingulate cortex in schizophrenia. Nature 1995; 378(6553): 180–2.

41. Emri M, Glaub T, Berecz R et al. Brain blood flow changes measured by positron emission tomography during an auditory cognitive task in healthy volunteers and in schizophrenic patients. Prog Neuropsychopharmacol Biol Psychiatry 2006; 30(3): 516–20.

42. Quintana J, Wong T, Ortiz-Portillo E, Marder SR, Mazziotta JC. Anterior cingulate dysfunction during choice anticipation in schizophrenia. Psychiatry Res 2004; 132(2): 117–30.

43. Carter CS, MacDonald AW 3rd, Ross LL, Stenger VA. Anterior cingulate cortex activity and impaired self-monitoring of performance in patients with schizophrenia: an event-related fMRI study. Am J Psychiatry 2001; 158(9): 1423–8.

44. Artiges E, Salame P, Recasens C et al. Working memory control in patients with schizophrenia: a PET study during a random number generation task. Am J Psychiatry 2000; 157(9): 1517–9.

45. Mulert C, Gallinat J, Pascual-Marqui R et al. Reduced event-related current density in the anterior cingulate cortex in schizophrenia. Neuroimage 2001; 13(4): 589–600.

46. Steen RG, Hamer RM, Lieberman JA. Measurement of brain metabolites by 1H magnetic resonance spectroscopy in patients with schizophrenia: a systematic review and meta-analysis. Neuropsychopharmacology 2005; 30(11): 1949–62.

47. Wood SJ, Yücel M, Wellard RM et al. Evidence for neuronal dysfunction in the anterior cingulate of patients with schizophrenia: a proton magnetic resonance spectroscopy study at 3 T. Schizophr Res 2007; 94(1–3): 328–31.

48. Benes FM, McSparren J, Bird ED, SanGiovanni JP, Vincent SL. Deficits in small interneurons in prefrontal and cingulate cortices of schizophrenic and schizoaffective patients. Arch Gen Psychiatry 1991; 48(11): 996–1001.

49. Cotter D, Landau S, Beasley C et al. The density and spatial distribution of GABAergic neurons, labelled using calcium binding proteins, in the anterior cingulate cortex in major depressive disorder, bipolar disorder, and schizophrenia. Biol Psychiatry 2002; 51(5): 377–86.

50. Benes FM, Vincent SL, Todtenkopf M. The density of pyramidal and nonpyramidal neurons in anterior cingulate cortex of schizophrenic and bipolar subjects. Biol Psychiatry 2001; 50(6): 395–406.

51. Todtenkopf MS, Vincent SL, Benes FM. A cross-study meta-analysis and three-dimensional comparison of cell counting in the anterior cingulate cortex of schizophrenic and bipolar brain. Schizophr Res 2005; 73(1): 79–89.

52. Benes FM, Vincent SL, Alsterberg G, Bird ED, SanGiovanni JP. Increased GABAA receptor binding in superficial layers of cingulate cortex in schizophrenics. J Neurosci 1992; 12(3): 924–9.

53. Benes FM. Model generation and testing to probe neural circuitry in the cingulate cortex of postmortem schizophrenic brain. Schizophr Bull 1998; 24(2): 219–30.

54. Benes FM. Emerging principles of altered neural circuitry in schizophrenia. Brain Res Brain Res Rev 2000; 31(2–3): 251–69.

55. Zavitsanou K, Ward PB, Huang XF. Selective alterations in ionotropic glutamate receptors in the anterior cingulate cortex in schizophrenia. Neuropsychopharmacology 2002; 27(5): 826–33.

56. Kubicki M, Westin CF, Nestor PG et al. Cingulate fasciculus integrity disruption in schizophrenia: a magnetic resonance diffusion tensor imaging study. Biol Psychiatry 2003; 54(11): 1171–80.

57. Buchsbaum MS, Friedman J, Buchsbaum BR et al. Diffusion tensor imaging in schizophrenia. Biol Psychiatry 2006; 60(11): 1181–7.

58. Hao Y, Liu Z, Jiang T et al. White matter integrity of the whole brain is disrupted in first-episode schizophrenia. Neuroreport 2006; 17(1): 23–6.

59. Rose SE, Chalk JB, Janke AL et al. Evidence of altered prefrontal-thalamic circuitry in schizophrenia: an optimized diffusion MRI study. Neuroimage 2006; 32(1): 16–22.

60. Seal ML, Yücel M, Wood SJ et al. Unravelling dysfunction in cingulate networks in schizophrenia: Evidence of selective white matter differences in chronic schizophrenia as determined by diffusion tensor imaging. Schizophr Res 2006; 81: 32.

61. Spence SA, Liddle PF, Stefan MD et al. Functional anatomy of verbal fluency in people with schizophrenia and those at genetic risk. Focal dysfunction and distributed disconnectivity reappraised. Br J Psychiatry 2000; 176: 52–60.

62. Yasuno F, Suhara T, Okubo Y et al. Abnormal effective connectivity of dopamine D2 receptor binding in schizophrenia. Psychiatry Res 2005; 138(3): 197–207.

63. Buchsbaum MS, Christian BT, Lehrer DS et al. D2/D3 dopamine receptor binding with [F-18]fallypride in thalamus and cortex of patients with schizophrenia. Schizophr Res 2006; 85(1–3): 232–44.

64. Suhara T, Okubo Y, Yasuno F et al. Decreased dopamine D2 receptor binding in the anterior cingulate cortex in schizophrenia. Arch Gen Psychiatry 2002; 59(1): 25–30.

65. Talvik M, Nordstrom AL, Olsson H, Halldin C, Farde L. Decreased thalamic D2/D3 receptor binding in drug-naive patients with schizophrenia: a PET study with [11C]FLB 457. Int J Neuropsychopharmacol 2003; 6(4): 361–70.
66. Hirvonen J, van Erp TG, Huttunen J et al. Brain dopamine d1 receptors in twins discordant for schizophrenia. Am J Psychiatry 2006; 163(10): 1747–53.
67. Okubo Y, Suhara T, Suzuki K et al. Decreased prefrontal dopamine D1 receptors in schizophrenia revealed by PET. Nature 1997; 385(6617): 634–6.
68. Abi-Dargham A, Mawlawi O, Lombardo I et al. Prefrontal dopamine D1 receptors and working memory in schizophrenia. J Neurosci 2002; 22(9): 3708–19.
69. Karlsson P, Farde L, Halldin C, Sedvall G. PET study of D(1) dopamine receptor binding in neuroleptic-naive patients with schizophrenia. Am J Psychiatry 2002; 159(5): 761–7.
70. Lapish CC, Kroener S, Durstewitz D, Lavin A, Seamans JK. The ability of the mesocortical dopamine system to operate in distinct temporal modes. Psychopharmacology (Berl) 2007; 191(3): 609–25.
71. Seamans JK, Gorelova N, Durstewitz D, Yang CR. Bidirectional dopamine modulation of GABAergic inhibition in prefrontal cortical pyramidal neurons. J Neurosci 2001; 21(10): 3628–38.
72. Trantham-Davidson H, Neely LC, Lavin A, Seamans JK. Mechanisms underlying differential D1 versus D2 dopamine receptor regulation of inhibition in prefrontal cortex. J Neurosci 2004; 24(47): 10652–9.
73. Seamans JK, Yang CR. The principal features and mechanisms of dopamine modulation in the prefrontal cortex. Prog Neurobiol 2004; 74(1): 1–58.
74. Alexander GE, DeLong MR, Strick PL. Parallel organization of functionally segregated circuits linking basal ganglia and cortex. Annu Rev Neurosci 1986; 9: 357–81.
75. Ferry AT, Ongur D, An X, Price JL. Prefrontal cortical projections to the striatum in macaque monkeys: evidence for an organization related to prefrontal networks. J Comp Neurol 2000; 425(3): 447–70.
76. Voorn P, Vanderschuren LJ, Groenewegen HJ, Robbins TW, Pennartz CM. Putting a spin on the dorsal-ventral divide of the striatum. Trends Neurosci 2004; 27(8): 468–74.
77. Ray JP, Price JL. The organization of projections from the mediodorsal nucleus of the thalamus to orbital and medial prefrontal cortex in macaque monkeys. J Comp Neurol 1993; 337(1): 131.
78. Xiaob D, Barbas H. Circuits through prefrontal cortex, basal ganglia, and ventral anterior nucleus map pathways beyond motor control. Thalamus & Related Systems 2004; 2: 325–43.
79. Zikopoulos B, Barbas H. Parallel driving and modulatory pathways link the prefrontal cortex and thalamus. PLoS ONE 2007; 2(9): e848.
80. Ongur D, Price JL. The organization of networks within the orbital and medial prefrontal cortex of rats, monkeys and humans. Cereb Cortex 2000; 10(3): 206–19.
81. Baleydier C, Mauguiere F. The duality of the cingulate gyrus in monkey. Neuroanatomical study and functional hypothesis. Brain 1980; 103(3): 525–54.
82. Floresco SB, Ghods-Sharifi S. Amygdala-prefrontal cortical circuitry regulates effort-based decision making. Cereb Cortex 2007; 17(2): 251–60.
83. Morecraft RJ, McNeal DW, Stilwell-Morecraft KS et al. Amygdala interconnections with the cingulate motor cortex in the rhesus monkey. J Comp Neurol 2007; 500(1): 134–65.
84. Morecraft RJ, Van Hoesen GW. Convergence of limbic input to the cingulate motor cortex in the rhesus monkey. Brain Res Bull 1998; 45(2): 209–32.
85. O'Donnell P, Grace AA. Synaptic interactions among excitatory afferents to nucleus accumbens neurons: hippocampal gating of prefrontal cortical input. J Neurosci 1995; 15(5 Pt 1): 3622–39.
86. Corson PW, Nopoulos P, Miller DD, Arndt S, Andreasen NC. Change in basal ganglia volume over 2 years in patients with schizophrenia: typical versus atypical neuroleptics. Am J Psychiatry 1999; 156(8): 1200–4.

87. Glenthoj A, Glenthoj BY, Mackeprang T et al. Basal ganglia volumes in drug-naive first-episode schizophrenia patients before and after short-term treatment with either a typical or an atypical antipsychotic drug. Psychiatry Res 2007; 154(3): 199–208.
88. Lieberman J, Chakos M, Wu H et al. Longitudinal study of brain morphology in first episode schizophrenia. Biol Psychiatry 2001; 49(6): 487–99.
89. Shihabuddin L, Buchsbaum MS, Hazlett EA et al. Dorsal striatal size, shape, and metabolic rate in never-medicated and previously medicated schizophrenics performing a verbal learning task. Arch Gen Psychiatry 1998; 55(3): 235–43.
90. Chakos MH, Lieberman JA, Alvir J, Bilder R, Ashtari M. Caudate nuclei volumes in schizophrenic patients treated with typical antipsychotics or clozapine. Lancet 1995; 345(8947): 456–7.
91. Chua SE, Cheung C, Cheung V et al. Cerebral grey, white matter and csf in never-medicated, first-episode schizophrenia. Schizophr Res 2007; 89(1–3): 12–21.
92. Corson PW, Nopoulos P, Andreasen NC, Heckel D, Arndt S. Caudate size in first-episode neuroleptic-naive schizophrenic patients measured using an artificial neural network. Biol Psychiatry 1999; 46(5): 712–20.
93. Jayakumar PN, Venkatasubramanian G, Gangadhar BN, Janakiramaiah N, Keshavan MS. Optimized voxel-based morphometry of gray matter volume in first-episode, antipsychotic-naive schizophrenia. Prog Neuropsychopharmacol Biol Psychiatry 2005; 29(4): 587–91.
94. Keshavan MS, Rosenberg D, Sweeney JA, Pettegrew JW. Decreased caudate volume in neuroleptic-naive psychotic patients. Am J Psychiatry 1998; 155(6): 774–8.
95. Levitt JJ, McCarley RW, Dickey CC et al. MRI study of caudate nucleus volume and its cognitive correlates in neuroleptic-naive patients with schizotypal personality disorder. Am J Psychiatry 2002; 159(7): 1190–7.
96. Salgado-Pineda P, Baeza I, Perez-Gomez M et al. Sustained attention impairment correlates to gray matter decreases in first episode neuroleptic-naive schizophrenic patients. Neuroimage 2003; 19(2 Pt 1): 365–75.
97. Cahn W, Hulshoff Pol HE, Bongers M et al. Brain morphology in antipsychotic-naive schizophrenia: a study of multiple brain structures. Br J Psychiatry Suppl 2002; 43: s66–72.
98. Gunduz H, Wu H, Ashtari M et al. Basal ganglia volumes in first-episode schizophrenia and healthy comparison subjects. Biol Psychiatry 2002; 51(10): 801–8.
99. Gur RE, Maany V, Mozley PD et al. Subcortical MRI volumes in neuroleptic-naive and treated patients with schizophrenia. Am J Psychiatry 1998; 155(12): 1711–7.
100. McCreadie RG, Thara R, Padmavati R, Srinivasan TN, Jaipurkar SD. Structural brain differences between never-treated patients with schizophrenia, with and without dyskinesia, and normal control subjects: a magnetic resonance imaging study. Arch Gen Psychiatry 2002; 59(4): 332–6.
101. Seidman LJ, Faraone SV, Goldstein JM et al. Reduced subcortical brain volumes in nonpsychotic siblings of schizophrenic patients: a pilot magnetic resonance imaging study. Am J Med Genet 1997; 74(5): 507–14.
102. Kreczmanski P, Heinsen H, Mantua V et al. Volume, neuron density and total neuron number in five subcortical regions in schizophrenia. Brain 2007; 130(Pt 3): 678–92.
103. Buchsbaum MS, Haier RJ, Potkin SG et al. Frontostriatal disorder of cerebral metabolism in never-medicated schizophrenics. Arch Gen Psychiatry 1992; 49(12): 935–42.
104. Cleghorn JM, Szechtman H, Garnett ES et al. Apomorphine effects on brain metabolism in neuroleptic-naive schizophrenic patients. Psychiatry Res 1991; 40(2): 135–53.
105. Juckel G, Schlagenhauf F, Koslowski M et al. Dysfunction of ventral striatal reward prediction in schizophrenia. Neuroimage 2006; 29(2): 409–16.
106. Morey RA, Inan S, Mitchell TV et al. Imaging frontostriatal function in ultra-high-risk, early, and chronic schizophrenia during executive processing. Arch Gen Psychiatry 2005; 62(3): 254–62.
107. Kumari V, Gray JA, Honey GD et al. Procedural learning in schizophrenia: a functional magnetic resonance imaging investigation. Schizophr Res 2002; 57(1): 97–107.

108. Zedkova L, Woodward ND, Harding I, Tibbo PG, Purdon SE. Procedural learning in schizophrenia investigated with functional magnetic resonance imaging. Schizophr Res 2006; 88(1–3): 198–207.

109. Kapur S, Mizrahi R, Li M. From dopamine to salience to psychosis--linking biology, pharmacology and phenomenology of psychosis. Schizophr Res 2005; 79(1): 59–68.

110. Agid O, Mamo D, Ginovart N et al. Striatal vs extrastriatal dopamine D2 receptors in antipsychotic response–a double-blind PET study in schizophrenia. Neuropsychopharmacology 2007; 32(6): 1209–15.

111. Kapur S, Zipursky R, Jones C, Remington G, Houle S. Relationship between dopamine D(2) occupancy, clinical response, and side effects: a double-blind PET study of first-episode schizophrenia. Am J Psychiatry 2000; 157(4): 514–20.

112. Abi-Dargham A, Gil R, Krystal J et al. Increased striatal dopamine transmission in schizophrenia: confirmation in a second cohort. Am J Psychiatry 1998; 155(6): 761–7.

113. Abi-Dargham A, Rodenhiser J, Printz D et al. Increased baseline occupancy of D2 receptors by dopamine in schizophrenia. Proc Natl Acad Sci U S A 2000; 97(14): 8104–9.

114. Breier A, Su TP, Saunders R et al. Schizophrenia is associated with elevated amphetamine-induced synaptic dopamine concentrations: evidence from a novel positron emission tomography method. Proc Natl Acad Sci U S A 1997; 94(6): 2569–74.

115. Laruelle M, Abi-Dargham A, van Dyck CH et al. Single photon emission computerized tomography imaging of amphetamine-induced dopamine release in drug-free schizophrenic subjects. Proc Natl Acad Sci U S A 1996; 93(17): 9235–40.

116. Talvik M, Nordstrom AL, Okubo Y et al. Dopamine D2 receptor binding in drug-naive patients with schizophrenia examined with raclopride-C11 and positron emission tomography. Psychiatry Res 2006; 148(2–3): 165–73.

117. Hirvonen J, van Erp TG, Huttunen J et al. Increased caudate dopamine D2 receptor availability as a genetic marker for schizophrenia. Arch Gen Psychiatry 2005; 62(4): 371–8.

118. Yeterian EH, Pandya DN. Corticothalamic connections of paralimbic regions in the rhesus monkey. J Comp Neurol 1988; 269(1): 130–46.

119. Sim K, Cullen T, Ongur D, Heckers S. Testing models of thalamic dysfunction in schizophrenia using neuroimaging. J Neural Transm 2006; 113(7): 907–28.

120. Gilbert AR, Rosenberg DR, Harenski K et al. Thalamic volumes in patients with first-episode schizophrenia. Am J Psychiatry 2001; 158(4): 618–24.

121. Byne W, Buchsbaum MS, Kemether E et al. Magnetic resonance imaging of the thalamic mediodorsal nucleus and pulvinar in schizophrenia and schizotypal personality disorder. Arch Gen Psychiatry 2001; 58(2): 133–40.

122. Kemether EM, Buchsbaum MS, Byne W et al. Magnetic resonance imaging of mediodorsal, pulvinar, and centromedian nuclei of the thalamus in patients with schizophrenia. Arch Gen Psychiatry 2003; 60(10): 983–91.

123. Ettinger U, Picchioni M, Landau S et al. Magnetic resonance imaging of the thalamus and adhesio interthalamica in twins with schizophrenia. Arch Gen Psychiatry 2007; 64(4): 401–9.

124. Pantelis C, Barnes TR, Nelson HE. Is the concept of frontal-subcortical dementia relevant to schizophrenia? Br J Psychiatry 1992; 160: 442–60.

125. Pantelis C, Brewer W. Neuropsychological and olfactory dysfunction in schizophrenia: relationship of frontal syndromes to syndromes of schizophrenia. Schizophr Res 1995; 17(1): 35–45.

126. Mitelman SA, Brickman AM, Shihabuddin L et al. Correlations between MRI-assessed volumes of the thalamus and cortical Brodmann's areas in schizophrenia. Schizophr Res 2005; 75(2–3): 265–81.

127. Lewis DA, Cruz DA, Melchitzky DS, Pierri JN. Lamina-specific deficits in parvalbumin-immunoreactive varicosities in the prefrontal cortex of subjects with schizophrenia: evidence for fewer projections from the thalamus. Am J Psychiatry 2001; 158(9): 1411–22.

128. Buchsbaum MS, Someya T, Teng CY et al. PET and MRI of the thalamus in never-medicated patients with schizophrenia. Am J Psychiatry 1996; 153(2): 191–9.

129. Hazlett EA, Buchsbaum MS, Kemether E et al. Abnormal glucose metabolism in the mediodorsal nucleus of the thalamus in schizophrenia. Am J Psychiatry 2004; 161(2): 305–14.

130. Kiehl KA, Liddle PF. An event-related functional magnetic resonance imaging study of an auditory oddball task in schizophrenia. Schizophr Res 2001; 48(2–3): 159–71.

131. Kiehl KA, Stevens MC, Celone K, Kurtz M, Krystal JH. Abnormal hemodynamics in schizophrenia during an auditory oddball task. Biol Psychiatry 2005; 57(9): 1029–40.

132. Crespo-Facorro B, Paradiso S, Andreasen NC et al. Recalling word lists reveals "cognitive dysmetria" in schizophrenia: a positron emission tomography study. Am J Psychiatry 1999; 156(3): 386–92.

133. Heckers S, Curran T, Goff D et al. Abnormalities in the thalamus and prefrontal cortex during episodic object recognition in schizophrenia. Biol Psychiatry 2000; 48(7): 651–7.

134. Lehrer DS, Christian BT, Mantil J et al. Thalamic and prefrontal FDG uptake in never medicated patients with schizophrenia. Am J Psychiatry 2005; 162(5): 931–8.

135. Mitelman SA, Byne W, Kemether EM, Hazlett EA, Buchsbaum MS. Metabolic disconnection between the mediodorsal nucleus of the thalamus and cortical Brodmann's areas of the left hemisphere in schizophrenia. Am J Psychiatry 2005; 162(9): 1733–5.

136. Yasuno F, Suhara T, Okubo Y et al. Low dopamine d(2) receptor binding in subregions of the thalamus in schizophrenia. Am J Psychiatry 2004; 161(6): 1016–22.

137. Grube BS, Bilder RM, Goldman RS. Meta-analysis of symptom factors in schizophrenia. Schizophr Res 1998; 31(2–3): 113–20.

138. Liddle PF, Barnes TR. Syndromes of chronic schizophrenia. Br J Psychiatry 1990; 157: 558–61.

139. Liddle PF, Friston KJ, Frith CD, Frackowiak RS. Cerebral blood flow and mental processes in schizophrenia. J R Soc Med 1992; 85(4): 224–7.

140. McGuire PK, Quested DJ, Spence SA et al. Pathophysiology of 'positive' thought disorder in schizophrenia. Br J Psychiatry 1998; 173: 231–5.

141. Lahti AC, Weiler MA, Holcomb HH et al. Correlations between rCBF and symptoms in two independent cohorts of drug-free patients with schizophrenia. Neuropsychopharmacology 2006; 31(1): 221–30.

142. Sabri O, Erkwoh R, Schreckenberger M et al. Correlation of positive symptoms exclusively to hyperperfusion or hypoperfusion of cerebral cortex in never-treated schizophrenics. Lancet 1997; 349(9067): 1735–9.

143. Kircher TT, Liddle PF, Brammer MJ et al. Neural correlates of formal thought disorder in schizophrenia: preliminary findings from a functional magnetic resonance imaging study. Arch Gen Psychiatry 2001; 58(8): 769–74.

144. Winterer G, Weinberger DR. Genes, dopamine and cortical signal-to-noise ratio in schizophrenia. Trends Neurosci 2004; 27(11): 683–90.

145. Suzuki M, Zhou SY, Hagino H et al. Morphological brain changes associated with Schneider's first-rank symptoms in schizophrenia: a MRI study. Psychol Med 2005; 35(4): 549–60.

146. Mamah D, Wang L, Barch D et al. Structural analysis of the basal ganglia in schizophrenia. Schizophr Res 2007; 89(1-3): 59–71.

147. Siegel BV Jr, Buchsbaum MS, Bunney WE Jr et al. Cortical-striatal-thalamic circuits and brain glucose metabolic activity in 70 unmedicated male schizophrenic patients. Am J Psychiatry 1993; 150(9): 1325–36.

148. Cleghorn JM, Garnett ES, Nahmias C et al. Regional brain metabolism during auditory hallucinations in chronic schizophrenia. Br J Psychiatry 1990; 157: 562–70.

149. Franck N, O'Leary DS, Flaum M, Hichwa RD, Andreasen NC. Cerebral blood flow changes associated with Schneiderian first-rank symptoms in schizophrenia. J Neuropsychiatry Clin Neurosci 2002; 14(3): 277–82.

150. Tamminga CA, Vogel M, Gao X, Lahti AC, Holcomb HH. The limbic cortex in schizophrenia: focus on the anterior cingulate. Brain Res Brain Res Rev 2000; 31(2–3): 364–70.

151. Spence SA, Brooks DJ, Hirsch SR et al. A PET study of voluntary movement in schizophrenic patients experiencing passivity phenomena (delusions of alien control). Brain 1997; 120 (Pt 11): 1997–2011.

152. Shergill SS, Brammer MJ, Williams SC, Murray RM, McGuire PK. Mapping auditory hallucinations in schizophrenia using functional magnetic resonance imaging. Arch Gen Psychiatry 2000; 57(11): 1033–8.

153. Shergill SS, Brammer MJ, Amaro E et al. Temporal course of auditory hallucinations. Br J Psychiatry 2004; 185: 516–7.

154. Silbersweig DA, Stern E, Frith C et al. A functional neuroanatomy of hallucinations in schizophrenia. Nature 1995; 378(6553): 176–9.

155. Berridge KC, Robinson TE. What is the role of dopamine in reward: hedonic impact, reward learning, or incentive salience? Brain Res Brain Res Rev 1998; 28(3): 309–69.

156. Shergill SS, Brammer MJ, Fukuda R et al. Engagement of brain areas implicated in processing inner speech in people with auditory hallucinations. Br J Psychiatry 2003; 182: 525–31.

157. Szechtman H, Woody E, Bowers KS, Nahmias C. Where the imaginal appears real: a positron emission tomography study of auditory hallucinations. Proc Natl Acad Sci USA 1998; 95(4): 1956–60.

158. Phillips PE, Walton ME, Jhou TC. Calculating utility: preclinical evidence for cost-benefit analysis by mesolimbic dopamine. Psychopharmacology (Berl) 2007; 191(3): 483–95.

159. Altman H, Collins M, Mundy P. Subclinical hallucinations and delusions in nonpsychotic adolescents. J Child Psychol Psychiatry 1997; 38(4): 413–20.

160. Peters ER, Joseph SA, Garety PA. Measurement of delusional ideation in the normal population: introducing the PDI (Peters et al. Delusions Inventory). Schizophr Bull 1999; 25(3): 553–76.

161. Preti A, Bonventre E, Ledda V, Petretto DR, Masala C. Hallucinatory experiences, delusional thought proneness, and psychological distress in a nonclinical population. J Nerv Ment Dis 2007; 195(6): 484–91.

162. Cosgrove GR, Rauch SL. Stereotactic cingulotomy. Neurosurg Clin N Am 2003; 14(2): 225–35.

163. Cohen RA, Kaplan RF, Zuffante P et al. Alteration of intention and self-initiated action associated with bilateral anterior cingulotomy. J Neuropsychiatry Clin Neurosci 1999; 11(4): 444–53.

164. Ochsner KN, Kosslyn SM, Cosgrove GR et al. Deficits in visual cognition and attention following bilateral anterior cingulotomy. Neuropsychologia 2001; 39(3): 219–30.

165. Cohen RA, Kaplan RF, Moser DJ, Jenkins MA, Wilkinson H. Impairments of attention after cingulotomy. Neurology 1999; 53(4): 819–24.

166. Yamasue H, Fukui T, Fukuda R et al. 1H-MR spectroscopy and gray matter volume of the anterior cingulate cortex in schizophrenia. Neuroreport 2002; 13(16): 2133–7.

167. Potkin SG, Alva G, Fleming K et al. A PET study of the pathophysiology of negative symptoms in schizophrenia. Positron emission tomography. Am J Psychiatry 2002; 159(2): 227–37.

168. Sabri O, Erkwoh R, Schreckenberger M et al. Regional cerebral blood flow and negative/positive symptoms in 24 drug-naive schizophrenics. J Nucl Med 1997; 38(2): 181–8.

169. Galeno R, Molina M, Guirao M, Isoardi R. Severity of negative symptoms in schizophrenia correlated to hyperactivity of the left globus pallidus and the right claustrum. A PET study. World J Biol Psychiatry 2004; 5(1): 20–5.

170. Liberman RP. The token economy. Am J Psychiatry 2000; 157(9): 1398.

171. Dickerson FB, Tenhula WN, Green-Paden LD. The token economy for schizophrenia: review of the literature and recommendations for future research. Schizophr Res 2005; 75(2-3): 405–16.

172. Kornhuber J, Riederer P, Reynolds GP et al. 3H-spiperone binding sites in post-mortem brains from schizophrenic patients: relationship to neuroleptic drug treatment, abnormal movements, and positive symptoms. J Neural Transm 1989; 75(1): 1–10.

173. Seeman P, Bzowej NH, Guan HC et al. Human brain D1 and D2 dopamine receptors in schizophrenia, Alzheimer's, Parkinson's, and Huntington's diseases. Neuropsychopharmacology 1987; 1(1): 5–15.

174. Silvestri S, Seeman MV, Negrete JC et al. Increased dopamine D2 receptor binding after long-term treatment with antipsychotics in humans: a clinical PET study. Psychopharmacology (Berl) 2000; 152(2): 174–80.

175. Lidow MS, Elsworth JD, Goldman-Rakic PS. Down-regulation of the D1 and D5 dopamine receptors in the primate prefrontal cortex by chronic treatment with antipsychotic drugs. J Pharmacol Exp Ther 1997; 281(1): 597–603.

176. Lidow MS, Goldman-Rakic PS. A common action of clozapine, haloperidol, and remoxipride on D1- and D2-dopaminergic receptors in the primate cerebral cortex. Proc Natl Acad Sci USA 1994; 91(10): 4353–6.

177. Holcomb HH, Cascella NG, Thaker GK et al. Functional sites of neuroleptic drug action in the human brain: PET/FDG studies with and without haloperidol. Am J Psychiatry 1996; 153(1): 41–9.

178. Miller DD, Andreasen NC, O'Leary DS et al. Effect of antipsychotics on regional cerebral blood flow measured with positron emission tomography. Neuropsychopharmacology 1997; 17(4): 230–40.

179. Conley RR, Kelly DL, Beason-Held LL, Holcomb HH, Richardson CM. The effects of clozapine and high-dose olanzapine on brain function in treatment-resistant schizophrenia: a case study. J Psychopharmacol 2004; 18(3): 429–31.

180. Lahti AC, Holcomb HH, Weiler MA et al. Clozapine but not haloperidol Re-establishes normal task-activated rCBF patterns in schizophrenia within the anterior cingulate cortex. Neuropsychopharmacology 2004; 29(1): 171–8.

181. Lahti AC, Holcomb HH, Weiler MA, Medoff DR, Tamminga CA. Functional effects of antipsychotic drugs: comparing clozapine with haloperidol. Biol Psychiatry 2003; 53(7): 601–8.

182. Mizrahi R, Bagby RM, Zipursky RB, Kapur S. How antipsychotics work: the patients' perspective. Prog Neuropsychopharmacol Biol Psychiatry 2005; 29(5): 859–64.

13 Neuropsychological markers and social cognition in schizophrenia

Jonathan Burns

INTRODUCTION

From the very outset a century ago, students of schizophrenia have emphasized the neurocognitive and social cognitive deficits that characterize the disorder. Emil Kraepelin named the disease *dementia praecox* or dementia of the young, defining it in terms of a progressive degeneration in cognitive function. His contemporary, Eugen Bleuler, who renamed the disease *schizophrenia*, identified autistic alienation as a core element essential for diagnosis. Bleuler's use of the term *autism* described a "detachment from outer reality and immersion in inner life"(1), thereby capturing the difficulties displayed by individuals with schizophrenia in engaging in social and interpersonal relationships. A 100 years after Kraepelin and Bleuler, we describe these neuropsychological features of schizophrenia in terms of neurocognitive or neuropsychological deficits and impairments of social cognition.

Despite the important early insights of these founding fathers of schizophrenia research, the orthodox view throughout the greater part of the 20th century was that cognitive dysfunction, if present in a patient, was secondary to the apathy and lack of volition associated with the disorder. *Feeblemindedness* was a term commonly ascribed. Later, with the advent of neuroleptic medication, deficits in cognitive functioning were commonly attributed to the drugs themselves—unfortunate but unavoidable side effects in the quest to control positive psychotic symptoms. Somehow, the recognition of cognitive dysfunction as a core aspect of the primary disease process was lost as clinicians focused on the more dramatic and intrusive positive symptoms and behavioral disturbances that commonly accompanied acute presentations. It is only within the past 20 years that neuropsychological and social cognitive dysfunction have again received attention as core elements of the schizophrenic disorder. In part, this rediscovery was a consequence of the introduction of atypical neuroleptics into the management of patients with schizophrenia. Improved control of positive symptoms in the absence of significant extrapyramidal side effects (EPSE's) clarified two issues: (a) Neuropsychological and social cognitive deficits were still evident and not attributable to EPSE's, and (b) Treatment with atypical neuroleptics resulted to some extent in improvements in both neuropsychological and social cognitive functioning. Thus, over the past decade, the major challenges within schizophrenia research and treatment discovery have been to identify the complex causes of neurodevelopmental impairment, develop strategies for early intervention and the prevention of cognitive and social decline, and preserve and optimize cognitive and social functioning.

In 2003, the National Institute of Mental Health (NIMH) established the measurement and treatment research to improve cognition in schizophrenia (MATRICS) consensus process (2, 3). This initiative was designed to support the development of pharmacological agents for improving the neurocognitive impairment associated with the disorder. The MATRICS process identified seven key cognitive domains as core problems in schizophrenia (speed of processing, attention/vigilance, working memory, verbal learning and memory, visual learning and memory, reasoning and problem solving, social cognition) and developed the MATRICS consensus cognitive battery to assess these domains.

A CORE FEATURE OF SCHIZOPHRENIA

There is good evidence that cognitive and social cognitive impairment are core features of schizophrenia (4) (See Table 13.1.) On average, patients perform 1.5 to 2.0 standard deviation below healthy controls on a variety of neurocognitive tasks, including those listed above (5). More important, these deficits can be considered trait markers rather than state markers as they appear relatively stable across changes in clinical state (6). For example, in a study of neuroleptic-naïve patients with schizophrenia, performance on a test of attention remained almost unchanged despite improvements in psychotic symptoms (7). Notably, schizophrenia has a modal profile in that individuals with the disorder have characteristic impairments across cognitive measures, although there are variations from person to person (6). A meta-analysis of 204 controlled studies showed a modal profile comprised of large cognitive impairments in memory, attention, and executive functions (8). Furthermore, cognitive deficits are present before the onset of clinical symptoms, having been demonstrated in adolescents at risk for schizophrenia (9) as well as in individuals with prodromal or "at risk mental states" (ARMS) (10, 11, 12). In patients presenting with a first-episode of psychosis in both developing- (13) and developed-world (14) contexts, deficits are present across most domains of cognitive functioning, especially in attention, processing speed, and working memory. It seems that cognitive impairment is relatively stable across the lifespan from the onset of the illness to at least 65 years of age (15). Finally, attenuated but significant deficits in attention, speed of processing, and executive functioning are present in healthy siblings of patients with schizophrenia (7, 16), demonstrating that this pattern of cognitive impairment is at least partially heritable and is intrinsic to the schizophrenic disorder.

NEUROCOGNITIVE ENDOPHENOTYPES

The heritability and stability of neurocognitive deficits in schizophrenia has given rise to the argument that neuropsychological markers should be considered suitable endophenotypes for genetic studies of the disorder (17). It is recommended that endophenotypes in psychiatry be associated with the illness, be heritable, be primarily state independent, and that they cosegregate within families (18). To this end, the Consortium on the Genetics of Schizophrenia (COGS) has selected neurocognitive measures according to these criteria, and Gur and colleagues have presented a strong case that these markers more than meet the criteria for endophenotypes in schizophrenia (17).

SPECIFIC NEUROCOGNITIVE IMPAIRMENTS

IQ

In terms of general intelligence, a number of studies support the finding of lower IQ in schizophrenia. For example, Frith and colleagues (19) assessed IQ in 283 patients with established diagnoses of schizophrenia and reported that current IQ was, on average, 16 points lower than controls. It appears that this decline occurs maximally within the first 5 years of illness (19, 20). Providing support to the fact that this is an

TABLE 13.1 Key findings on Neurocognition in Schizophrenia: summary, evidence and literature review

Neurocognition (Nc)	Evidence	Literature
NC is a core feature of schizophrenia	Widely prevalent among patients with schizophrenia Independent of clinical state (i.e. trait rather than state marker) A modal profile of deficits Present before onset of psychosis Stable across the lifespan Present in healthy 1st degree relatives (i.e. heritable)	4, 5, 6, 7, 8, 9, 15, 16
NC is a useful endophenotype for genetic studies of schizophrenia	Largely familial basis	17, 18
NC is more specific for schizophrenia than for affective psychoses (i.e. "increases the point of rarity")	Modal profile	6, 8
NC correlates well with structural and functional anatomical deficits in schizophrenia	Deficits in PFC, OFC, STG, PHG, hippocampus, amygdala, striatum, cerebellum, thalamus and IPC	4, 34, 37, 38, 39, 40, 41, 42, 43, 45, 46, 47, 48, 49, 50, 51, 52, 53, 54, 55, 56, 57, 58, 60
NC is a better predictor (than psychotic symptoms) of functional outcome in schizophrenia	NC impairment predicts ability to maintain social and work connections, live independently and acquire skills in PSR programmes	6, 79, 80
NC is considered an important treatment target in schizophrenia	Novel psychotropics, psychotherapeutic and rehabilitative techniques	2, 5, 6, 15

inherent feature of the disorder (rather than a consequence of institutionalization or medication, etc.) is the findings of the Edinburgh High Risk Study (EHRS) that healthy first-degree relatives who are at enhanced genetic risk of developing schizophrenia generally perform less well on IQ tests than controls (21). Furthermore, follow-up of the same high-risk individuals revealed that those who subsequently developed psychosis had an increased decline in IQ compared with their premorbid assessment (22). These findings suggest that some intellectual decline precedes the onset of psychosis in schizophrenia.

EXECUTIVE FUNCTIONING

A meta-analysis identified 38 controlled studies, with data from 2,671 patients with schizophrenia, reporting performance on tasks of executive functioning (including the Stroop, WCST, and Trail-Making tests) (23). Patients performed significantly worse on tasks of executive functioning (effect size: –.49.) Executive impairments are also evident in high-risk first-degree relatives, although in an attenuated form (see 21 using the Hayling Sentence Completion test.) A meta-analysis by Sitskoorn and colleagues

(24) of 34 studies found that relatives of patients perform worse than controls on executive tasks, with significant mean effect sizes being in the moderate range. This supports a genetic contribution to prefrontal lobe dysfunction in schizophrenia.

WORKING MEMORY

Problems with working memory are one of the most consistent findings in schizophrenia and have been reported in patients with an established diagnosis (25, 26), in neuroleptic-naïve first-episode patients (27), in individuals with an at-risk mental state (10) and in high-risk, first-degree relatives (21). The EHRS found impaired performance on learning and memory tasks using the Rivermead Behavioral Memory Test (RBMT) in high-risk subjects (21) with a greater degree of impairment in those who subsequently developed psychotic symptoms (22).

ATTENTION

Attentional deficits have long been considered central features of schizophrenia (17) and include problems with sustained focused attention (28), selective attention (29), and cognitive control of attention (30). Meta-analyses of neurocognition in schizophrenia report moderate-to-large effect sizes for tests of attention such as continuous performance tests (CPT) (8, 23). CPT deficits are also present in first-degree relatives (31), including the children (32), siblings, and parents (7, 33) of patients with schizophrenia. Furthermore, attentional deficits have been shown to be independent of clinical state (17).

THE ANATOMY OF COGNITIVE IMPAIRMENT

In a review of neurocognition and its relation to brain structure in schizophrenia, Antonova and colleagues identify the prefrontal cortex (PFC), superior temporal gyrus (STG) and medial temporal lobe (MTL), the thalamus, basal ganglia, and cerebellum as the primary sites of cognitive impairment (34). However, they stress the point that these regions comprise nodes within a distributed functional neural network linking the PFC to posterior cortical and subcortical regions.

WHOLE-BRAIN VOLUME

Generally whole-brain volume (WBV) tends to correlate positively with a range of cognitive domains in a nonspecific manner. This is particularly true in female patients where IQ correlates closely with a number of regional brain volumes including left- and right-cerebral hemispheres, hippocampus, and cerebellum (34). These relationships may be disrupted in male schizophrenic patients (35). More important, significant correlations between WBV and cognition have been related to the presence of deficit symptomatology in schizophrenia (36).

FRONTAL LOBE

Reductions in total frontal volume (FV) do not necessarily correlate with deficits in neurocognitive testing in schizophrenic patients (37). However, volumetric abnormalities of the dorsal PFC have been correlated with a range of cognitive deficits including abstraction, attention, verbal memory, and psychomotor speed (38, 39). Sanfilipo and colleagues (39) found that greater prefrontal white-matter volume (WMV) was associated with increased cognitive flexibility in patients. Working-memory deficits have been correlated with reductions in both prefrontal grey- (GMV) and white- (WMV) matter volumes (40), while volume reductions in the left frontal lobe have been associated with thought and language disturbances in first-episode patients (41).

When considering the subregions of the PFC, deficits in executive functioning such as attention, abstraction, and flexibility correlate with grey-matter reductions in the dorsolateral (DLPFC) and dorsomedial (DMPFC) prefrontal cortex, while verbal and spatial memory deficits correlate with grey-matter reductions of the orbitofrontal cortex (OFC) (38). Working-memory deficits routinely correlate with structural (34, 37) and functional (4, 42) deficits in the DLPFC. It seems that DLPFC activation only fails when working-memory load (or task difficulty) increases (43).

TEMPORAL LOBE

While a few studies have found reductions in total temporal-lobe volume (TLV) in relation to executive-functioning deficits in both chronic (41) and first-episode (44) patients, the majority have found no such associations. The evidence for superior temporal gyrus (STG) and medial temporal lobe (MTL) involvement in neurocognitive impairment is however much greater. In healthy controls, greater STG volume is associated with better processing speed, spatial memory, and attention (38, 39). In patients with schizophrenia, reductions in STG volume (especially grey-matter volume) correlate with poorer verbal fluency, picture naming, abstraction and categorization, and verbal memory (40, 41). The findings of Nestor and colleagues (40) are interesting as their correlation of poor semantic processing with grey-matter reductions in the posterior STG (encompassing Wernicke's area) provides one insight into the anatomical basis of language disorder in schizophrenia. The STG also shows functional abnormalities during graded memory tasks with a failure of normal inhibition (43). Structures in the medial temporal lobe (MTL) are commonly associated with memory, semantic processing, and executive functioning. Impaired memory for stories correlates with volume reductions of the hippocampus in chronic patients (45) and the parahippocampal gyrus (PHG) in first-episode patients (46), while verbal and spatial memory deficits are associated with hippocampal volume reductions (38, 39). Functional imaging reveals impaired recruitment of the hippocampus during memory tasks (47). Impaired executive functioning is correlated with reduced anterior hippocampal volume in first-episode men (48) and with reduced PHG volume in chronic patients (49). PHG volume reductions are also associated with deficits in cognitive functions related to the semantic system, and this association seems to be specific for schizophrenia (46, 49). Finally, impaired emotional learning is associated with a reduction of the right amygdala volume (50).

OTHER REGIONS

There is some evidence that reduced volume of the corpus striatum correlates with impaired goal-directed behavior and executive functioning in schizophrenia (51); however, there is no evidence for an association with learning and memory, and functional deficits are evident during verbal learning tasks (52). Reduced thalamic volume is associated with attentional deficits (53) and impaired executive functioning (54) in first-episode patients, while reduced thalamic glucose metabolism is evident during verbal learning (55). With respect to the cerebellum, Nopoulos and colleagues found a reduction in anterior vermal volume that correlated with reduced full-scale and verbal

IQ in male patients (56). Interestingly, Levitt and colleagues also found an association between cognitive functioning (verbal memory) and vermal volume (57). However, in this study, patients had increased vermal WMV as compared with controls. During functional imaging, decreased blood flow in the cerebellum is detected during memory tasks (58). Finally, reduced parietal-lobe volume has only been correlated weakly in one study with deficits in working memory and executive functioning (59). On the contrary, functional abnormalities of the inferior parietal cortex (IPC) during working-memory and attentional tasks have been well replicated (43, 60).

NEUROCOGNITIVE MODELS OF SCHIZOPHRENIA
A number of models have been proposed to describe the mechanisms by which dysfunction in different regions of the brain might lead to the neuropsychological deficits and symptoms characteristic of schizophrenia.

ABERRANT LATERALIZATION
Schizophrenia has been related to a failure in the development of normal brain asymmetry (61). There is good evidence for lateralized structural and functional abnormalities in the disorder, and it has been postulated that impaired callosal connectivity gives rise to a lack of interhemispheric integration that results in deficits in semantic processing.

THE DISCONNECTION HYPOTHESIS
The disconnection hypothesis attributes neurocognitive and social cognitive abnormalities as well as symptoms in schizophrenia to a breakdown in the normal functional integration of activity between the PFC and posterior cortical and subcortical regions (62, 63). There is good evidence for both functional (62) and structural (64) disconnectivity in prefrontal-temporal and prefrontal-parietal tracts. Frith and others have argued that disconnection leads to a failure of prefrontal self-monitoring so that stimuli in the temporal and parietal cortices are attributed to an external source.

COGNITIVE DYSMETRIA
Drawing on evidence for both thalamic and cerebellar impairment in schizophrenia, Andreasen and colleagues have proposed a model of "cognitive dysmetria" whereby misconnection in the corticocerebellar–thalamiccortical circuit gives rise to symptoms of the disorder through a problem in the coordination of cognitive functions (65).

SOCIAL COGNITION IN SCHIZOPHRENIA
Social cognition refers to the mental operations underlying social interactions and includes processes involved in perceiving, interpreting, and generating responses to the intentions, dispositions, and behaviors of others (66, 67). It is a concept that attracts multidisciplinary interest with research emanating from fields as diverse as cognitive neuroscience, social psychology, and primatology. Within psychiatry, it has been examined primarily in relation to autism and schizophrenia, where deficits in interpersonal communication and relationship can be regarded as central features of

TABLE 13.2 Key findings on Social Cognition in Schizophrenia: summary, evidence and literature review

Social cognition (sc)	Evidence	Literature
SC is a core feature of schizophrenia	SC is widely prevalent in schizophrenia Theory of Mind (ToM) is a trait (rather than state) marker Facial affect recognition (FAR) seems to be stable, independent of state	67, 68, 70, 71, 73, 74
SC is functionally and anatomically distinct from NC in schizophrenia	Deficits in medial PFC, OFC, ACC, STS, IPC and amygdala	72, 73, 74, 76, 77, 78
SC is an independent predictor of functional and social outcome	SC predicts social skills, social behaviour in the milieu and community functioning	67, 68, 79, 80
NC is considered an important treatment target in schizophrenia	Novel psychotropics, psychotherapeutic and rehabilitative techniques	2, 5, 15

these disorders (See Table 13.2.) There is good evidence that social cognition may be functionally and anatomically distinct from traditional neurocognitive domains (68) and, therefore, should be assessed using specific tasks sensitive to the individual cognitive components of social function. In schizophrenia, all of these components are impaired. This has led to the inclusion of social cognition as one of the seven domains represented in the MATRICS consensus cognitive battery (67).

COMPONENTS OF SOCIAL COGNITION IN SCHIZOPHRENIA

The study of social cognition in schizophrenia has focused particularly on components such as theory of mind, social perception, and attributional style.

THEORY OF MIND

The term "theory of mind" (ToM) was coined by Premack and Woodruff in 1978 in relation to chimpanzee's capacity for deception (69). ToM refers to the ability to represent the mental states of others and to make inferences about others' intentions (68). Patients with schizophrenia perform poorly on a range of ToM tasks in comparison to control subjects (see 70 for a review). Specifically, impairments are most profound in individuals with negative features, passivity, and paranoid symptoms and behavioral disturbance (71). Most of the evidence seems to support the stability of ToM as a trait marker, although this issue remains controversial (70). Frith developed a cognitive model of schizophrenia based on ToM dysfunction (72). He suggested that ToM never develops in autism, while in schizophrenia the deficit involves the breakdown of an initially intact ToM, where mental state inferences are still being made but are faulty. Impaired self-monitoring leads to externalized attribution of self-generated stimuli (e.g., voices); while false inferences about the intentions of others lead to persecutory delusions.

SOCIAL PERCEPTION

Research on social perception in schizophrenia has focused on two main areas: facial affect recognition (FAR) and social cue perception (SCP). Individuals with schizophrenia have deficits in FAR compared with controls, and these impairments are more evident for the perception of negative emotional displays (e.g., for fearful faces) (73). Furthermore, FAR seems to be a stable deficit, although some studies suggest improved performance with remission of an acute episode. Tasks that assess SCP use more dynamic stimuli that require multiple sensory modalities and the impairments of SCP characteristic of schizophrenia appear to be more pronounced for abstract relative to concrete social cues (74).

ATTRIBUTIONAL STYLE

Bentall has argued that individuals who experience hallucinations are biased toward attributing internal perceptual events to an external source, whereas individuals who experience paranoid delusions tend to attribute negative outcomes to others and positive outcomes to themselves (75).

THE ANATOMY OF SOCIAL COGNITION IN SCHIZOPHRENIA

Numerous studies have now confirmed the central role of the medial prefrontal cortex (MPFC), especially Brodmann's areas 8 and 9, in social cognition (see 76 for a review). Impaired ToM performance in schizophrenia correlates with lower activation of the MPFC as compared with healthy controls (77). Other regions implicated in ToM include the orbitofrontal cortex (OFC), the paracingulate cortex (ACC), the superior temporal sulcus (STS), the inferior parietal cortex (IPC), and the amygdala. The IPC seems to play a special role in the attribution of agency.

FAR, SCP, and the processing of emotionally laden stimuli are associated with activity in a network of regions including the lateral fusiform gyrus, the STS, the amygdala, and the OFC. Disturbed FAR in schizophrenic patients correlates with hypoactivity in fusiform, prefrontal, anterior temporal, and inferior parietal regions (78).

NEUROCOGNITION, SOCIAL COGNITION, AND FUNCTIONAL OUTCOME

Neurocognitive and social cognitive deficits contribute to poor functional outcome (6). Cognitive impairment correlates strongly with longitudinal ability to maintain social and work connections, live independently, and acquire skills in psychosocial rehabilitation programs (79). Furthermore, cognitive impairment is a better predictor of functional outcome than psychotic symptoms (80). This has important implications for strategies to prevent the long-term disability associated with schizophrenia. More important, cognitive deficits strongly predict the ease with which individuals acquire skills as they progress through skills training and rehabilitation programs (79). The effectiveness of psychosocial rehabilitation, therefore, depends in part on cognitive status, making cognitive impairment an important treatment target in schizophrenia (6).

There is good evidence that social cognition is related to social impairments and functional outcome in schizophrenia, even after controlling for performance on neurocognitive tasks (68). Thus, social cognition can be considered an independent predictor of functional outcome. A review by Couture and colleagues (80) found that social perception is significantly associated with most measures of functional outcome; emotional perception correlates strongly with community functioning, social behavior in the milieu, and social skills, and there is growing evidence that theory of mind (ToM) relates to social skills, community functioning, and social behavior in the milieu.

NEUROCOGNITION, SOCIAL COGNITION, AND DSM-V
Based upon the accumulated evidence that cognitive impairment is a core, stable feature of schizophrenia, is more specific for the disorder than for the affective psychoses, correlates well with structural and functional anatomical deficits and is predictive of functional outcome, Keefe and Fenton have presented a sound argument for the inclusion of cognitive impairment as a specific criterion for the diagnosis and subtypology of schizophrenia in *DSM-V* (5). The MATRICS consensus process indicates that this proposal is receiving serious consideration. The clinical importance of neurocognitive and social cognitive impairment lies in the fact that it is widely prevalent among patients with schizophrenia, seemingly independent of clinical state, has a largely familial basis, may increase the "point of rarity" with affective psychoses, is predictive of functional outcome, and is increasingly considered an important treatment target in management of the disorder. Keefe and Fenton suggest that its inclusion as a criterion in *DSM-V* may increase clinicians' awareness of cognitive impairment and thereby lead to more accurate prognosis and better treatment outcomes. The development of accessible and reliable tools for the evaluation of neurocognitive and social impairment in schizophrenia within clinical and research settings is, therefore, a priority. If we are to overcome the pessimistic views of Kraepelin and Bleuler and their successors, of schizophrenia as a chronic deteriorating disorder associated with serious functional disability, then it is imperative that we develop novel and effective strategies for detecting and managing cognitive and social cognitive impairment in patients with schizophrenia.

REFERENCES

1. Stanghellini G. Psychopathology of common sense. Philosophy, Psychology and Psychiatry 2001; 8: 201–18.
2. Green MF, Neuchterlein K. The MATRICS initiative: developing a consensus cognitive battery for clinical trials. Schizophr Res 2004; 72: 1–3.
3. Green MF, Neuchterlin KH, Gold JM et al. Approaching a consensus cognitive battery for clinical trials in schizophrenia: the NIMH-MATRICS conference to select cognitive domains and test criteria. Biol Psychiatry 2004; 56: 301–7.
4. Kuperberg G, Heckers S. Schizophrenia and cognitive function. Curr Opin Neurobiol 2000; 10: 205–10.
5. Keefe RSE, Fenton WS. How should DSM-V criteria for schizophrenia include cognitive impairment? Schizophr Bull 2007; 33(4): 912–20.
6. Green MF. Cognitive impairment and functional outcome in schizophrenia and bipolar disorder. J Clin Psychiatry 2006; 67(suppl 9): 3–8.
7. Finkelstein JR, Cannon TD, Gur RE et al. Attentional dysfunctions in neuroleptic- naïve and neuroleptic-withdrawn schizophrenic patients and their siblings. J Abnorm Psychol 1997; 106: 203–12.
8. Heinrichs RW, Zakzanis KK. Neurocognitive deficit in schizophrenia: a quantitative review of the evidence. Neuropsychology 1998; 12: 426–45.
9. Mohamed S, Paulsen JS, O'Leary D et al. Generalized cognitive deficits in schizophrenia: as study of first-episode patients. Arch Gen Psychiatry 1999; 56: 749–54.
10. Pflueger MO, Gschwandtner U, Stieglitz RD et al. Neuropsychological deficits in individuals with an at risk mental state for psychosis – Working memory as a potential trait marker. Schizophr Res 2007; 97: 14–24.

11. Eastvold AD, Heaton RK, Cadenhead KS. Neurocognitive deficits in the (putative) prodrome and first episode of psychosis. Schizophr Res 2007; 93: 266–77.

12. Pukrop R, Ruhrmann S, Schutze-Lutter F et al. Neurocognitive indicators for a conversion to psychosis: Comparison of patients in a potentially initial prodromal state who did or did not convert to a psychosis. Schizophr Res 2007; 92: 116–25.

13. Ayres AM, Busatto GF, Menezes PR et al. Cognitive deficits in first-episode psychosis: A population-based study in São Paulo, Brazil. Scizophr Res 2007; 90: 338–43.

14. Albus M, Hubmann W, Mohr F et al. Neurocognitive functioning in patients with first-episode schizophrenia. Eur Arch Psychiatry Clin Neurosci 2006; 256: 442–51.

15. Gold JM. Cognitive deficits as treatment targets in schizophrenia. Scizophr Res 2004; 72: 21–8.

16. Kuha A, Tuulio-Henriksson A, Eerola M et al. Impaired executive performance in healthy siblings of schizophrenia patients in a population-based study. Schizophr Res 2007; 92: 142–50.

17. Gur RE, Calkins ME, Gur RC et al. The consortium on the genetics of schizophrenia: neurocognitive endophenotypes. Schizophr Bull 2007; 33(1): 49–68.

18. Gottesman II, Gould TD. The endophenotype concept in psychiatry: etymology and strategic intentions. Am J Psychiatry 2003; 160: 636–45.

19. Frith CD, Leary J, Cahill C, Johnstone EC. Disabilities and circumstances of schizophrenic patients – a follow-up study. IV. Performance on psychological tests: demographic and clinical correlates of the results of these tests. Br J Psychiatry 1991; 159(suppl 13): 26–9.

20. Nelson HE, Pantelis C, Carruthers K et al. Cognitive functioning and symptomatology in chronic schizophrenia. Psychol Med 1990; 20: 357–65.

21. Byrne M, Hodges A, Grant E et al. Neuropsychological assessment of young people at high genetic risk for developing schizophrenia compared with controls: preliminary findings of the Edinburgh High Risk Study (EHRS). Psychol Med 1999; 29: 1161–73.

22. Cosway R, Byrne M, Clafferty R et al. Neuropsychological change in young people at high risk for schizophrenia: results from the first two neuropsychological assessments of the Edinburgh High Risk Study. Psychol Med 2000; 30: 1111–21.

23. Fioravanti M, Carlone O, Vitale B et al. A meta-analysis of cognitive deficits in adults with a diagnosis of schizophrenia. Neuropsychol Rev 2005; 15(2): 73–95.

24. Sitskoorn M, Aleman A, Ebisch S et al. Cognitive deficits in relatives of patients with schizophrenia: a meta-analysis. Schizophr Res 2004 71: 285–95.

25. Aleman A, Hijman R, de Haan EHF, Kahn RS. Memory impairment in schizophrenia: a meta-analysis. Am J Psychiatry 1999; 156: 1358–66.

26. Lee J, Park S. Working memory impairments in schizophrenia: a meta-analysis. J Abnorm Psychol 2005; 114: 599–611.

27. Saykin AJ, Shtasel DL, Gur RE et al. Neuropsychological deficits in neuroleptic-naïve patients with first-episode schizophrenia. Arch Gen Psychiatry 1994; 51: 124–31.

28. Cornblatt BA, Keilp JG. Impaired attention, genetics, and the pathophysiology of schizophrenia. Schizophr Bull 1994; 20: 31–46.

29. Nestor PG, Han SD, Niznikiewicz M et al. Semantic disturbance in schizophrenia and its relationship to the cognitive neuroscience of attention. Biol Psychol 2001; 57: 23–46.

30. Cohen JD, Braver TS, O'Reilly RC. A computational approach to prefrontal cortex, cognitive control and schizophrenia: recent developments and current challenges. Philos Trans R Soc Lond B Biol Sci 1996; 351: 1515–27.

31. Snitz BE, Macdonald AW III, Carter CS. Cognitive deficits in unaffected first-degree relatives of schizophrenia patients: a meta-analytic review of putative endophenotypes. Schizophr Bull 2006; 32: 179–94.

32. Rutschmann J, Cornblatt B, Erlenmeyer-Kimling L. Sustained attention in children at risk for schizophrenia. Arch Gen Psychiatry 1977; 34: 571–75.

33. Chen WJ, Chang CH, Liu SK et al. Sustained attention deficits in nonpsychotic relatives of schizophrenia patients: a recurrence risk ratio analysis. Biol Psychiatry 2004; 55: 995–1000.

34. Antonova E, Sharma T, Morris R, Kumari V. The relationship between brain structure and neurocognition in schizophrenia: a selective review. Schizophr Res 2004; 70: 117–45.

35. Flaum M, Andreasen NC, Swayze VW et al. IQ and brain size in schizophrenia. Psychiatry Res 1994; 53: 243–57.
36. Kareken DA, Gur RC, Mozley PD et al. Cognitive functioning and neuroanatomic volume measures in schizophrenia. Neuropsychology 1995; 9: 211–9.
37. Crespo-Facorro B, Barbadillo L, Pelayo-Teran JM et al. Neuropsychological functioning and brain structure in schizophrenia. Int Rev Psychiatry 2007; 19(4): 325–36.
38. Gur RE, Cowell PE, Latshaw A et al. Reduced dorsal and orbital prefrontal grey matter volumes in schizophrenia. Arch Gen Psychiatry 2000; 57: 761–8.
39. Sanfilipo M, Lafargue T, Rusinek H et al. Cognitive performance in schizophrenia: relationship to regional brain volumes and psychiatric symptoms. Psychiatry Res 2002; 116: 1–23.
40. Nestor PG, O'Donnell BF, McCarley RW et al. A new statistical method for testing hypotheses of neuropsychological/MRI relationships in schizophrenia: partial least squares analysis. Schizophr Res 2002; 53: 57–66.
41. Vita A, Dieci M, Giobbio GM et al. Language and thought disorder in schizophrenia: brain morphological correlates. Schizophr Res 1995; 15: 243–51.
42. Goldman-Rakic PS. The physiological approach: functional architecture of working memory and disordered cognition in schizophrenia. Biol Psychiatry 1999; 46: 650–61.
43. Fletcher PC, McKenna PJ, Frith CD et al. Brain activations in schizophrenia during a graded memory task studied with functional neuroimaging. Arch Gen Psychiatry 1998; 55: 1001–8.
44. Hoff AL, Riordan H, O'Donnell D et al. Anomalous lateral sulcus asymmetry and cognitive function in first-episode schizophrenia. Schizophr Bull 1992; 18: 257–72.
45. Goldberg TE, Torrey EF, Berman KF et al. Relations between neuropsychological performance and brain morphological and physiological measures in monozygotic twins discordant for schizophrenia. Psychiatry Res 1994; 55: 51–61.
46. De Lisi LE, Hoff AL, Schwartz JE et al. Brain morphology in first-episode schizophrenic-like psychotic patients: a quantitative magnetic resonance imaging study. Biol Psychiatry 1991; 29: 159–75.
47. Heckers S, Rauch SL, Goff D et al. Impaired recruitment of the hippocampus during conscious recollection in schizophrenia. Nat Neurosci 1998; 1: 318–23.
48. Szeszko PR, Strous RD, Goldman RS et al. Neuropsychological correlates of hippocampal volumes in patients experiencing a first episode of schizophrenia. Am J Psychiatry 2002; 159: 217–26.
49. Krabbendam L, Derix MM, Honig A et al. Cognitive performance in relation to MRI temporal lobe volume in schizophrenic patients and healthy control subjects. J Neuropsychiatry Clin Neurosci 2000; 12: 251–56.
50. Exner C, Boucsein K, Degner D et al. Impaired emotional learning and reduced amygdala size in schizophrenia: a 3-month follow-up. Schizophr Res 2004; 71: 93–503.
51. Stratta P, Mancini F, Mattei P et al. Association between striatal reduction and poor Wisconsin card sorting test performance in patients with schizophrenia. Biol Psychiatry 1997; 42: 816–20.
52. Shihabuddin L, Buchsbaum MS, Hazlett EA et al. Dorsal striatal size, shape, and metabolic rate in never-medicated and previously medicated schizophrenics performing a verbal learning task. Arch Gen Psychiatry 1998; 55: 235–43.
53. Salgado-Pineda P, Baeza I, Perez-Gomez M et al. Sustained attention impairment correlates to gray matter decreases in first episode neuroleptic-naïve schizophrenic patients. Neuroimage 2003; 19: 365–75.
54. Crespo-Facorro B, Roiz-Santianez R, Pelayo-Teran JM et al. Reduced thalamic volume in first-episode non-affective psychosis: correlations with clinical variables, symptomatology and cognitive functioning. Neuroimage 2007; 35: 1613–23.
55. Hazlett EA, Buchsbaum MS, Byne W et al. Three-dimensional analysis with MRI and PET of the size, shape, and function of the thalamus in the schizophrenia spectrum. Am J Psychiatry 1999; 156: 1190–9.
56. Nopoulos PC, Ceilley JW, Gailis EA et al. An MRI study of cerebellar vermis morphology in patients with schizophrenia: evidence in support of the cognitive dysmetria concept. Biol Psychiatry 1999; 46: 703–11.

57. Levitt JJ, McCarley RW, Nestor PG et al. Quantitative volumetric MRI study of the cerebellum and vermis in schizophrenia: clinical and cognitive correlates. Am J Psychiatry 1999; 156: 1105–7.
58. Andreasen NC, Nopoulos P, O'Leary DS et al. Defining the phenotype of schizophrenia: cognitive dysmetria and its neural mechanisms. Biol Psychiatry 1999; 46: 908–20.
59. Laywer G, Nyman H, Agartz I et al. Morphological correlates to cognitive dysfunction in schizophrenia as studied with Bayesian regression. BMC Psychiatry 2006; 6: 31.
60. Cleghorn JM, Kaplan RD, Nahmias C et al. Inferior parietal region implicated in neurocognitive impairment in schizophrenia. Arch Gen Psychiatry 1989; 46: 758–60.
61. Crow TJ. Is schizophrenia the price that Homo sapiens pays for language? Schizophr Res 1997; 28: 127–41.
62. Friston KJ, Frith CD. Schizophrenia: a disconnection syndrome? Clin Neurosci 1995; 3: 89–97.
63. Dolan RJ, Fletcher PC, McKenna P et al. Abnormal neural integration related to cognition in schizophrenia. Acta Psychiatr Scand 1999; (Suppl), 395: 58–67.
64. Burns J, Job D, Bastin ME et al. Structural disconnectivity in schizophrenia: a diffusion tensor magnetic resonance imaging study. Br J Psychiatry 2003; 182: 439–43.
65. Andreasen NC. A unitary model of schizophrenia: Bleuler's "fragmented phrene" as schizencephaly. Arch Gen Psychiatry 1999; 56: 781–7.
66. Brothers L. The neural basis of primate social communication. Motiv Emotion 1990; 14: 81–91.
67. Green MF, Olivier B, Crawley JN et al. Social cognition in schizophrenia: recommendations form the Measurement and Treatment Research to Improve Cognition in Schizophrenia New Approaches Conference. Schizophr Bull 2005; 31(4): 882–7.
68. Pinkham AE, Penn DL, Perkins DO et al. Implications for the neural basis of social cognition for the study of schizophrenia. Am J Psychiatry 2003; 160: 815–24.
69. Premack D, Woodruff G. Does the chimpanzee have a 'theory of mind'? Behav Brain Sci 1978; 4: 515–26.
70. Harrington L, Siegert RJ, McClure J. Theory of mind in schizophrenia: a critical review. Cogn Neuropsychiatry 2005; 10(4): 249–86.
71. Pickup GJ, Frith CD. Theory of mind impairments in schizophrenia: symptomatology, severity, and specificity. Psychol Med 2001; 31: 207–20.
72. Frith CD. The cognitive neuropsychology of schizophrenia. Hove, UK: Psychology Press, 1992.
73. Mandal MK, Pandey R, Prasad AB. Facial expressions of emotion and schizophrenia: a review. Schizophr Bull 1998; 24: 399–412.
74. Leonhard C, Corrigan PW. Social perception in schizophrenia. In: Corrigan PW, Penn DL, eds. Social Cognition in Schizophrenia. Washington DC: American Psychological Association, 2001: 73–95.
75. Bentall RP. The illusion of reality: a review and integration of psychological research on hallucinations. Psychol Bull 1990; 107: 82–95.
76. Amodio DM, Frith CD. Meeting of minds: the medial frontal cortex and social cognition. Nat Rev Neurosci 2006; 7: 268–77.
77. Russell TA, Rubia K, Bullmore ET et al. Exploring the social brain in schizophrenia: left prefrontal underactivation during mental state attribution. Am J Psychiatry 2000; 157: 2040–2.
78. Streit M, Ioannides A, Sinnemann T et al. Disturbed facial affect recognition in patients with schizophrenia associated with hypoactivity in distributed brain regions: a magnetoencephalographic study. Am J Psychiatry 2001; 158: 1429–36.
79. Green MF, Kern RS, Heaton RK. Longitudinal studies of cognition and functional outcome in schizophrenia: implications for MATRICS. Schizophr Res 2004; 72: 41–51.
80. Green MF. What are the functional consequences of neurocognitive deficits in schizophrenia? Am J Psychiatry 1996; 153: 321–30.

14 An update of meta-analyses on second-generation antipsychotic drugs for schizophrenia

Stefan Leucht, Caroline Corves, Werner Kissling, and John M Davis

INTRODUCTION

There is continuing debate about the superiority of second-generation ("atypical") antipsychotic drugs (SGA) compared to conventional neuroleptics (first-generation antipsychotic drugs, FGA) which is mainly driven by the higher cost of the former. A number of meta-analyses on this question have been published (6, 4, 1). Limitations of these meta-analyses were that most of them analyzed only overall efficacy, although SGAs are thought to be especially effective for negative symptoms and depression associated with schizophrenia. Cochrane reviews on single SGAs are available (1), but, because they were published in different reports, it is difficult to form a gestalt. The older meta-analyses also failed to thoroughly assess side effects, although these are important criteria in drug choice. Furthermore, the number of randomized controlled trials (RCT) in this area is continually increasing, which made new meta-analyses necessary. In the current chapter, we summarize the findings of three updated syatematic reviews on the effects of second-generation antipsychotics in schizophrenia (13, 14, 17), compare the results with other meta-analyses (6, 4, 1) and the results of the recent effectiveness studies, CATIE, CUtLASS, and EUFEST (19, 9, 18, 10).

METHOD

We summarize and comment on the results of our previous meta-analyses comparing SGAs with placebo (13), with first-generation antipsychotics (FGAs) (14), and SGAs head to head (17). What follows is a discussion in the context of other reviews and recent effectiveness studies.

RESULTS

SGAs versus placebo (meta-analysis based on 38 studies with 7,323 participants (13)):

Efficacy

All SGAs and haloperidol were more efficacious than placebo for overall symptoms of schizophrenia as measured by the PANSS or BPRS total score or the number of responders (see Figure 14.1). However, the effects were of only medium size and ranged from 0.41 (aripiprazole) to 0.59 (risperidone), and the pooled effect size across drugs was 0.51. Only a single old clozapine study yielded an effect size of 1.64. Numbers needed to treat ranged between 4 and 7 and were 6 overall. We found in a meta-regression that in the past decades the drug–placebo difference decreased over time.

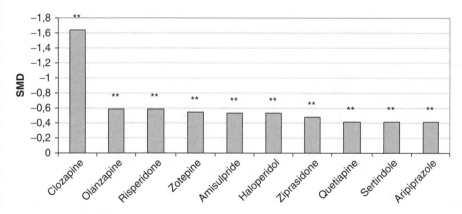

FIGURE 14.1 Second generation antipsychotic drugs and haloperidol versus placebo (data from Leucht et al. 2008a).

The bars are the mean effect sizes for the primary outcome overall symptoms (PANSS or BPRS total score reduction from baseline to endpoint) of the various antipsychotic drugs compared to placebo. It should be noted that the clozapine effect size was based on a single, small and old study (n = 22), SMD = standardised mean difference (Hedges's g), ** = p < 0.01.

Most SGAs have also been shown to reduce relapse rates more than placebo, although true maintenance studies were only available for aripiprazole, olanzapine, ziprasidone, and zotepine. Overall, 5 participants had to be treated for approximately 6 months instead of placebo to avoid one relapse (NNT = 5).

All second-generation antipsychotic drugs also reduced the positive and negative symptoms more than placebo (concerning positive symptoms except for amisulpride and zotepine that have not been examined in relevant patient populations). It should be noted that negative symptoms were generally reduced less than positive symptoms (pooled effect size across drugs: –.39 for negative symptoms compared to –.48 for positive symptoms). The likely reason is that almost all studies were conducted in participants with predominant positive symptoms. Therefore, floor effects may have limited the drug–placebo difference in negative symptoms. Furthermore, haloperidol successfully reduced negative symptoms, as well, and the effect size (–.30) was similar to that of the SGAs (range –.26 to –.44). An even more surprising finding was that not only some SGAs but also haloperidol reduced depressive symptoms more than placebo. It has been described that haloperidol can induce depression ("pharmacogenic depression"; (25)). It is possible that in the short-term haloperidol improves depressive symptoms associated with schizophrenia and that in the long-term dopamine blockade and extrapyramidal side effects (EPS) induce depression.

Side effects
There were no significant differences in EPS between SGA's and placebo, whereas haloperidol induced clearly more EPS. Only risperidone had a nonsignificant trend (p = 0.07) to produce more EPS than placebo. We believe that some SGAs do induce more EPS than placebo (although on a clearly lower level than haloperidol for which 48% of the participants needed antiparkinson medication). For example, 32% of

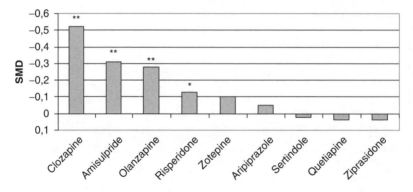

FIGURE 14.2 Second generation antipsychotic drugs versus first generation antipsychotic drugs (data from Leucht et al. 2008b).

The bars are the mean effect sizes for the primary outcome overall symptoms (PANSS or BPRS total score reduction from baseline to endpoint) of the various second generation antipsychotic drugs compared to first generation antipsychotic drugs. SMD = standardised mean difference (Hedges's g), * = $p < 0.05$, ** = $p < 0.01$.

risperidone patients received antiparkinsonian medication (compared to 26% of the patients in its placebo groups). The high EPS rate in the placebo group may have made it impossible to show a difference, when compared to risperidone. It can probably be explained by carry-over effects from prestudy treatment due to too short wash-out phases that typically lasted only a few days.

There were only a few SGAs that were more sedating than placebo, but the assessment of this outcome is difficult because concomitant benzodiazepines are allowed in all these trials.

Surprisingly, there were no differences in dropouts due to adverse events (except sertindole using the risk as an effect size). We stressed that not only efficacy-related events (e.g., a "psychotic exacerbation") but also side effects are considered as adverse events (13). Therefore, "dropout due to adverse events" is unfortunately not a pure measure of tolerability.

SGAs versus first-generation antipsychotics (14):

This meta-analysis was based on 215 studies, but when we found that open-label studies significantly favored the SGAs, we based all results only on the 150 double-blind trials with 21,533 participants (14).

Efficacy

Amisulpride, clozapine, olanzapine, risperidone were more efficacious than FGAs with small-to medium-effect sizes in terms of primary outcome and overall symptoms (PANSS/BPRS total score, range: risperidone ES 0.13 to clozapine ES 0.52, NNT range 6 to 15). The other SGAs were as efficacious as FGAs (see Figure 14.2).

When we analyzed specific symptoms of schizophrenia, we found that the four, overall more efficacious SGAs were also more efficacious for positive symptoms and negative symptoms. The other SGAs were again (only) as efficacious as FGAs, and quetiapine was indeed less effective for positive symptoms. As only four SGAs were significantly superior for negative symptoms, we concluded that high efficacy for negative symptoms cannot be a core component of "atypicality" (14).

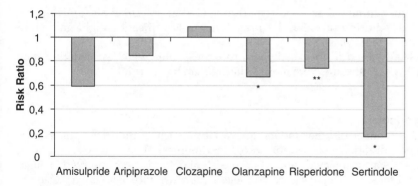

FIGURE 14.3   Relapse (data from Leucht et al. 2008b).

The bars are the mean risk ratios for the outcome relapse of the various second generation antipsychotic drugs compared to first generation antipsychotic drugs. It should be noted that for the other second generation antipsychotic drugs relevant data were not available. * = p < 0.05, ** = p < 0.01.

Fewer data available on depression showed a slightly different pattern: In addition to amisulpride, clozapine, and olanzapine, aripiprazole and quetiapine were more efficacious, while risperidone was not. This finding was interesting because aripiprazole and quetiapine have been shown to be efficacious for major depression. A methodological limitation was that the results were usually based on depression subscores of the PANSS or the BPRS, whereas only a few studies applied validated depression rating scales.

Although second-generation antipsychotic drugs are marketed as being especially beneficial for quality of life, very few studies on this concept were available. Only amisulpride, clozapine, and sertindole proved superior to FGAs. As "no evidence of effect does not mean evidence of no effect," more studies are needed (14).

Similarly, only a few long-term studies with heterogeneous designs are available that showed a reduction of relapses for olanzapine, risperidone, and sertindole (the NNT ranged between 11 and 17 (14)).

Side effects
We found that all SGAs induced fewer EPS than haloperidol, most even when the latter was used in low doses below 7.5mg/day. In single studies, a one-time daily dosage of 3 to 4 mg haloperidol produced more EPS than risperidone and sertindole (26, 23). The finding that even in low doses haloperidol induces more EPS than SGAs has recently also been replicated by the EUFEST study that limited the upper haloperidol dose range to 4 mg/day (10).

The difference in EPS between SGAs and so-called low-potency FGAs (e.g., chlorpromazine, thioridazine, perazine) was less clear. A limitation of this comparison was the smaller number of RCTs. Nevertheless, it is possible that not all SGAs produce more EPS than FGAs, or at least the difference may be smaller.

But low-potency FGAs are known to be associated with weight gain and sedation, and indeed, we did not find a significant difference in weight gain between any SGA and low-potency FGAs. On the other hand, compared to haloperidol, the weight-gain pattern was similar to that found by Allison et al. 2000: Clozapine (3.4 kg), olanzapine (3.3 kg), sertindole (3.3 kg), and zotepine (2.7 kg) induced the most weight gain; quetiapine (1.7 kg) and risperidone (1.4kg), intermediate; amisulpride (0.9 kg), little; and aripiprazole and ziprasidone, no significant weight gain compared to haloperidol (14).

The SGAs differed in their sedative properties, some were less sedating than low-potency FGAs, but some were more sedating than haloperidol.

Moderator variables

We analyzed a number of other moderator variables such as industry sponsorship, chronicity, study duration, comparator dose, EPS differences between SGA and FGA, prophylactic anti-Parkinson medication. No consistent patterns were observed in meta-regressions and sensitivity analyses. Nevertheless, the sensitivity of meta-regression to detect significant differences is low because it addresses these moderators on a study level rather than on and individual-patient level (14).

SGAs versus SGAs head to head (meta-analysis of 78 studies with 13,558 participants (17))

People frequently interpret meta-analyses comparing SGAs with FGAs in a problematic way; for example, the fact that amisulpride was more efficacious than haloperidol while aripiprazole was only as efficacious has often been interpreted as amisulpride is better than aripiprazole. This conclusion could be wrong due to multiple confounders. For example, the amisulpride studies have all been conducted in Europe and earlier than the aripiprazole studies. Therefore, head-to-head comparisons were needed to compare the various SGAs.

The first meta-analysis comparing all SGAs head to head found a similar efficacy pattern as it was observed in the meta-analysis with FGA as comparator (17), see Table 14.1). Olanzapine turned out to be more efficacious than aripiprazole, quetiapine, risperidone, and ziprasidone; risperidone was more efficacious than quetiapine and ziprasidone. Amisulpride was not statistically different from olanzapine or risperidone but more efficacious than ziprasidone in dropout due to inefficacy. The surprise of this analysis was that clozapine was not generally more efficacious than other SGAs, although it is thought to be the most effective compound and the meta-analysis of (11). Clozapine proved superior only to zotepine and to risperidone in dropout due to inefficacy (for discussion see the following).

We have not yet published our results on comparative side effects of the various SGAs, but preliminary analyses showed that the data are compatible with those of the indirect analyses (data not shown).

DISCUSSION

Currently, at least 38 double-blind, randomized controlled trials (RCT) compared SGAs with placebo; 150 double-blind studies compared SGAs with FGAs; and 78 blinded studies compared SGAs head to head with other SGAs. In our opinion, it is impossible to summarize this incredible amount of studies with conventional review methods, which makes updated meta-analyses necessary. Furthermore, we have illustrated that the debate about the SGAs is more driven by values than by objective data (16). Some think that efficacy is most important and highlight efficacy differences between the compounds. Others are interested in weight gain and its resulting metabolic problems and, therefore, stress the weight gain associated with some SGAs. Many are concerned

TABLE 14.1 Brief summary of results in terms of the primary outcome PANSS total score of the meta-analysis comparing second-generation antipsychotic drugs head to head (modified from (Leucht et al. 2008d)).

	Amisulpride	Aripiprazole	Clozapine	Olanzapine	Quetiapine	Risperidone	Sertindole	Ziprasidone	Zotepine
Aripiprazole									
Clozapine									
Olanzapine	↔ 701	OLA ↑ 794	↔ 619						
Quetiapine			↔ 232	OLA ↑ 1449					
Risperidone	↔ 291	↔ 372	↔ 466	OLA ↑ 2404	RIS ↑ 1953				
Sertindole						↔ 493			
Ziprasidone	↔ 122		↔ 146	OLA ↑ 1291	↔ 710	RIS ↑ 1016			
Zotepine			CLO ↑ 59						

Blank fields indicate that no study is available. ↑ Statistically significantly superior, ↔ no significant difference between groups. CLO = clozapine. OLA = olanzapine. RIS = risperidone.
The numbers below the arrows represent the number of participants included in the comparison.

with EPS and tardive dyskinesia. Again, others question the high cost of the SGAs. We think that very often the debate is rather political and the arguments are not always based on evidence. Meta-analyses can partly overcome this subjectivity by objectively summarizing the data in a uniform way.

There is relatively little controversy about the side-effect profiles of the different drugs: All second-generation antipsychotic drugs produced fewer extrapyramidal side effects than haloperidol, even if the latter is used in relatively small doses (10, 13). The difference in EPS between SGAs and low-potency FGAs such as chlorpromazine is smaller and may be absent for some SGAs. Not all SGAs are completely free of EPS. This is shown by a meta-analysis on SGAs for bipolar mania where aripiprazole, risperidone, and ziprasidone ($p = 0.06$) did induce some EPS (22). Furthermore, in a study on adolescents with schizophrenia, aripiprazole clearly produced EPS (5). It should also be noted that compared to placebo, amisulpride has only been studied in low doses (maximum 300mg/day(13), at higher doses EPS can occur.

Most SGAs induce more weight gain than haloperidol. But more important, the degree of weight gain differs between SGAs and not all of them are affected. Just as discussed in the work by (2), clozapine, olanzapine, zotepine, and sertindole caused the most weight gain, followed by quetiapine and risperidone, while amisulpride had little effect, and there was no significant difference between aripiprazole or ziprasidone and haloperidol. What is often forgotten in the debate is that low-potency FGAs induce considerable weight gain as well. Furthermore, low-potency FGAs are quite sedating, and the SGAs also differ in their sedating properties.

Prolactin increase is another important side effect that was not addressed by the meta-analyses. While the prolactin increase of most SGAs is small, for amisulpride and risperidone, however, it is larger compared to haloperidol (12). Potentially dangerous prolongations of the QTc interval have been mainly associated with sertindole and ziprasidone.

Whether there are relevant efficacy differences between SGAs and FGAs is more controversial. We found that amisulpride, clozapine, olanzapine, and risperidone were significantly more efficacious than FGAs, while the other SGAs were only as efficacious (15). Figure 14.4 shows that the results of large meta-analyses by (6, 4, 15) and the current versions of the Cochrane reviews (1) are quite consistent. However, these reviews differed in interpretation. Ways to more consistently interpret meta-analyses must be found, if not, then the method may be called into question.

In the meta-analysis of RCTs comparing the SGAs head to head, we found a by and large compatible efficacy pattern. Olanzapine was superior to aripiprazole, quetiapine, risperidone, and ziprasidone. Risperidone was more efficacious than quetiapine and ziprasidone. Clozapine proved superior to zotepine, and to risperidone, when it was used in doses higher than 400mg/day (17). The only unexpected finding was the lack of a general superiority of clozapine. We discussed that probably too low doses of clozapine explain this surprising finding (17). The clozapine doses were usually well below 400mg/day (in five studies, even under 210mg/day), which is in contrast to the pivotal studies proving clozapine's superiority, compared to FGAs (11, 21); 600mg/day and 523mg/day, respectively), and lower than the optimum dose found in the only true dose-finding study (24, 3). We add that a sufficient number of trials is currently only available for the comparison of clozapine with olanzapine and risperidone, the more efficacious among SGAs. Nevertheless, we concluded that a definitive study comparing clozapine versus other SGAs trial is still needed (17).

The results are not identical, but at least in part compatible with the recent effectiveness studies CATIE (19), CUtLASS (18), and EUFEST (10). In CATIE-I, olanzapine

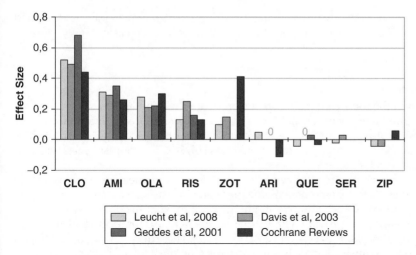

FIGURE 14.4 The results of meta-analysis comparing SGAs with FGAs are consistent. The bars are the mean effect sizes (Hedges's adjusted g) for the primary outcome overall symptoms of schizpohrenia in the various reviews. CLO = clozapine, AMI = amisulpride, OLA = olanzapine, RIS = risperidone, ZOT = zotepine, ARI = aripiprazole, QUE = quetiapine, SER = sertindole, ZIP = ziprasidone. Modified from Leucht et al. 2009.

was significantly better than perphenazine in its primary efficacy measure dropout due to inefficacy and time on effective treatment, and (open label) clozapine was better than other SGAs in CATIE-II (20). As in the meta-analysis comparing SGAs with FGAs quetiapine and ziprasidone were not more efficacious. The difference between CATIE and the meta-analyses was a lack of superiority of risperidone. We discussed that a relatively low risperidone dose may have played a role (16). Furthermore, it should be noted that in the meta-analysis comparing SGAs with FGAs (15) the effect size of risperidone was statistically significant, but numerically very small. The differences in weight gain and metabolic side effects were very consistent with previous knowledge. While perphenazine was associated with most dropouts due to EPS and most frequent anti-Parkinson medication use, there was no difference in scale for derived EPS. Whether this relatively small difference can be simply explained by perphenazine being a mid-potency FGA is unclear. In a Cochrane review on perphenazine, we did not find clear differences in EPS between perphenazine and other FGAs (8).

The CUtLASS study found no significant difference between SGAs and FGAs. This finding was not entirely unexpected because, in this study, clinicians could choose among SGAs and FGAs, and we found not all SGAs are more efficacious. Furthermore, 60% of the participants of the FGA group were started on sulpiride, a drug with a similar receptor binding as amisulpride. Although CUtLASS suggests that patients can be treated reasonably well when carefully chosen among old drugs, there is the problem that in many countries neither sulpiride nor perphenazine was the mainstay of treatment. If CUtLASS were interpreted such that all drugs are equal, psychiatrists might return to high-dose haloperidol (16).

The EUFEST study was randomized, but being open label, not included in our meta-analysis (14). It found a similar rank order in that olanzapine and amisulpride were best in discontinuation due to inefficacy. However, unlike the meta-analysis, haloperidol did significantly worse than ziprasidone, which may in part be explained by lack of blinding. The resultant side effects were again very consistent with previous knowledge.

CONCLUSION

We have drawn the following main conclusions from the meta-analyses:

SGAs differ in many properties including: efficacy, side effects (even in the occurrence of EPS), cost (some are becoming generic), and pharmacology (amisulpride is not a 5-HT2 blocker) and are, therefore, not a class (14, 16). The confusing classification may, therefore, be abandoned.

Overall, the results are relatively consistent. Therefore, the debate appears to be driven more by values than by data: Some place an emphasis on cost, others focus on EPS, weight gain, or efficacy (16). We should go back to what the data say.

The meta-analyses provide data that clinicians may use for individualized treatment based on efficacy, side effects, and cost (13, 14, 17). These decisions should be shared with the patients because, after all, it is the patients who must take the drugs (7).

ACKNOWLEDGMENT

Conflict of interest: Stefan Leucht has received speaker and/or consultancy honoraria from SanofiAventis, BMS, EliLilly, Janssen/Johnson and Johnson, Lundbeck and Pfizer, and he has received funding for research projects from EliLilly and SanofiAventis. Werner Kissling has received speaker and/or advisory board/consultancy honoraria from Janssen, Sanofi-AVentis, Johnson and Johnson, Pfizer, Bayer, BMS, Astra Zeneca, Lundbeck, Novartis, and EliLilly. Caroline Corves: none to declare. John M Davis: none to declare.

Grant support: Financial support was provided by a grant from the German Federal Ministry of Education and Research, no FKZ: 01KG 0606, GZ: GFKG01100506 (SL), and a grant from the National Institute of Mental Health, Advanced Center for Intervention and Services Research Center (MH-68580), Grant No. 1 P01MH68580-01 CFDA #93.242, the Maryland Psychiatric Research Center (JD).

REFERENCES

1. Adams C.E, Coutinho E, Davis J.Met al. Cochrane Schizophrenia Group. In: "The Cochrane Library", John Wiley & Sons Ltd, Chichester, UK, 2008.
2. Allison DB, Mentore JL, Heo M et al. Antipsychotic-induced weight gain: A comprehensive research synthesis. Am J Psychiatry 1999; 156: 1686–96.
3. Davis JM, Chen N. Dose-response and dose equivalence of antipsychotics. J Clin Psychopharmacol 2004; 24: 192–208.
4. Davis JM, Chen N, Glick ID. A meta-analysis of the efficacy of second-generation antipsychotics. Arch Gen Psychiatry 2003; 60: 553–64.
5. Findling RA, Robb A, Nyilas M et al. A multi-center, randomized, double-blind, placebo-controlled study of oral aripiprazole for treatment of adolescents with schizophrenia. Am J Psychiatry 2008; epub ahead of print.
6. Geddes J, Freemantle N, Harrison P, Bebbington P. Atypical antipsychotics in the treatment of schizophrenia: systematic overview and meta-regression analysis. BMJ 2000; 321: 1371–6.
7. Hamann J, Leucht S, Kissling W. Shared decision making in psychiatry. Acta Psychiatrica Scandinavica 2003; 107: 403–9.

8. Hartung B, Wada M, Laux G, Leucht S. Perphenazine for schizophrenia. Cochrane Database of Systematic Reviews 2005; CD003443.

9. Jones PB, Barnes TRE, Davies L et al. Randomized controlled trial of the effect on quality of life of second- vs first-generation antipsychotic drugs in schizophrenia – cost utility of the latest antipsychotic drugs in schizophrenia study (CUtLASS 1). Arch Gen Psychiatry 2006; 63: 1079–86.

10. Kahn RS, Fleischhacker WW, Boter H et al. Effectiveness of antipsychotic drugs in first-episode schizophrenia and schizophreniform disorder: an open randomised clinical trial. Lancet 2008; 371: 1085–97.

11. Kane JM, Honigfeld G, Singer J , Meltzer H, and the Clozaril Collaborative study group.. Clozapine for the treatment-resistant schizophrenic. A double-blind comparison with chlorpromazine. Arch Gen Psychiatry 1988; 45: 789–96.

12. Kleinberg DL, Davis JM, de Coster R, Van Baelen B, Brecher M. Prolactin levels and adverse events in patients treated with risperidone. Journal of Clinical Psychopharmacology 1999; 19: 57–61.

13. Leucht S, Arbter D, Engel RR, Kissling W, Davis JM . How effective are second-generation antipsychotic drugs? A meta-analysis of placebo-controlled trials. Mol Psychiatry 2008a; Epub ahead of print.

14. Leucht S, Corves C, Arbter D et al. A meta-analysis comparing second-generation and first-generation antipsychotics for schizophrenia. Lancet 2009 Jan 3; 373(9657): 31–41.

15. Leucht S, Corves C, Arbter D et al. Second-generation versus first-generation antipsychotic drugs for schizophrenia: a meta-analysis. Lancet 2008c; epub ahead of print.

16. Leucht S, Kissling W, Davis JM. Second-generation antipsychotic drugs for schizophrenia: can we resolve the conflict? Psychol Med 2009; epub ahead of print.

17. Leucht S, Komossa K, Rummel-Kluge C et al. A meta-analysis of head to head comparisons of second generation antipsychotics in the treatment of schizophrenia. American Journal of Psychiatry 2009 Feb; 166(2): 152–63.

18. Lewis SW, Barnes TR, Davies L et al. Randomized controlled trial of effect of prescription of clozapine versus other second-generation antipsychotic drugs in resistant schizophrenia. Schizophr Bull 2006; 32: 715–23.

19. Lieberman JA, Stroup TS, McEvoy JP et al. Effectiveness of antipsychotic drugs in patients with chronic schizophrenia. N Engl J Med 2005; 353: 1209–23.

20. McEvoy JP, Lieberman JA, Stroup TS et al. Effectiveness of clozapine versus olanzapine, quetiapine, and risperidone in patients with chronic schizophrenia who did not respond to prior atypical antipsychotic treatment. Am J Psychiatry 2006; 163: 600–10.

21. Rosenheck R, Cramer J, Xu WC et al. A comparison of clozapine and haloperidol in hospitalized patients with refractory schizophrenia. N Engl J Med 1997; 337: 809–15.

22. Scherk H, Pajonk FG, Leucht S. Second generation antipsychotics in the treatment of acute mania: a systematic review and meta-analysis of randomized, controlled trials. Arch Gen Psychiatry 2007; 64: 442–55.

23. Schooler N, Rabinowitz J, Davidson M et al. Risperidone and haloperidol in first-episode psychosis: A long-term randomized trial. Am J Psychiatry 2005; 162: 947–53.

24. Simpson GM, Josiassen RC, Stanilla JK et al. Double-blind study of clozapine dose response in chronic schizophrenia. Am J Psychiatry 1999; 156: 1744–50.

25. Van Putten T. Akinetic depression in schizophrenia. Arch Gen Psychiatry 1978; 35: 1101–7.

26. Zimbroff DL, Kane JM, Tamminga CA et al. Controlled, dose response study of sertindole and haloperidol in the treatment of schizophrenia. Am J Psychiatry 1997; 154: 782–91.

15 Maintenance pharmacotherapy in schizophrenia

Siegfried Kasper, Elena Akimova, Martin Fink, and
Rupert Lanzenberger

INTRODUCTION

The long-term maintenance treatment of schizophrenic patients with antipsychotic/
neuroleptic medication is still limited by treatment dissatisfaction and discontinuation in daily practice (1). From a treatment perspective it is important to focus on the
course of schizophrenia, which is characterized by a wide spectrum of symptoms,
including hallucination, delusions, hostility (positive symptoms), negative symptoms (flattened affect, anhedonia, avolition), cognitive deficits, depression, and anxiety symptoms (2) (see Table 15.1). Naturalistic long-term studies indicate that 4–6
years before an acute breakdown with positive symptoms, there are already negative, cognitive, and affective symptoms (3, 4). Long-term studies in schizophrenia
are indicative that some positive symptoms decline over the long-term, however
reality distortions become more prominent and disorganization becomes disassembled to alternative elements (5). Negative symptoms become more prominent and
sharply delineated (6) and are correlated with low self-esteem (7) (see Table 15.2).
Since schizophrenia is a life-long illness, it therefore requires long-term treatment
for the different symptom domains (see Figure 15.1). The treatment aims include the
control of acute psychotic and hostility symptoms, and for the long-term treatment
phase improved outcomes in patient functions and quality of life are required (8, 9).
While in older treatment studies the focus was solely on the psychotic and so-called
positive manifestations of the disorder, there is now growing evidence that negative,
affective, and cognitive symptoms are important predictors for the long-term treatment outcome. It is apparent that an effective treatment regiment must address the
full spectrum of symptoms and not impair patient functions as this often leads to a
decrease of patient compliance in treatment.

It is also well known that approximately 40% of patients with schizophrenia are
poorly compliant to their antipsychotics at any given time and the impact of this is
seen in treatment outcomes. Therefore, addressing partial or noncompliance should
be considered when planning schizophrenia treatment (10, 11, 12).

LONG-TERM EFFICACY OF ANTIPSYCHOTICS

After the introduction of neuroleptic treatment in the 50s of the past century, it
was soon apparent that maintenance treatment can significantly reduce the risk of
schizophrenia relapse and improve long-term symptom control (13, 14). However,
field studies indicated that as many as 60% of the patients experienced relapses within
one year of therapy (15, 16, 17) and a high rate of 80% of the patients was estimated to be
noncompliant with treatment (18). Whereas the so-called "typical" neuroleptics (older
or first generation antipsychotics, FGAs) were able to treat positive symptoms, the introduction of the so-called "atypical" antipsychotics (newer or second generation antipsychotics, SGAs) treated the full range of symptoms with a low incidence of adverse
events (AEs) thereby facilitating long-term adherence and patient satisfaction.

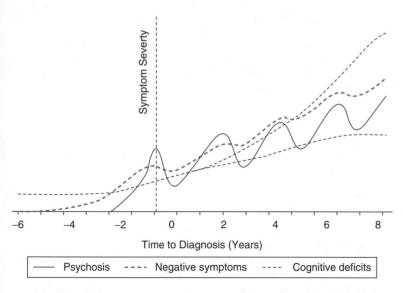

FIGURE 15.1   Long-term pattern of symptom development in schizophrenia (Davidson, 2001, personal communication).

TABLE 15.1   Five symptom domains of schizophrenia

Positive	Negative	Cognitive	Affective
Hallucinations	Flattened affect	Learning	Dysphoria
Delusions	Anhedonia	Memory	Depression
Bizarre behavior	Avolition	Attention	Aggression
Thought disorder	Social withdrawal	Executive function	Anxiety
Agitation	Alogia	Language skills	Psychomotor activiation
	Aggressivity, hostility		

TABLE 15.2   Long-term experience of schizophrenia

Positive symptoms

Decline over the long term: reality distortion becomes altered and disorganisation becomes
  disassembled to alternative elements (Source: Ref.5)

Negative symptoms

Psychomotor poverty becomes more dominant and sharply delineated (Source: Ref.5)
Correlated with low self-esteem (Source: Ref.6)
In a comparison with non-deficit patients, patients with primary negative symptoms experienced:
  Increased anhedonia and negative affectivity
  Reduction in ability to experience positive emotions (Source: Ref.7)

Owing to the specific pharmacodynamic properties, affecting not only the dopaminergic, but also the serotonergic and noradrenergic system, SGAs are able to treat patients with a low side-effect profile and are additionally effective regarding negative, cognitive as well as affective symptoms.

TABLE 15.3   Possible long-term consequences of relapse of schizophrenia

Accelerated rate of deterioration
Increased resistance to treatment
Enhanced impairment of cognitive and neuropsychological function
Failure to recover full functionality after relapse
Longer to recovery after each event
Worsened outcome

TABLE 15.4   Predictors of relapse (Source: Ref.27)

Medication status is the strongest predictor of relapse
Lack of psychosocial intervention
Poor social adaptation and social withdrawal
Discontinuation of medication increases relapse risk five-fold

Rehospitalization rates as well as symptom reappearance could be substantially lowered with the introduction of depot formulations, which could reduce hospitalization rates within one year from approximately 60% to 40% (19, 20).

The results from the study by Law et al. indicated that higher hospitalization rates due to disruptions in medication adherence usually occur within the first 10 days without therapy (21). This study suggested that immediate action to support re-initiation of treatment early in a possible gap in therapy could potentially prevent relapse and re-hospitalization.

The majority of evidence indicates that long-acting injectable medications can increase compliance and reduce relapse rates. Furthermore, treatment guidelines recommend the use of long-acting injectable medications for patients who are suspected of noncompliance with oral medication (22, 23, 24, 25, 26).

The possible long-term consequences of relapse in schizophrenia include an accelerated rate of deteriorization, increased resistance to treatment, enhanced impairment of cognitive and neuropsychological functions and failure to recover full functionality after relapse, longer recovery after each relapse and altogether a worsened outcome (see Table 15.3).

The predictors for relapse are of course poor social adaptation and social withdrawal as well as lack of psychosocial intervention (see Table 15.4). However, it has emerged that medication status is the strongest predictor of relapse meaning that discontinuation of medication increases the relapse risk 5-fold (27). It is therefore evident that psychosocial variables are secondary to the fact if a patient takes the medication or not.

EFFICACY AND TOLERABILITY – A CLINICAL BALANCE
In the long-term treatment of schizophrenia, clinicians must seek a balance between efficacy and tolerability. If however higher efficacy is only achieved with a higher side-effect profile such as extrapyramidal motor symptoms (EPS), patients are not willing to take the medication. Furthermore, the risk of tardive dyskinesia increases with the duration of the illness, since patients most likely take medication from the time the diagnosis is established (2). A recent investigation of 7,648 patients indicated a 10% risk of tardive dyskinesia in schizophrenic patients treated predominantly with FGAs over a 20-year time span (2).

The relationship between compliance and discontinuation of antipsychotic therapy with SGA and one FGA (perphenazine) has been recently studied in an investigation known as CATIE (Clinical Antipsychotic Trials of Intervention Effectiveness) in 1,493 patients treated in the USA (28). 64–82% of the patients discontinued the medication in the CATIE study before 18 months of treatment and the main reasons for discontinuation were inefficacy and intolerable side-effects. The time period until discontinuation for any reason was significantly longer in the olanzapine group than in the quetiapine or risperidone group. The time for discontinuation due to intolerable side-effects was lowest in risperidone while in olanzapine it was highest. Although olanzapine had the lowest rates of discontinuation for any cause, it was still associated with a significant rate of discontinuation due to weight gain and metabolic side-effects. This illustrates the difficulty of balancing efficacy and tolerability. However, the results of this study should be viewed critically, since a number of methodological limitations, such as non-equivalent dosing of treatment groups and an overrepresentation of patients with tardive dyskinesia randomized to SGAs and further points have been raised (29). But most importantly, this and also another phase IV study named CUtLASS (30) cannot falsify previously performed phase III-studies on the grounds of the above-mentioned methodological limitations.

Long-term efficacy for positive symptoms

Therapy approaches using both FGAs and SGAs have been shown to improve positive symptoms in patients suffering from schizophrenia in the long-term perspective (31). Long-term trials are being carried out comparing FGAs, SGAs, and also placebo treatment. There is no study to date in which newer agents have been compared to each other in a long-term double-blind approach. However, short-term studies such as the one published by Conley and Mahmoud (32) indicate that both positive and negative symptoms can be successfully treated with different SGAs. Regarding positive symptoms, further studies demonstrate that the effectiveness within the groups of SGAs is similar, although differences may exist in the side-effect profiles (33, 34, 1).

One example of long-term efficacy in treating of positive symptoms is a 52-week study in which the efficacy and safety of aripiprazole was compared with haloperidol in long-term maintenance treatment following acute relapses of schizophrenia (35). This is currently the largest available long-term study and indicates that there is no difference between aripiprazole and haloperidole with regard to positive symptoms. Additionally, a placebo-controlled study comparing aripiprazole (15 mg/d) over a 26-week period demonstrated that aripiprazole was significantly different to placebo with regard to PANSS-Total Score and PANSS-Positive Score (36). Comparisons of olanzapine and haloperidole in a 12-month controlled trial revealed that there were no significant overall differences between treatment modalities suggesting similar effects of SGAs and FGAs on this symptom domain of positive symptoms (37), a finding, which has also been demonstrated by Leucht (38) in a metaanalytic approach.

The newer agent paliperidone extended release (ER) has been studied in a randomized, double-blind, placebo controlled, multicenter study. The initial open-label treatment revealed a significantly improved symtomatology, and this improvement was maintained with continued treatment, as were functioning and quality-of-life measures (39). This finding was also obtained in pooled data from 52-week open label extension (OLE) phases of three 6-week, placebo controlled, double-blind trials involving 1,083 schizophrenia patients (40). Outcome measures included Positive and Negative Syndrome Scale and Personal and Social Performance scale score. The improvement observed in active treatment groups during the double-blind phases were maintained during the OLE phase.

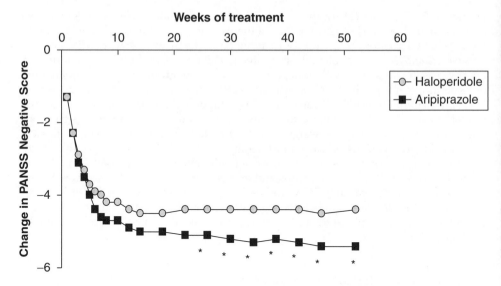

FIGURE 15.2 Aripiprazole vs haloperidole long-term trial: reduction in negative symptoms. Aripiprazole significantly greater improvement (52 weeks): $p<0.05$, ANCOVA Baseline PANSS scores: aripiprazole 24.7 ($n=853$); haloperidol 24.7 ($n=430$): Reproduction with permission of Cambridge University Press (Kasper S, Lerman MN, McQuade RD, et al. Efficacy and safety of aripiprazole vs, haloperidol for long-term treatment following acute relapse in schizophrenia. Int. J. Neuropsychopharmacol. 2003, 325–337).

Long-term efficacy for negative symptoms

The impact of negative symptoms on functional wellbeing, disability, mortality and occupational impairment as well as persistent cognitive effects is well documented in the literature. For instance, negative psychopathology has been linked to reduced ratings of affect and show significant negative correlation with self-esteem (6); social anhedonia and a reduced ability to experience positive emotions have been documented in patients with primary negative symptoms (7). Furthermore, delay in treatment has been discussed as leading to a worsening of the condition in the long-term (41) and the concept of prolonged untreated psychosis includes the fact that dominant negative symptoms worsen the outcome of the disease (42).

The comparative study between olanzapine and risperidone in a randomized prospective double-blind 28-week trial revealed that olanzapine exhibited significant superiority in effect, avolition and anhedonia in the Scale for Assessment of Negative Symptoms (SANS) (42). The comparison of haloperidole and aripiprazole in a long-term 52-week study demonstrated that aripiprazole was superior to haloperidole across all symptom measures of PANSS Negative Subscale Score (35) (See Figure 15.2). This is important in so far as a similar therapeutic benefit was documented for the relief of positive symptoms compared with haloperidole as mentioned above; however negative symptoms were significantly ameliorated with the SGA aripiprazole.

LONG-TERM EFFICACY FOR COGNITIVE SYMPTOMS

Cognitive deficits are a core feature of schizophrenia and seem to be relatively stable following the onset of illness despite fluctuations in other symptoms (43, 44). In the early days of psychosocial rehabilitation programs, cognition in antipsychotic therapy was not considered to be of great importance, a view, which changed with the introduction of SGAs. Later with the availability of SGAs it became apparent that cognitive functions are strong patient-related predictors of relapse (45, 46, 47).

A number of studies including research on SGAs have been conducted which indicate that antipsychotic therapy may improve cognition in patients with schizophrenia. There seems to be a differential effect of various agents on thought processing and learning abilities. A recent metaanalysis provides evidence that cognitive improvement is associated with SGA treatment and to a lower degree also with FGAs (48). To be included in this metaanalysis the following criteria had to be fulfilled by the individual study: First, it had to examine cognitive change following treatment with either clozapine, olanzapine, quetiapine, or risperidone prospectively. Second, a commonly used neuropsychological test battery had to be performed. Third, it was necessary to provide data for which relevant effect sizes could be calculated. A total number of 41 studies met these criteria and the analysis revealed that SGAs were superior to FGAs in improving overall cognitive functions. The specific improvements were observed in learning and speech domains. The inclusion of anticholinergic agents in the group of FGAs, which are known to impair cognition, might be one of the reasons why FGAs have worse improvement rates than SGAs. The comparison between SGAs revealed that all cognitive domains (vigilance and selective attention, working memory, learning, processing speech, cognitive flexibility and abstraction, verbal fluency, visuo-spatial processing, motor skills and delayed recall) improved significantly with SGAs, with subtle differences between specific compounds.

Comparative studies investigating the effects of olanzapine and aripiprazole on cognition have furthermore lent support to the evidence for improved neurocognition with SGAs as well (49). In this 26-week open-label randomized study significant improvements have been achieved in working memories with both treatment modalities. However, distinct differences were observed in verbal learning, for example, which was significantly improved in the aripiprazole, but not in the olanzapine group. Double-blind treatments for assessment of cognitive parameters within the group of SGAs are necessary in a long-term approach, which might elucidate the distinct clinical difference between individual SGA compounds.

The role of cognition in long-acting injectable medication has been studied for long-acting risperidone in stable patients with schizophrenia or schizoaffective disorder for one year (50). The domains assessed included processing speed, attention and impulsivity, working memory, verbal learning and memory, visual memory, executive function and social cognition. The patients who entered the trial with stable clinical profiles continued to improve throughout the study in their clinical status, as well as in their cognitive functioning and quality of life.

Long-term efficacy for affective and anxiety symptoms

Affective symptoms are widespread in schizophrenia (3) and it has been discussed that more than 40% of the patients experienced depressive symptoms during the illness (51). The presence of affective symptoms is associated with poorer patient outcome and patients with depressive symptoms show increased likelihood of hospitalization (52) and increased risk of suicide (53). SGAs have been shown to have significantly greater improvements in depression/anxiety symptoms compared to haloperidole (54, 55, 56) (see Table 15.5).

Pooled analyses of data from six double-blind trials of risperidone versus haloperidol showed that anxious/depressive clusters of the PANSS were significantly

TABLE 15.5   Affective symptoms in schizophrenia

Affective symptoms are widespread in schizophrenia
>40% of patients experience depressive symptoms during their illness (Source: Ref.51 and 3)
Affective symptoms are associated with poorer patient outcome
Patients with depressive symptoms show increased likelihood of hospitalisation (Source: Ref.52)
and increased risk of suicide (Source: Ref.53)
Atypical antipsychotics shown to improve affective symptoms in short-term trials
Second generation antipsychotics have shown significantly greater improvements in depression/
anxiety symptoms compared with haloperidol (Source: Ref.35, 54, 55)

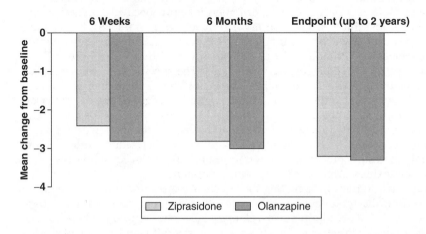

FIGURE 15.3   Ziprasidone/Olanzapine in a long-term study: Depression Scores (Calgary Depression Scale Reduction from baseline (LOCF data). Data from responders to a 6-week acute study of olanzapine and ziprasidone during a blinded 6-month continuation study and optional (2-year) extension study (Source: Ref.58). Reproduction with permission of Elsevier Press (Kasper S. Optimisation of long-term treatment in schizophrenia: treating the true spectrum of symptoms. Eur. Neuropsychopharmacol. 2006,16, S135–141).

better with the SGA risperidone than the FGA haloperidol. Subanalysis of patients with an anxious/depressive cluster scores larger than 2 at baseline also indicated that risperidone was superior to haloperidol (54). This is of importance since anxiety has been linked both to EPS and suicidality. In a short-term study Tollefson et al. (55) demonstrated that anxiety/depression improved significantly after treatment with olanzapine. Similar results have also been shown in the study by Kasper et al. (57) in which haloperidole was compared to aripiprazole, with a clear advantage of aripiprazole for its efficacy in relieving depressive symptomatology.

A 2-year extension study comparing ziprasidone and olanzapine indicated long-term improvements of depressive symptomatology as measured with the Calgari Depression Scale for schizophrenia (58) (see Figure 15.3). From a pharmacodynamic perspective, the 5-HT2 blockade, as well as other mechanisms, like norepiphrenine reuptake inhibition, or a 5HT1A agonistic property, may be responsible for the clear advantages of SGAs over FGAs in the treatment of mood and anxiety symptoms. This is in so far of importance, since also lower dosages of FGAs are not able to achieve the same efficacy as SGAs in this domain.

TOLERABILITY FROM A LONG-TERM PERSPECTIVE

Besides efficacy, tolerability is in schizophrenia, like in other treatment indications most important for patient adherence to the treatment regime. Newer agents are less likely to cause extrapyramidal symptoms (EPS) than FGAs and therefore are better tolerated (59, 60). However, SGAs are associated with other adverse effects (1, 61). The most distressing non-EPS side effects from SGAs include weight gain and sedation (62). Weight gain and/ or metabolic disturbances (63) are mainly associated with treatment employing olanzapine and clozapine, and are significantly lower with risperidone and quetiapine, while almost negligible with aripiprazole, ziprasidone, and amisulpride. Sedation is an undesired side-effect of long-term use of the medication and mainly stems from its antihistaminergic properties. A comparative study between aripiprazole and olanzapine revealed higher sedation and somnolence rates for olanzapine compared to aripiprazole (64).

The long-term efficacy, tolerability, and safety of paliperidone extended-release were evaluated in pooled data from 52-week open label extension (OLE) phases of three 6-week, placebo controlled, double-blind trials involving 1,083 schizophrenia patients. Most commonly ($\geq$ 10% patients) reported Adverse Events (AE) were insomnia, headache, and akathisia. Since metabolic issues are now discussed with atypical compounds it is worthwhile to mention that the baseline to endpoint change was 1.1 kg across treatment groups and there were no clinically meaningful changes for plasma glucose, insulin, or lipid levels. This analysis shows that paliperidone ER is generally well tolerated for up to 52 weeks in schizophrenia patients (40).

SUMMARY

Schizophrenia is a life-long disorder and therefore requires long-term treatment. Achieving the treatment goals for effective maintenance of symptom control, treatment compliance while minimising adverse effects can be a difficult balance to achieve. Compared to the past, treatment nowadays should focus on the whole spectrum of symptoms including the "positive", the "negative" and the affective symptoms as well as aggression and hostility. Treatment needs to minimize side-effects, that contribute to discontinuation or deficits in patient functionality. SGAs have low liability in EPS; however other side-effects, including weight gain and metabolic disturbances, have important clinical implications with respect to long-term health. For patients who are noncompliant or partially compliant, long-acting injectable formulations need also to be considered in countries where this treatment approach is not widely accepted. In the future, a more specific pharmacogenetic approach should enable clinicians to administer antipsychotics more specifically with regard to their efficacy and side-effect profile and thereby optimise long-term treatment in schizophrenia.

REFERENCES

1. Tandon R, Belmaker RH, Gattaz WF et al. World Psychiatry Association Pharmacopsychiatry Section statement on comparative effectiveness of antipsychotics in the treatment of schizophrenia. Schizophr Res 2008; 100: 20–38.
2. Kasper S, Lowry A, Hodge A et al. Tardive dyskinesia: Analysis of outpatients with schizophrenia from Latin America, Asia, Central and Eastern Europe, and Africa and the Middle East. Schizophr Res 2006; 81: 139–43.
3. Häfner H, Maurer K, Trendler G et al. The early course of schizophrenia and depression. Eur Arch Psychiatry Clin Neurosci 2005; 255: 167–73.

4. Häfner H, an der Heiden W, Maurer K. Evidence for separate diseases: Stages of one disease or different combinations of symptom dimensions? Eur Arch Psychiatry Clin Neurosci 2008; Suppl 2: 85–96.

5. Meagher DJ, Quinn, JF, Bourke S. Longitudinal assessment of psychopathological domains over late-stage schizophrenia in relation to duration of initially untreated psychosis: 3-year prospective study in a long-term inpatient population. Psychiatry Res 2004; 126: 217–27.

6. Hofer A, Kemmler G, Eder U et al. Quality of life in schizophrenia: the impact of psychopathology, attitude toward medication, and side effects. J Clin Psychiatry 2004; 65: 932–9.

7. Horan WP, Blanchard JJ. Neurocognitive, social, and emotional dysfunction in deficit syndrome schizophrenia. Schizophr Res 2003; 65: 125–37.

8. Altamura C, Bobes J, Cunningham Owens D et al. Schizophrenia: diagnosis and continuing treatment. Principles of practice from the European Think Tank on the contemporary treatment of schizophrenia. Int J Psychiat Clin 2000; 4: S1–S11.

9. Van Os J, Altamura AC, Bobes J et al. 2-COM: an instrument to facilitate patient-professional communication in routine clinical practice. Acta Psychiat Scand 2002; 106: 446–52.

10. Kane JM. Treatment Adherence and Long-Term Outcomes. CNS Spectr 2007; 12: 21–6.

11. Keith SJ, Kane LM. Partial compliance and patient consequences in schizophrenia: our patients can do better. J Clin Psychiatry 2003; 64: 1308–15.

12. Llorca PM. Partial compliance in schizophrenia and the impact on patient outcomes. Psychiatry Res 2008; 161: 235–47.

13. Hogarty GE, Goldberg SC, Schooler NR et al. Drug and sociotherapy in the aftercare of schizophrenic patients. II. Two-year relapse rates. Arch Gen Psychiatry 1974; 31: 603–8.

14. Schooler NR, Keith SJ, Severe JB et al. Relapse and rehospitalization during maintenance treatment of schizophrenia. The effects of dose reduction and family treatment. Arch Gen Psychiatry 1997; 54: 453–63.

15. Kane JM. Schizophrenia. N Engl J Med 1996; 334: 34–41.

16. Crow TJ, MacMillan JF, Johnson AL et al. A randomized controlled trial of prophylactic neuroleptic treatment. Br J Psychiatry 1986; 148: 20–127.

17. Weiden P, Glazer W. Assessment and treatment selection for "revolving door" inpatients with schizophrenia. Psychiatr Q 1997; 68: 377–92.

18. Corrigan PW, Liberman RP, Engel JD. From noncompliance to collaboration in the treatment of schizophrenia. Hosp Commun Psychiatry 1990; 41: 1203–11.

19. Kasper S, Lehofer M, Bach M et al. Schizophrenie. Medikamentöse Therapie. Konsensus-Statement - State of the art 2008. CliniCum neuropsy Sonderausgabe November 2008.

20. Remington G, Kwon J, Collins A et al. The use of electronic monitoring (MEMS) to evaluate antipsychotic compliance in outpatients with schizophrenia. Schizophr Res 2007; 90: 229–37.

21. Law MR, Soumerai SB, Ross-Degnan D et al. A longitudinal study of medication nonadherence and hospitalization risk in schizophrenia. J Clin Psychiatry 2008; 69: 47–53.

22. Gerlach J. Oral versus depot administration of neuroleptics in relapse prevention. Acta Psychiatr Scand Suppl 1994; 382: 28–32.

23. Davis J, Metalon L, Watanabe M et al. Depot antipsychotic drugs: Place in therapy. Drugs 1994; 47: 741–73.

24. Klingberg S, Schneider S, Wittorf A et al. Collaboration in outpatient antipsychotic drug treatment: Analysis of potentially influencing factors. Psychiatry Res 2008; 161: 225–34.

25. Kikkert MJ. Assessment of medication adherence in patients with schizophrenia: the Aquilles heel of adherence research. J Nerv Ment Dis 2008; 196: 4.

26. American Psychiatric Association. Practice guideline for the treatment of patients with schizophrenia. Am J Psychiatry 1997; 154: 1–65.

27. Robinson D, Woerner MG, Alvir JM et al. Predictors of Relapse Following Response From a First Episode of Schizophrenia or Schizoaffective Disorder. Arch Gen Psychiatry 1999; 56: 241–7.

28. Lieberman JA, Stroup TS, McEvoy JP et al. Effectiveness of antipsychotic drugs in patients with chronic schizophrenia. N Engl J Med 2005; 353: 1209–23.

29. Kasper S, Winkler D. Addressing the limitations of the CATIE study. World J of Biol Psychia 2006; 7: 126–7.

30. Jones PB, Davies L, Barnes TR et al. Randomized controlled trial of effect on quality of life of second-generation versus first generation antipsychotic drugs in schizophrenia. Arch Gen Psychiatry 2006; 63: 1079–87.

31. Falkai P, Wobrock T, Lieberman J et al. World Federation of Societies of Biological Psychiatry (WFSBP) guidelines for biological treatment of schizophrenia, part 2: long-term treatment of schizophrenia. World J of Biol Psychia 2006; 7: 1–40.

32. Conley RR, Mahmoud R. A randomized double-blind study of risperidone and olanzapine in the treatment of schizophrenia or schizoaffective disorder. Am J Psychiatry 2001; 158: 765–74.

33. Schooler NR. Maintaining symptom control: review of ziprasidone long-term efficacy data. J Clin Psychiatry 2003; 64: 26–32.

34. Glick ID, Marder SR. Long-term maintenance therapy with quetiapine versus haloperidol decanoate in patients with schizophrenia or schizoaffective disorder. J Clin Psychiatry 2005; 66: 638–41.

35. Kasper S, Lerman MN, McQuade RD et al. Efficacy and safety of aripiprazole vs. haloperidol for long-term maintenance treatment following acute relapse of schizophrenia. Int J Neuropsychopharmacol 2003; 6: 325–37.

36. Pigott TA, Carson WH, Saha AR et al. Aripiprazole for the prevention of relapse in stabilized patients with chronic schizophrenia: a placebo-controlled 26-week study. J Clin Psychiatry 2003; 64: 1048–56.

37. Rosenheck R, Perlick, D, Bingham S et al. Effectiveness and cost of olanzapine and haloperidol in the treatment of schizophrenia: a randomized controlled trial. Jama 2003; 290: 2693–702.

38. Leucht S, Corves C, Kissling W, Davis JM. An update of meta-analyses on second-generation antipsychotic drugs for schizophrenia. In: Kasper S, Papadimitriou G, eds. Schizophrenia: Biopsychosocial Approaches and Current Challenges. 2nd ed. Place: Informa Healthcare, 2009; 43: 164–173.

39. Kramer M, Simpson G, Maciulis V et al. Paliperidone Extended-Release Tablets for Prevention of Symptom Recurrence in Patients With Schizophrenia: A Randomized, Double-Blind, Placebo-Controlled Study. J Clin Psychopharmacology 2007; 27: 6–14.

40. Emsley R, Berwaerts J, Eerdekens M et al. Efficacy and safety of oral paliperidone extended-release tablets in the treatment of acute schizophrenia: pooled data from three 52-week open-label studies. Int. Clin. Psychopharmacol 2008; 23: 343–56.

41. McCreadie RG. Managing the first episode of schizophrenia: the role of new therapies. Eur. Neuropsychopharmacol 1996; 6: S3–5.

42. Tran PV, Hamilton SH, Kuntz AJ et al. Double-blind comparison of olanzapine versus risperidone in the treatment of schizophrenia and other psychotic disorders. J Clin Psychopharmacol 1997; 17: 407–18.

43. Weinberger DR, Gallhofer B. Cognitive function in schizophrenia. Int Clin Psychopharmacol 1997; 12: S29–36.

44. Green MF, Kern RS, Braff DL, Mintz J. Neurocognitive deficits and functional outcome in schizophrenia: are we measuring the "right stuff"? Schizophr Bull 2000; 26: 119–36.

45. Green MF. What are the functional consequences of neurocognitive deficits in schizophrenia? Am J Psychiatry 1996; 153: 321–30.

46. Velligan DI, Bow-Thomas CC, Mahurin RK et al. Do specific neurocognitive deficits predict specific domains of community function in schizophrenia? J Nerv Ment Dis 2000; 188: 518–24.

47. Jeste DV, Barak Y, Madhusoodanan S et al. International multi-site double-blind trial of the atypical antipsychotics risperidone and olanzapine in 175 elderly patients with chronic schizophrenia. Am J Geriatr Psychiatry 2003; 11: 638–47.

48. Woodward ND, Purdon SE, Meltzer HY et al. A meta-analysis of neuropsychological change to clozapine, olanzapine, quetiapine, and risperidone in schizophrenia. Int J Neuropsychopharmacol 2005; 8; 457–72.

49. Cornblatt B, Kern RS, Carson WH et al. Neurocognitive effects of aripiprazole versus olanzapine in stable psychosis. Int J Neuropsychopharmacol 2002; 5: S185.
50. Simpson GM, Mahmoud RA, Lasser RA et al. A 1-year double-blind study of 2 doses of long-acting risperidone in stable patients with schizophrenia or schizoaffective disorder. J Clin Psychiatry 2006; 67: 1194–203.
51. Markou P. Depression in schizophrenia: a descriptive study. Aust N Z J Psychiatry 1996; 30: 354–7.
52. Roy A, Thompson R, Kennedy S. Depression in chronic schizophrenia. Br J Psychiatry 1983; 142; 465–70.
53. Roy A. Depression, attempted suicide, and suicide in patients with chronic schizophrenia. Psychiatr. Clin North Am 1986; 9; 193–206.
54. Peuskens J, Van Baelen B, De Smedt C et al. Effects of risperidone on affective symptoms in patients with schizophrenia. Int Clin Psychopharmacol 2000; 15: 343–9.
55. Tollefson GD, Sanger TM, Lu Y et al. Depressive signs and symptoms in schizophrenia: a prospective blinded trial of olanzapine and haloperidol. Arch Gen Psychiatry 1998; 55: 250–8.
56. Kasper S. Quetiapine is effective against anxiety and depressive symptoms in long-term treatment of patients with schizophrenia. Depress. Anxiety 2004; 20: 44–7.
57. Kasper S. Optimisation of long-term treatment in schizophrenia - treating the true spectrum of symptoms. Eur Neuropsychopharmacol 2006; 16: S135–41.
58. Simpson GM, Weiden P, Pigott T et al. Six-month, blinded, multicenter continuation study of ziprasidone versus olanzapine in schizophrenia. Am J Psychiatry 2005; 162: 1535–8.
59. Kerwin RW. The new atypical antipsychotics. A lack of extrapyramidal side-effects and new routes in schizophrenia research. Br J Psychiatry 1994; 164: 141–8.
60. Geddes J, Freemantle N, Harrison P et al. Atypical antipsychotics in the treatment of schizophrenia: a systematic overview and meta-regression analysis. BMJ 2000; 321: 1371–6.
61. Möller HJ. Side effect burden of antipsychotic medication. In: Kasper S, Papadimitriou G, eds. Schizophrenia: Biopsychosocial Approaches and Current Challenges. 2nd ed. Place: Informa Healthcare, 2009; 43: 231–259.
62. Weiden PJ, Miller AL. Which side effects really matter? Screening for common and distressing side effects of antipsychotic medications. J Psychiatr Prac 2001; 7: 41–7.
63. Franciosi LP, Kasper S, Garber AJ et al. Advancing the treatment of people with mental illness: A call to action in the management of metabolic issues. J Clin Psychiatry 2005; 66: 790–8.
64. McQuade RD, Stock E, Marcus R et al. A comparison of weight change during treatment with olanzapine or aripiprazole.: results from a randomized, double-blind study. J Clin Psychiatry 2004; 65: 47–56.

16 Evaluation and medication therapy for treatment resistance in schizophrenia

Robert R Conley

One fifth to one third of all people with schizophrenia have core positive symptoms (such as hallucinations, delusions, and thought disorder) which are resistant to antipsychotic treatment. This finding has been consistent over time (1–4). Treatment of patients in this group has remained a persistent public health problem. These patients are highly symptomatic and require extensive periods of hospital care (5). Their care comprises a disproportionately high share of the total cost of treating schizophrenia (6). These facts were the basis for the enthusiasm of clinicians following the demonstration of clozapine's efficacy in inpatients with treatment-resistant schizophrenia (7). However, clozapine treatment carries with it significant morbidity from serious side metabolic and cardiovascular effects, and the need for continual blood monitoring. There are now many new antipsychotics available. While none have the demonstrated the superior efficacy of clozapine in schizophrenia, a thoughtful approach to use of these agents will maximize their potential benefit for people who do not easily and robustly respond to their first drug treatment strategy.

CHRONIC ILLNESS VERSUS TREATMENT RESISTANCE

Studies of treatment resistance in schizophrenia have long been hampered by a lack of consistency in definition. Commonly, treatment resistance was considered to be roughly equivalent to chronic or frequent hospitalization (8–13). The likely cause of this serious problem is however, poor drug compliance and/or tolerance and a relative lack of efficacy with current antipsychotic drugs in regard to the cognitive and social deficits associated with schizophrenia. Persistent positive symptoms of psychosis and at least moderate overall severity of illness should be present in order for treatment resistance to be diagnosed (14). It is now generally recognized that chronic illness alone is not accurate in predicting likelihood of response to an antipsychotic trial (15, 16).

For various reasons, many people with schizophrenia who have been chronically or frequently hospitalized may not be truly resistant to drug treatment.

Factors other than choice of medication that may influence a patient's recovery include individual factors relating to the patient, the illness and the treatment. These include poor compliance with drug therapy, concurrent illicit substance use (especially cannabis and psychostimulants), psychosocial stressors, home environment, physical comorbidity, associated organic abnormality, prominent negative symptoms and neuropsychological deficits or a history of committing violence. An optimized medication and treatment trial should be employed before a patient's illness is considered nonresponsive. In addition, the effects of drug noncompliance, dysphoria associated with antipsychotic therapy and extrapyramidal side effects can mimic true treatment resistance (17, 18). At least a one- to two-year course of persistent symptoms should also be a criterion for treatment resistance in schizophrenia.

DEFINITION OF TREATMENT RESISTANCE

There are a number of reasons to consider replacing the term *treatment resistance* when describing response in schizophrenia. The use of the *word resistance* suggests that nothing can be done to improve symptoms and conveys the thought that the patient is resisting treatment rather than the illness itself being resistant to treatment. The treatment resistance label is no also not in line with current therapeutic alternatives or with more recent understandings of the basis of schizophrenia. Therefore, treatment resistance is better viewed as *incomplete response*, a term reflecting the potential for improved therapeutic outcomes.

The most accepted current criteria for treatment resistance in schizophrenia were first widely used by Kane et al. (7) and collaborators in the Multicenter Clozapine Trial (MCT). Originally, these criteria were:

1. Persistent positive psychotic symptoms: (Item score > 4 (moderate) on at least two of four positive symptom items (rated on a 1–7 scale) on the Brief Psychiatric Rating Scale (BPRS) (19)—hallucinatory behavior, suspiciousness, unusual thought content and conceptual disorganization);
2. Current presence of at least a moderately severe illness as rated by the total BPRS score (score > 45 on the 18 item scale) and a score of > 4 (moderate) on the Clinical Global Impression (CGI) (20);
3. Persistence of illness: no period of good social and/or occupational functioning within the last five years; and
4. Drug-refractory condition: at least three periods of treatment in the preceding 5 years with conventional antipsychotics (from at least two chemical classes) at doses > 1000 mg per day of chlorpromazine for 6 weeks, each without significant symptom relief, and failure to improve by at least 20% in total BPRS score or intolerance to a 6-week prospective trial of haloperidol at a dose of 10–60 mg per day.

These criteria meet the test of persistent illness with continuing positive symptomatology in the face of adequate current treatment. Their usefulness was shown in the MCT, where subjects who met them, when randomized to chlorpromazine treatment showed only a 4% rate of response and no significant changes on total BPRS score or positive symptoms. Clozapine's superior efficacy has now been replicated using similar criteria (21, 22).

DEFINING ADEQUATE DRUG TRIALS

The fourth criterion for treatment resistance, regarding drug trials, has been modified since it was first proposed. The fact that there was only a 3% response rate to prospective haloperidol treatment and a 4% response rate to double-blind chlorpromazine treatment in the MCT led to the belief that two retrospective drug trial failures would be as effective as three in screening for treatment resistance. Kane's group showed that subjects not responsive to two adequate antipsychotic trials (one retrospective and one prospective) have less than a 7% chance of responding to another trial (23). The FDA guidelines for clozapine's use state that people should fail to respond to two separate trials of antipsychotics, before being treated with clozapine (24). The evidence that second generation antipsychotics are somewhat more effective than traditional medication has reopened the question of the type of drug a patient should fail.

There have also been other changes regarding the definition of an adequate drug trial. It is generally recognized that a 4- to 6-week period (rather than strictly a

6-week one) is adequate for a treatment trial of an antipsychotic (25). Recommended dosage has also been revised. The dose used during conventional antipsychotic trial was first proposed to be at least 1000 mg per day of chlorpromazine, or its equivalent. However, doses of ≥ 400 mg per day of chlorpromazine have been shown to be adequate to block 80–90% of dopamine receptors (thought to be the target of this drug action; 26). Higher doses produce no direct therapeutic benefit even in patients not responsive to therapy (27, 23) and do not have greater efficacy in acute treatment than lower doses (28–30). Therefore, a 4- to 6-week trial of 400–600 mg of chlorpromazine is now accepted as a standard for an adequate trial (31). These modified criteria have been used to define treatment resistance in recent clinical trials (17, 18). They are also the basis for a recently proposed treatment strategy that allows a clear progression of drug therapy in any patient with schizophrenia to optimize the likelihood of response throughout the course of drug treatment (31). The issue of dosing is also certainly crucial to defining adequate trials of newer antipsychotics. There is good evidence that an optimal trial of risperidone is in the 2 mg to 6 mg per day range (32), ziprasidone should be dosed at its maximal FDA recommended dose, 160 mg per day, if tolerated. The optimal doses of olanzapine, quetiapine and aripiprazole are less clear.

PREVALENCE OF TREATMENT RESISTANCE IN SCHIZOPHRENIA

The prevalence of treatment resistance is hard to determine given the lack of agreement on defining the term. It has been estimated that 20%–45% of people with schizophrenia of over 2 years duration are only partially responsive to antipsychotic medication (33) and 5%–10% of patients derive no benefit at all (34). Two independent groups have estimated the prevalence of treatment resistance in current treatment populations. Juarez-Reyes et al. (35) used a broad interpretation of the FDA-approved Clozaril package insert to determine treatment resistance rates in a county mental health system in California. They sampled a random, stratified group of people with schizophrenia ($n = 293$) consisting of all those served by a county mental health system in 1991 (inpatients and outpatients). Patients were considered treatment-resistant if they were older than 16, had a diagnosis of schizophrenia or schizoaffective disorder, had failed two drug trials of 4 weeks in length at 600 mg per day or greater, or had tardive dyskinesia and had a Global Assessment of Functioning score of less than 61. The estimate of treatment resistance based on these broad criteria was 42.9 ± 5.9 percent. (This estimate was lowered to 12.9 ± 2.7 percent when the criteria of Kane et al. (7) were used, primarily because of a lack of ability to document three drug trial failures.) Essock et al. (3) used the criteria of failure of two six-week drug trials of 1000 mg per day chlorpromazine equivalents, inpatient status of at least 4 months and a total hospitalization of at least 24 months in the preceding 5 years. They estimated that 48% of all Connecticut State hospital inpatients with a diagnosis of schizophrenia or schizoaffective disorder were treatment-resistant from a total sample of 803 inpatients. These estimates of the prevalence of treatment resistance are similar to those made when clozapine was first marketed (36). They would extrapolate to a total of 200,000–500,000 people with treatment-resistant schizophrenia currently living in the United States.

NEUROBIOLOGY OF TREATMENT RESISTANCE IN SCHIZOPHRENIA

Until the arrival of standardized criteria for defining treatment resistance, research into the neurobiological nature of the problem had been scant (37). However, with the use of more objective criteria some consistent findings have been seen. People with treatment-resistant schizophrenia appear to have increased cortical atrophy on MRI compared to those with responsive illness (38, 39). This was particularly true if they had predominant negative symptoms (40). People with persistent negative symptoms also have a tendency to have abnormal cell migration in their prefrontal cortex (41). Lack of response to early treatment is also predictive of nonresponse (38, 42). Delay in first treatment may also be associated with a higher likelihood of resistance, also (43). These people also appear to have lower catecholamine levels in the CSF (44). Clozapine response has been associated with low ratios of CSF homovanillic acid to 5-hydroxy-indoleacetic acid (45). These findings suggest that drugs with low dopamine antagonism and high serotonergic antagonism may be useful in treatment-resistant schizophrenia.

VIOLENCE ASSOCIATED WITH TREATMENT RESISTANCE IN SCHIZOPHRENIA
Violence in schizophrenia has long been considered a problem (46). People with schizophrenic symptoms have a markedly increased rate of perpetrating serious violence toward others (47). Patients with refractory schizophrenia also have an increased likelihood of being victims of violence, probably due primarily to their rate of chronic hospitalization (48).

There has recently been some therapeutic optimism regarding this problem. Several groups have noted that clozapine is effective in reducing violent behavior and hostility compared to standard antipsychotic therapy (49, 50, 51, 52). Risperidone treatment has also been seen to decrease hostility (53). This raises the question of whether effectiveness against hostility, rather than being a particular property of clozapine, or rather a phenomenon of the reduced EPS liability or other effects shared by the second generation antipsychotics. It has been recognized that treatment with low potency antipsychotics (with reduced EPS liability) is associated with improvement in violent behavior rates compared to haloperidol therapy (46). However, this finding may have been due to the increased sedation seen with these drugs.

DRUG THERAPY FOR TREATMENT RESISTANCE
Historically, drug therapy for treatment-resistant schizophrenia centered either on the use of different dose strategies of conventional antipsychotics, or the use of adjunct agents such as lithium, β-blocking drugs, anticonvulsants, and benzodiazepines. These strategies have been well reviewed elsewhere (16, 54), and thus will be only briefly reviewed here. Since the arrival of clozapine, attention in the field has shifted to a greater focus on the use of newer antipsychotics for treatment resistance in schizophrenia.

CONVENTIONAL ANTIPSYCHOTIC DRUGS
Conventional antipsychotic drugs had long been the first line drug therapy for treating schizophrenia. These drugs were considered interchangeable in terms of efficacy as in over 100 studies comparing them to each other in schizophrenia, only one showed a differential effect (55, 56). In controlled trials in people with drug-resistant symptoms, fewer than 5% responded after having their drug therapy changed from one conventional antipsychotic to another (7, 57). The primary reason for choosing

between these drugs was to reduce side effects and to provide different dosing strategies. High potency drugs, such as haloperidol and fluphenazine have high extrapyramidal side effects, but cause less sedation and postural hypertension than low potency drugs such as chlorpromazine or thioridazine. Haloperidol and fluphenazine are the only two conventional antipsychotics available as injectable depot medication, a formulation that can assure drug delivery and sometimes optimize response. This strategy is sometime useful in patients who show a lack of response, but it is important to note that unless the patient has a positive therapeutic effect from a drug and associates the drug with that effect, the likelihood of long-term therapeutic benefit and compliance is low.

DATA WITH NEWER DRUGS
Clozapine
Clozapine was approved for use by the Food and Drug Administration in 1990 specifically for the treatment of patients whose symptoms do not adequately respond to conventional antipsychotic therapy, e ither because therapy was not effective or because it cannot be continued secondary to intolerable side effects. It is still the only drug with proven efficacy in rigorously defined treatment-resistant schizophrenia (58). Clozapine has also been useful in reducing violent behavior (59, 57), tardive dyskinesia (60), and the risk of suicide (49, 61). Despite this efficacy profile, clozapine has been relatively underused (62).

This phenomenon of relative under usage of clozapine probably relates to the costs and complexities of clozapine therapy. These arise from the need for long term hematological monitoring for agranulocytosis and persistent serious side effects, such as weight gain, sialorrhea, tachycardia and sedation present with this clozapine. Despite the robust clinical effects of clozapine in long-term use (63, 49, 57), benefits that translate into improved living situations and decreased cost of care have not always been shown in large public health sector populations (64, 65), particularly in the first year of use (3, 66). Partly this is because clozapine is still frequently being reserved for only the most difficult to treat (and discharge) segment of the population with schizophrenia (67) or only being used by a select subset of clinicians comfortable with the drug. With longer term follow up clozapine benefits become more evident to patients, health care providers and families (68).

The optimal dose strategy for clozapine is slow dose escalation. Patients should be evaluated for response at dose plateaus of 200–400 mg per day and 500–600 mg per day. Only patients with few side effects to clozapine should be titrated to doses higher than 600 mg per day. Patients should not be titrated to a higher dose of clozapine if myoclonus is present, as this side effect may precede the development of seizures (69). Patients who respond to clozapine will usually begin to respond within 8 weeks of reaching their response dose (33, 70). However, the total time course of clozapine response is still controversial (71, 61).

Risperidone, paliperidone ER
Risperidone has been approved for use in schizophrenia since 1994. It is indicated for the treatment of positive and negative symptoms of this disorder. Clinical trials show that risperidone is an effective treatment for positive psychotic symptoms (72, 73).

There were early reports of patients with poorly responsive schizophrenia who showed some improvement with risperidone (74, 75), but these studies were open-labeled, retrospective, or not controlled. There is one well controlled double-blind study of risperidone versus haloperidol in this group (76). Risperidone is more effective and better tolerated than haloperidol in this study, but the differential efficacy is not as large as what is usually seen with clozapine. There are two studies in which risperidone shows similar efficacy to clozapine in chronic poorly responsive schizophrenic patients (77, 78). In these studies the patients were not categorized by typical treatment resistant criteria. Also, the studies were not large enough to truly test a noninferiority hypothesis. Also risperidone therapy was more effective than prior conventional therapy, but not as effective as clozapine in well categorized patients in one open study (79). In contrast, it has been widely recognized that risperidone treatment is usually not effective in clozapine responders (80, 81). Risperidone may be more tolerable to those with schizophrenia than older antipsychotics and has some benefits in terms of superior clinical improvement. Benefits this drug must be balanced against its increased tendency to cause side effects such as weight gain and hyperprolactinemia (82). Paliperidone, which is the active metabolite of risperidone in humans, has recently been introduced to the clinic. However, there are some relevant differences in the metabolism and pharmacokinetics of Paliperidone ER compared to risperidone. Paliperidone ER is predominantly excreted by the kidney (59% excreted unchanged in the urine) and therefore not expected to cause clinically important interactions with drugs metabolized by the CYP450 pathway. No dosage adjustment is required for patients with relevant comedications and comorbidities, for example, mild to moderate hepatic impairment or smokers. In addition, paliperidone ER as an antipsychotic uses an innovative delivery technology, the OROS® (Osmotic Release Oral Delivery) system. The OROS® formulation provides minimal fluctuations in plasma concentrations of paliperidone over a 24-h period. By reducing the amplitude of peaks and troughs, which are associated with IR oral therapies, and providing smoother plasma profiles similar to those achieved with long-acting injectable antipsychotic agents, it is anticipated that paliperidone ER could potentially reduce the risk of adverse effects and improve tolerability. (R Conley; Current Medical research and Opinion 2006, Vol 22, N°10: 1879–1892). Overall it appears to have similar efficacy and safety to risperidone (83), although further research on this is currently being undertaken.

Olanzapine

Olanzapine was approved for the treatment of schizophrenia in 1996. It has a receptor binding profile that is very similar to clozapine, leading to hopes that it would show similar efficacy. There were several open reports of possible efficacy in this group (84, 85). On reanalysis of double-blind comparative data showed olanzapine to have a better effect than haloperidol in people with poorly responsive schizophrenia (86), but this effect was not as great as one would have expected with clozapine. This was confirmed by several other studies. Conley et al. (87) in 1998, in a double-blind trial, and Sanders and Mossman in 1999 (88), in an open study, both failed to demonstrate a clozapine-like effect in well-characterized patients with treatment resistant illness. Furthermore, the olanzapine resistant patients from the Conley 1998 trial did respond to a subsequent trial of clozapine at about the rate that would have been expected in any other treatment resistant group (89). There is evidence that olanzapine may be more efficacious in schizophrenia than other antipsychotics, except for clozapine (90, 91) and that doses higher than those labeled for use in schizophrenia may show some increased efficacy. However this benefit must be balanced against the substantial weight gain and metabolic disturbances seen on many people treated with this drug (92).

Quetiapine

Quetiapine has been shown to be effective in treatment-responsive schizophrenia (93). It has a pharmacological profile that includes high serotonin (5HT1a) receptor affinity compared to dopamine receptor affinity. It is also a low-potency compound. The most effective doses in clinical studies are 300 mg to 450 mg per day, similar dose potency to clozapine (93). There was no difference between placebo and quetiapine in the amount of EPS or akathisia in published trials to date. There are several reports of beneficial effects of quetiapine in treatment resistance (94, 95), but no published controlled trials to date. Overall, quetiapine is effective for the treatment of schizophrenia, but it is not much different from older antipsychotics or risperidone with respect to treatment withdrawal and efficacy (96). It may be less effective than olanzapine (97, 91), therefore a quetiapine trial should not be the only antipsychotic trial given to a patient before clozapine therapy is considered.

Aripiprazole

Aripiprazole differs little from typical antipsychotic drugs with respect to efficacy; however, it presents significant advantages in terms of tolerability (98). This may present an advantage when people are being treated for a refractory condition which may be due to drug intolerance. It also may be less effective than olanzapine (91), therefore a quetiapine trial should not be the only antipsychotic trial given to a patient before clozapine therapy is considered.

Ziprasidone

The short-term efficacy of ziprasidone for core positive symptoms of schizophrenia appears to be comparable to other antipsychotics. The safety database suggests that the overall risk associated with ziprasidone therapy is lower than with other many other antipsychotics, with notably lower risk of drug-related increases in weight, glucose, or lipids. The data also suggest a modestly increased risk of QTc prolongation that is not dose related or linked to torsades de pointes. Switching to ziprasidone from other drugs, such as olanzapine and risperidone, appears to improve metabolic parameters (99).

Sulpiride

Sulpiride is an effective antipsychotic, which is used widely, but is not marketed in the United States. It belongs to the same drug class as remoxipride, a drug that may have been effective in treatment resistant schizophrenia (100). There is one well-controlled double-blind study showing a positive effect of adjunct sulpiride in clozapine partial responders (101). A separate open study suggested efficacy in olanzapine partial responders(102). These findings should be more fully explored.

OTHER TREATMENTS
Lithium

Adjunct lithium therapy has been seen to be beneficial in some older studies in patients with treatment-resistant schizophrenia (103, 12, 9). These patients were often not defined by the rigorous criteria of later studies. A 4-week trial of medication appears adequate to define response. The response seen may be more prominent in those patients with affective symptoms, but patients who do respond do so in many areas of functioning (104). There are reports that lithium has been helpful in reducing hostility in patients with treatment-resistant schizophrenia, and thus may be helpful in some violent patients (16).

The published trials of adjunct lithium, though positive, have been conducted with small numbers of patients, and often the criteria for defining treatment resistance were not clear, or were over inclusive. The size of the clinical effect in these trials was limited (54). Therefore, definitive evidence of the benefit of lithium is not yet present (105). Lithium should be used with caution in combination with conventional antipsychotics or clozapine because of the recognized dangers of delirium, encephalopathy, and neurotoxicity that have been reported with these combinations (106, 107).

Anticonvulsants

Carbamazepine and valproic acid have been observed to be effective in bipolar affective disorder (108, 109), and are often considered as an adjunct therapy in patients with schizophrenia. There have only been controlled trials in schizophrenia with adjunct carbamazepine. These trials have been consistently positive (110, 111, 61). However, these trials have had relatively few subjects. The positive effects seen have been modest and usually involved nonspecific improvement in areas such as behavior and social adjustment.

Carbamazepine needs to be used with caution because of reports of disorientation and ataxia associated with its use (112, 113). It can also reduce the blood level of haloperidol by as much as 50% (114). Valproic acid should be used with caution because of the possibility of hepatic toxicity.

Benzodiazepines

There have been several reports on the use of adjunct benzodiazepines in treatment-resistant schizophrenia. Results have been mixed, with some double-blind studies showing a treatment effect (10, 115), while other studies are negative (8, 116, 11, 117). Given that patients with schizophrenia often have anxiety and irritability, it is not surprising that benzodiazepines are often useful agents in the treatment of this disorder. However, there is no firm evidence for a specific adjunct antipsychotic effect with these agents. They should be used with caution because of the risks of chronic sedation, fatigue ataxia, and dependence. There are some reports of behavioral disinhibition (117) with these drugs, and the possibility of synergistic toxicity with clozapine (118). While these reports have not been systematically confirmed, they also suggest caution with this drug combination.

Electroconvulsive Therapy (ECT)

There have been no controlled studies of ECT to date in treatment-resistant schizophrenic patients. Before the use of clozapine there was some evidence from uncontrolled trials that ECT provided benefit for treatment-resistant patients (119), but usually the effect of ECT has been the most robust in patients with a short duration of illness (120). There were two open trials of added ECT in patients who had an inadequate clozapine response (121, 122). Both trials showed some benefit from ECT. Also there are some reports of maintenance ECT continuing efficacy and preventing relapse (123). Overall evidence suggests that ECT, combined with treatment with antipsychotic drugs, may be considered an option for people with schizophrenia who show limited response to medication alone. However, initial beneficial effect may not last beyond the short term (124).

Miscellaneous therapies

There are historical studies suggesting that β-blockers and reserpine may be useful in refractory schizophrenia (16). However, there are no available controlled studies, with current diagnostic criteria. There is very limited evidence that long-term therapy with either of these strategies is beneficial.

SUMMARY

A defined approach to patients with treatment-resistant schizophrenia is critical. Clinician must first ensure that the patient truly meets criteria. Most guidelines for treating schizophrenia suggest that patients should have undergone a minimum of two trials in which they received 300–600 mg chlorpromazine equivalents/day of chlorpromazine for 4–6 week with adequate adherence. The use of an intramuscular depot antipsychotic can be useful when compliance has been confirmed to be problem. Also importantly side effects need to be minimized. Patients should be treated with at least two trials of appropriately dosed antipsychotics. At least one trial should be of either risperidone or olanzapine, if these can be tolerated as they may be at least somewhat more effective than other drugs.

Although the importance of affective symptoms in schizophrenia is starting to be recognized, optimal dosage and duration of drug therapy for treating affective disturbance are not yet established. However, the treatment of depressive symptoms should be undertaken if clearly present in the case. The outcome of drug therapy may be a subtle stabilization of mood or improvement in behavior rather than a major change in affective symptoms.

If there is no response to these measures, clozapine therapy should be attempted. Clozapine remains unique in its ability to improve outcomes in patients with treatment-resistant positive symptoms. However, the drug's benefits must be weighed against its serious potential risks.

Finally, there are those whose positive symptoms ultimately do not respond even to an adequate trial of clozapine. At this stage, adjunctive drug treatment such as mood stabilizers (lithium and valproate), sulpiride or risperidone may be considered. There is some evidence for efficacy of all of these adjunctive therapies, but it is not strong. They should be considered on an individual basis, with goals of treatment carefully defined and subsequently monitored so that ineffective polypharmacy is avoided. The use of electroconvulsive therapy (ECT) should also be considered for patients who have failed to respond to all other treatments.

Pharmacotherapy should not be given in isolation or without careful thought and monitoring. The following practices should maximize the likelihood of a successful outcome in an antipsychotic drug trial:

1. Identification of defined target symptoms. Antipsychotics are most helpful for the positive symptoms of psychosis: hallucinations, delusions and thought disorder. Newer medications may also be helpful in reducing negative symptoms, such as poor socialization, withdrawal and affective blunting, particularly if

these are secondary to extrapyramidal side effects of conventional antipsychotics. Clozapine has been shown to be effective in hostile, aggressive psychotic patients. Understanding the target symptoms for a specific drug trial will allow for greater clarity in defining the parameters of success and failure.

2. The systematic use of drugs at sufficient dosages and for a sufficient duration to establish efficacy. This is particularly critical before adjunct drugs are used as these may complicate the therapeutic situation to the point where defining the optimal drug treatment for a patient is not possible.

3. Consideration that medication intolerance, noncompliance, inadequate social support, and inadequate psychosocial treatment may create the appearance of treatment resistance. A consideration of these factors should precede the declaration of any drug therapy to be a failure. Although therapeutic ranges of most antipsychotics are not well established, measuring blood levels may be useful to establish compliance and to rule out the unlikely event of poor medication absorption.

4. Exhausting the utility of single agents before using multiple agents. There is tremendous pressure for the clinician to find a drug to rapidly treat every psychological problem manifest in a patient. It is important to remember that no adjunct agent has ever been shown to robustly improve antipsychotic response. Hostility, irritability, insomnia, and withdrawal can all be secondary to psychosis and may resolve only after a patient has had a good antipsychotic drug effect.

5. Aggressively preventing EPS through the appropriate choice of primary therapy. With the arrival of antipsychotic agents that are clearly effective at doses that do not produce extrapyramidal symptoms in the vast majority of patients, we should be able to almost eliminate persistent side effects as a reason for therapeutic failure.

6. Maintaining a positive therapeutic attitude. There are more choices now for antipsychotic therapy than ever before, with new drugs appearing annually. Patients should be encouraged to think that there is good reason to be optimistic that some therapy will be found that will be beneficial to them, even if they have had a history of severe illness.

As the antipsychotics being introduced today have different mechanisms of action than older antipsychotics and than each other, clinicians will need to explore the possibility of response with each of these new agents in turn with their patients with persistently refractory symptoms. Some newer antipsychotics, such as risperidone and olanzapine may be somewhat more effective than other antipsychotics. However to date, clozapine is the only medication with demonstrated efficacy in well-defined treatment resistance.

ACKNOWLEDGMENT
This work is the independent product of Robert R Conley, MD. As such, it does not represent the official opinion of the Eli Lilly & Company in any matter.

REFERENCES
1. Prien RF, Cole JO. High dose chlorpromazine therapy in chronic schizophrenia. Arch Gen Psychiatry 1968; 18(4): 482–95.
2. Davis JM, Casper R. Antipsychotic drugs: clinical pharmacology and therapeutic use. Drugs 1977; 12: 260–82.
3. Essock SM, Hargreaves WA, Dohm FA et al. Clozapine eligibility among state hospital patients. Schizophr Bull 1996; 22(1): 15–25.

4. Elkis H, Treatment-resistant schizophrenia. Psychiatr Clin North Am 2007; 30(3): 511–33.
5. McGlashan TH. A selective review of recent North American long-term follow-up studies of schizophrenia. Schizophr Bull 1988; 14(4): 515–42.
6. Revicki DA, Luce BR, Weschler JM, Brown RE, Adler MA. Economic grand rounds: cost-effectiveness of clozapine for treatment-resistant schizophrenic patients. Hosp Community Psychiatry 1990; 41(8): 850–4.
7. Kane J, Honigfeld G, Singer J, Meltzer H and the Clozaril Collaborative Study Group. Clozapine for the treatment-resistant schizophrenic. Arch Gen Psychiatry 1988; 45: 789–96.
8. Holden JM, Itil TM, Keskiner A, Fink M. Thiordazine and chlordiazepoxide, alone and combined, in the treatment of chronic schizophrenia. Compr Psychiatry1968; 9: 633–43.
9. Small JG, Kellams JJ, Milstein V, Moore J. A placebo-controlled study of lithium combined with neuroleptics in chronic schizophrenic patients. Am J Psychiatry 1975; 132: 1315–7.
10. Lingjaerde O, Engstrand E, Ellingsen P, Stylo DA, Robak OH. Antipsychotic effect of diazepam when given in addition to neuroleptics in chronic psychotic patients: a double-blind clinical trial. Curr Ther Res 1979; 26: 505–12.
11. Ruskin P, Averbukh I, Belmaker RH, Dasberg H. Benzodiazepines in chronic schizophrenia. Biol Psychiatry 1979; 14: 557–8.
12. Carmen JS, Bigelow LB, Wyatt RJ. Lithium combined with neuroleptics in chronic schizophrenic and schizoaffective patients. J Clin Psychiatry1981; 42: 124–8.
13. Wolkowitz OM, Pickar D, Doran AR et al. Combination alprazolam-neuroleptic treatment of the positive and negative symptoms of schizophrenia. Am J Psychiatry 1986; 143: 85–7.
14. Meltzer HY, Burnet S, Bastani B, Ramirez LF. Effects of six months of clozapine treatment on the quality of life of chronic schizophrenic patients. Hosp Community Psychiatry 1990; 141: 892–7.
15. Brenner HD, Dencker SJ, Goldstein MJ et al. Defining treatment refractoriness in schizophrenia. Schizophr Bull 1990; 16(4): 551–61.
16. Christison GW, Kirch DG, Wyatt RJ. When symptoms persist: choosing among alternative somatic treatments for schizophrenia. Schizophr Bull 1991; 17(2):217–45.
17. Kinon BJ, Kane JM, Johns C et al. Treatment of neuroleptic-resistant schizophrenia relapse. Psychopharmacol Bull 1993; 29: 309–14.
18. Shalev A, Hermesh H, Rothberg J, Munitz H. Poor neuroleptic response in acutely exacerbated schizophrenic patients. Acta Psychiatra Scandinavica 1993; 87: 86–91.
19. Overall JE, Gorham DE. The brief psychiatric rating scale. Psychol Rep 1961; 10: 799–812.
20. Guy W. ECDEU assessment manual for psychopharmacology. US Dept. of Health and Human Services publication (ADM) 1976; 76(338): 534–5.
21. Pickar D, Owen RR, Litman RE et al. Clinical and biologic response to clozapine in patients with schizophrenia. Crossover comparison with fluphenazine. Arch Gen Psychiatry 1992; 49(5): 345–53.
22. Buchanan RW, Breier A, Kirkpatrick B, Ball P, Carpenter WT Jr. Positive and negative symptom response to clozapine in schizophrenic patients with and without the deficit syndrome. Am J Psychiatry 1998; 155(6): 751–60.
23. Kinon B, Kane JM, Perovish R, Ismi, M, Koreen A. "Influence of neuroleptic dose and class in treatment-resistant schizophrenia relapse." Presented at the 32nd Annual Meeting of the New Clinical Drug Evaluation Unit, Key Biscayne, FL, May 1992.
24. Physicians Desk Reference, Medical Economics Data Production Company, Publisher, Montvale, N.Y, 2007.
25. Kane JM, Marder SR. Psychopharmacologic treatment of schizophrenia. Schizophr Bull 1993; 19(2): 113–28.
26. Farde L, Norstrom A-L, Wiesel F-A et al. Positron emission tomographic analysis of central D_1 and D_2 dopamine receptor occupancy in patients treated with classical neuroleptics and clozapine: relation to extrapyramidal side effects. Arch Gen Psychiatry 1992; 49: 538–44.
27. Wolkin A, Barouche F, Wolf AP et al. Dopamine blockade and clinical response: evidence for two biological subgroups of schizophrenia. Am J Psychiatry 1989; 146: 905–8.

28. Rifkin A, Quitkin F, Rabiner CJ, Klein DF. Fluphenazine decanoate, fluphenazine hydrochloride given orally, and placebo in remitted schizophrenics: I. relapse rates after one year. Arch Gen Psychiatry 1977; 34(1): 43–7.
29. Baldessarini RJ, Cohen BM, Teicher M. Significance of neuroleptic dose and plasma level in the pharmacological treatment of psychoses. Arch Gen Psychiatry1988; 45: 79–91.
30. Van Putten T, Marder SR, Mintz J. A controlled dose comparison of haloperidol in newly admitted schizophrenic patients. Arch Gen Psychiatry 1990; 47: 754–8.
31. Dixon LB, Lehman AF, Levine J. Conventional antipsychotic medications for schizophrenia. Schizophr Bull 1995; 21(4): 567–77.
32. Love RC, Conley RR, Kelly DL, Bartko JJ. A dose-outcome analysis of risperidone. J Clin Psychiatry 1999; 60(11): 771–5.
33. Conley RR, Carpenter WT, Tamminga CA. Time to response and response-dose in a 12-month clozapine trial. Am J Psychiatry 1997; 154(9): 1243–7.
34. Pantelis C, Barnes TR. Drug strategies and treatment-resistant schizophrenia. Aust N Z J Psychiatry 1996; 30: 20–37.
35. Juarez-Reyes MG, Shumway M, Battle C et al. Effects of stringent criteria on eligibility for clozapine among public mental health clients. Psychiatr Serv 1995; 46(8): 801–6.
36. Terkelsen KG, Grosser RC. Estimating clozapine's cost to the nation. Hosp Community Psychiatry 1990; 41(8): 863–9.
37. Dencker SJ, Kulhanet F. eds. Treatment Resistance in Schizophrenia._Braunschweig/ Wiesbaden: Vieweg Verlag, 1988.
38. Stern RG; Kahn RS, Davidson M. Predictors of response to neuroleptic treatment in schizophrenia. Psychiatric Clinic of North Am 1993; 16(2): 313–38.
39. Bilder RM, Wu H, Chakos MH et al. Cerebral morphometry and clozapine treatment in schizophrenia. J Clin Psychiatry1994; 55(Suppl B): 53–6.
40. Ota P, Maeshiro H, Ishido H et al. Treatment resistant chronic psychophathology and CT scans in schizophrenia. Acta Psychiatrica Scandinavica 1987; 75: 415–27.
41. Kirkpatrick B, Conley RR, Kakoyannis A, Reep RL, Roberts RC. Interstitial cells of the white matter in the inferior parietal cortex in schizophrenia: an unbiased cell-counting study. Synapse 1999; 34(2): 95–102.
42. Lieberman JA. Prediction of outcome in first-episode schizophrenia. J Clin Psychiatry 1993; 54(13): 7.
43. Edwards J, Maude D, McGorry PD, Harrigan SM, Cocks JT. Prolonged recovery in first-episode psychosis. Br J Psychiatry 1998; Suppl 172(33): 107–16.
44. Van Kammen DP, Schooler N. Are biochemical markers for treatment-resistant schizophrenia state dependent or traits? Clin Neuropharmacol 1990; 13(1): 516–28.
45. Pickar D, Breier A, Keisoe J. Plasma homovanillic acid as an index of central dopaminergic activity: studies in schizophrenic patients. Ann N Y Acad Sci 1988; 537: 339–46.
46. Herrera JN, Sramek JJ, Costa JF et al. High potency neuroleptics and violence in schizophrenics.J Nerv Ment Dis 1988; 176(9): 558–61.
47. Eronen M, Hakola P, Tiihonen J. Mental disorders and homicidal behavior in Finland. Arch Gen Psychiatry 1996; 53: 497–501.
48. Malone ML, Thompson L, Goodwin JS. Aggressive behavior among the institutionalized elderly. J Am Geriatr Soc 1993; 41(8): 853–6.
49. Wilson WH. Clinical review of clozapine treatment in a state hospital. Hosp Community Psychiatry 1992; 43: 700–3.
50. Ratey JJ, Leveroni C, Kilmer D, Gutheil C, Swartz B. The effects of clozapine on severely aggressive psychiatric inpatients in a state hospital. J Clin Psychiatry 1993; 54(6): 219–23.
51. Volavka J, Zito JM, Vitrai J, Czobar P. Clozapine effects on hostility and aggression in schizophrenia (Letter to Editor). J Clin Psychopharmacol 1993; 13(4): 287–9.
52. Bellus SB, Stewart D, Kost PP. Clozapine in aggression (Letter to Editor).Psychiatr Serv 1995; 46(2): 187.

53. Czobor P, Volavka J, Meibach RC. Effect of risperidone on hostility in schizophrenia. J Clin Psychopharmacol 1995; 15(4): 243–9.
54. Kane JM. Schizophrenia. N Engl J Med 1996; 334(1): 34–41.
55. Klein DF, Davis JM. Diagnosis and drug treatment of psychiaric disorders. Baltimore: Williams & Wilkins; 1969.
56. Janicak PG, Davis JM, Preskorn SH, Ayd FJ Jr. Principles and Practice of Psychopharmacotherapy. Baltimore: Williams & Wilkins, 1993: 104–6.
57. Breier A, Buchanan RW, Irish D, Carpenter WT Jr. Clozapine treatment of outpatients with schizophrenia: outcome and long-term response patterns. Hosp Community Psychiatry 1993; 44(12): 1145–9.
58. Essali A, Al-Haj Haasan N, Li C, Rathbone J. Clozapine versus typical neuroleptic medication for schizophrenia. Cochrane Database Syst Rev 2009; (1): CD000059.
59. Mallya AR, Roos PD, Roebuck-Colgan K. Restraint, seclusion, and clozapine. J Clin Psychiatry 1992; 53: 395–7.
60. Tamminga CA, Thaker GK, Moran M, Kakigi T, Gao XM. Clozapine in tardive dyskinesia: observations from human and animal model studies. Journal of Clinical Psychiatry 1994; 55: 102–6.
61. Meltzer HY, Okayli G. Reduction of suicidality during clozapine treatment in neuroleptic-resistant schizophrenia: impact on risk-benefit assessment. Am J Psychiatry 1995; 152: 183–90.
62. Bustillo JR, Lauriello J, Keith SJ. Schizophrenia: improving outcome. Harv Rev Psychiatry 1999; 6(5): 229–40.
63. Meltzer HY. Commentary: defining treatment refractoriness in schizophrenia. Schizophr Bull 1990; 16(4): 563–5.
64. Zito JM, Volavka J, Craig TJ et al. Pharmacoepidemiology of clozapine in 202 inpatients with schizophrenia. Ann Pharmacother 1993; 27: 1262–9.
65. Rosenheck RA, Leslie DL, Doshi JA. Second-generation antipsychotics: cost-effectiveness, policy options, and political decision making. Psychiatr Serv 2008; 59(5): 515–20.
66. Rosenheck R, Cramer J, Allan E et al. Cost-effectiveness of clozapine in patients with high and low levels of hospital use. Department of Veterans Affairs Cooperative Study Group on Clozapine in Refractory Schizophrenia. Arch Gen Psychiatry 1999; 56(6): 565–72.
67. Safferman A, Lieberman JA, Kane JM, Szymanski S, Kinon B. Update on the clinical efficacy and side effects of clozapine. Schizophr Bull 1991; 17(2): 247–61.
68. Rosenheck R, Cramer J, Jurgis G et al. Clinical and psychopharmacologic factors influencing family burden in refractory schizophrenia. J Clin Psychiatry 2000; 61(9): 671–6.
69. Bak TH, Bauer M, Schaub RT, Hellweg R, Reishiss FM. Myoclonis in patients treated with clozapine. J Clin Psychiatry 1995; 56(9): 418–22.
70. Rosenheck R, Evans D, Herz L et al. How long to wait for a response to clozapine: a comparison of time course of response to clozapine and conventional antipsychotic medication in refractory schizophrenia. Schizophr Bull 1999b; 25(4): 709–19.
71. Carpenter WT, Conley RR, Buchanan RW, Breier A, Tamminga CA. Patient response and resource management: another view of clozapine treatment of schizophrenia. Am J Psychiatry 1995; 152: 6.
72. Chouinard G, Jones B, Remington G et al. A Canadian multicenter placebo-controlled study of fixed doses of risperidone and haloperidol in the treatment of chronic schizophrenic patients. J Clin Psychopharmacol 1993; 13(1): 25–39.
73. Marder SR, Meiback RC. Risperidone in the treatment of schizophrenia. Am J Psychiatry 1994; 151: 825–35.
74. Chouinard G, Vainer JL, Belanger MC et al. Rispridone and clozapine in the treatment of drug-resistant schizophrenia and neuroleptic-induced supersensitivity psychosis. Prog Neuropsychopharmacol Biol Psychiatry 1994; 18(7): 1129–41.
75. Keck PE Jr, Wilson DR, Strakowski SM et al. Clinical predictors of acute risperidone response in schizophrenia, schizoaffective disorder, and psychotic mood disorders. J Clin Psychiatry 1995; 56(10): 455–70.

76. Wirshing DA, Marshall BD Jr, Green MF et al. Risperidone in treatment-refractory schizophrenia. Am J Psychiatry 1999; 156(9): 1374–9.
77. Klieser E, Lehmann E, Kinzler E, Wurthmann C, Heinrich K. Randomized, double-blind, controlled trial of risperidone versus clozapine in patients with chronic schizophrenia. J Clin Psychopharmacol 1995; (1suppl 1): 45S–51S.
78. Bondolfi G, Dufour H, Patris M et al. Risperidone versus clozapine in treatment-resistant chronic schizophrenia: a randomized double-blind study. The Risperidone Study Group. Am J Psychiatry 1998; 155(4): 499–504.
79. Flynn SW, MacEwan GW, Altman S et al. An open comparison of clozapine and risperidone in treatment-resistant schizophrenia. Pharmacopsychiatry 1998; 31(1): 25–9.
80. Lacey RL, Preskorn S.H, Jerkovich GS. Is risperidone a substitute for clozapine for patients who do not respond to neuroleptics? (Letter to Editor). Am J Psychiatry 1995; 152(9): 1401.
81. Shore D. Clinical implications of clozapine discontinuation: Report of an NIMH workshop. Schizophr Bull 1995; 21(2): 333–7.
82. Hunter RH, Joy CB, Kennedy E, Gilbody SM, Song F. Risperidone versus typical antipsychotic medication for schizophrenia. Cochrane Database Syst Rev 2003; (2): CD000440.
83. Nussbaum A, Stroup TS. Paliperidone for schizophrenia. Cochrane Database Syst Rev 2008; (2): CD006369.
84. Thomas SG, Labbate LA. Management of treatment-resistant schizophrenia with olanzapine. Can J Psychiatry 1998; 43(2): 195–6.
85. Tollefson GD, Kuntz AJ. Review of recent clinical studies with olanzapine. Br J Psychiatry 1999; (37): 30–5.
86. Breier A, Hamilton SH. Comparative efficacy of olanzapine and haloperidol for patients with treatment-resistant schizophrenia. Biol Psychiatry 1999; 45(4): 403–11.
87. Conley RR, Tamminga CA, Bartko JJ et al. Olanzapine compared with chlorpromazine in treatment-resistant schizophrenia. Am J Psychiatry 1998; 155(7): 914–20.
88. Sanders RD, Mossman D. An open trial of olanzapine in patients with treatment-refractory psychoses. J Clin Psychopharmacol 1999; 19(1): 62–6.
89. Conley RR, Tamminga CA, Kelly DL, Richardson CM. Treatment-resistant schizophrenic patients respond to clozapine after olanzapine non-response. Biol Psychiatry 1999; 46(1): 73–7.
90. Lieberman JA. Effectiveness of antipsychotic drugs in patients with chronic schizophrenia: efficacy, safety and cost outcomes of CATIE and other trials. J Clin Psychiatry 2007; 68(2): e04.
91. Leucht S, Komossa K, Rummel-Kluge C et al. A meta-analysis of head-to-head comparisons of second-generation antipsychotics in the treatment of schizophrenia. Am J Psychiatry Nov 17, 2008.
92. Daumit GL, Goff DC, Meyer JM et al. Antipsychotic effects on estimated 10-year coronary heart disease risk in the CATIE schizophrenia study. Schizophr Res 2008; 105(1–3): 175–87.
93. Arvanitis LA, Miller BG. Multiple fixed doses of „Seroquel" (quetiapine) in patients with acute exacerbation of schizophrenia: a comparison with haloperidol and placebo. The Seroquel Trial 13 Study Group. Biol Psychiatry 1997; 42(4): 233–46.
94. Szigethy E, Brent S, Findling RL. Quetiapine for refractory schizophrenia. J Am Acad Child Adolesc Psychiatry 1998; 37(11): 1127–8.
95. Reznik I, Benatov R, Sirota P. Seroquel in a resistant schizophrenic with negative and positive symptoms. Harefuah 1996; 130(10): 675–7.
96. Srisurapanont M, Maneeton B, Maneeton N. Quetiapine for schizophrenia. Cochrane Database Syst Rev 2004; (2): CD000967.
97. Lieberman JA, Stroup TS, McEvoy JP et al. Clinical Antipsychotic Trials of Intervention Effectiveness (CATIE) Investigators. Effectiveness of antipsychotic drugs in patients with chronic schizophrenia. N Engl J Med 2005; 353(12): 1209–23.
98. Bhattacharjee J, El-Sayeh HG. Aripiprazole versus typical antipsychotic drugs for schizophrenia. Cochrane Database Syst Rev 2008; (3): CD006617.

99. Nemeroff CB, Lieberman JA, Weiden PJ et al. From clinical research to clinical practice: a 4-year review of ziprasidone. CNS Spectr 2005; 10(11Suppl 17): 1–20.

100. Conley R, Tamminga CA, Nguyen JA. Clinical action of remoxipride. Arch Gen Psychiatry 1994; 51(12): 1001.

101. Shiloh R, Zemishlany Z, Aizenberg D et al. Sulpiride augmentation in people with schizophrenia partially responsive to clozapine. A double-blind, placebo-controlled study. Br J Psychiatry 1997; 171: 569–73.

102. Raskin S, Durst R, Katz G, Zislin J. Olanzapine and sulpiride: a preliminary study of combination/augmentation in patients with treatment-resistant schizophrenia. J Clin Psychopharmacol 2000; 20(5): 500–3.

103. Growe GA, Crayton JW, Klass DB, Evans H, Strizich M. Lithium in chronic schizophrenia. Am J Psychiatry 1979; 136: 454–5.

104. Delva NJ, Letemendia FJ. Lithium treatment in schizophrenia and schizoaffective disorders. Edited by Kerr A, Snaith P. In Contemporary Issues in Schizophrenia. London: Royal college of Psychiatrists, 1986: 381–96.

105. Johns CA, Thompson JW. Adjunctive treatments in schizophrenia: pharmacotherapies and electroconvulsive therapy. Schizophr Bull 1995; 21: 607–19.

106. Cohen WJ, Cohen NH. Lithium carbonate, haloperidol and irreversible brain damage. JAMA 1974; 230: 1283–7.

107. Miller F, and Menninger J. Lithium-neuroleptic neurotoxicity is dose-dependent. J Psychopharmacol 1987; 7: 89–91.

108. Post RM. Non-lithium treatment for bipolar disorder. J Clin Psychiatry 1900; 51: 9–16.

109. Freeman TW, Clothier JL, Pazzaglia P, Lesem MD, Swann AC. A double-blind comparison of valproate and lithium in the treatment of acute mania. Am J Psychiatry 1992; 149: 108–11.

110. Schulz SC, Kahn EM, Baker RW, Conley RR. Lithium and carbamazepine augmentation in treatment-refractory schizophenia. In:Angrist, B.; Schulz, S.C. eds. The Neuroleptic-Nonresponsive Patient:Characterization and Treatment. Washington, D.C.: American Psychiaric Press, 1990: 109–36.

111. Simhandl C, Meszaros K. The use of carbamazepine in the treatment of schizophrenia and schizoaffective psychosis: a review. J Psychiatry Neurosci 1992; 17: 1–14.

112. Kanter GL, Yerevsanian BI, Ciccone JR. Case report of a possible interaction between neuroleptics and carbamazepine. Am J Psychiatry 1984; 14: 1101–2.

113. Yerevanian BI, Hodgman CH. A haloperidol-carbamazepine interaction in a patients with rapid-cycling bipolar disorder (Letter). Am J Psychiatry 1985; 142: 785–6.

114. Kahn EM, Schulz SC, Perel JM, Alexander JE. Change in haloperidol level due to carbamazepine: a complicating factor in combined medication for schizophrenia. J Clin Psychiatry 1990; 10: 54–57.

115. Wolkowitz OM, Turetsky N, Reus VI, Hargreaves WA. Benzodiazepine agmentation of neuroleptics in treatment-resistant schizophrenia. Psychopharmacol Bull 1992; 28: 291–5.

116. Halon TE, Ota KY, Burland AA. Comparative effects of fluphenazine, fluphenazine-chlordiazepoxide and fluphenazine-imipramine. Disorders Nerv Syst 1970; 31: 171–7.

117. Pato CN, Wolkowitz OM, Rapaport M, Schulz SC, Pickar D. Benzodiazepine augmentation of neuroleptic treatment in patients with schizophrenia. Psychopharmacol Bull 1989; 25: 263–6.

118. Meltzer HY. New drugs for the treatment of schizophrenia. Psychiatr Clin North Am 1993; 16: 365–85.

119. Friedel RO. The combined use of neuroleptics and ECT in drug-resistant schizophrenic patients.Psychopharmacol Bull 1986; 22: 928–30.

120. Small JG. Efficacy of electroconvulsive therapy in schizophrenia, mania, and other disorders. I. Schizophrenia. Convuls Ther 1985; 1: 263–70.

121. Remington GJ, Addington D, Collins EJ et al. Clozapine: current status and role in the pharmacotherapy of schizophrenia. Can J Psychiatry 1996; 41(3): 161–6.

122. Benatov R, Sirota P, Megged S. Neuroleptic-resistant schziophrenia treated with clozapine and ECT. Convuls Ther 1996; 12(2): 117–21.

123. Chanpattana W. Maintenance ECT in treatment-resistant schizophrenia. J Med Assoc Thai 2000; 83(6): 657–62.
124. Tharyan P, Adams CE. Electroconvulsive therapy for schizophrenia. Cochrane Database Syst Rev 2005; (2): CD000076.
125. American Psychiatric Association. DSM-III: Diagnosis and Statistical manual of Mental Disorders. 3d ed. Washington, DC: The Association, 1980.

BIBLIOGRAPHY

Beasley CM, Tollefson G, Tran P. Olanzapine versus placebo and haloperidol. Neuropsychopharmacology 1996; 14: 111–23.
Buckley PF, Buchanan RW. Catching up on schizophrenia. Arch Gen Psychiatry 1996; 53: 456–62.
Dursun SM, Gardner DM, Bird DC, Flinn J. Olanzapine for patients with treatment-resistant schizophrenia: a naturalistic case-series outcom e study. Can J Psychiatry 1999; 44(7): 701–4.
Lindstrom E, Eriksson B, Hellgren A, von Knorring L, Eberhard G. Efficacy and safety of risperidone in the long-term treatment of patients with schizophrenia. Clin Ther 1995; 17(3): 402–12.
Migler BM, Warawa EJ, Malick JB. Seroquel: behavioral profile of a potential atypical antipsychotic. Psychopharmacology 1993; 112: 299–307.
Reich J. Use of high-dose olanzapine in refractory psychosis. Am J Psychiatry 1999; 156(4): 661.
Smith TE, Docherty JP. Standards of care and clinical algorithms for treating schizophrenia. Psychiatr Clin North Am 1998; 21(1): 203–20.

17

First episode schizophrenia: Considerations on the timing, selection, and duration of antipsychotic therapies

Brian J Miller and Peter F Buckley

In recent years, there has been an encouraging and accelerated growth in research in First Episode Psychosis (FEP). The growth in FEP research results from a confluence of findings pointing to the early (even in-utero) origins of schizophrenia. There is also a broadening appreciation that while it is not yet possible to "spot" schizophrenia from a variety of nonspecific and subtle "impairments" in social, linguistic, and cognitive performance, it is nevertheless evident that people later diagnosed with schizophrenia have been "ill" for (in many instances) several years before they actually present for care (1). Moreover, there is now intriguing and provocative information from several high risk studies which suggests that effective, early intervention might (at least) forestall the onset of FEP (2, 3). Such a perspective is important because it offers a glimpse of the potential for primary prevention of schizophrenia. Heretofore this was largely considered an unrealistic proposition. There is evidence now of early cognitive and structural brain neurodegenerative changes even at (or close to) the onset of FEP (4, 5). Thus, appropriate (and even "aggressive") management of schizophrenia at its first presentation might result in a more favorable trajectory over the course of subsequent care. While both of these suppositions are just that—suppositions—nevertheless they form an important and heuristic "backdrop" when considering the pharmacologic management of FEP.

The purpose of this chapter, framed within the context and set against the other findings illuminated in this comprehensive text on schizophrenia, is to give a current account of both the guiding principles and the current "state-of-play" of the treatment of FEP. For completeness sake, the reader is also referred to a previous chapter that, while now older, gives an excellent historical perspective on FEP (6).

WHEN TO INITIATE MEDICATION TREATMENT

Consider the following "all-too-familiar" scenario: A 19-year-old man presents for the first time to the Emergency Department with a 12 month history of apparently irrational fears that his college roommates are spying on him. He is convinced that they are plotting to get him thrown out of school. He tells the emergency department doctor that he has even overheard them say, "Let's put arsenic in his coffee". He is agitated when interviewed, shouting aloud that, "There is nothing wrong," and claiming, "I need a lawyer. The police should have arrested my friends and not brought me here in handcuffs. I will sue all of you for violating my rights". He refuses to answer questions from the doctor. The doctor talks with the police who confirm that his residence was a total mess, and that his family said he had been not caring for himself for months.

This is a fairly straightforward and typical presentation of FEP. The presence of florid (and already pretty systematized) delusions, hallucinations, impaired functioning, and self-neglect all suggest that this patient has been ill for some time. Also, he is now agitated and lacking insight. Things could easily escalate further in the emergency department, given his lack of insight, refusal to accept treatment, and threatening behavior. Starting some treatment with an antipsychotic (as well, of course, as completing a thorough diagnostic workup) now seems an entirely appropriate strategy. Indeed, if things worsen, it seems that there is a fair chance that this patient's first exposure to antipsychotic medications will be with a short-acting formulation given involuntarily by injection. This will be followed by a period of inpatient stabilization. Then there will be the "back and forth" process of negotiating with the patient to continue on this new medication ("you want to give me an antipsychotic, but I'm not psychotic") once he is discharged to outpatient care.

Consider this alternative scenario: the same patient is brought by his mother to their family practitioner. She is worried that he is not adjusting well at college. His mother reports that he seems to spend too much time in his room instead of being with his friends who are out partying. He tells the doctor that there is nothing wrong with him. In his "defense", he also tells the doctor that he thinks his friends have something against him. He admits, but is not quite sure, to considering that he overheard them on one occasion saying that he was "no fun to be with". His mother tells the doctor she is worried because she had a cousin who committed suicide in his first year of college.

So, what should we do now—treat or not treat? It may seem obvious, in light of the first scenario. But if you did not know that he was going to become psychotic and he was (just) presenting with these vague features and worries, would you start treatment? And which treatment would you give? It's a very complex question, especially since you might expose this person to powerful, "mind altering" drugs that also have serious—as well as distressing—side effects. And, if you treated now, would it make the psychosis "go away" or just "prolong the inevitable"? These are tough questions, too (Table 17.1). Recent prodromal studies provide some guidance here (7, 8). Several studies of patients who are at risk to progress toward full-blown psychosis suggest that intervening early with a medication is associated with a lower conversion rate to psychosis over the period of observation. In a seminal study, McGorry and colleagues (9) found that 19% of patients with prodromal features of psychosis who were treated with low doses of risperidone converted to frank psychosis over 6 months. This contrasted favorably with a 39% conversion rate in the placebo control group. McGlashan and colleagues (10) found a similar effect for olanzapine over a longer period of observation, although the "drop out" rate from the study and the inherent difficulty in following people for any length of time that are "not sick" moderates the conclusions from this important study. Interestingly, another more naturalistic study of high-risk young people observed a similar effect with antidepressant medications alone (11). Moreover, a British study suggests that even counseling/cognitive behavioral therapy can have a powerful effect (to forestall psychosis) in this vulnerable patient group (12).

FIRST GENERATION ANTIPSYCHOTICS FOR FEP

There is ample evidence that first generation antipsychotics (FGAs) are an appropriate and effective treatment option for patients with FEP. Oosthuizen and colleagues (13) compared low dose haloperidol (2 mg/day) with moderate doses of haloperidol (8 mg/day) in $N = 40$ FEP patients. Symptomatic response was similar between both groups, with 74% of patients completing the 6 week trial. However, low doses of haloperidol produced less EPS overall. In a seminal study of FEP, Lieberman and

TABLE 17.1 Should You Intervene With Patients in Suspected Psychotic Prodrome?

Arguments for:

Early treatment may prevent psychosocial decline.

Treatment may delay or ameliorate psychosis onset.

Treatment may improve patient awareness and acceptance of diagnosis.

Antipsychotics are effective for symptoms and may be neuroprotective.

Medications may improve overall outcome.

Neuroimaging findings may predict psychosis.

Outcome scales have improved diagnosis.

Treatment may reduce prodrome duration and improve prognosis.

Arguments against:

Treatment would likely be given to persons who would not develop psychosis.

Treatment would unnecessarily stigmatize individuals who do not have schizophrenia.

Exposing patients with uncertain diagnosis to treatment risks is an ethical dilemma.

Antipsychotics are associated with side effects.

Psychotic prodrome studies are inconclusive, with small sample sizes and short follow-up.

No biologic markers exist to predict psychosis.

colleagues (14) showed that these medications achieved resolution of acute symptoms in approximately 85% of FEP patients. The time that it took to achieve this was, on average, 36 weeks. This is a long time, and FEP patients often will not stay on medications long enough during this first treatment experience. Indeed, as Dr. Nina Schooler explains in an astute analogy (personal communication 2/21/08), patients tend to take a viewpoint that taking antipsychotics to treat schizophrenia is akin to taking a short course of antibiotics for a respiratory infection, "I took the medication. My symptoms got better. I am 'cured'." In addition, the side effect profile of FGAs, especially sedation and akathisia, reinforce to the patient that these are not medications that he or she wants to be taking any longer than is absolutely necessary. Because the drugs are effective in treating (especially) the positive symptoms for which the patient might have some insight, ironically the good initial response reinforces the patient's opinion that the powerful drugs have done their work and that prolonged treatment makes no sense. In attempting to "broker" with the patient to stay on these medications, the clinician can take support from evidence that low doses of FGAs can be used effectively and with less side effects (15). However, these drugs are still "toxic" and tardive dyskinesia is still a concern. Indeed, studies have even cited a 17% rate of extrapyramidal signs in patients with FEP who are neuroleptic-naïve (16).

Schooler and colleagues conducted several years ago a pivotal study called the "Treatment Strategies in Schizophrenia (TSS)". This study found that, even with low doses of an FGA in a stable, restricted group of patients early in their course of illness, there was a high (almost 50%) chance of relapse during 2 years of treatment. And so the idea that you can treat acute schizophrenia like a respiratory infection is incorrect and patients do need to maintain on treatment to reduce the risk of relapse. How long a patient with FEP should continue on an antipsychotic is discussed later in this chapter.

TABLE 17.2 Clinical Studies of Second-Generation Antipsychotics in First-Episode Psychosis

SGA	Authors	Year	Type of Trial	Duration	Subjects N	Diagnosis	Comparator	Primary Efficacy Measure
Risperidone	Emsley	1999	RCT	6 weeks	183	DSM-III-R Schizophrenia or Schizophreniform	Haloperidol	≥50% decrease in PANSS
	Gutierrez et al.	2002	Open-label	104 weeks	436	DSM-IV First Episode Psychosis	None	PANSS, CGI
	Harvey et al.	2005	RCT	12 weeks	338	DSM-IV SSD	Haloperidol	Cognitive testing battery, PANSS
	Kopala et al.	1997	Case series	7.1 weeks (mean)	22	DSM-IV Schizophrenia or Schizophreniform	None	PANSS, CGI, GAF
	Kopala et al.	1998	Open-label	9.6 weeks (mean	41	DSM-IV Schizophrenia or Schizophreniform	None	PANSS, CGI, GAF
	Lane et al.	2001	Randomized Fixed-dose	6 weeks	24	DSM-IV	Risperidone (3mg vs 6 mg)	PANSS
	Malla et al.	2001	Cohort study (post-hoc analysis)	52 weeks (minimum)	38	DSM-III-R/IV Schizophrenia	FGA	BPRS, SANS, SAPS Rehospitalization
	Merlo et al.	2002	Randomized Fixed-dose	8 weeks	49	DSM-IV SSD	Risperidone (2mg vs 4 mg)	BPRS, SANS, CGI, SOFAS
	Schooler et al.	2005	RCT	30 weeks (median)	555	DSM-IV SSD	Haloperidol	≥20% decrease in PANSS
	Yap et al.	2001	Open-label	8 weeks	24	DSM-IV Schizophrenia or Schizophreniform	None	≥20% decrease in PANSS CGI, GAF
	Yoshimura et al.	2003	Open-label	2 weeks	34	DSM-IV Schizophrenia	None	≥50% decrease in PANSS

		Year	Design	Duration	N	Diagnosis	Comparator	Outcome measures
Paliperidone	None							
Olanzapine	Bobes et al.	2003	Open-label	Not specified	158	ICD-10 Schizophrenia	FGA	≥ 40% decrease in BPRS plus end BPRS <18 or CGI <3
	Green et al.	2006	RCT	104 weeks	263	DSM-IV SSD	Haloperidol	PANSS, CGI, MADRS
	Keefe et al.	2004	RCT	12 weeks	167	DSM-IV SSD	Haloperidol	Cognitive testing battery
	Lieberman et al.	2003	RCT	12 weeks	263	DSM-IV SSD	Haloperidol	PANSS, CGI, MADRS
	Montes et al.	2003	Open-label	24 weeks	182	ICD-10 Schizophrenia	FGA	CGI, GAF
	Sanger et al.	1999	RCT subpopulation	6 weeks	83	DSM-IV SSD	Haloperidol	≥ 40% decrease in BPRS
	Tollefson et al.	1997	RCT (post-hoc analysis)	Not specified	1996	DSM-III-R SSD	Haloperidol	≥ 40% decrease in BPRS
Quetiapine	Good et al.	2002	Open-label	104 weeks	34	Not specified	None	Cognitive testing battery
	Ohlsen et al.	2004	Open-label	48 weeks	33	Not specified	None	PANSS, BPRS, CDSS
	Tauscher-Wisniewski et al.	2002	Open label	12 weeks	14	DSM-IV SSD	None	
Aripiprazole	Saha et al.	2004	Open-label	4 weeks	20	Not specified	None	PANSS, CGI
Ziprasidone	None							

BPRS=Brief Psychiatric Rating Scale
PANSS=Positive and Negative Syndrome Scale
CDSS=Calgary Depression Scale for Schizophrenia
RCT=Randomized-Controlled Trial
CGI=Clinical Global Impressions Scale
SANS=Scale for the Assessment of Negative Symptoms
FEP=First Episode Psychosis
SAPS=Scale for the Assessment of Positive Symptoms
FGA=First-Generation Antipsychotic
SGA=Second-Generation Antipsychotic
GAF=Global Assessment of Functioning Scale
SSD=Schizophrenia Spectrum Disorders (Schizophrenia, Schizophreniform,and Schizoaffective)
MADRS=Montgomery-Asberg Depression Rating Scale

EVIDENCE THAT SECOND GENERATION ANTIPSYCHOTICS WORK IN FEP

The advent of SGAs has led naturally to their use in patients with FEP. Yet in spite of such a shift in clinical practice (more evident in the United States than in Europe where FGAs are still often the first choice medicines), there is still relatively little known about the impact of these drugs in FEP. This is particularly so in considering the relative impact across SGAs in this population. A systematic review of the literature identified 22 published studies between 1997 and 2007, including five randomized trials, which describe the efficacy of SGAs in first-episode psychosis. The general characteristics of these studies are outlined in Table 17.2. Details of several studies for each drug are given below.

Risperidone and paliperidone ER

Risperidone has been the most widely studied SGA to date in first episode psychosis, with 11 published studies, including four randomized trials. Emsley and the Risperidone Working Group (17) conducted a 6-week international, multicenter, double-blind, randomized trial in $N = 183$ patients with FEP, using flexible doses of either risperidone or haloperidol (mean daily dose 6.1 mg vs. 5.6 mg, respectively). At the end of the study, 63% of risperidone-treated patients (vs. 56% of haloperidol-treated patients) were clinically improved, measured by a $\geq 50\%$ decrease in Positive and Negative Syndrome Scale total scores. The authors also found significantly lower severity of extrapyramidal symptoms, measured by Extrapyramidal Symptom Rating Scale scores, and less use of antiparkinsonian medications in patients receiving lower doses (≤ 6 mg/day) than higher doses (> 6 mg/day) doses of risperidone or haloperidol.

Lane and colleagues (18) compared fixed doses of risperidone in $N = 24$ antipsychotic-naïve patients hospitalized with first-episode schizophrenia in a 6-week trial. They found comparable efficacy between 3 mg/day and 6 mg/day dosing, measured by a $\geq 20\%$ decrease in Positive and Negative Syndrome Scale total scores in 64% versus 67% of patients, respectively. There was also a trend toward fewer adverse events, including EPS, in the 3 mg/day group. Merlo and colleagues (19) also compared fixed doses of risperidone in $N = 49$ patients with FEP in an 8-week trial. They found a significant reduction in positive and negative symptoms at both 2 mg/day and 4 mg/day doses. Although there were no significant difference between the two groups in motor side effects, as measured by the Barnes Akathisia Scale and the Simpson-Angus Scale, the 2 mg/day group showed significantly less dysfunction on a computerized fine motor assessment.

Schooler et al. (20) conducted a double-blind, randomized, controlled, flexible-dose, relapse-prevention trial in $N = 555$ patients with FEP between risperidone and haloperidol (mean modal daily dose 3.3 mg vs. 2.9 mg, respectively). The median length of treatment in this study was 206 days. The authors found significant improvements in Positive and Negative Syndrome Scale and Clinical Global Impression scores at 12 weeks relative to baseline, with no significant difference between risperidone and haloperidol. Among the three-quarters of patients in this study with clinical improvement, as defined by a $\geq 20\%$ decrease in Positive and Negative Syndrome Scale scores, the median time to relapse was significantly longer for patients treated with risperidone than haloperidol. Furthermore, patients in the risperidone group showed greater improvements than patients in the haloperidol group on a range of cognitive tests over the course of the study (21).

Several other nonrandomized trials have studied the efficacy of risperidone in FEP. In a case series by Kopala et al. (22), risperidone was effective for both positive and negative symptoms in $N = 22$ patients with first-episode psychosis. The average daily dose in these patients was 6 mg, and some extrapyramidal symptoms were reported. Kopola and colleagues (23) also showed improvements in Clinical Global Impression and Global Assessment of Functioning scores in patients treated with risperidone. In an open-label study of $N = 24$ patients with first-episode psychosis by Yap and colleagues (24), the response rate ($\geq 20\%$ decrease in PANSS) was 87.5%. The mean dose of risperidone in this study was 2.7 mg/day. Several long-term studies have reported fewer hospitalizations, shorter hospitalizations, longer duration of clinical improvement, and fewer extrapyramidal symptoms in first-episode patients treated with risperidone versus first-generation antipsychotics (25, 26). Another study of $N = 34$ patients with FEP by Yoshimura and colleagues (27) found higher pre-treatment plasma homovanillic acid levels in patients responding to risperidone.

There is, as yet, no information on the use of paliperidone in FEP. One could speculate that its adverse effect profile (28) might make it a more advantageous choice over risperidone (from which it is derived) in this patient group.

Concerning Long Acting Injectable (LAI) risperidone, Emsley and colleagues (29) conducted an open-labelled study of 25-50 mg every 2 weeks for 2 years in 50 FEP patients. A clinical response of at least 20% reduction on PANSS total scores was obtained by 46 patients and a reduction of at least 50% was obtained by 42 (84%) of the patients. A total of 32 (64%) patients achieved remission at some stage in this study. Of these 32 patients, 31 (97%) maintained this status throughout the study.

Olanzapine

Published data for the use of olanzapine in FEP come from five studies, including three randomized trials. Sanger and colleagues (30) reported on a subpopulation of $N = 83$ patients with FEP from a large prospective, multicenter, international, double blind, 6 week acute treatment study of olanzapine versus haloperidol (mean modal daily dose 11.6 mg versus 10.8 mg respectively). They found a significantly higher clinical response, as defined by a $\geq 40\%$ decrease in Brief Psychiatric Rating Scale scores, in olanzapine-treated (67.2%) versus haloperidol-treated (29.2%) patients. Patients in the olanzapine group also had significant improvements in Simpson-Angus scale and Barnes Akathisia Scale scores, while patients in the haloperidol group showed a worsening on both measures. Furthermore, olanzapine-treated first-episode patients had significantly higher clinical response rates compared to olanzapine-treated patients with multiple episodes of psychosis in the parent study.

Lieberman and colleagues (31) completed a randomized, double-blind trial in $N = 263$ first-episode patients followed for up to 2 years of olanzapine versus haloperidol (mean modal daily doses 9.1 mg vs. 4.4 mg, respectively). In the first 12 weeks of this study, patients in the olanzapine group were more likely than patients in the haloperidol group to complete the first 12 weeks of the study (67% vs. 54%, respectively). Patients receiving olanzapine showed greater improvement in positive, negative, and depressive symptoms than patients receiving haloperidol. However, patients receiving olanzapine also had weight gain than patients receiving haloperidol (7.3 kg vs. 2.6 kg) over the course of the study. Patients in both the olanzapine and haloperidol groups had significant improvements in neurocognitive function, but there was not a significant difference between the groups based on an unweighted, composite score (32). Green and colleagues (33) presented the 2-year data from this trial. They found that while olanzapine and haloperidol were associated with similar, significant reductions in symptom severity, patients were less likely to discontinue treatment with olanzapine than with haloperidol. Furthermore, remission rates were greater for olanzapine-treated (57.25%) versus haloperidol-treated (43.94%) patients. In this study, extrapyramidal side effects were more common with haloperidol, while increased weight gain, cholesterol, and liver function tests were more common with olanzapine.

Several other nonrandomized trials have studied the efficacy of olanzapine in FEP. In an open-label, prospective, naturalistic study of $N = 158$ patients with FEP, Bobes and colleagues (34) found significantly higher clinical response, as measured by a ≥40% decrease in Brief Psychiatric Rating Scale scores plus and endpoint BPRS <18 or CGI <3, in olanzapine-treated patients (76.7%) compared to patients treated with first-generation antipsychotics (54.4%). The mean modal daily doses of olanzapine and haloperidol in this study were 15.8 mg and 15.3 mg, respectively. The frequency of new or worsening of existing extrapyramidal symptoms was less in the olanzapine group (13.5%) than in the group receiving FEP (55.1%). In an open-label, observational, naturalistic study of $N = 182$ patients with first-episode psychosis, Montes and colleagues (35) found similar improvements in CGI and GAF scale scores in patients treated with olanzapine versus first-generation antipsychotics. By contrast, olanzapine-treated patients had greater quality of life improvements compared to patients treated with FEP. In a post-hoc analysis of patients with first-episode psychosis from a larger randomized trial, Tollefson and colleagues (36) found a significantly higher response rate and greater reduction in symptom severity scores in olanzapine-treated compared to haloperidol-treated patients.

Quetiapine

There are three open-label studies of quetiapine in the treatment of FEP. Good and colleagues (37) reported on an interim analysis of a 2-year study of the effects of quetiapine (mean dose = 517.9 mg/day) on cognition in $N = 34$ patients with first-episode schizophrenia. The authors found significant improvement on measures of attention (Continuous Performance Test) after 3, 6, and 12 months of treatment, and measures of verbal productivity (Verbal Fluency Test) and executive function (Object Alternation Test) after 6 and 12 months of treatment. In a study of $N = 14$ patients with FEP treated with quetiapine (mean daily dose 427 mg) for 12 weeks, Tauscher-Wisniewski and colleagues (38) found a clinical response, defined by a Clinical Global Impressions improvement scale score of "much improved" or greater, in 71% of patients. The mean weight gain for the $N = 10$ subjects completing the trial was 4.2 kg, and no clinically relevant motor side effects occurred. Ohlsen and colleagues (39) studied $N = 33$ patients with FEP treated with quetiapine (mean dose 431.8 mg/day) for 48 weeks. They found significant symptomatic and functional improvements on multiple rating scales, including the Positive and Negative Syndrome, Brief Psychiatric Rating Scale, Calgary Depression in Schizophrenia Scale, Global Assessment of Functioning scale, and Schizophrenia Quality of Life Scale. There were negligible treatment-emergent extrapyramidal symptoms and no cases of tardive dyskinesia.

Aripiprazole

There is only one published study of aripiprazole in the treatment of FEP. Saha and colleagues (40) completed a 4-week, multicenter, open-label, fixed-dose trial in twenty patients with first-episode schizophrenia (mean daily dose = 17 mg). They reported improvement in Positive and Negative Syndrome Scale and Clinical Global Impression scores across all doses. The most frequently reported adverse events during the study were anxiety, akathisia, tachycardia, and dizziness. Furthermore, the authors note that there were no significant laboratory findings, and minimal change in body weight.

Ziprasidone

At present there are no published studies that characterize the efficacy and tolerability of ziprasidone in patients with FEP.

EVIDENCE FOR COMPARATIVE EFFICACY OF SECOND GENERATION ANTIPSYCHOTICS IN FEP

Three additional clinical studies have compared the relative efficacy of SGAs in FEP. Robinson and colleagues (41) compared 4-month treatment outcomes in $N = 112$ patients with schizophrenia spectrum disorders treated with olanzapine and risperidone (mean modal daily doses 11.8 mg and 3.9 mg, respectively). They found that the clinical response rate did not significantly differ between olanzapine (43.7%) and risperidone (54.3%). Negative symptom outcomes and measures of extrapyramidal symptoms did not differ between medications. Olanzapine-treated patients gained significantly more weight relative to baseline than risperidone-treated patients (17.3% versus 11.3%, respectively).

In the Comparison of Atypicals for First Episode (CAFE) study, McEvoy and colleagues (42) completed a 52-week randomized, double-blind, flexible-dose, multi-center study of the efficacy (measured by rates of treatment discontinuation) of olanzapine, quetiapine, and risperidone (mean modal daily doses 11.7 mg, 506 mg, and 2.4 mg, respectively) in $N = 400$ patients with first-episode psychosis. There were no differences in all-cause treatment discontinuation rates for olanzapine (68.4%), quetiapine (70.9%), and risperidone (71.4%). Parenthetically, the overall discontinuation rate is remarkably similar to that of the CATIE trial, a "big sister" trial in patients with chronic schizophrenia. While reductions in Positive and Negative Syndrome Scale total scores were similar for the three treatment groups, reduction in PANSS positive subscales scores were greater in the olanzapine group (at 12 and 52 weeks or withdrawal) and the risperidone group (at 12 weeks). Results of analyses of metabolic disturbances show some benefits for risperidone, with the largest and most frequent weight gain occuring in olanzapine-treated patients.

Kahn and colleagues (43) conducted a key study—the European First Episode Schizophrenia Trial (EUFEST)—comparing treatment with amisulpride, quetiapine, olanzapine, and ziprasidone to a low dose of haloperidol in an unselected sample of patients with first episode schizophrenia and minimal prior exposure to antipsychotics. 498 patients aged 18-40 were randomized to 1-year of treatment with one of the study drugs. The primary outcome measure of the study was all-cause treatment discontinuation. While 725 of patients on haloperidol discontinued treatment compared with 53% for quetiapine, 45% for ziprasidone, 40% for amisulpride, and 33% for olanzapine-treated patients, there were, no differences between drugs in terms of actual symptom improvements. In addition, the high discontinuation rate bears resemblance to the similarly rate in the 1-year CAFE first-episode study. Thus, medication nonadherence itself is a *major* treatment issue right from the first episode. In addition, the findings from EUFEST do not endorse the preferential "lead off" with any particular agent and they perhaps support the case for wide availability and choice of antipsychotic medications, rather than confining to a selective FGA first or A drug before trying B among the SGAs. With respect to the issue of nonadherence and the potential benefit of a LAI formulation from the beginning of treatment, Weiden and colleagues (44) have recently completed a comparative study of LAI risperidone versus oral GSAs. They found a good acceptance of this LAI in FEP patients. Surprisingly, however, the rate of nonaderence with treatment was comparable between both groups.

METABOLIC DISTURBANCES WITH SECOND GENERATION ANTIPSYCHOTICS IN FEP

The metabolic syndrome, a constellation of disturbances involving obesity, impaired glucose tolerance, and lipid abnormalities that is a risk factor for cardiovascular disease and diabetes, is highly prevalent in patients with schizophrenia. In the CATIE trial, McEvoy and colleagues (45) found that overall 40% of patients met criteria at baseline for metabolic syndrome. Given the myriad of other concerns in FEP, do we need to worry about the metabolic syndrome in these patients, too? The evidence supports that managing the risk of metabolic disturbances in FEP is an important consideration. In a study of $N = 263$ FEP patients treated with either olanzapine or haloperidol, Zipursky and colleagues (46) found that mean weight gain after 2 years of treatment was for 10.2 kg for olanzapine and 4.0 kg for haloperidol. In $N = 400$ FEP patients from the CAFÉ study, Patel and colleagues (47) found that 4.3% of patients met criteria for metabolic syndrome at baseline, increasing to 13.4% after 52 weeks of treatment.

Although antipsychotic medications contribute to the risk of metabolic syndrome, as exhaustively reviewed by Newcomer (48), several lines of evidence suggest people with schizophrenia may also have an increased risk of Type 2 diabetes mellitus independent of antipsychotic use (49). For example, studies predating the advent of antipsychotics suggested that impaired glucose tolerance has an increased prevalence within schizophrenia (50, 51). Three family studies have found that the relatives of patients with schizophrenia have an increased risk of Type 2 diabetes (52, 53, 54). Lastly, two studies found impaired fasting glucose tolerance in antipsychotic-naïve patients with schizophrenia, compared to well-matched controls (55, 56).Thus, FEP patients may have heightened risk at baseline for metabolic syndrome, and interventions to address this risk from the onset of antipsychotic treatment are warranted.

OTHER TREATMENT OPTIONS IN FEP

Clozapine is not a "first line" treatment option for the patient population. However, that is not to say that all FEP patients are treatment responsive. Indeed, there is a small subset of patients who have such a bad illness that clozapine might be a "third" line choice relatively quickly in their illness. There are some studies that provide guidance and context in consideration of this issue. Patients in the Hillside First Episode study who proved refractory over the course of treatment and then became candidate for clozapine showed a good response to clozapine (57). In another first-episode study from the same center (58), 66% of patients who were treated with clozapine responded within 13 weeks. Hofer and colleagues (59) from Austria studied clozapine use in $N = 39$ patients with first-episode schizophrenia and reported a responder rate of 51%. There is also a 1-year, double-blind comparative trial of clozapine versus chlorpromazine in $N = 160$ first-episode patients (60). In this study, first-episode patients on clozapine remitted more quickly and remained stable longer. However, the overall outcome for both treatments was similar at the end of one year. More recently, Kumra and colleagues (61) reported a comparable response between clozapine and olanzapine in children with early-onset schizophrenia. Thus, clozapine is not a first choice but, at the same time, should not be delayed indefinitely for the FEP patient who is not responding.

In the United States (at least), long acting injectable (LAI) formulations of antipsychotics are generally considered for patients at a more chronic stage of their illness. This is especially the case if their care is also hampered by medication noncompliance. However, there are some data on LAI antipsychotics in FEP patients. Goldstein and colleagues (62) compared 6 weeks of low-dose FGA (fluphenazine 6.25 mg given alternate weeks) with moderate doses (25 mg). They found a high relapse in the low dose group, particularly among those patients whose family was not also receiving family therapy more recently. Weiden and colleagues have presented (see earlier; 44) information on the use of LAI risperidone microspheres in FEP patients. It appears that the drug is acceptable and well tolerated among this group.

The study by Cornblatt and colleagues (11) cited earlier in this chapter is noteworthy that it showed a benefit for use of an antidepressant alone in a prodromal patient population. While there is no evidence or clinical support to endorse the use of antidepressant as monotherapy in FEP, this drug class is still an important treatment strategy in FEP patients. Many patients develop clear-cut depression—so called post psychotic depression—early on in the course of illness. Indeed, this is associated with a heightened risk of suicide in this population. In contrast to some other psychotic conditions (e.g., alcoholism), this risk of suicide is seen early on in the illness. Thus, clinicians may need (in spite of the concern of using too many medications in these patients) to take consideration of the selection of an antidepressant. Of note, there is no recent research to guide this approach. There is also no evidence for the efficacy (or indication for the use) of electroconvulsive therapy in FEP.

A variety of antipsychotic augmentation strategies have been tried—with inconsistent results—in patients with chronic schizophrenia (63). There is no information on the use of these strategies in FEP. Accordingly, there is no indication for this approach early in the treatment of schizophrenia. A more provocative question—also uniformed by data—is whether we should be considering (either preemptively or early on in treatment) the use of cholesterol-lowering and/or antiobesity agents during treatment of FEP. A recent Chinese study of patients with FEP showed benefits of metformin (especially when given in combination with a behavioral approach) in reducing weight in patients who had gained weight during their first antipsychotic treatment (64).

DURATION OF ANTIPSYCHOTIC TREATMENT IN FEP

The efficacy of antipsychotic medications in the treatment of FEP is well-documented. A logical question that follows—for clinicians, as well patients and their families—is for how long should patients with FEP be treated with antipsychotics? We must attempt to balance factors including response to treatment, patient preferences, risk of relapse, risk of movement disorders and/or metabolic disturbances, and aspects of informed consent with these medications. Going back to the scenario described at the beginning of the chapter, given a patient who is otherwise healthy, believes that "nothing is wrong", and is acutely agitated, how and when do we discuss with the patient (and their family) that they may need to take antipsychotic medication indefinitely, and that doing so might increase their risk of developing obesity, diabetes, and high cholesterol? This is yet another complex series of questions.

According to the Texas Medication Algorithm Project (TMAP) for schizophrenia (63), "A trial period off antipsychotics may be reasonable for some patients early in the course of illness. This, an individualized decision, depends on a number of factors that do not lend themselves to an algorithmic approach. Thus, the schizophrenia algorithm contains no guidelines for antipsychotic medication discontinuation, which is anticipated to be a rare event in the typical mental health clinic patient population." Similarly, the *American Psychiatric Association Practice Guidelines for the Treatment of Patients with Schizophrenia*, 2nd edition (65), conclude "Unfortunately there is no reliable indicator to differentiate the minority who will not from the majority who will relapse with drug discontinuation. Indefinite maintenance antipsychotic medication is recommended for patients who have had multiple prior episodes or two episodes within five years." Thus, the optimal duration of treatment in FEP is not explicitly clear.

CONCLUSIONS

Treatment of FEP presents a window of opportunity, assuming that there is ease of access to expert care and also good medication compliance. These are big assumptions. Two recent meta-analyses confirm the long delay to treatment in FEP (averaged 124 and 74 weeks) (66, 1). In an effort to reduce this delay, some centers (especially in Australia), have set up dedicated First Episode programs to help patients who are becoming psychotic to gain ready access to specialist care (2).

The choice of antipsychotic in FEP patients is still open to debate. Pros and cons for the use of FGAs and SGAs are listed in Table 17.3. The most recent iteration of the Texas Medication Algorithm Project (63) does not preferentially endorse any particular antipsychotic. What is probably of greater importance than any individual medication selection is to ensure (through close monitoring) that the drug is effective. In addition, it is crucial that side effects be minimized and effectively dealt with when they occur. If these circumstances do not prevail, then the chance that the patient will stop his or her their medication is inordinately high. Thereupon, the chances of a relapse for that patient are five times that of the FEP patient at who is medication compliant (67). There is presently no consensus on how long a patient should remain on an antipsychotic medication once the episode is resolved. It is debatable whether a FEP patient now stable and in remission should remain on medication for one year, for 3 to 5 years, or even

TABLE 17.3 Factors Influencing the Choice of Antipsychotic (FGA versus SGA) in FEP

Potential neuroprotective effect associated with SGAs.

Acute EPS—especially dystonia—is a major turnoff for therapeutic engagement, and it's a major risk factor for noncompliance.

Acute EPS is a risk factor for TD, and rates of TD appear higher with FGAs.

FGAs may induce dysphoria, and post-psychotic depression is common in FEP as symptoms abate.

CATIE shows equal effectiveness of typicals versus atypicals.

In studies where SGAs appear to have a broader range of efficacy including cognitive effects, FGAs were dosed incorrectly.

Acute EPS can be avoided by correct dosing of FGAs.

Compliance is not different in the unbiased studies between drug groups.

indefinitely (68). Given the broader context of recovery and functional improvement rather than just symptomatic control with medications, as a healthcare policy and the federal research agenda is how focusing on more concerted, multimodal approaches can sustain and enhance remission and functional recovery in FEP.

REFERENCES

1. Perkins DO, Gu H, Boteva K, Lieberman JA. Relationship between duration of untreated psychosis and outcome in first-episode schizophrenia: a critical review and meta-analysis. Am J Psychiatry 2005; 162: 1785–1804.
2. McGorry PD, Killackey E, Yung AR. Early intervention in psychotic disorders: detection and treatment of the first episode and the critical early stages. Med J Aust 2007(a); 197(7): S8.
3. McGorry PD, Purcell R, Hickie IB et al. Clinical staging: a heuristic model for psychiatry and youth mental health. Med J Aust 2007(b); 187(7): S42.
4. Pantelis C, Velakoulis D, Wood SJ et al. Neuroimaging and emerging psychotic disorders: the Melbourne ultra-high risk studies. Int Rev Psychiatry Rev 2007; 19(4): 371–81.
5. Pantelis C, Velakoulis D, McGorry PD et al. Neuroanatomical abnormalities before and after onset of psychosis: a cross-sectional and longitudinal MRI comparison. Lancet 2003 Jan; 361(9354): 281–8.
6. Miyamoto S, Stroup TS, Duncan GE, Aoba A, Lieberman JA. Acute pharmacological treatment of schziophrenia. In: Schizophrenia, Eds. Hirsch SR and Weinberger DR. Backwell Publishers, Oxford, England, 2003.
7. Addington J, Cadenhead KS, Cannon TD et al. North American Prodrome Longitudinal Study. North American Prodrome Longitudinal Study: a collaborative multisite approach to prodromal schizophrenia research. Schizophr Bull 2007; 33(3): 665–72.
8. McGlashan TH, Addington J, Cannon T et al. Recruitment and treatment practices for help-seeking "prodromal" patients. Schizophr Bull 2007; 33(3): 715–26.
9. McGorry PD, Yung AR, Phillips LJ et al, Yue. Randomized controlled trial of interventions designed to reduce the risk of progression to first-episode psychosis in a clinical sample with subthreshold symptoms. Arch Gen Psychiatry. 2002 Oct;59(10):921–8.
10. McGlashan TH, Zipursky RB, Perkins D et al. Randomized, double-blind trial of olanzapine versus placebo in patients prodromally symptomatic for psychosis. Am J Psychiatry 2006; 163(5): 790–9.
11. Cornblatt BA, Lencz T, Smith CW et al. Can antidepressants be used to treat the schizophrenia prodrome? Results of a prospective, naturalistic treatment study of adolescents. J Clin Psychiatry. 2007; 68(4): 546–57.
12. French P, Shryane N, Bentall RP, Lewis SW, Morrison AP. Effects of cognitive therapy on the longitudinal development of psychotic experiences in people at high risk of developing psychosis. Br J Psychiatry Suppl 2007; 51: s82–7.
13. Oosthuizen P, Emsley R, Jadri Turner H, et al. A randomized, controlled comparison of the efficacy and tolerability of low and high doses of haloperidol in the treatment of first-episode psychosis. Int J Neuropsychopharmacol 2004; 7(2): 125–31.
14. Lieberman J, Jody D, Geisler S et al. Time course and biologic correlates of treatment response in first-episode schizophrenia. Arch Gen Psychiatry. 1993; 50(5): 369–76.
15. Ossthuizen P, Emsley R, Jadri Turner H, Keyter N. A randomized, controlled comparison of the efficacy and tolerability of low and high doses of haloperidol in the treatment of first-episode psychosis. Int J Neuropsychopharmacol 2004; 7(2): 125–31.
16. Chatterjee A, Chakos M, Koreen A et al. Prevalence and clinical correlates of extrapyramidal signs and spontaneous dyskinesia in never-medicated schizophrenic patients. Am J Psychiatry. 1995; 152(12): 1724–9.
17. Emsley RA. Risperidone in the treatment of first-episode psychotic patients: a double-blind multicenter study. Risperidone Working Group. Schizophr Bull 1999; 25: 721–9.

18. Lane HY, Chang WH, Chiu CC et al. A pilot double-blind dose-comparison study of risperidone in drug-naïve, first-episode schizophrenia. J Clin Psychiatry 2001; 62: 994–5.
19. Merlo MC, Hofer H, Gekle W et al. Risperidone, 2 mg/day vs. 4 mg/day, in first-episode, acutely psychotic patients: treatment efficacy and effects on fine motor functioning. J Clin Psychiatry 2002; 63(10): 885–91.
20. Schooler N, Rabinowitz J, Davidson M, et al. Risperidone and haloperidol in first-episode psychosis: a long-term randomized trial. Am J Psychiatry 2005;162(5): 947–53.
21. Harvey PD, Rabinowitz J, Eerdekens M, Davidson M. Treatment of cognitive impairment in first episode psychosis: a comparison of risperidone and haloperidol. Am J Psychiatry 2005; 162(10): 1888–95.
22. Kopala LC, Good KP, Honer WG. Extrapyramudal signs and clinical symptoms in first episode schizophrenia: response to low dose risperidone. J Clin Psychopharmacol 1997; 17: 308–13.
23. Kopala LC, Good KP, Fredrikson D et al. Risperidone in first-episode schizophrenia: improvement in symptoms and pre-existing extrapyramidal signs. Int J Psychiatry Clin Pract 1998; 2: S19–S25.
24. Yap HL, Mahendran R, Lim D et al. Risperidone in the treatment of first episode psychosis. Singap Med J 2001; 42: 170–3.
25. Gutierrez FM, Segarra ER, Gonzalez-Pinto AA, Martinez JG. Risperidone in the early treatment of first-episode psychosis: a two-year follow-up study. Actas Esp Psiquiatr 2002; 30: 142–52.
26. Malla AK, Norman RMG, Scholten DJ, Zirul S, Kotteda V. A comparison of long-term outcome in first-episode schizophrenia following treatment with risperidone or a typical antipsychotic. J Clin Psychiatry 2001; 62: 179–84.
27. Yoshimura R, Ueda N, Shinkai K et al. Plasma levels of homovanillic acid and the response to risperidone in first episode untreated acute schizophrenia. Int Clin Psychopharmacol 2003; 18(2): 107–11.
28. Dolder C, Nelson M, Deyo Z. Paliperidone for schizophrenia. Am J Health Syst Pharm Rev 2008; 65(5): 403–13.
29. Emsley R,Medori R, Koen L et al. "Long acting injectable risperidone in the treatment of subjects with recent onset psychosis-a preliminary study". J Clin Psychopharmacol 2008; 28(2):210–3.
30. Sanger TM, Lieberman JA, Tohen M et al. Olanzapine versus haloperidol treatment in first-episode psychosis. Am J Psychiatry 1999; 156: 79–87.
31. Lieberman JA, Tollefson G, Tohen M et al. HGDH Study Group. Comparative efficacy and safety of atypical and conventional antipsychotic drugs in first-episode psychosis: a randomized, double-blind trial of olanzapine versus haloperidol. Am J Psychiatry 2003; 160(8): 1396–404.
32. Keefe RS, Seidman LJ, Christensen BK et al. Comparative effect of atypical and conventional antipsychotic drugs on neurocognition in first-episode psychosis: a randomized, double-blind trial of olanzapine versus low doses of haloperidol. Am J Psychiatry. 2004; 161(6): 985–95.
33. Green AI, Lieberman JA, Hamer RM et al HGDH Study Group. Olanzapine and haloperidol in first episode psychosis: two-year data. Schizophr Res. 2006; 86(1–3): 234–43.
34. Bobes J, Gibert J, Ciudad A et al. Safety and effectiveness of olanzapine versus conventional antipsychotics in the acute treatment of first-episode schizophrenic patients. Prog Neuropsychopharmacol Biol Psychiatry 2003; 27(3): 473–81.
35. Montes JM, Ciudad A, Gomez JC; EFESO Study Group. Safety, effectiveness, and quality of life of olanzapine in first-episode schizophrenia: a naturalistic study. Prog Neuro-Psychopharmacol Biol Psychiatry 2003; 27: 667–74.
36. Tollefson GD, Beasley Jr CM, Tran PV et al. Olanzapine versus haloperidol in the treatment of schizophrenia and schizoaffective and schizophreniform disorders: results of an international collaborative trial. Am J Psychiatry 1997; 154: 457–65.

37. Good KP, Kiss I, Buiteman C et al. Improvement in cognitive functioning in patients with first-episode psychosis during treatment with quetiapine: an interim analysis. Br J Psychiatry 2002; 181(243): 45–9.

38. Tauscher-Wisniewski S, Kapur S, Tauscher J et al. Quetiapine: an effective antipsychotic in first-episode schizophrenia despite only transiently high dopamine-2 receptor blockade. J Clin Psychiatry 2002; 63(11): 992–7.

39. Ohlsen RI, O'Toole MS, Purvis RG et al. Clinical effectiveness in first-episode patients. Eur Neuropsychopharmacol Rev 2004; 14(Suppl 4): S445–51.

40. Saha AR, Brown D, McEvoy J et al. Tolerability and efficacy of aripiprazole in patients with first-episode schizophrenia: an open-label pilot study. Schizophr Res 2004; 67S: S158.

41. Robinson DG, Woerner MG, Napolitano B et al. Randomized comparison of olanzapine versus risperidone for the treatment of first-episode schizophrenia: 4-month outcomes. Am J Psychiatry 2006; 163(12): 2096–102.

42. McEvoy JP, Lieberman JA, Perkins DO et al. Efficacy and tolerability of olanzapine, quetiapine, and risperidone in the treatment of early psychosis: a randomized, double-blind 52-week comparison. Am J Psychiatry 2007; 164(7): 1050–60.

43. Kahn RS, Fleischhacker WW, Boter H et al. Effectiveness of antipsychotic drugs in first-episode schizophrenia and schizophreniform disorder: an open ramdomised trial Lancet 2008; 371(9618): 1085–97.

44. Weiden PJ, Schooler NR,Sunakawa A et al. New research on pharmacologic interventions for adherence; A prospective study of long-acting risperidone VS oral second-generation antipsychotic in first-episodeschizophrenia. Schizophren Bull 2009; 35(1): 353.

45. McEvoy JP, Meyer JM, Goff DC et al. Prevalence of the metabolic syndrome in patients with schizophrenia: baseline results from the Clinical Antipsychotic Trials of Intervention Effectiveness (CATIE) schizophrenia trial and comparison with national estimates from NHANES III. Schizophr Res 2005; 80(1): 19–32.

46. Zipursky RB, Gu H, Green AI et al. HGDH Study Group. Course and predictors of weight gain in people with first-episode sychosis treated with olanzapine or haloperidol. Br J Psychiatry 2005; 187: 537–43.

47. Patel JK, Buckley PF, Woolson S, et al. Metabolic profiles of second-generation antipsychotics in early psychosis: findings from the CAFE study. Schizophr Res 2009; 111(1-3): 9–16.

48. Newcomer JW. Antipsychotic medications: metabolic and cardiovascular risk. J Clin Psychiatry 2007; 68(Suppl 4): 8–13.

49. Dixon L, Weiden P, Delahanty J et al. Prevalence and correlates of diabetes in national schizophrenia samples. Schizophr Bull 2000; 26(4): 903–912.

50. Kasanin J. The blood sugar curve in mental disease, II: the schizophrenic (dementia praecox) group. Arch Neurol Psychiatry 1926; 16; 414–19.

51. Robinson GW, Shelton P. Incidence and interpretation of diabetic-like dextrose tolerance curves in nervous and mental patients. JAMA 1940; 1142279.

52. Fernandez-Egea E, Miller B, Bernardo M, Donner T, Kirkpatrick B. Parental history of Type 2 diabetes in patients with nonaffective psychosis. Schizopr Res 2008; 98: 302–6.

53. Mukherjee S, Schnur DB, Reddy R. Family history of type 2 diabetes in schizophrenic patients (letter). Lancet 1989; 1: 495.

54. Spelman LM, Walsh PI, Sharifi N, Collins P, Thakore JH. Impaired glucose tolerance in first-episode drug-naive patients with schizophrenia. Diabet. Med 2007; 24(5): 481–5.

55. Ryan MC, Collins P, Thakore JH. Impaired fasting glucose tolerance in first-episode, drug-naive patients with schizophrenia. Am J Psychiatry 2003; 160(2): 284–69.

56. Fernandez-Egea E, Bernardo M, Parellada E et al. Abnormal Cardiovascular Function in Antipsychotic-Naïve, Newly Diagnosed Patients with Nonaffective Psychosis, Manuscript submitted for publication.

57. Lieberman JA, Alvir JM, Woerner MG et al. Prospective study of psychobiology in first-episode schizophrenia at Hillside Hospital. Schizophr Bull 1992; 18: 351–71.

58. Woerner MG, Robinson DG, Alvir JM et al. Clozapine as a first treatment for schizophrenia. Am J Psychiatry 2003; 160(8): 1514–6.

59. Hofer A, Hummer M, Kemmler G et al. The safety of clozapine in the treatment of first- and multiple-episode patients with treatment-resistant schizophrenia. Int J Neuropsychopharmacol 2003; 6(3): 201–6.

60. Lieberman JA, Tollefson G, Tohen M et al. HGDH Study Group. Comparative efficacy and safety of atypical and conventional antipsychotic drugs in first-episode psychosis: a randomized, double-blind trial of olanzapine versus haloperidol. Am J Psychiatry 2003; 160(8): 1396–404.

61. Kumra S, Kranzler H, Gerbino-Rosen G et al. Clozapine and "high-dose" olanzapine in refractory early-onset schizophrenia: A 12-week randomized and double-blind comparison. Biol Psychiatry 2008; 63: 524–9.

62. Goldstein MJ, Rodnick EH, Evans JR, May PR, Steinberg MR. Drug and family therapy in the aftercare of acute schizophrenics. Arch Gen Psychiatry 1978; 35(10): 1169–77.

63. Cornblatt BA, Lencz T, Smith CW et al. Can antidepressants be used to treat the schizophrenia prodrome? Results of a prospective, naturalistic treatment study of adolescents. J Clin Psychiatry. 2007; 68(4): 546–57.

64. Moore TA, Buchanan RW, Buckley PF et al. The Texas Medication Algorithm Project antipsychotic algorithm for schizophrenia: 2006 update. J Clin Psychiatry 2007; 68(11): 1751–62.

65. Wu RR, Zhao JP, Jin H et al. Lifestyle intervention and metformin for treatment of antipsychotic-induced weight gain: a randomized controlled trial. JAMA 2008; 299(2): 185–93.

66. Lehman AF, Lieberman JA, Dixon LB et al. Work Group on Schizophrenia. American Psychiatric Association Practice Guideline for the Treatment of Patients With Schizophrenia, second edition; 2004.

67. Marshall M, Lewis S, Lockwood A et al. Association between duration of untreated psychosis and outcome in cohorts of first-episode patients: a systematic review. Arch Gen Psychiatry 2005; 62: 975–83.

68. Robinson D, Woerner MG, Alvir JM et al. Predictors of relapse following response from a first-episode of schizophrenia or schizoaffective disorder. Arch Gen Psychiatry 1999(b); 56: 241–7.

69. Lieberman JA, Perkins DO, Jarskog LF. Neuroprotection: a therapeutic strategy to prevent deterioration associated with schizophrenia. CNS Spectr 2007; 12(Suppl 4): 1–13.

70. Addington J, Van Mastrigt S, Hutchinson J, Addington D. Pathways to care: help seeking behavior in first episode psychosis. Acta Psychiatr Scand 2002; 106(5): 358–64.

71. Hafner H, Löffler W, Maurer K, Hambrecht M, an der Heiden W. Depression, negative symptoms, social stagnation and social decline in the early course of schizophrenia. Acta Psychiatr Scand 1999; 100(2): 105–18.

72. Albus M. Hubmann W, Mohr F et al. Neurocognitive functioning patients with first-episode schizophrenia: results of a prospective 5-year follow-up study. Eur Arch Psychiatry Clin Neurosci 2006; 256(7): 442051.

73. Emsley R, Rabinowitz J, Medori R. Time course for antipsychotic treatment response in first-episode schizophrenia. Am J Psychiatry 2006; 163(4): 743–5.

74. McEvoy JP, Hogarty GE, Steingard S. Optimal dose of neuroleptic in acute schizophrenia. A controlled study of the neuroleptic threshold and higher haloperidol dose. Arch Gen Psychiatry 1991; 48(8): 739–45.

75. Patel JK, Buckley PF, Woolson S et al. CAFE investigators. Changes in metabolic parameters in first episode schizophrenia following treatment with atypical antipsychotics for 52 weeks: subset analysis from the CAFE Study. Schizophr Bull 2007; 33(2): 504.

76. Penn DL, Waldheter EJ, Perkins DO, Mueser KT, Lieberman JA. Psychosocial treatment for first-episode psychosis: a research update. Am J Psychiatry 2005; 162(12): 2220–32.

77. Robinson DG, Woerner MG, Alvir JM et al. Predictors of treatment response from a first episode of schizophrenia or schizoaffective disorder. Am J Psychiatry 1999(a); 156(4):544–9.

78. Robinson DG, Woerner MG, Alvir JM et al. Predictors of medication discontinuation by patients with first-episode schizophrenia and schizoaffective disorder. Schizophr Res 2002; 57: 209–19.
79. Robinson DG, Woerner MG, McMeniman M, Mendelowitz A, Bilder RM. Symptomatic and functional recovery from a first episode of schizophrenia or schizoaffective disorder. Am J Psychiatry 2004; 161(3): 473–9.
80. Schooler NR, Keith SJ, Severe JB et al. Relapse and rehospitalization during maintenance treatment of schizophrenia: the effects of dose reduction and family treatment. Arch Gen Psychiatry 1997; 54: 453–63.
81. Schooler N, Rabinowitz J, Davidson M et al. Early Psychosis Global Working Group. Reduced rates of relapse in risperidone versus haloperidol in the long term treatment of recent onset schizophrenia patients. Annual meeting of American College of Neuropsychopharmacology, Puerto Rico, December, 2003.
82. Tarrier N, Lewis S, Haddock G et al Cognitive-behavioral therapy in first-episode and early schizophrenia. 18 month follow-up of a randomized controlled trial. Br J Psychiatry 2004; 184: 231–9.
83. Weiden PJ, Buckley PF, Grody M. Understanding and treating "first-episode" schizophrenia. Psychiatr Clin N Am 2007; 30(3): 481–510.

18

Pharmacological profile and pharmacogenetic approaches of antipsychotics

Min-Soo Lee and Hun Soo Chang

INTRODUCTION

Since the antipsychotic effects of chlorpromazine have been found in 1950s, many antipsychotics have been introduced. They enabled psychiatrists to use various strategies of pharmacotherapies against schizophrenia (1). The first generation antipsychotics induced many side-effects such as sedation and involuntary movements. The development of atypical antipsychotics was regarded as the major advance primarily because these drugs reduced such side-effects. "Atypical antipsychotics" can be defined as the antipsychotics that have 'low extrapyramidal symptoms' and 'good for negative symptoms'. Since various atypical antipsychotics, however, have different pharmacological profile, understanding those diverse profiles helps to make more accurate choices of drugs in clinical practice.

While the side-effect profile of antipsychotics has continued to improve, their efficacy seems to remain poor. The remission after antipsychotic treatment in the previous studies reached only up to 50 to 60% (2). Since the antipsychotic effect in schizophrenia tends to appear later on, it takes 6 to 8 weeks to decide such effect in schizophrenia. The response to medication such as above can be influenced by several physiological and environmental factors, including age, renal function, liver function, nutritional status, smoking and alcohol consumption. Such responses can also be affected by biological factors, among which is the genetic factor. Pharmacogenetics, firstly defined by Vogel as a sphere of study for the interaction between genes and drugs (3), has been growing in many pharmacological fields for various diseases. This field has tremendously progressed after completion of the first draft of Human Genome Project in 2005. In addition, with the development of large-scale DNA sequencing and genotyping technology, several thousands of reports on these subjects have been submitted every year. In psychiatric field, there have been many efforts to investigate the relationship between candidate genes and antipsychotic drug responses.

This chapter will overview the pharmacological profiles of antipsychotics, and will introduce pharmacogenetic approaches to the effects of antipsychotics in individuals with different genotypes.

PHARMACOLOGICAL PROFILES OF ANTIPSYCHOTICS

Conventional antipsychotics

Many studies for chlorpromazine suggested that dopamine pathway plays critical roles in the pathophysiology of schizophrenia, which triggered the development of drugs which targeted dopamine receptors, especially the dopamine (DA) D2 receptor. These kinds of antipsychotics, so-called the 'conventional' antipsychotics, showed dramatic effects on the treatment of schizophrenia and became the most popular strategy for schizophrenia therapy. Motivated by their effects, a number of antipsychotics have been developed since the introduction of chlorpromazine. While they are not

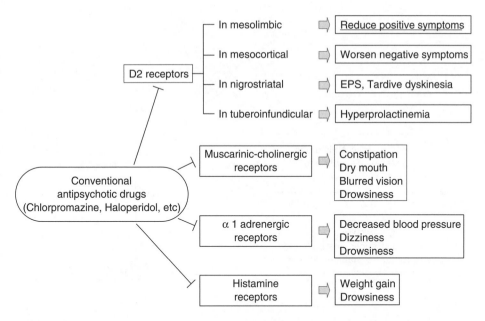

FIGURE 18.1 The action of the conventional antipsychotic drugs and possible outcomes.

as widely used as before since the introduction of atypical antipsychotics, the typical antipsychotics such as haloperidol, molindone, perphenazine, sulpride, or trifluoperazine are still used.

Although the blockade of D2 receptors by the conventional antipsychotics dramatically reduces positive symptoms of schizophrenic patients through inhibition of the mesolimbic dopamine pathway, the conventional antipsychotics can inhibit nonspecifically all D2 receptors in other dopamine pathways, which results in many side-effects. The inhibition of D2 receptors in mesocortical dopamine pathway can cause negative and cognitive symptoms, which are called the neuroleptic-induced deficit syndrome. When D2 receptors are inhibited in nigrostriatal DA pathway, which is known to be involved in the extrapyramidal system; it can result in extrapyramidal symptoms (EPS) or tardive dyskinesia (TD). To make matters worse, the conventional antipsychotics can block the D2 receptors in tuberoinfundibular DA pathway, which results in the hyperprolactinemia. Nonspecific blockade of D2 receptors by the conventional antipsychotics can cause other side-effects such as convulsion and orthostatic hypotension as well as sudden death. Furthermore, conventional antipsychotic drugs are known to inhibit other neurotransmission systems including muscarinic cholinergic receptor, alpha 1 adrenergic receptors, and histamine receptors. The blockade of muscarinic cholinergic receptor causes constipation, dry mouth, blurred vision, and drowsiness. The conventional antipsychotics also can result in decreased blood pressure and dizziness through alpha 1 adrenergic receptor inhibition and in weight gain through the blockade of histamine receptor (Figure 18.1).

Atypical antipsychotics
Due to the disadvantages of the conventional antipsychotics described above, the atypical antipsychotics are rapidly replacing conventional ones in treatment of schizophrenia. From

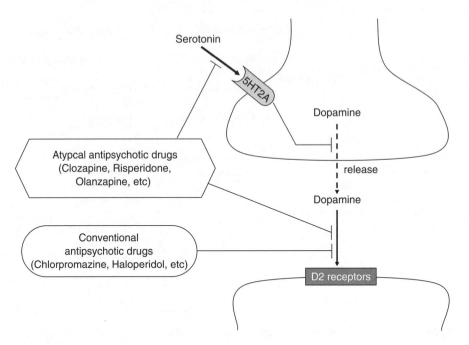

FIGURE 18.2 Comparison of action between conventional antipsychotics and atypical antipsychotics.

the pharmacological perspective, the atypical antipsychotics as a class may be defined in at least three ways: as 'serotonin dopamine antagonists (SDA)', as 'D2 antagonists with rapid dissociation', or as 'D2 partial agonists (DPA)' (4).

A key biological background of atypical antipsychotics is that secretion of dopamine from dopaminergic neurons is inhibited by serotonin binding to serotonin 2A (5HT2A) receptors. Most of the atypical antipsychotics have dual mode of actions; antagonizing both D2 receptor and 5HT2A receptor (Figure 18.2). In nigrostriatal pathway, the SDA block D2 receptors and 5HT2A receptor which is followed by facilitation of dopamine release. Then, in synapse, dopamine which was released through serotonin receptor blockade can compete with SDA for the D2 receptor, which causes reverse of D2 antagonism of SDA. Finally, those activities of SDA attenuate EPS or TD, which is a side-effect of the conventional antipsychotics that are caused by the blockade of D2 in nigrostriatal DA pathway. Relatively low levels of dopamine and an excessive amount of serotonin are known to exist in mesocortical dopamine pathway of schizophrenic patients. In this circumstance, SDA dominantly inhibits the serotonin receptor, which results in the release of dopamine followed by the improvement of negative and cognitive symptoms. Furthermore, in tuberoinfundibular pathway, pituitary lactoroph cells release prolactin which is inhibited by dopamine, while induced by serotonin. Thus, the conventional antipsychotics induce prolactin secretion through the blockade of D2, which causes hyperprolactinemia. Reversely, comparing to the conventional antipsychotic drugs, SDA is deemed to be able to reduce prolactin secretion via its 5HT2A antagonism which is followed by the alleviation of hyperprolactinemia.

The feature of recently developed atypical antipsychotics is not restricted to D2 and 5HT2A antagonism. One of the important properties of the atypical antipsychotics is the ability to dissociate rapidly from D2 receptors. Rapid dissociation from the

D2 receptor enables antipsychotics to leave prior to causing any extrapyramidal side-effects, but these antipsychotics are able to stay at D2 receptors long enough for antipsychotic action. The antipsychotics with low potency such as clozapine and quetiapine show faster dissociation than high-potency agents. DPA also makes any antipsychotics atypical. DPAs bind to D2 receptor in intermediary manner (neither too antagonizing, nor too stimulating). Therefore, DPAs have unique mode of action. DPAs reduce the hyperactivity of D2 in mesolimbic dopamine pathway. DPAs rarely cause EPS because the blocking of dopamine in the nigrostriatal pathway is insufficient to cause EPS. Aripiprazole, bifeprunox, and amisulpride are known to have DPA action (4). Atypical antipsychotics can also inhibit dopamine D1, D3, D4, serotonin 5HT1A, 5HT1D, 5HT2C, 5HT3, 5HT6, and 5HT7. These multiple pharmacologic actions of atypical antipsychotics should be considered in the treatment of schizophrenia and in pharmacological and pharmacogenetic studies about atypical antipsychotics.

Pharmacological profiles of each atypical antipsychotics

Clozapine is recognized to be the prototypical atypical antipsychotic and is known to have SDA. However, it has very complex pharmacological profiles. Clozapine is polyreceptor antagonist. It has the affinity for D1, D2, D3, D4, 5HT2A, 5HT2C, 5HT3, 5HT6, 5HT7, muscarinic M1, M2, M3, α1, α2, and histamine H1 receptors (5). Clozapine has good clinical efficacy, but it is not prescribed as the first-line treatment due to its side-effects including agranulocytosis and seizures. The exact mechanism for these side-effects is not known.

The chemical structure of olanzapine is related to that of clozapine. Olanzapine is capable of strong binding with receptors such as D2, D3, D4, α1, H1, 5HT2A, 5HT2C, 5HT6, and M1 (6). Its action on the 5HT2 receptor is known to be related with the alleviation of affective and cognitive symptoms and the reduction of negative symptoms and EPS.

Quetiapine also has very similar receptor-binding pattern as clozapine does. It acts as an antagonist to many receptors including 5HT1A, 5HT2A, D1, D2, H1, α1, and α2 receptors and has particularly high affinity for 5HT2A and medium affinity for D2 receptor (6). Unlike clozapine or olanzapine, however, quetiapine does not have particularly strong affinity for muscarine receptor, which is presumed to be the reason that quetiapine has positive effect on cognitive function (7).

Risperidone has potent blocking effects for the 5HT2 and the D2 receptor. While it is considered an atypical antipsychotics in that it has a high 5HT2A/D2 receptor binding ratio, it also displays certain characteristics of the conventional antipsychotics in that it produces much EPS at high doses. While risperidone has an affinity for D2, 5HT2A, 5HT7, α1, and α2, it has simpler pharmacological receptor profile than other atypical antipsychotics such as clozapine.

A long-acting form of risperidone (Risperidone Long Acting Injectable, RLAI) became available in Europe from August 2002 and is now broadly available for the treatment of schizophrenia. Although long-acting risperidone has the advantage of depot formulations for conventional antipsychotics, it is not considered a depot because it differs in several important ways from traditional decanoates; 1) Conventional depot antipsychotics are esterified to a fatty acid by a hydroxyl group on the antipsychotic molecule, forming a prodrug that is soluble in oil, which are injected in a highly viscous oil-based vehicle. In contrast, because risperidone does not have a hydroxyl group for esterification, the molecules are encapsulated in a carbohydrate polymer, which forms microspheres, approximately 25–150 microns in diameter, containing risperidone. These microspheres are suspended in an aqueous vehicle for injection. 2) While release of conventional decanoate antipsychotics into the body occurs by enzyme-mediated hydrolysis of the prodrug, risperidone is released from microspheres by hydrolysis of the polymer. 3) End products of conventional decanoate release are the drug, the fatty acid, and the oil vehicle, which can cause tissue damage at the injection site. In contrast, the final products of microsphere hydrolysis are risperidone, carbon dioxide, and water, which are formed by normal metabolic processes (Kreb's cycle) for degradation of lactide and glycolide, which are released as the microspheres dissolve (8). As the polymer is hydrolyzed, risperidone is released and provides its clinical effects. Less than 1% of risperidone is released initially upon injection. The main period of risperidone release occurs approximately 3 weeks later.

Paliperidone is a 9-hydroxy-risperidone and an active metabolite of risperidone, predominantly excreted by the kidney (59% excreted unchanged in the urines). Accordingly, paliperidone shares many pharmacological profiles with risperidone. As a metabolite, however, paliperidone does not compete, unlike risperidone, for metabolism with other medications, and it causes no cytochrome inhibition or induction that could lead to a drug interaction. Moreover, the unique extended-release delivery system of paliperidone made the one a day administration possible, and no dosage adjustment is required for patients with relevant co-medications and co-morbidities, e.g., mild to moderate hepatic impairment or smokers (9).

Paliperidone ER consists of an osmotically active tri-layer core, composed of two drug layers and a push layer, which is designed to ensure a gradual rise in the blood concentrations. This allows treatment to begin with a therapeutically effective starting dose from day 1 without the need for initial dose titration. The OROS formulation also provides minimal fluctuations in plasma concentrations of paliperidone over a 24-hour period. By reducing the amplitude of peaks and troughs, which are associated with IR oral therapies, and providing smoother plasma profiles similar to those achieved with long-acting injectable antipsychotic agents, it is anticipated that paliperidone ER could potentially reduce the risk of adverse effects and improve tolerability(10).

Paliperidone depot formulation for 4 weeks has been recently developed and is soon to be released, which is expected to improve patients' compliance and ultimately the overall treatment results.

Ziprasidone has a high affinity for human D2 receptor. It is a strong antagonist at 5HT2A, 5HT2C, and 5HT1D receptors. Ziprasidone is a strong agonist at 5HT1A and thus has an anti-anxiety and antidepressant effect (11). The major advantage of ziprasidone is that it has little propensity for weight gain. It is probably because ziprasidone has the 5HT2C-antagonist actions while it does not have the antihistamine property (4).

Aripiprazole is the first DPA. Its major unique feature is the silent antagonism to D2 receptors. In addition, aripiprazole has the 5HT2A antagonist property, which is deemed to contribute to its tolerability profile and antidepressant effect (12). Aripiprazole does not have α1, M1, or H1 antagonism that is related to sedation, which sometimes results in activation, mild agitation, or akathisia in some patients (4).

As explained above, many antipsychotics have similar profiles to each other but, at the same time, have unique pharmacological profiles on their own. Accordingly, it will be the clinician's duty to know the characteristics of various antipsychotics and to choose the appropriate antipsychotics for the patients.

PHARMACOGENETICS OF ANTIPSYCHOTICS

Antipsychotics have a multiple mechanism of action and their treatment responses can be affected by several different genes. In pharmacokinetic aspects, most pharmacogenetic investigations into antipsychotics have been conducted on candidate genes which are involved in drug metabolism. Therefore, many studies have been performed for genes which are related cytochrome P450 system including CYP2D6 and CYP1A2 genes. In a standpoint of pharmacodynamics, antipsychotics are also deemed to regulate monoaminergic neurotransmission including serotonergic and dopaminergic pathways. This chapter reviews the pharmacogenetic studies into the effects on the action of antipsychotics of the genes that are related to the pathways, such as receptors or transporters for dopamine, serotonin, tryptophan hydroxylase, the ß3 subunit of G protein (GNB3) and brain-derived neurotrophic factor (BDNF).

Pharmacogenetics in pharmacokinetics

There have been many studies concerning the relationships between treatment responses and genes that that encode cytochrome P450 such as CYP1A2, CYP2C9, CYP2C19, and CYP3A4, which are major enzymes that metabolize most of the antipsychotics. The activities of these enzymes influence the susceptibility and the responses to drugs, which varies between individuals. Such diversity is thought to be determined by genetic properties of each person. Thus, the effectiveness and side-effect of medications might be affected by polymorphisms on these genes.

Based on their drug responses, individuals can be separated to several groups; poor metabolizer (PMs), extensive metabolizers (EMs), and ultrarapid metabolizers (UMs), which are genetically characterized as carrying defective, normal or duplicate copies of CYP genes, respectively (13, 14). The frequencies of each group are known to be different between ethnics. For example, the frequencies of PMs against debrisoquine/sparteine have been reported to be 5–10% in European population, in contrast, only 2 % in Asians (15, 16). PMs are inferred to have higher risk of side-effect because of the high concentration of drugs in their blood. In fact, it was reported that PMs against debrisoquine showed higher levels of antipsychotics such as perphenazine or thioridazine and had higher risk of side-effect caused by these drugs than EMs did (17). In addition, patients treated with antipsychotics showed some relationship between PM phenotype and side-effect such as sedation, postural hypotension, and extrapyramidal symptoms in early period of their drug treatment (18–20). In contrast, it has been controversial that there is the association of CYP2D6 gene polymorphism with the long-term response to antipsychotics (21–25).

It is also reported that functional polymorphisms on CYP1A2 gene, which mediates clozapine metabolism (26, 27), are associated with the TD in subjects with schizophrenia (28). However, there has been no clear evidence to the association between these polymorphisms and the response to antipsychotics. Although there are some evidence for association between other kinds of drugs and the polymorphisms on other CYP genes including CYP2C9 (29), CYP2C19 (30), and CYP3A4 (31), the relationships between these polymorphisms and the antipsychotics response still remain unknown.

The lack of evidence for the associations between polymorphisms on CYP genes and drug-responses could be explained in a couple of ways; 1) side-effects of drugs might not be entirely reflected by their blood concentrations, 2) loss of function in an enzyme could be compensated by others because most of drugs are metabolized by diverse enzymes.

Nevertheless, in case of enzymes which regulate the main stream of drug metabolisms such as rate limiting enzymes or drugs which are metabolized by specific enzyme subfamily, the relationships between side-effect or efficacies of drugs and genetic polymorphisms are expected to be revealed in time due to a rapid growth of the quality and the quantity of information about pharmacogenetics in psychiatry.

Pharmacogenetics in pharmacodynamics

Most pharmacogenetics studies on antipsychotics have involved the prototype atypical neuroleptic clozapine. Many investigations of the influences of dopaminergic (D2, D3, and D4) receptors and serotonergic (5HT2A, 5HT2C, and 5HT6) receptor genes on the effect of clozapine action have produced conflicting results (Table 18.1).

Dopamine receptors

To date, five subtypes of dopamine receptors (DR) have been found; DRD1, 2, 3, 4, and 5. Among them, DRD2 has been known to be the target of the conventional antipsychotic drugs. It has been reported that there are functional polymorphisms in promoter region and coding region of DRD2 gene; however, the relationships between these polymorphisms and drug response have not been elucidated.

In other hands, the DRD3 subtype has received considerable attention due to its localization within limbic structures and its affinity to classical and atypical neuroleptics. The Ser9Gly polymorphism of the D3 receptor is associated with the action of classical neuroleptics and clozapine (32, 33). Moreover, an association between the Ser9Gly polymorphism and the development of TD has been demonstrated, suggesting that the Ser9 allele protects against the development of this disabling adverse effect (34). A major candidate gene for clozapine action is the D4 receptor gene, since this receptor is located on the prefrontal cortex, a brain region that is thought to be linked to cognitive dysfunction in schizophrenia (35).

Serotonin receptors

At least two polymorphisms in the 5HT2A receptor gene (a silent T102C exchange and a structural His452Tyr substitution) appear to play a role in the clozapine response (36); the frequency of minor allele homozygote on T102C is known to be higher in poor responders to clozapine (37) or typical neuroleptics (38) than in good responders, although the polymorphism is synonymous SNP.

Furthermore, a structural variant in the 5HT2C receptor that leads to a Cys23Ser substitution might be important for responses and, more importantly, may be associated with the weight gain that is observed with several atypical neuroleptics (39). Cys23Ser polymorphism on 5HT2C has been reported to affect the affinity with m-chlorophenylpiperazine (MCPP), which is considered to cause some difference in drug response (40). Indeed, the minor allele frequency of this polymorphism was reported to be higher in nonresponder to clozapine than in responder (41). However, replication of this observation has been failed in other population (42, 43). Similarly, although the association of various polymorphisms on serotonin receptors genes such as 5HT6 or 5HT3A with the responses to antipsychotics has been investigated (44–46), clear relationships have not been established yet.

Pharmacogenetics in side-effect of antipsychotic drugs

There are no significant differences in the clinical efficacy among various antipsychotics, therefore, it is important to prevent and predict the adverse effects of antipsychotics. Therefore, many pharmacogenetic studies concerning antipsychotics have focused on the side-effects of antipsychotics.

TABLE 18.1 Pharmacogenetics studies on the effects of antipsychotic drugs.

Authors	Gene	Locus	Drug	Findings	Sample	Ethnicity
Hwu et al. (56)	DRD4	48-bp repeat	Variable antipsychotics	Homozygous for 48-bp repeats in both is associated with good neuroleptic response during acute treatment	Schizophrenia	Asian
Rao et al. (57)	DRD4	48-bp repeat	Clozapine	No association	Schizophrenia	Caucasian
Shaikh et al. (58)	DRD4	48-bp repeat	Clozapine	No association	Schizophrenia	Caucasian
Kaiser et al. (59)	DRD4	48-bp repeat	Typical antipsychotics, clozapine	No association	Schizophrenia	Caucasian
Shaikh et al. (60)	DRD3	S9G	Clozapine	s/s genotype more frequent among nonresponders	Schizophrenia	Caucasian
Malhotra et al. (30)	DRD3	S9G	Clozapine	No association	Schizophrenia	Caucasian
Scharfetter et al. (31)	DRD3	S9G	Clozapine	G allele is associated with clozapine response	Schizophrenia	Asian
Lin et al. (61)	5HTR2A	T102C	Clozapine	No association	Schizophrenia	Asian
Lane et al. (62)	5HTR2A	T102C	Risperidone	C102/C102 genotype associated with a better response	Schizophrenia	Asian
Joober et al. (36)	5HTR2A	T102C	Typical antipsychotic drugs	Trend toward association between C/C genotype and poor response among men	Schizophrenia	Caucasian
Arranz et al. (63)	5HTR2A	G-1438A	Clozapine	GG genotype more common in nonresponders	Schizophrenia	Caucasian
		H452T	Clozapine	Frequency of T allele higher in nonresponders	Schizophrenia	Caucasian
Arranz et al. (64)	5HTR2A	H452T	Clozapine	T allele associated with poor response	Schizophrenia	Caucasian
Arranz et al. (35)	5HTR2A	T102C	Clozapine	C/C genotype associated with poor response	Schizophrenia	Caucasian

(continued)

TABLE 18.1 (*Continued*)

Authors	Gene	Locus	Drug	Findings	Sample	Ethnicity
Malhotra et al. (65)	5HTR2A	T102C	Clozapine, typical antipsychotics	No association	Schizophrenia or schizoaffective disorder	Caucasian
		H452T	Clozapine, typical antipsychotics	No association	Schizophrenia or schizoaffective disorder	Caucasian
Nimgaonkar et al. (66)	5HTR2A	T102C	Clozapine	No association	Schizophrenia	Caucasian
Nöthen et al. (67)	5HTR2A	T102C	Clozapine	No association	Schizophrenia	Caucasian
		H452T	Clozapine	No association	Schizophrenia	Caucasian
		T25N	Clozapine	No association	Schizophrenia	Caucasian
Malhotra et al. (40)	5HTR2C	C23S	Clozapine	No association	Schizophrenia	Caucasian
Sodhi et al. (39)	5HTR2C	C23S	Clozapine	S allele associated with clozapine response	Schizophrenia	Caucasian
Rietschel et al. (68)	5HTR2C	C23S	Clozapine	No association	Schizophrenia	Caucasian
Yu et al. (44)	5HTR6	C276T	Clozapine	Homogeneous 267T/T genotype associated with better response	Schizophrenia	Asian
Masellis et al. (43)	5HTR6	C276T	Clozapine	No association	Schizophrenia	Caucasian

DRD4: dopamine receptor D4, 5HT: serotonin

Among pharmacogenetic studies concerning the side-effect of antipsychotics, the most popular topic has been TD. Since TD is a serious and potentially irreversible side-effect and the development of TD requires genetic vulnerability, TD is an important topic in the pharmacogenetic study. The candidate genes in a research on TD are the dopamine-related genes such as dopamine receptor genes, dopamine transporter gene, and catecholamine-O-methyl transferase gene, serotonin receptor genes such as 5HT2A and 5HT2C, and some other genes that are related to metabolism such as CYP 2D6, 1A2, and 3A4. Due to the recent hypothesis that TD is caused from an oxidative stress and that neurotrophic factor prevents TD, nitric oxide synthase gene, glutathione S-transferase genes, manganese superoxide gene, or BDNF gene are also deemed to be prominent candidate genes as well (47). One of the most replicated studies is the one concerning Ser9Gly polymorphism on DRD3 gene, and Gly-type homozygotes of Ser9Gly polymorphism on DRD3 gene have been reported to be susceptible for the risk of TD (48–50).

Recently, as atypical antipsychotics are being prescribed more often than before, the weight gain as their side-effects draw more attention. Weight gain is the major reason for noncompliance of patients, damages their self esteem, and causes metabolic sequelae. Particularly, while clozapine and olanzapine have high efficacy, they cause the weight gain issue in some patients so seriously that it substantially aggravates the treatment of such patients. In addition, the weight gain issue indicates considerable variability among patients, which is due to the biological susceptibility including genetic factors. A large number of pharmacogenetic studies have been conducted based on the above hypothesis. The genes that suggested to be related to antipsychotics-induced weight gain include adrenergic 2A receptor gene (51, 52), GNB3 gene (53), leptin gene (54, 55), and 5HT2C gene (56).

The pharmacogenetic studies have also been conducted regarding antipsychotics-induced metabolic syndrome, restless legs syndrome, agranulocytosis, and akathisia. These pharmacogenetic studies would suggest the usefulness of genotype determination for the purpose of predicting side-effect of individuals as genetic biomarkers.

Future of pharmacogenetics in psychiatry

Response to antipsychotics is considered as complex traits, which are regulated complicatedly by various factors including environment and genetic properties. Many factors such as gender, ethnics, age, severity of disease, dietary status, functions of liver or kidney and interaction between drugs could influence on drug responses. Thus, the confounding factors should be strictly adjusted in pharmacogenetic and pharmacogenomic research. In addition, genetic interaction between individual genes or polymorphisms should be considered. To achieve the above, adequately large size of population and well-designed approach are necessary. Also, the replication of association and the evaluation of molecular or cellular functions of each associated polymorphism should be achieved in order to discover the 'true' genetic effects. Pharmacogenetic studies for antipsychotics have used candidate gene approaches. Although these approaches have been successful in some cases, it is difficult to identify the susceptible locus or gene which is involved in the differences of treatment responses. Recently, the high-throughput methods for genotype determination that are based on DNA microarray have been developed by various manufacturers, which helps save time for pharmacogenetic study. Furthermore, the epigenetic approaches are also necessary because the epigenetic alterations of treatment responses have been previously suggested in dopamine- and serotonin-related genes (57). Through these approaches to pharmacogenetic studies, our knowledge in this field will undoubtedly improve and "Personalized Medicine" might come true sooner or later.

REFERENCES

1. Cabana MD, Rand CS, Powe NR et al. Why don't physicians follow clinical practice guidelines? A framework for improvement. JAMA 1999; 282(15): 1458–65.
2. Gasquet I, Haro JM, Tcherny-Lessenot S, Chartier F, Lepine JP. Remission in the outpatient care of schizophrenia: 3-Year results from the Schizophrenia Outpatients Health Outcomes (SOHO) Study in France. Eur Psychiatry 2008; 23(7): 491–6.
3. Weber WW. Pharmacogenetics. New York: Oxford University Press; 1997.
4. Stahl SM. Stahl's essential psychopharmacology : Neuroscientific Basis and Practical Applications. 3rd ed. New York: Cambridge University Press; 2008.
5. Baldessarini RJ, Frankenburg FR. Clozapine. A novel antipsychotic agent. N Engl J Med 1991; 324(11): 746–54.
6. Naber D. Atypical antipsychotics in the treatment of schizophrenic patients. 1. Aufl. ed. Bremen: Uni-Med; 2002.
7. Saller CF, Salama AI. Seroquel: biochemical profile of a potential atypical antipsychotic. Psychopharmacology (Berl) 1993; 112(2-3): 285–92.

8. Davis JM, Matalon L, Watanabe MD et al. Depot antipsychotic drugs. Place in therapy. Drugs 1994; 47(5): 741–73.
9. Dlugosz H, Nasrallah HA. Paliperidone: a new extended-release oral atypical antipsychotic. Expert Opin Pharmacother 2007; 8(14): 2307–13.
10. Conley R, Gupta SK, Sathyan G. Clinical spectrum of the osmotic-controlled release oral delivery system (OROS), an advanced oral delivery form Current Medical research and Opinion 2006; 22(10): 1879–92.
11. Schmidt AW, Lebel LA, Howard HR Jr et al. Ziprasidone: a novel antipsychotic agent with a unique human receptor binding profile. Eur J Pharmacol 2001; 425(3): 197–201.
12. Goodnick PJ, Jerry JM. Aripiprazole: profile on efficacy and safety. Expert Opin Pharmacother 2002; 3(12): 1773–81.
13. Lin KM, Poland RE, Wan Y-JY et al. The evolving science of pharmacogenetics: clinical and ethnic perspectives. Psychopharmacol Bull 1996; 21: 205–17.
14. Meyer UA. Pharmacogenetics: the slow, therapid, and the ultrarapid. Proc Natl Acad Sci U S A 1994; 91(6): 1983–4.
15. Cholerton S, Daly AK, Idle JR. The role of individual human cytochromes P450 in drug metabolism and clinical response. Trends Pharmacol Sci 1992; 13(12): 434–9.
16. Gaedigk A, Blum M, Gaedigk R et al. Deletion of the entire cytochrome P450 CYP2D6 gene as a cause of impaired drug metabolism in poor metabolizers of the debrisoquine/sparteine polymorphism. Am J Hum Genet 1991; 48(5): 943–50.
17. Meyer JW, Woggon B, Baumann P et al. Clinical implications of slow sulphoxidation of thioridazine in a poor metabolizer of the debrisoquine type. Eur J Clin Pharmacol 1990; 39(6): 613–4.
18. Spina E, Ancione M, Di Rosa AE et al. Polymorphic debrisoquine oxidation and acute neuroleptic-induced adverse effects. Eur J Clin Pharmacol 1992; 42(3): 347–8.
19. Spina E, Campo GM, Calandra S et al. Debrisoquine oxidation in an Italian population: a study in healthy subjects and in schizophrenic patients. Pharmacol Res 1992; 25(1): 43–50.
20. Vandel P, Haffen E, Vandel S et al. Drug extrapyramidal side effects. CYP2D6 genotypes and phenotypes. Eur J Clin Pharmacol 1999; 55(9): 659–65.
21. Andreassen OA, MacEwan T, Gulbrandsen AK et al. Non-functional CYP2D6 alleles and risk for neuroleptic-induced movement disorders in schizophrenic patients. Psychopharmacology 1997; 131(2): 174–9.
22. Armstrong M, Daly AK, Blennerhassett R et al. Antipsychotic drug-induced movement disorders in schizophrenics in relation to CYP2D6 genotype. Br J Psychiatry 1997; 170: 23–6.
23. Arthur H, Dahl ML, Siwers B et al. Polymorphic drug metabolism in schizophrenic patients with tardive dyskinesia. J Clin Psychopharmacol 1995; 15(3): 211–6.
24. Kapitany T, Meszaros K, Lenzinger E et al. Genetic polymorphisms for drug metabolism (CYP2D6) and tardive dyskinesia in schizophrenia. Schizophr Res 1998; 32(2): 101–6.
25. Ohmori O, Kojima H, Shinkai T et al. Genetic association analysis between CYP2D6*2 allele and tardive dyskinesia in schizophrenic patients. Psychiatry Res 1999; 87(2-3): 239–44.
26. Bertilsson L, Carrillo JA, Dahl ML et al. Clozapine disposition covaries with CYP1A2 activity determined by a caffeine test. Br J Clin Pharmacol 1994; 38(5): 471–3.
27. Pirmohamed M, Williams D, Madden S et al. Metabolism and bioactivation of clozapine by human liver in vitro. J Pharmacol Exp Ther 1995; 272(3): 984–90.
28. Basile VS, Ozdemir V, Masellis M et al. A functional polymorphism of the cytochrome P450 1A2 (CYP1A2) gene: association with tardive dyskinesia in schizophrenia. Mol Psychiatry 2000; 5(4): 410–7.
29. Gill HJ, Tjia JF, Kitteringham NR et al. The effect of genetic polymorphisms in CYP2C9 on sulphamethoxazole N-hydroxylation. Pharmacogenetics 1999; 9(1): 43–53.
30. Ibeanu GC, Blaisdell J, Ferguson RJ et al. A novel transversion in the intron 5 donor splice junction of CYP2C19 and a sequence polymorphism in exon 3 contribute to the poor metabolizer phenotype for the anticonvulsant drug S-mephenytoin. J Pharmacol Exp Ther 1999; 290(2): 635–40.

31. Coutts RT, Urichuk LJ. Polymorphic cytochromes P450 and drugs used in psychiatry. Cell Mol Neurobiol 1999; 19(3): 325–54.

32. Malhotra AK, Goldman D, Buchanan RW et al. The dopamine D3 receptor (DRD3) Ser9Gly polymorphism and schizophrenia: a haplotype relative risk study and association with clozapine response. Mol Psychiatry 1998; 3(1): 72–5.

33. Scharfetter J, Chaudhry HR, Hornik K et al. Dopamine D3 receptor gene polymorphism and response to clozapine in schizophrenic Pakastani patients. Eur Neuropsychopharmacol 1999; 10(1): 17–20.

34. Masellis M, Basile VS, Ozdemir V et al. Pharmacogenetics of antipsychotic treatment: lessons learned from clozapine. Biol Psychiatry 2000; 47(3): 252–66.

35. Seeman MV. Schizophrenia: D4 receptor elevation. What does it mean? J Psychiatry Neurosci 1994; 19(3): 171–6.

36. Wilffert B, Zaal R, Brouwers JR. Pharmacogenetics as a tool in the therapy of schizophrenia. Pharm World Sci 2005; 27(1): 20–30.

37. Arranz M, Collier D, Sodhi M et al. Association between clozapine response and allelic variation in 5-HT2A receptor gene. Lancet 1995; 346(8970): 2812.

38. Joober R, Benkelfat C, Brisebois K et al. T102C polymorphism in the 5HT2A gene and schizophrenia: relation to phenotype and drug response variability. J Psychiatry Neurosci 1999; 24(2): 141–6.

39. Reynolds GP, Zhang Z, Zhang X. Polymorphism of the promoter region of the serotonin 5-HT(2C) receptor gene and clozapine-induced weight gain. Am J Psychiatry 2003; 160(4): 677–9.

40. Okada M, Northup JK, Ozaki N et al. Modification of human 5-HT(2C) receptor function by Cys23Ser, an abundant, naturally occurring amino-acid substitution. Mol Psychiatry 2004; 9(1): 55–64.

41. Sodhi MS, Arranz MJ, Curtis D et al. Association between clozapine response and allelic variation in the 5-HT2C receptor gene. Neuroreport 1995; 7(1): 169–72.

42. Malhotra AK, Goldman D, Ozaki N et al. Clozapine response and the 5HT2C Cys23Ser polymorphism. Neuroreport 1996; 7(13): 2100–2.

43. Rietschel M, Kennedy JL, Macciardi F et al. Application of pharmacogenetics to psychotic disorders: the first consensus conference. The Consensus Group for Outcome Measures in Psychoses for Pharmacological Studies. Schizophr Res 1999; 37(2): 191–6.

44. Arranz MJ, Munro J, Birkett J et al. Pharmacogenetic prediction of clozapine response. Lancet 2000; 355(9215): 1615–6.

45. Masellis M, Basile VS, Meltzer HY et al. Lack of association between the T-->C 267 serotonin 5-HT6 receptor gene (HTR6) polymorphism and prediction of response to clozapine in schizophrenia. Schizophr Res 2001; 47(1): 49–58.

46. Yu YW, Tsai SJ, Lin CH et al. Serotonin-6 receptor variant (C267T) and clinical response to clozapine. Neuroreport 1999; 10(6): 1231–3.

47. Lee HJ. Pharmacogenetic studies investigating the adverse effects of antipsychotics. Psychiatry Invest 2007; 4: 66–75.

48. Rietschel M, Krauss H, Müller DJ et al. Dopamine D3 receptor variant and tardive dyskinesia. Eur Arch Psychiatry Clin Neurosci 2000; 250(1): 31–5.

49. Segman R, Neeman T, Heresco-Levy U et al. Genotypic association between the dopamine D3 receptor and tardive dyskinesia in chronic schizophrenia. Mol Psychiatry 1999; 4(3): 247–53.

50. Steen VM, Løvlie R, MacEwan T et al. Dopamine D3-receptor gene variant and susceptibility to tardive dyskinesia in schizophrenic patients. Mol Psychiatry 1997; 2(2): 139–45.

51. Park YM, Chung YC, Lee SH et al. Weight gain associated with the alpha2a-adrenergic receptor -1,291 C/G polymorphism and olanzapine treatment. Am J Med Genet B Neuropsychiatr Genet 2006; 141B(4): 394–7.

52. Wang YC, Bai YM, Chen JY et al. Polymorphism of the adrenergic receptor alpha 2a -1291C>G genetic variation and clozapine-induced weight gain. J Neural Transm 2005 112(11): 1463–8.
53. Wang YC, Bai YM, Chen JY et al. C825T polymorphism in the human G protein beta3 subunit gene is associated with long-term clozapine treatment-induced body weight change in the Chinese population. Pharmacogenet Genomics 2005; 15(10): 743–8.
54. Kang SG, Lee HJ, Park YM et al. Possible association between the -2548A/G polymorphism of the leptin gene and olanzapine-induced weight gain. Prog Neuropsychopharmacol Biol Psychiatry 2008; 32(1): 160–3.
55. Zhang ZJ, Yao ZJ, Mou XD et al. [Association of -2548G/A functional polymorphism in the promoter region of leptin gene with antipsychotic agent-induced weight gain]. Zhonghua Yi Xue Za Zhi 2003; 83(24): 2119–23.
56. Reynolds GP, Zhang ZJ, Zhang XB. Association of antipsychotic drug-induced weight gain with a 5-HT2C receptor gene polymorphism. Lancet 2002; 359(9323): 2086–7.
57. Abdolmaleky HM, Thiagalingam S, Wilcox M. Genetics and epigenetics in major psychiatric disorders: dilemmas, achievements, applications, and future scope. Am J Pharmacogenomics 2005; 5(3): 149–60.

19 | Side effect burden of antipsychotic medication

Hans-Jürgen Möller and Michael Riedel

INTRODUCTION

Antipsychotics are relatively well tolerable substances with a broad therapeutic index. Severe complications are extremely rare. Tardive dyskinesia is to be considered a specifically impairing side effect of First Generation Antipsychotics (FGAs) due to frequency and chronicity. Since the introduction of the Second Generation Antipsychotics (SGAs) weight gain and the associated metabolic syndrome are considered important also. In terms of a risk-benefit analysis these, as well as all other side effects, have to be put in relation to the severity of the basic disease and are considered justifiable regarding the aspect of disadvantageous prognosis of many patients with schizophrenic diseases. In case of indications outside schizophrenia, for example affective disorders, the weighing should respectively be different. A number of other frequently occurring side effects, for example xerostomia, are subjectively annoying rather than clinically relevant. For the recording of important clinical side effects such as change in the blood picture or cardiovascular disorders, regular check-ups are necessary.

Differences in the risk of specific side effects of antipsychotic medications are often predictable from the receptor binding profiles of the various agents. Some side effects result from receptor mediated effects (Figure 19.1) within the central nervous system (e.g., extrapyramidal side effects, hyperprolactinemia, sedation)

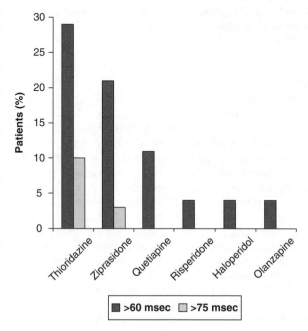

FIGURE 19.1 Comparison of six antipsychotics in patients with a QTc prolongation > 60 msec and >75 msec.

Source: http://www.fda.gov/ohrms/dockets/ac/backgrd/3619b1b.pdf

or outside the central nervous system (e.g., constipation, hypotension), whereas other side effects are of unclear or very complex pathophysiology (e.g., weight gain, metabolic syndrome). Shared side effects of FGAs and SGAs include neurological effects (i.e., acute and chronic extrapyramidal effects, neuroleptic malignant syndrome), sedation, cardiovascular effects (i.e., hypotension, tachycardia, and conduction abnormalities), anticholinergic and antiadrenergic effects, weight gain and glucose and lipid metabolic abnormalities, and sexual dysfunction, all in a class- and substance-specific (often dose-related) frequency and intensity. Table 19.1 gives an overview of the estimated frequency of some important side effects of several SGAs and haloperidol. Table 19.2 gives recommendations for monitoring. The clinical decision making should be based in all cases on the individual disposition for side effects of the respective patient as well as on the relative potential of individual antipsychotic drugs to cause extrapyramidal side effects and metabolic side effects including weight gain and other side effects (including unpleasant subjective experience). The most recent clinical guidelines issued by NICE (National Institute for Health and Clinical Excellence) provide indications in terms of pharmacological interventions. For people with newly diagnosed schizophrenia, offer oral antipsychotic medication. Provide information and discuss the benefits and side-effect profile of each drug with the service user. The choice of drug should be made by the service user and healthcare professional together, considering:

– The relative potential of individual antipsychotic drug to cause extrapyramidal side effects (including akathisia), metabolic side effects (including weight gain) and other side effects (including unpleasant subjective experience).

In the following the spectrum of unwanted effects under treatment with antipsychotics will be presented with special focus on extrapyramidal symptoms as well as weight gain and related metabolic syndrome. An adequate management of side effects may contribute to increased treatment adherence and better outcome. Therefore strategies for the management of disabling side effects are reviewed and recommended in the following sections. A short overview of therapeutic options for managing relevant side effects is given in Tables 19.3 and 19.4.

EXTRAPYRAMIDAL SIDE EFFECTS
Extrapyramidal side effects (EPS) pose a high burden for the respective patient, which can affect the subjective quality of life and compliance immensely (Awad et al. 1997; Hellewell 2002; Naber and Karow 2001; Naber and Lambert 2004; Oehl et al. 2000). In times of the antipsychiatry movement neuroleptics were therefore denigrated to being a "chemical straitjacket". Even from an objective point of view it cannot be ignored, that EPS do stigmatize the patients additionally to the disease with parkinsonism as well as dyskinesia, making them peculiar and unattractive in public. From a clinical point of view it should be emphasized, that EPS are not only relevant per se, but that they can secondarily lead to a depressive symptomatic (pharmacogenetic depression, akinetic depression), to a similarly negative symptomatic and to cognitive impairment. All these are important reasons to save the patient from EPS. Contrary to common statements, a low dose of haloperidol is not sufficient to keep the risk of EPS respectively low, so impressively shown by a randomized double-blind 7-arm study on sertindole and haloperidol (Zimbroff et al. 1997), and recently confirmed by a double-blind randomized comparison study on risperidone versus haloperidol (Möller et al. 2008), among others. All consecutively mentioned extrapyramidal side

TABLE 19.1 Selected side effects of commonly used antipsychotics

Side effect	Antipsychotic medication							
	Haloperidol	Amisulpride	Clozapine	Olanzapine	Risperidone	Queriapine	Ziprasidone	Aripiprazole
Akathisia/Parkinsonism	++	0–+	0	0–+	0–++	0–+	0–+	+
Tardive dyskinesia	++	(+)	0	(+)	(+)	?	?	?
Seizures	+	0	++	0	0	0	0	(+)
QTc Prolongation	+	(+)	(+)	(+)	(+)	(+)	+	0(?)
Glucose abnormalities	(+)	(+)	+++	+++	++	++	0	0
Lipid abnormalities	(+)	(+)	+++	+++	++	++	0	0
Constipation	+	++	+++	++	++	+	0	0
Hypotension	++	0	(+)	(+)	++	++	0	0
Agranulocytosis	0	0	+	0	0	0	0	0
Weight gain*	+	+	+++	+++	++	++	0–+	+
Prolactin elevation	+++	+++	0	(+)	++	(+)	(+)	0
Galaktorrhoea	++	++	0	0	++	0	0	0
Dysmenorrhoea/Amenorrhoea	+++	++	0	0	++	(+)	0	0
Sedation	++	0-(+)	+++	+-++	+	++	0-(+)	0
Malignant neuroleptic syndrome	(+)	?	(+)	(+)	(+)	(+)	?	(+)

Note: Frequency and severity of side effects refers to information obtained by drug companies, FDA, additional literature and other guidelines (e.g., APA 2004).

0=no risk; (+)=Occasionally, may be no difference to placebo; +=mild (less 1%); ++=Sometimes (less 10%); +++=frequently (>10%); ?= no statement possible due to lacking data.

*Weight gain during 6–10 weeks: +=low (0–1.5 kg); ++=medium (1.5–3 kg); +++=high (> 3 kg).

Source: Falkai et al. (156)

TABLE 19.2 Monitoring for Patients on Second Generation Antipsychotics*

	Baseline	4 Weeks	8 Weeks	12 Weeks	Quarterly	Annually
Personal/family history	X					x
Weight (BMI)	X	x	x	X	x	x
Waist circumference	X					x
Blood pressure	X	x		X		x
Fasting plasma glucose	X			X		x
Fasting lipid profile	X			X		x
Blood cell count	X	x		X		x
ECG	X					

BMI = body mass index; ECG = electrocardiogram.
*More frequent assessments may be warranted based on clinical status.
Note: Assessments refer mainly to American Diabetes Association and American Psychiatric Association (2004), Diabetes Care 27: 596–601.
Source: Falkai et al.(156)

effects appear much less under treatment with SGAs than under classical neuroleptics (Tandon et al. 2008). Clozapine seems to have almost no extrapyramidal risks. Studies provided evidence that clozapine-and probably quetiapine-induced EPS are not dose dependent (Buchanan 1995; Cheer and Wagstaff 2004). Due to the extremely low frequency of EPS with quetiapine and particularly clozapine, these can possibly be considered spontaneously appearing EPS (McCreadie et al. 1996; McCreadie et al. 2002; McCreadie et al. 2005).

Extrapyramidal side effects can be divided into acute and chronic categories. Acute extrapyramidal side effects are signs and symptoms that occur in the first days and weeks of antipsychotic medication administration. They are dose dependent and are reversible with medication dose reduction or discontinuation (Goetz and Klawans 1981). Chronic extrapyramidal side effects occur under chronic treatment with antipsychotics and often persist even after withdrawal of antipsychotic treatment. Tardive dyskinesia is the most important chronic extrapyramidal side effect.

Early dyskinesia
Intermittent or permanent muscle spasm and posture anomalies occur. Most commonly affected are the muscles of the eyes, the face, the neck, and the pharynx: blepharospasm, trismus, hyoglossus spasm, grimacing. Acute diskinetic syndromes occur in the first hours or days of the neuroleptic treatment. The incidence is shown in a range of 5–10%. Acute dystonia typically occurs with high potency FGAs and more frequently in young, male patients, but has also been reported in association with SGAs, e.g., risperidone (Leucht et al. 1999; Rupniak et al. 1986).

Acute dystonic reactions respond immediately to the administration of anticholinergic or antihistaminic medication (American Psychiatric Association 1997). Parenteral administration will have a more rapid onset of action than oral administration.

Parkinsonism
Parkinsonism occurs with akinesia, rigor tremor and a respective posture disorder. Akinesia is in the foreground. The incidence depends strongly on the type of

TABLE 19.3 Therapeutic options to manage antipsychotic side effects

Side effect	Prevention	Treatment
EPS:		
Acute dystonic reactions	– Selecting SGA with low rate of EPS – Start with low dose – Increase dose slowly and stepwise	– Oral or intravenous application of anticholinergic drug, e.g., 2.5–5 mg biperiden, if necessary repeating procedure after 30 minutes, continuing biperiden orally (maximal 12 mg/d) – Switching to SGA
Parkinsonism	– Selecting SGA – Increase dose slowly and stepwise	– Dose reduction – Oral application of anticholinergic drug (e.g., biperiden 4–12 mg/d) – Switching to SGA
Akathisia	– Selecting SGA – Increase dose slowly and stepwise	– Dose reduction – 1. Oral application of beta blocking agent (e.g., propranolol 30–90 mg/d) – 2. Oral application of benzodiazepines (e.g., diazepam) – 3. Try anticholinergic drug (e.g., biperiden, max. 12 mg/d) – Switiching to SGA
Tardive Dyskinesia	– Selecting SGA – Evaluating risk factors for TD – Supplementing vitamin E	– Switching to clozapine (alternatively to other SGA, e.g., olanzapine, quetiapine, aripiprazole) – Oral application of tiapride – Oral application of baclofen (20–120 mg/d) or valproate (500–1200 mg/d) – Try supplementing with vitamin E (400–1600 IE/d)
NMS:		
Neuroleptic Malignant Syndrome	– Selecting SGA	– Intensive care management – Stopping antipsychotic treatment – Application of dantrolene i.v. (2.5–10 mg/kg body weight daily) – Application of lorazepam 4–8 mg i.v. /d – Alternatively bromocriptine, lisurid, amantadine or clonidine – In single cases ECT

Source: Falkai et al.(157)

neuroleptics used as well as on predisposing factors, for example age beyond 40 years. Antipsychotic-induced parkinsonism is thought to affect 10–80% (depending on population and doses) of patients undergoing therapy with high-potency FGAs (Bollini et al. 1994).

TABLE 19.4 Therapeutic options to manage antipsychotic side effects

Side effect	Prevention	Treatment
Weight gain	– Selecting antipsychotic with lower risk of weight gain	– Dietary supplementation, physical activity – CBT or psychoeducation – Switching to another antipsychotic – Adding a H2-receptor blocker (e.g., nizatidine, ranitidine) – Combine with topiramate
Hyperlipidemia	– Screening for risk factors, cholesterol and triglycerides (TG) – Selecting antipsychotic with low risk of inducing hyperlipidemia	– Dietary management, weight reduction – Specific pharmacological treatment (e.g., cholesterol and TG reducer) – Switching to an antipsychotic with lower risk of hyperlipidemia
Diabetes	– Screening for diabetes risk factors, fasting blood glucose, in some cases hemoglobin A1c – Selecting antipsychotic with low risk of inducing diabetes	– Dietary management – Referring to a diabetologist for special pharmacological treatment of diabetes – Switching to an antipsychotic with lower risk of diabetes
Orthostatic hypotension	– Starting with low dose, increase dose slowly and stepwise – Selecting antipsychotic with low alpha-adrenergic receptor-blocking profile	– Physical activity – Application of oral dihydroergotamine (max. 6 mg/d) or etilefrine (20–60 mg/d) – Switching to other antipsychotics (due to receptor profile)
QTc Prolongation	– Selecting antipsychotic with low risk of QTc Prolongation – Evaluation of cardiac risk factors – Control for pharmacological interactions – Control of ECG	– If QTc > 480–520 ms or has increased more than 60 ms switching to an other antipsychotic is indicated
Dry Mouth	– Prescribing low doses – Selecting antipsychotic with lower risk	– Drinking small amounts frequently – Using sugarfree drops or chewing gum – Dose reduction
Sialorrhea	– Selecting antipsychotic with lower risk	– Application of pirenzepine 25–50 mg/d – Dose reduction (e.g., of clozapine)
Sexual dysfunction	– Selecting antipsychotic with no or minimal prolactin elevation Evaluating prolactin level	– Switching to another antipsychotic with lower risk of prolactin elevation
Constipation	– Selecting antipsychotic with lower risk	– Dietary supplementation, physical activity – Lactulose 5–10 g/d, or macrogol 13–40 g/d, or natriumpicosulfat 5 – 10 mg/d

(continued)

TABLE 19.4 Continued

Side effect	Prevention	Treatment
Urinary retention	– Selecting antipsychotic with low anticholinergic side effects	– Dose reduction – Switching to another antipsychotic – Application of carbachole 1–4 mg/d orally; if necessary 0.25 mg i.m. or s.c. – Application of distigmine 2.5–5 mg/d orally
Leukopenia	-controlling white blood cell count (WBC)	– In case of agranulocytosis (< 1000 granulocytes) immediately stopping antipsychotic treatment – Cooperate with an hematologist – Prevent infections, monitoring WBC – In some cases application of GM-CSF/G-CSF – Clozapine treatment has to be stopped if leukocytes < 3500 or granulocytes < 1500

Source: Falkai et al.(157)

Antipsychotic-induced parkinsonism generally resolves after discontinuation of antipsychotic medication, although some cases of persisting symptoms have been reported (Melamed et al. 1991). The primary treatment of drug-induced parkinsonism consists of preventative and therapeutic dose reductions or the administration of atypical antipsychotic medications. If this is not possible, administration of anticholinergic agents or dopamine agonists should be considered. However, dopamine agonists carry a potential risk of exacerbating psychosis, and anticholinergic drugs can cause anticholinergic side effects. Thus, excessive doses and chronic use of these agents should be avoided or minimized.

Akathisia

The patients complain that they are unable to sit, stand, or lie still. The symptoms mostly occur during the first months of treatment. Akathisia occurs with a mean frequency of approximately 20–25% in patients undergoing treatment with FGAs (Braude et al. 1983; Grebb 1995), while the incidence under treatment with second generation antipsychotics is much lower.

Several strategies have been used to decrease akathisia. Treatment of akathisia consists of a dose reduction of antipsychotics or administration of beta-blockers. In contrast to FGAs, the newer atypical antipsychotic medications are far less likely to trigger akathisia. They are thus the drugs of choice in intolerable akathisia occurring with typical FGA medications. Effective treatments for akathisia include centrally acting beta-blockers, such as a low dose of propranolol (e.g., 30–90 mg/day) (Fleischhacker et al. 1990). When these medications are administered, blood pressure and pulse rate should be monitored with dose changes. Benzodiazepines such as lorazepam –1.0 –2.5 mg/day and clonazepam are also effective in decreasing symptoms of akathisia. (American Psychiatric Association 1997; Kutcher et al. 1989; Pujalte et al. 1994).There is no randomized, controlled trial which provides evidence for the use of anticholinergic drugs for treatment of akathisia. Should a person suffer from distressing akathisia as an experimental approach despite other treatment strategies, a trial of an anticholinergic drug may be warranted (Lima et al. 2004).

Neuroleptic malignant syndrome

Very rare but particularly severe manifestations of parkinsonism are catatonic reactions and neuroleptic malignant syndrome (NMS) characterized by a central dysregulation or impaired consciousness.

NMS is characterized by dystonia, rigidity, fever, autonomic instability such as tachycardia, delirium, myoglobinuria and increased levels of creatine kinase, leukocytes and hepatic enzymes. The prevalence of NMS is uncertain; it probably occurs in less than 1% of patients treated with FGAs (Adityanjee et al. 1999) and is even more rare among patients treated with SGAs (Caroff et al. 2000). Risk factors for NMS include acute agitation, young age, male gender, preexisting neurological disability, physical illness, dehydration, rapid escalation of antipsychotic dose, use of high-potency medications, and use of intramuscular preparations (Pelonero et al. 1998).

If NMS occurs, antispychotic treatment should immediately be terminated, vital functions stabilized under close monitoring and hyperthermia adequately treated.

Dantrolen showed success (dosage 2.5–10 mg/kg body weight daily, intravenously applied) and provided the greatest reduction in mortality compared to the treatment with bromocriptine and amantadine (Sakkas et al. 1991). There are several case reports for successful treatment with amantadine in doses of 200–400 mg/day (Susman 2001). Dopaminergic agents, e.g., L-Dopa itself, in combination with and without carbidopa and apomorphine show some efficacy in treating NMS in case reports (Wang and Hsieh 2001). Case reports recommend the use of bromocriptine in doses of 7.5–45 mg/day (Susman 2001). Lisurid was also reported to be effective and may have some advantages compared to bromocriptine, because it can be administered additionally intravenously and subcutaneously. Benzodiazepines are recommended traditionally and were used particularly if MNS could not be distinguished from catatonia ("catatonic dilemma"). Especially in less severe cases there were no adverse effects when treatment with benzodiazepines was initiated, for example, lorazepam in doses of 4–8 mg/day was recommended (Susman 2001). Treatment with clonidine demonstrated success and improved the course of NMS (e.g., reduced stay in an intensive care unit) (Gregorakos et al. 2000). Administration of anticholinergics was reported to be beneficial, but may cause hyperthermia itself. Therefore anticholinergics are not recommended in the treatment of NMS (Caroff et al. 2000).

Treatment with ECT demonstrated efficacy in NMS in open studies and case reports (Davis et al. 1991) compared to a control group. Prior to ECT, an attempt with dantrolene may be useful (Nisijima and Ishiguro 1999). After the treatment of NMS, reintroduction of antipychotic therapy is recommended, whereby an atypical agent not relevantly associated with a risk of NMS should be preferred.

Tardive dyskinesia

This is a hyperkinetic motor disturbance that appears at the earliest after 3 to 6 months of treatment—usually after longer treatment—with neuroleptics. It is characterized by orofacial dyskinesia such as lip-smacking, masticating, and tongue-rolling movements, and sometimes choreatic movements of the extremities. Typically, the disorder becomes more severe when the neuroleptic dose is decreased or the medication discontinued. The incidence of the disorder is described very differently depending on the clientele being examined. An average of approximately 20% following many years of antipsychotic treatment is often given as an estimate for orientation. The frequency increases with increasing length of treatment, with an incidence rate of 4.8% (Glazer 2000; Kane et al. 1986). In about 50% of affected patients the disorder is irreversible. After 4 years of therapy with high-potency FGAs, approximately 20% of patients have tardive dyskinesia and the rate is higher (up to 50%) in elderly patients (Fenton 2000; Glazer 2000; Jeste 2000) Risk factors are age, female gender, the presence of drug-induced parkinsonian symptoms, diabetes mellitus, affective disturbances and higher dose and longer duration of antipsychotic therapy (Morgenstern and Glazer 1993). SGAs induce fewer extrapyramidal symptoms (EPS) in a therapeutic dose range than FGAs and show a significant reduction in the risk of tardive dyskinesia compared to FGAs (Correll et al. 2004; Woods et al. 2008).

Despite the fact that neuroleptic cessation is frequently a first-line recommendation, there were no RCT-derived data to support this (McGrath and Soares-Weiser 2004). Two studies found a reduction in TD associated with neuroleptic reduction (Cookson 1987; Kane et al. 1983), although the risk of psychotic relapse should be taken into consideration when lowering the neuroleptic dose (Gilbert et al. 1995).

Due to the serious burden which TD puts on a patient, several approaches were tried to help these patients. Administration of clozapine is recommended in severe forms, as an antidyskinetic effect of this agent is under discussion, as well as the possible avoidance of further risk accumulation. No randomized, controlled trial-derived data were available to clarify the role of neuroleptics as treatments for tardive dyskinesia (TD). This includes the newer atypical antipsychotics and clozapine, although there is some preliminary evidence derived from nonrandomized, controlled trials that clozapine is an effective treatment for TD (McGrath and Soares-Weiser 2004).

The use of cholinergic agents like lecithin, deanol or meclofenoxate for treatment of neuroleptic-induced tardive dyskinesia is not recommended because of the lack of evidence and due to adverse effects (Tammenmaa et al. 2004). There is no compelling evidence that benzodiazepines decrease tardive dyskinesia in a sufficient manner (Walker and Soares 2004). The two randomized, controlled trials with small sample sizes showed no clinically relevant advantage for benzodiazepines (diazepam mean dose 12–48 mg/day and alprazolam mean dose 7.2 mg/day) compared with no treatment on top of standard care or placebo (Csernansky et al. 1988; Weber et al. 1983).

In the absence of reliable evidence, the possible benefits of calcium channel blockers in the treatment of tardive dyskinesia have to be balanced against the potential adverse effects, for example, lowering of blood pressure and even causing symptoms of tardive dyskinesia to increase (Soares-Weiser and Rathbone 2004).

A tendency for reduced TD symptoms was reported for treatment with GABA-agonist drugs (baclofen, progabide 20–40 mg/kg per day, sodium valproate 500–1,200 mg/day, or tetrahydroisoxazolopyridine, THIP), but a clinically important improvement (reduction of more than 50% on any TD scale) could not be demonstrated in three randomized, controlled trials compared with placebo (Soares et al. 2004). In cross-over trials a significant improvement was reported in two studies with baclofen 20–120 mg/day (Ananth 1987; Gerlach et al. 1978), one with sodium valproate 900 mg/day (Linnoila et al. 1976) and one with THIP 60–120 mg/day (Thaker et al. 1987), but these trials also showed a range of moderate to severe side effects. In one cross-over study neither improvement nor side effects with baclofen up to 90 mg/day during the follow-up period were described (Nair et al. 1978). Levetiracetam, an ethyl analogon of the nootropic pracetam, and already on the market for several years, appears to have a favorable effect on TD.

In several open studies and a randomized placebo-controlled study levetirac-etam in a dosage of 500–3,000 mg/day proved to be effective in the treatment of TD. Levetiracetam has shown a favorable side-effect profile (Konitsiotis et al. 2006; Meco et al. 2006; Woods et al. 2008).

Small trials with uncertain quality of randomization indicate that vitamin E pro-tects against deterioration of TD but there is no evidence that vitamin E improves symptoms of TD (Soares and McGrath 2000).

Cognitive side effects

Although antipsychotic medications can effectively improve cognitive functions in schizophrenic patients, memory problems and cognitive disorders represent possible side effects of antipsychotic therapy, which are particularly associated with the anti-cholinergic effect of antipsychotic medications and the use of anticholinergic agents such as biperiden. Drug-induced cognitive disorders have been more frequently reported in treatment with typical antipsychotic medications (Bilder et al. 2002; Buchanan and Sharpe 1994; Green et al. 2002; Harvey and Keefe 2001; Keefe et al. 1999; Meltzer and McGurk 1999; Purdon et al. 2000; Velligan et al. 2002).

2. WEIGHT GAIN AND METABOLIC SIDE EFFECTS
Obesity and weight gain

Individuals with schizophrenia are more likely to be overweight or obese than the average population (De Hert et al. 2009; Marder et al. 2004). Combined with other risk factors like smoking, reduced physical activity, diabetes, and hyperlipidemia the risk for cardiovascular morbidity and mortality is increased. Besides lifestyle factors, such as poor diet and lack of exercise, treatment with FGAs and SGAs can contribute to weight gain and related metabolic risks (Marder and Fenton 2004; Marder et al. 2004; Nasrallah 2008; Newcomer 2007; Sentissi et al. 2007; Tschoner et al. 2007). Weight gain is a multifactorial occurrence during treatment with neuroleptic agents. According to a meta-analysis, the mean weight gain associated with SGAs is highest with clozapine and olanzapine, and lower with risperidone, whereas ziprasidone hardly affects body weight (Allison et al. 1999; Allison and Casey 2001); American Diabetes Association et al. 2004). It can be derived from this meta-analysis that also FGAs carry a risk of weight gain, especially for example chlorpromazine and to a lesser degree haloperi-dol. The side effect of weight gain has to be given due consideration, as it affects ther-apy adherence, somatic sequelae, mortality, stigmatization and quality of life (Allison and Weber 2003; De Hert et al. 2009). Therefore clinicians should sensitize patients and their caregivers to the health risk associated with excess weight and should encourage patients to self-monitor their weight. Body mass index (BMI) and waist size can serve as useful risk indicators (Marder et al. 2004). Recently positive data were published on paliperidone, demonstrating a relatively low risk of weight gain induction (Meltzer et al. 2008). For the recommended 6 mg daily dose, the observed weight gain was 0.6 +/- 3.2 in a pooled analysis of 3 similarly designed 6-week, multicenter, double-blind study, while it was 1.1 +/- 5.47 kg across treatment groups in a 25- week open label study (Emsley et al. 2008).

The causes of the relative frequent occurrence of weight gain under neurolep-tic treatment (Allison and Casey 2001) are probably the effect of the medication on the systems in the interbrain that regulate eating behavior on the one hand, and on the other a general sedation and reduction in motor activity. In a well-known consensus paper, the American Diabetes Association (ADA) and the American Psychiatric Association (APA) (American Diabetes Association et al. 2004) suggested measures for dealing with the problem, as does currently a joint statement of the European Psychiatric Association (EPA) together with the European Association for the Study of Diabetes (EASD) and the European Society of Cardiology (ESC) (de Hert 2009). It is important that weight gain and if possible the changes in metabolic parameters connected with it be carefully recorded. The decision as to whether or not an antipsychotic should be changed or continued to be used for treatment depends on the extent of the weight gain and the extent of the changes in metabolic laboratory parameters, as well as on the risk factors that should also be taken into account when treatment with the antipsychotic is begun. It must be borne in mind that any changes in neuroleptic treatment will be accompanied by a potential risk that the patient will be destabilized (Table 19.1).

Patients should be made aware of potential weight gain during antipsychotic treatment by continuous assessments. Management of drug-induced weight gain in schizophrenic patients has to refer to the multifactorial pathophysiology of this phenomenon. Behavior and lifestyle are an important part of weight maintenance in psychiatric patients. Therefore, physicians should encourage patients to increase their physical activity gradually and stepwise in combination with dietary restriction to obtain negative energy balance (Ananth et al. 2004b). Several dietary, counseling and behavior therapy programmes were suggested and some of them were evaluated. The results are not congruent, but at least altogether they give a positive signal that such an approach might be meaningful (Aquila and Emanuel 2000; Ball et al. 2001; Birt 2003; Littrell et al. 2003; Menza et al. 2004; Umbricht et al. 2001; Werneke et al. 2003).

Unfortunately the effectiveness of psychological interventions for weight reduction in schizophrenic patients seems to be low, although five earlier dietary and cognitive behavior trials predating the availability of SGAs suggested that patients with mental illness may change their lifestyle and display weight loss (Birt 2003). Factors affecting management of weight gain are negative symptoms, cognitive impairment, low income level, preference of high-calorie food, impaired satiety, level of sedation, and reduced ability to handle daily hassles (e.g., shopping and cooking) (Sharpe and Hills 2003). In hospitalized, clozapine-treated patients with preexisting physical or metabolic defects, dietary restriction led to mean weight loss of 7.1 kg in men and 0.5 kg in women compared to weight gain of 2.0 kg in men and 6.1 kg in women not dieting over 6 months (Heimberg et al. 1995). In a residential setting, a low-fat, low-calorie diet was not able to change average body weight in more than 2 years, but clozapine-and olanzapine-treated patients who gained weight were able to lose it during this nutrition counseling programme (Aquila and Emanuel 2000). A community-based educational programme failed to induce weight loss in patients with clozapine, whereas olanzapine-treated patients had some benefits (Wirshing et al. 1999). In a small sample of olanzapine-treated outpatients, a Weight Watchers programme with 10 weekly sessions provided moderate weight loss in men, but rarely in women participating in this intervention (Ball et al. 2001). Successful reversal of antipsychotic-induced weight gain in 6 months was described in a sample of patients receiving a weight loss programme designed for the mentally ill with respect to dietary counseling, exercise programme, and self-monitoring (Centorrino et al. 2002).

The effectiveness of a multimodal intensive weight management programme consisting of exercise, nutrition and behavioral interventions could be demonstrated by significant weight loss and increase of nutrition knowledge at the 12-months outcome in patients receiving different atypicals compared to a matched control group (Menza et al. 2004). In a randomized, experimental design an intensive psychoeducational programme with weekly 1-hour sessions, focusing on nutrition and fitness, for a total of 4 months demonstrated superiority in preventing olanzapine-induced weight gain compared to standard care consisting of diet counseling and exercise (Littrell et al. 2003). A cognitive behavioral approach including seven to nine individual and 10 bi-weekly group sessions followed by six group sessions on weight maintenance led to a significant drop in mean body mass index in a small sample of clozapine-and olanzapine-rated outpatients, but long-term success was not assessed (Umbricht et al. 2001). A systematic review of behavioral interventions in cases of antipsychotic weight gain, which included 13 studies, stated that calorie restriction in a controlled ward environment, structured counselling combined with CBT, counselling on life style and provision of rewards may potentially lead to weight loss. This result is limited due to the weak methodology used in the studies; furthermore, of seven trials with a control group only two yielded significant results (Werneke et al. 2003).

Also pharmacological approaches such as dosage reduction or switching to an SGA with a lower weight gain liability promise to be successful interventions for weight loss; however, this strategy has to be weighed against the potentially higher risk of relapse when changing an effective agent (Sharpe and Hills 2003). In an open, 8-week study, switching from other antipsychotics to aripiprazole resulted in significant weight loss (Casey et al. 2003). In an open-label study including 12 psychiatrically stable schizophrenic, schizoaffective and bipolar patients displaying excessive weight gain with olanzapine, switching to quetiapine led to a decline in mean weight of 2.25 kg in 10 weeks (Gupta and Masand 2004). In an open-label, parallel-group, 6-week trial, switching to ziprasidone led to a significant reduction of the mean body weight under risperidone (mean change 0.9 kg) and olanzapine (mean change 1.8 kg), but to a slight increase from FGAs (mean change 0.3 kg) in a large sample of stable outpatients with persistent symptoms or troublesome side effects (Weiden et al. 2003). In all these studies no worsening of psychopathology was observed.

In a nonpsychiatric population specific drug therapy for obesity is recommended exclusively as part of an integral treatment plan in patients with a BMI above 30, or in combination with obesity related risk factors or diseases with a BMI above 27 (Zimmermann et al. 2003). It seems meaningful to test such an intervention in psychiatric patients who have gained weight under neuroleptic treatment even before they reach a BMI of above 30, especially if in a particular case there are no other alternatives like changing the antipsychotic. There is one case report suggesting moderate weight loss after adding orlistat, a lipase inhibitor reducing intestinal fat absorption, to amisulpride (Anghelescu et al. 2000). An open study in 19 paediatric patients treated with olanzapine, risperidone, quetiapine or valproate revealed a decrease of mean body weight (2.9 kg after 12 weeks) after adding metformine 500 mg three times daily, an antidiabetic drug (Morrison et al. 2002). In contrast, no effect of metformine was reported in five patients on long-term treatment with haloperidol, fluphenazine, trifluperazine or risperidone (Baptista et al. 2001). Weight reduction was reported with open-label add-on treatment of amantadine after 2 weeks in 10 patients taking FGAs (Correa et al. 1987). The effect of weight loss could be confirmed by add-on treatment with 100–300 mg/day amantadine for 3–6 months in 12 patients who gained excessive weight while taking olanzapine (Floris et al. 2001), and in a double-blind, 16-week trial in 60 patients with schizophrenia, schizophreniform, or bipolar disorder compared to placebo (Deberdt et al. 2005). Amantadine, a dopamine agonist, has a risk of worsening psychosis (Ananth et al. 2004a) . Nizatidine , a peripheral H2-receptor blocker, which probably acts by inducing early satiety related to increased cholecystokinine and reduced production of gastric acid, has been reported to reduce weight gain in doses of 300 mg/day in a patient taking olanzapine (Sacchetti et al. 2000). In 8-week, randomized, double-blind, placebo-controlled studies, nizatidine confirmed its weight-losing effect in patients treated with olanzapine (mean weight decrease 1.0 kg) (Atmaca et al. 2003), and stopped weight gain in patients treated with quetiapine (Atmaca et al. 2004). A further double-blind RCT in patients treated with olanzapine (5–20 mg/day) demonstrated significantly less weight gain after 4 weeks add-on treatment with doses of 300 mg nitazidine twice daily without presenting significant differences in adverse events (Cavazzoni et al. 2003), but the difference was not statistically significant at 16 weeks. In a 16-week, randomized, open-label trial, positive effects in preventing weight gain were observed with treatment of ranitidine (300–600 mg/day) added to olanzapine (Lopez-Mato et al. 2003), whereas famotidine failed to show significant effects in a double-blind placebo-controlled study (Poyurovsky et al. 2004). There have been four case reports published indicating that the anticonvulsant topiramate added to valproate, carbamazepine, quetiapine, and olanzapine demonstrates benefits in weight loss (Birt 2003). In addition, topiramate, given at a dose of 125 mg/day over 5 months, led to weight loss in a patient taking clozapine (Dursun and Devarajan 2000). Cautious use in people with mental illness is warranted for anorecting agents like phentermine, chlorphentermine, sibutramine, or phenylpropanolamine due to exacerbation of psychotic symptoms. For this reason these agents cannot be recommended in patients with schizophrenia. Furthermore, adding phentermine and chlorphentermine in patients with chlorpromazine-associated weight gain (Sletten et al. 1967) and phenylpropanolamine to clozapine therapy (Borovicka et al. 2002) failed to show any significant positive effects on weight gain. Combinations of fluoxetine (20 mg/day in one RCT and 60 mg/day in another RCT) with olanzapine demonstrated no significant weight loss or prevention of weight gain compared to placebo (Bustillo et al. 2003; Poyurovsky et al. 2002). An RCT augmentation of fluvoxamine (50 mg/day) to clozapine (dosage up to 250 mg/day) revealed significantly less weight gain compared to clozapine monotherapy (dosage up to 600 mg/day), controlled for similar clozapine levels in both groups (Lu et al. 2004). Add-on treatment with reboxetine led to a significant reduction of mean body weight in olanzapine-treated patients compared to placebo in a randomized, controlled study (Poyurovsky et al. 2003).

Metabolic side effects

Diabetes

There is evidence that schizophrenia itself is an independent risk factor for impaired glucose tolerance, which is a known risk factor for developing type 2 diabetes, regardless of whether patients receive antipsychotic medication (Bushe and Holt 2004; De Hert et al. 2009; Ryan et al. 2003). The interactions between schizophrenia and diabetes are likely to be multifactorial and include genetic and environmental factors. Besides endocrine stress sytems like the sympathetic-adrenal-medullary system and the hypothalamic-pituitary-adrenal axis, lifestyle factors such as poor diet, obesity, and lack of exercise are involved in the genesis of diabetes (Dinan et al. 2004; Marder et al. 2004). An increase in blood sugar and inhibition of insulin secretion as well as a reduced glucose tolerance were already reported in the early neuroleptic literature under low doses of chlorpromazine (below 100 mg/day).

Pharmaco-epidemiological studies revealed a higher rate of diabetes in patients receiving SGAs compared with those not receiving antipsychotics or with those receiving FGAs (Haddad 2004). Studies attempting to establish whether the association with diabetes varies between different SGAs are inconclusive (Bushe and Leonard 2004; Haddad 2004; Koro CE et al. 2002; Wirshing et al. 2002b). Nevertheless, clozapine and olanzapine are thought to be the agents most commonly associated with diabetes (Marder et al. 2004).

A baseline measure of (fasting) plasma glucose level should be collected for all patients before starting a new antipsychotic, or alternatively hemoglobin A1c should be measured (Marder et al. 2004). Patients and their caregivers should be informed about the symptoms of diabetes, and patients should be monitored at regular intervals for the presence of these symptoms. The risks and consequences of diabetes have to be weighed against the control of psychotic symptoms if switching to another agent with an assumed lower risk of diabetes is considered. An internist should be involved in the treatment of diabetes.

Hyperlipidemia
Retrospective reports and pharmacoepidemiological studies found a significantly greater extent of elevations of lipids (trigylcerides) in patients taking certain SGAs (olanzapine and clozapine) than in patients receiving other antipsychotics (e.g., haloperidol, quetiapine, risperidone) (Wirshing et al. 2002a; Koro CE et al. 2002) . Similar to diabetes, hyperlipidemia is linked to a multifactorial genesis and is associated with obesity and lifestyle factors like poor diet and lack of exercise. Elevated triglyceride and cholesterol levels are associated with coronary heart disease, including ischaemic heart disease and myocardial infarction. Therefore total cholesterol, low-density lipoprotein (LDL) and HDL cholesterol, and triglyceride levels should be measured (Marder et al. 2004). If the LDL level is greater than 130 mg/dl the patient should be referred to an internist to evaluate whether treatment with a cholesterol-lowering drug should be initiated.

3. OTHER SIDE EFFECTS
Impairment of thermoregulation
Neuroleptics cause a central disturbance or blockage of thermoregulation which under adequate heat exposure can lead to complications (e.g., heatstroke).

Pharmacogenic depression
Treatment with FGAs can lead to pharmacogenic depression. Apart from a reduction in the neuroleptic dose, before treatment with antidepressives at least one (parenteral) treatment attempt with an anticholinergic should be carried out. This treatment approach is sensible, since sometimes with administration of an anticholinergic the depressive syndrome subsides very quickly, if this is a symptom associated with a more or less obvious parkinsonism ("akinetic depression"; also see (Möller and von Zerssen 1986) The risk of a pharmacogenic depression can be avoided by the primary administration of an SGA (Möller 2005).

Epileptic seizures

Epileptic seizures occur in an average of 0.5–0.9% of patients receiving antipsychotic medications, whereby treatment with clozapine and zotepine is dose-dependently associated with the highest incidence rate (up to 17%). Seizures can be effectively treated with benzodiazepines, as well as anticonvulsant agents such as phenytoin or valproic acid) (American Psychiatric Association 1997). Carbamazepine should not be used in combination with clozapine due to its potentiation of neutropenia and agranulocytosis. In general, in the presence of seizures a dose reduction is recommended, or a switch from clozapine or zotepine to another antipsychotic medication if the former option is not justified for clinical and psychopathological reasons.

Cognitive side effects

Although antipsychotic medications can effectively improve cognitive functions in schizophrenic patients, memory problems and cognitive disorders represent possible side effects of antipsychotic therapy, due to antihistamines with anticholinergic effects. Drug-induced cognitive disorders have been more frequently reported during treatment with SGAs (Buchanan 1995; Harvey and Keefe 2001). The most extreme case of cognitive side effects is a delirious state.

Sedation

Sedation is a common side effect of FGAs, as well as of several SGAs, due to antagonist effects of those drugs on histaminergic, adrenergic and serotonergic receptors. Sedation occurs more frequently with low-potency typical antipsychotic medications and clozapine. Sedation is most pronounced in the initial phases of treatment, since most patients develop some tolerance to the sedating effects with continued administration. Lowering of the daily dose, consolidation of divided doses into one evening dose, or changing to a less-sedating antipsychotic medication may be effective in reducing the severity of sedation. There are no systematic data on specific pharmacological interventions for sedation, but caffeine may be a relatively safe option. Some forms of psychostimulants (e.g., modafinil) have also been used to treat daytime drowsiness. However, there have been case reports of clozapine toxicity associated with modafinil and other stimulant treatments of sedation, and thus this drug combination should be carefully considered and used with caution. If anticholinergic treatment is required to prevent or improve EPS (e.g., under treatment with FGAs), and cognitive side effects may result from this treatment, switching to SGAs has to be considered.

Cardiovascular side effects

Hypotension and orthostatic hypotension are related to the antiadrenergic effects of antipsychotic medications, and are therefore particularly associated with low-potency FGAs and some SGAs, e.g., clozapine (Buchanan 1995). Tachycardia is particularly relevant in pre-existing cardiac disease. Tachycardia can result from the anticholinergic effects of antipsychotic medications, but may also occur as a result of postural hypotension. Tachycardia unrelated to orthostatic blood pressure changes that result from anticholinergic effects may occur in up to 25% of patients treated with clozapine (American Psychiatric Association 2004). Management strategies for orthostatic hypotension include decreasing or dividing doses of an antipsychotic, or switching to an antipsychotic without antiadrenergic effects. Gradual dose titration, starting with a low dose, and monitoring of orthostatic signs minimizes the risk of complications due to orthostatic hypotension. Tachycardia due to anticholinergic effects without hypotension can be managed with low doses of a peripherally acting beta-blocker (e.g., atenolol) (Miller 2000). Supportive measures include the use of support stockings, increased dietary salt and cautioning patients who experience severe postural hypotension against getting up quickly and without assistance, as falls can result in hip fractures and other accidents, particular in elderly patients.

Cardiac side effects
Cardiac side effects of antipsychotic medications registered as ECG-abnormalities include prolongation of the QT interval, abnormal T-waves, prominent U-waves and widening of the QRS complex (Haddad and Anderson 2002). The average QTc interval in healthy adults is approximately 400 ms. QTc prolongation (QTc intervals above 450–500 ms) is associated with an increased risk of torsade de pointes and transition to ventricular fibrillation (Glassman and Bigger, Jr. 2001). At varying rates, all antipsychotics may cause (dose dependent) cardiac side effects; of the FGAs, this predominantly applies to tricyclic neuroleptic agents of the phenothiazine type (e.g., chlorpromazine, promethazine, perazine and, especially, thioridazine) and to pimozide. In addition, high-dose intravenous haloperidol has been associated with a risk of QTc prolongation (Al Khatib et al. 2003). Of the SGAs, sertindole and ziprasidone were found to lengthen the QT interval in a significant manner (Glassman and Bigger 2001; Marder et al. 2004).

Experience with ziprasidone has shown that the risk linked to it was overestimated. Even sertindole (Kasper 2008), which had to be taken off the market temporarily on order of the drug approval agency, because the risk was considered too high, was reapproved in 2006 with the agreement of the European approval agency, after extensive studies had proven its safety.

Prior to commencement, and at subsequent increases of dose, of antipsychotic therapy with thioridazine, mesoridazine and pimozide, ECG monitoring is obligatory. This recommendation also applies to ziprasidone and sertindole if cardiac risk factors, like known heart disease, congenital long QT syndrome, personal history of syncope and family history of sudden death at an early age, are present. If the latter risk factors are present, thioridazine, mesoridazine and pimozide should not be given (Marder et al. 2004). The application of two or more antipsychotics or other adjunctive agents could increase the risk of cardiac side effects (e.g., QTc prolongation). If this occurs under neuroleptic treatment, the medication should be discontinued and switched to an antipsychotic with a lower risk of cardiac conduction disturbances (Marder et al. 2004).

Case reports indicate that the use of clozapine is associated with a risk of myocarditis in 1 per 500 to 1 per 10,000 treated patients (Killian et al. 1999; La Grenade et al. 2001; Warner et al. 2000). If the diagnosis is probable, clozapine should be stopped immediately and the patient referred urgently to a specialist for internal medicine (Marder et al. 2004).

Anticholinergic side effects
Anticholinergic side effects predominantly arise with the use of low-potency tricylic neuroleptics: dryness of the mouth, difficulty in focusing, disturbance of urinary

bladder function, constipation—in severe cases with paralytic bowel obstruction. If severe anticholinergic side effects appear the dose has to be reduced or a butyrophenone-type antipsychotic administered. In the case of life-threatening side effects a cholinergic is administered.

Dry mouth and eyes, and constipation may result from adrenergic and anticholinergic effects, but also from adrenergic effects of antipsychotics. Patients may be advised to use sugar free chewing gum or drops against dry mouth. To treat constipation, patients should be advised to drink more, and in some cases administration of lactulose may be useful. Usually patients mostly suffer from the described autonomic side effects when antipsychotic treatment is introduced or doses are increased.

Urinary tract problems
Urinary tract problems such as urinary retention and urinary incontinence may be particularly provoked by antipsychotic medications with marked anticholinergic components such as phenothiazines and those with cholinergic effects. Acute urinary retention problems may be treated with low dose carbachole.

Sialorrhea
Sialorrhea and drooling occur relatively frequently with clozapine treatment and are most likely due to decreased saliva clearance related to impaired swallowing mechanisms, or possibly to muscarinic cholinergic antagonist activity at the M4 receptor or to a-adrenergic agonist activity (Rabinowitz et al. 1996). Therapeutic options for sialorrhea include the application of pirenzepine 25–50 mg/day and dose reduction of clozapine, if possible.

Disturbance of liver function
Hepatic effects, such as elevated hepatic enzymes, may be triggered by a number of antipsychotic medications, whereby this is usually asymptomatic. Direct hepatotoxicity or cholestatic jaundice occur extremely rarely and are particularly associated with low-potency phenothiazines (American Psychiatric Association 2004). In studies involving olanzapine, reversible, mainly slight elevations in hepatic enzymes have been reported. (Beasley, Jr. et al. 1996).

Hematological effects
Temporary changes in blood count are often observed. Of clinical importance are rare cases of leukopenia/agranulocytosis, which are also known to be a problem in treatment with antidepressants. The latency period given for the appearance of agranulocytosis varies, but it can be expected from the third week onward. The decrease in the leukocyte count is usually gradual rather than abrupt, and with short enough periods between laboratory checks (1 week) and the immediate discontinuation of the medication it can often be reversed. Hematological effects, like inhibition of leukopoiesis, occur in patients being treated with chlorpromazine, for example, as benign leukopenia in up to 10% and as agranulocytosis in approximately 0.3% of patients (American Psychiatric Association 2004). The risk of agranulocytosis (defined as an absolute neutrophil count less than $500/mm^3$) has been estimated at 0.05– 2.0% of patients per year of treatment with clozapine (Buchanan 1995). The risk is highest in

the first 6 months of treatment, and therefore weekly white blood cell (WBC) and neutrophil monitoring is required. After 18 weeks, the monitoring rate may be reduced to every 2– 4 weeks, as the risk of agranulocytosis appears to diminish considerably (an estimated rate of three cases per 1000 patients). WBC counts must remain above 3,000/ mm3 during clozapine treatment, and absolute neutrophil counts must remain above 1,500/ mm^3. With maintenance treatment, patients should be advised to report any sign of infection immediately (e.g., sore throat, fever, weakness or lethargy) (American Psychiatric Association 2004).

Agranulocytosis is the most severe side effect of clozapine and some other FGAs (e.g., chlorprothixen). In rare cases, however, the condition may also occur in association with other antipsychotic medications. During clozapine treatment, WBC count B 2,000/mm^3 or absolute neutrophil count (ANC) B 1,000/mm^3 indicates impending or current agranulocytosis; the clinician should stop clozapine treatment immediately, check WBC and differential counts daily, monitor for signs of infection, and consider bone marrow aspiration and protective isolation if granulopoiesis is deficient. A WBC count of 2,000–3,000/mm^3 or ANC of 1,000–1,500/mm^3 indicates a high risk of agranulocytosis, and the clinician should stop clozapine treatment immediately, check the WBC and differential counts daily, and monitor for signs of infection. If the subsequent WBC count is 3,000–3,500/mm^3 and the ANC is <1,500/mm^3, the WBC count has to be repeated with a differential count twice a week until the WBC count is >3,500/mm^3.

Dermatological and allergic effects

Allergic and dermatological effects, including photosensitivity, occur infrequently but are most common with low-potency phenothiazine medications. Patients should be instructed to avoid excessive sunlight and use sunscreen (American Psychiatric Association 2004).

The most frequent side effects are maculopapular rashes. The skin reactions subside when treated symptomatically, often with continuation of the medication suspected of causing them. Very rarely, severe allergic reactions can occur – for example, exfoliative dermatitis or angioedema. In rare cases following long-term treatment with phenothiazines permanent grey or reddish pigmentation on skin areas usually exposed to light have been observed.

Ophthalmological effects

To prevent pigmentary retinopathies, corneal opacities and cataracts, patients maintained on thioridazine and chlorpromazine should have periodic ophthalmological examinations (approximately every 2 years for patients with a cumulative treatment of more than 10 years), and a maximum dose of 800 mg/day of thioridazine is recommended (American Psychiatric Association 2004). As cataracts were observed in beagles that were given quetiapine, psychiatrists should ask about the quality of distance vision and about blurry vision, and should refer to an ocular evaluation yearly or every 2 years (Marder et al. 2004).

Hyperprolactinemia and sexual dysfunction

Antipsychotics—particularly FGAs, amisulpride and risperidone—can cause hyperprolactinemia by blocking dopamine D2 receptors (Marder et al. 2004; Mota et al. 2003). Hyperprolactinemia can lead to galactorrhoea, menstrual, cyclical and sexual disturbances in women, and reproductive and sexual dysfunction and galactorrhoea/ gynaecomastia in men (Dickson and Glazer 1999). Plasma prolactin concentrations may remain elevated for up to 2 weeks after the cessation of oral therapy with a conventional antipsychotic, and for up to 6 months after cessation of depot therapy (Cutler 2003). Studies of SGAs (with the exception of amisulpride and risperidone) suggested that the transiently elevated prolactin levels tended to return to the normal range within a few days (Marder et al. 2004). Effects on dopaminergic, adrenergic, cholinergic and serotonergic mechanisms may also lead to sexual dysfunction, whereby it is difficult to distinguish between this and disease-related impairment of sexual activity (Baldwin and Birtwistle 1997; Fortier et al. 2000). Peripheral a-adrenergic blockade can be responsible for priapism (Cutler 2003). Of the SGAs, clozapine, olanzapine and ziprasidone were associated with only little or modest prolactin elevation (Cutler 2003). Aripiprazole and quetiapine did not lead to hyperprolactinemia (Arvanitis and Miller 1997) (Shim et al. 2007). A clear association between prolactin elevation and sexual dysfunction has not been established. Rather, besides an increase in prolactin there also has to be a decrease in sexual hormones before a causal link to sexual dysfunction can be drawn (Aizenberg et al. 1995; Kleinberg et al. 1999). There is still an ongoing debate as to whether hyperprolactinemia increases the risk of breast cancer, and the studies are inconclusive to date (Marder et al. 2004). Hyperprolactinemia is suspected to cause osteoporosis if it impairs sex steroid production.

If hyperprolactinemia is suspected in a schizophrenic patient, prolactin levels should be measured and the cause, if not explained by the use of neuroleptic medication, should be determined (e.g., exclusion of a pituitary tumor) (Marder et al. 2004). When antipsychotic-induced hyperprolactinemia is associated with menstrual and sexual dysfunction, consideration should be given to changing the medication to a prolactin-sparing agent. If the signs and symptoms disappear and the prolactin level decreases, an endocrine workup can be avoided. The treatment of choice is a switch of medication and administration of bromocriptine. Gynaecomastia and priapism are rare events.

5. INTERACTIONS AND CONTRAINDICATIONS

Interactions

As with antidepressants, the administration of antipsychotics can lead to numerous interactions when prescribed together with other substances. Such comedications are often unavoidable. However, the physician treating the patient should be familiar with the problems of interaction in order, for example, to be able to adjust the dose of the medication involved accordingly.

Interactions can develop on different levels such as the pharmacodynamic level and on the other side the pharmacokinetic level. Regarding pharmacodynamic interactions the binding receptors and the efficacy as well as the side-effect profile are affected. These interactions are based on agonistic and antagonistic actions of different substances on similarly working receptors and receptor systems. The pharmacodynamic interactions can be of therapeutic advantage. For example, in the case of continuing positive symptoms while treating a patient suffering from schizophrenia with a clozapine monotherapy, the additional administration of amisulpride could be a beneficial and effective choice due to the distinctive antagonistic properties at the dopamine-D2-receptor.

However, also unwanted side-effects can be induced or potentiated, as most psychotropic substances bind to more than one receptor system. The combination of substances with, for example, high affinity on histaminergic receptors can induce or potentiate sedation or weight gain (e.g., the combination of olanzapine and promethazine).

In addition, with applied polypharmacy pharmacokinetic interactions can occur generally relating to the hepatic metabolism of substances. Most drugs are lipophilic substances, which are reabsorbed after glomerular filtration. In order to eliminate external substances more easily, they are metabolized into hydrophilic substances by the liver's phase-I and phase-II reactions, during phase I the mircosomale monooxigenase is of great importance with its inhibitor proteine cytochrome P450. The P450 is not one single enzyme, but a super-genetically coded group of enzymes. The P450 system can be altered by different inhibiting or inducing compounds resulting in an increased or decreased enzyme activity. The often applied mood stabilizer carbamazepine induces the isoenzymes CYP1A2 and CYP3A4. Isoenzyme substrates such as olanzapine (CYP1A2), clozapine (CYP1A2, CYP3A4) or quetiapine (CYP3A4) are then metabolized more rapidly, and efficient plasma levels might not be achieved.

The combination of SSRIs with typical as well as atypical antipsychotics is often performed in daily clinical routine in order to enhance treatment response, especially when negative symptoms are prominent. Well researched and documented is the additional SSRI administration with clozapine. Through the inhibitory property of some SSRIs the plasma level of the active metabolite norclozapin can be increased up to threefold. In this way, the administration is supposed to lead to a satisfying antipsychotic effect with comparatively low dosages and a favorable side-effect profile (Centurio F, Baldisarini AJ, Frankenburg FR, Gando JC; Volpizelli SA, Flott JG 1994: Serum levels of clozapin and norclozapine and its major metabolites: effects of code treatment with fuoxetine or valproate. Am. J. Psychiatry 151:820–822). In this context, fluvoxamine was often applied as inhibitor at the CYP1A2, CYP2C9, CYP2C10 and fluoxetine as inhibitor at CYP2D6 and CYP3A4.

Apart from the fact that the increased efficacy of clozapine and norclozapine respectively could not be confirmed by current data, such an approach also bears significant risks, since the regulation of plasma levels while using enzyme inhibition is hardly calculable. With polypharmacy, next to the inhibition and induction of the mentioned enzymes, there is also the possibility of substrate inhibition. Applying at the same time two similar compounds, metabolized by the same isoenzymes, the metabolization can be hampered causing an elevation of the plasma levels.

Even though treatment guidelines recommend monotherapy, combination therapy is often indispensable in daily clinical routine. For this reason antipsychotics are increasingly administered in combination therapy. Antipsychotics are mainly renally eliminated and are only to a certain degree hepatically metabolized, such as amisulpride or paliperidone. Paliperidone is in the broadest sense the active metabolite of risperidone so that only around 4% of the applied dosages are hepatically metabolized and approximately 60% renally eliminated. Apart from parenteral application, these antipsychotics are of special importance when patients feature different P450 polymorphisms. Several studies showed that around 10% of Europeans have a genetically determined reduced activity of the CYP 2D6 (poor metabolizer), resulting in unwanted side-effects even when low dosages are applied. Around 1% (CYP2D6) of the population are so-called rapid metabolizers. These patients feature an increased enzyme activity which can in turn lead to insufficient plasma levels of drugs metabolized by these isoenzymes.

Another important aspect is the pharmacokinetic interaction in the context of the distribution of the binding potency, such as the competition of binding sites at the plasma proteins. Drugs with a higher affinity to plasma proteins can eliminate drugs with a lower binding potency. This is of special importance when the eliminated drugs only hold a small therapeutic window. For example, if a patient is treated with an anticoagulant (e.g., phenprocoumon) and additionally with an antipsychotic with a high protein affinity (e.g., olanzapine), the anticoagulant can be eliminated out of its protein binding and thereby induce a higher plasma level with the risk of an increased tendency toward hemorrhage. Less importance is given to interactions and secretion, as for example changes in the ph-value or the competition at carrier binding points.

Contraindications

Strict contraindications under neuroleptics are very seldom. In particular intoxication under centrally sedating medications and alcohol, as well as complications in the hematopoietic system, especially agranulocytosis, are among the exceptions. The relative contraindications are based on the interactions between neuroleptics and the receptors of the various transmitter systems and are consequently closely connected to the frequent motor, sedating and anticholinergic side effects of this group of substances.

- With regard to components having anticholinergic effects care must be taken if there is a risk of glaucoma, hypertrophy of the prostate, stenosis in the gastrointestinal area, and previous cerebro-organic damage.
- Regarding components with sympatholytic effects, restrictions in the case of hypotension and cardiac arrhythmias are necessary.
- Due to the lowering of the convulsion threshold, patients suffering from cerebral convulsions should only be given neuroleptica in lower doses, if at all.
- If a substance has antidopaminergic effects, restrictions may also be necessary in patients with Parkinson's disease.

Pregnancy and Lactation

During pregnancy, the risk the primary disorder holds for the mother always has to be weighed against possible pharmacogenic damage to the child (Rohde and Schaefer 2006; Trixler et al. 2005). With regard to mutagenic and teratogenic effects, phenothiazines are the best studied neuroleptics. A prospective study on more than 50,000 pregnant women and their children (among whom were 1309 children whose mothers had taken phenotiazines) showed no evidence of mutagenic or teratogenic effects (Slone et al. 1977). No definite results are available on a possible risk from other neuroleptics, particularly SGAs, can be made, since the studies carried out so far in this regard have been too small (Elia et al. 1987; McKenna et al. 2005).

If antipsychotic treatment is necessary, the minimum effective dose should be used and special attention paid to lowering the dose during the month before delivery or terminating 5–10 days before anticipated delivery (American Psychiatric Association 1997; Working Group for the Canadian Psychiatric Association and the Canadian Alliance for Research on Schizophrenia 1998). Because there is still more experience with FGAs in pregnancy, no advantages of SGAs in this condition has been demonstrated (Gentile 2004). Some high-potency agents appear to be safe (e.g., haloperidol), and they should be used preferentially but as briefly as possible, and the dose should be low enough to avoid EPS and therefore the necessity of antiparkinson medications. Antiparkinson medication should especially be avoided in the first trimester (American Psychiatric Association 1997) and treatment with phenothiazines should not be conducted (Deutsche Gesellschaft für Psychiatrie 1998) After delivery, resumption of the full dose of FGA or SGA has to be considered, because there may be an increased risk of psychosis postpartum (American Psychiatric Association 1997; Working Group for the Canadian Psychiatric Association and the Canadian Alliance for Research on Schizophrenia 1998).

Because antipsychotics can accumulate in breast milk, especially observed with clozapine medication, and based on only sparse literature reports, *breast feeding* could not be recommended for women taking antipsychotic drugs (Gentile 2004). There is consensus among different guidelines to avoid breast feeding during psychotropic treatment of the mother (American Psychiatric Association 1997; Deutsche Gesellschaft für Psychiatrie 1998; Working Group for the Canadian Psychiatric Association and the Canadian Alliance for Research on Schizophrenia 1998).

REFERENCES

1. Adityanjee, Aderibigbe YA, Mathews T. Epidemiology of neuroleptic malignant syndrome. Clin Neuropharmacol 1999; 22: 151–8.
2. Aizenberg D, Zemishlany Z, Weizman A. Cyproheptadine treatment of sexual dysfunction induced by serotonin reuptake inhibitors. Clin Neuropharmacol 1995; 18: 320–4.
3. Al Khatib SM, LaPointe NM, Kramer JM, Califf RM. What clinicians should know about the QT interval. JAMA 2003; 289: 2120–7.
4. Allison DB, Casey DE. Antipsychotic-induced weight gain: a review of the literature. J Clin Psychiatry 2001; 62(Suppl 7): 22–31.
5. Allison DB, Mentore JL, Heo M et al. Antipsychotic-induced weight gain: a comprehensive research synthesis. Am J Psychiatry 1999; 156: 1686–96.
6. Allison DB, Weber MT. Treatment and prevention of obesity: what works, what doesn't work, and what might work. Lipids 2003; 38: 147–55.
7. American Psychiatric Association. Practice guideline for the treatment of patients with schizophrenia. Am J Psychiatry 1997; 154(Suppl 4): 1–63.
8. American Psychiatric Association. Practice guidelines for the treatment of patients with schizophrenia. 2nd ed. Am J Psychiatry 2004; 161(Suppl 2): 1–114.
9. Ananth J. Benzodiazepines: selective administration. J Affect Disord 1987; 13: 99–108.
10. Ananth J, Parameswaran S, Gunatilake S, Burgoyne K, Sidhom T. Neuroleptic malignant syndrome and atypical antipsychotic drugs. J Clin Psychiatry 2004a; 65: 464–70.
11. Ananth J, Venkatesh R, Burgoyne K et al. Atypical antipsychotic induced weight gain: pathophysiology and management. Ann Clin Psychiatry 2004b; 16: 75–85.
12. Anghelescu I, Klawe C, Benkert O. Orlistat in the treatment of psychopharmacologically induced weight gain. J Clin Psychopharmacol 2000; 20: 716–7.
13. Aquila R, Emanuel M. Interventions for weight gain in adults treated with novel antipsychotics. Prim Care Companion J Clin Psychiatry 2000; 2: 20–3.
14. Arvanitis LA, Miller BG. Multiple fixed doses of "Seroquel" (quetiapine) in patients with acute exacerbation of schizophrenia: a comparison with haloperidol and placebo. The Seroquel Trial 13 Study Group. Biol Psychiatry 1997; 42: 233–46.
15. Atmaca M, Kuloglu M, Tezcan E, Ustundag B. Nizatidine treatment and its relationship with leptin levels in patients with olanzapine-induced weight gain. Hum Psychopharmacol 2003; 18: 457–61.
16. Atmaca M, Kuloglu M, Tezcan E, Ustundag B, Kilic N. Nizatidine for the treatment of patients with quetiapine-induced weight gain. Hum Psychopharmacol 2004; 19: 37–40.

17. Awad AH, Shin GS, Rosenbaum AL, Goldberg RL. Autogenous fascia augmentation of a partially extirpated muscle with a subperiosteal medial orbitotomy approach. J AAPOS 1997; 1: 138–42.
18. Baldwin DS, Birtwistle J. Schizophrenia, antipsychotic drugs and sexual function. Prim Care Psychiatry 1997; 3: 117–22.
19. Ball K, Owen N, Salmon J, Bauman A, Gore CJ. Associations of physical activity with body weight and fat in men and women. Int J Obes Relat Metab Disord 2001; 25: 914–9.
20. Baptista T, Hernandez L, Prieto LA, Boyero EC, de Mendoza S. Metformin in obesity associated with antipsychotic drug administration: a pilot study. J Clin Psychiatry 2001; 62: 653–5.
21. Beasley CM Jr, Sanger T, Satterlee W et al. Olanzapine versus placebo: results of a double-blind, fixed-dose olanzapine trial. Psychopharmacology (Berl) 1996; 124: 159–67.
22. Bilder RM, Goldman RS, Volavka J et al. Neurocognitive effects of clozapine, olanzapine, risperidone, and haloperidol in patients with chronic schizophrenia or schizoaffective disorder. Am J Psychiatry 2002; 159: 1018–28.
23. Birt J. Management of weight gain associated with antipsychotics. Ann Clin Psychiatry 2003; 15: 49–58.
24. Bollini P, Pampallona S, Orza MJ, Adams ME, Chalmers TC. Antipsychotic drugs: is more worse? A meta-analysis of the published randomized control trials. Psychol Med 1994; 24: 307–16.
25. Borovicka MC, Fuller MA, Konicki PE et al. Phenylpropanolamine appears not to promote weight loss in patients with schizophrenia who have gained weight during clozapine treatment. J Clin Psychiatry 2002; 63: 345–8.
26. Braude WM, Barnes TR, Gore SM. Clinical characteristics of akathisia. A systematic investigation of acute psychiatric inpatient admissions. Br J Psychiatry 1983; 143: 139–50.
27. Buchanan N, Sharpe C. Clonazepam withdrawal in 13 patients with active epilepsy and drug side effects. Seizure 1994; 3: 271–5.
28. Buchanan RW. Clozapine: efficacy and safety. Schizophr Bull 1995; 21: 579–91.
29. Bushe C, Holt R. Prevalence of diabetes and impaired glucose tolerance in patients with schizophrenia. Br J Psychiatry 2004; (Suppl 47): S67–71.
30. Bushe C, Leonard B. Association between atypical antipsychotic agents and type 2 diabetes: review of prospective clinical data. Br J Psychiatry 2004; (Suppl 47):S87–93.
31. Bustillo JR, Lauriello J, Parker K et al. Treatment of weight gain with fluoxetine in olanzapine-treated schizophrenic outpatients. Neuropsychopharmacology 2003; 28: 527–9.
32. Caroff SN, Mann SC, Keck PE Jr, Francis A. Residual catatonic state following neuroleptic malignant syndrome. J Clin Psychopharmacol 2000; 20: 257–9.
33. Casey DE, Carson WH, Saha AR et al. Switching patients to aripiprazole from other antipsychotic agents: a multicenter randomized study. Psychopharmacology (Berl) 2003; 166: 391–9.
34. Cavazzoni P, Tanaka Y, Roychowdhury SM, Breier A, Allison DB. Nizatidine for prevention of weight gain with olanzapine: a double-blind placebo-controlled trial. Eur Neuropsychopharmacol 2003; 13: 81–5.
35. Centorrino F, Eakin M, Bahk WM et al. Inpatient antipsychotic drug use in 1998, 1993, and 1989. Am J Psychiatry 2002; 159: 1932–5.
36. Cheer SM, Wagstaff AJ. Quetiapine. A review of its use in the management of schizophrenia. CNS Drugs 2004; 18: 173–99.
37. Cookson IB. The effects of a 50% reduction of cis(z)-flupenthixol decanoate in chronic schizophrenic patients maintained on a high dose regime. Int Clin Psychopharmacol 1987; 2: 141–9.
38. Correa N, Opler LA, Kay SR, Birmaher B. Amantadine in the treatment of neuroendocrine side effects of neuroleptics. J Clin Psychopharmacol 1987; 7: 91–5.
39. Correll CU, Leucht S, Kane JM. Lower risk for tardive dyskinesia associated with second-generation antipsychotics: a systematic review of 1-year studies. Am J Psychiatry 2004; 161: 414–25.

40. Csernansky JG, Tacke U, Rusen D, Hollister LE. The effect of benzodiazepines on tardive dyskinesia symptoms. J Clin Psychopharmacol 1988; 8: 154–5.

41. Cutler AJ. Sexual dysfunction and antipsychotic treatment. Psychoneuroendocrinology 2003; 28(Suppl 1): 69–82.

42. Davis JM, Janicak PG, Sakkas P, Gilmore C, Wang Z. Electroconvulsive therapy in the treatment of the neuroleptic malignant syndrome. Convuls Ther 1991; 7: 111–20.

43. De Hert M, Dekker J, Wood D, Kahl K, Möller HJ. Cardiovascular disease and diabetes in people with severe mental illness: position statement from the European Psychiatric Association (EPA), supported by the European Association for the Study of Diabetes (EASD) and the European Society of Cardiology (ESC). J Euro Psychiatry 2009; in press.

44. Deberdt W, Winokur A, Cavazzoni PA et al. Amantadine for weight gain associated with olanzapine treatment. Eur Neuropsychopharmacol 2005; 15: 13–21.

45. Deutsche Gesellschaft für Psychiatrie PuND. Deutsche G (ed). Praxisleitlinien in der Psychiatrie und Psychotherapie. Band 1, Behandlungsleitlinie Schizophrenia ed. 1998.

46. Dickson RA, Glazer WM. Hyperprolactinemia and male sexual dysfunction. J Clin Psychiatry 1999; 60: 125.

47. Dinan T, Peveler R, Holt R. Understanding schizophrenia and diabetes. Hosp Med 2004; 65: 485–8.

48. Dursun SM, Devarajan S. Clozapine weight gain, plus topiramate weight loss. Can J Psychiatry 2000; 45: 198.

49. Elia J, Katz IR, Simpson GM. Teratogenicity of psychotherapeutic medications. Psychopharmacol Bull 1987; 23: 531–86.

50. Emsley R, Berwaerts J, Eerdekens M et al. Efficacy and safety of oral paliperidone extended-release tablets in the treatment of acute schizophrenia: pooled data from three 52-week open-label studies. Int Clin Psychopharmacol 2008; 23: 343–56.

51. Fenton WS. Prevalence of spontaneous dyskinesia in schizophrenia. J Clin Psychiatry 2000; 61(Suppl 4):10–4.

52. Fleischhacker WW, Roth SD, Kane JM. The pharmacologic treatment of neuroleptic-induced akathisia. J Clin Psychopharmacol 1990; 10: 12–21.

53. Floris M, Lejeune J, Deberdt W. Effect of amantadine on weight gain during olanzapine treatment. Eur Neuropsychopharmacol 2001; 11: 181–2.

54. Fortier AH, Grella DK, Nelson BJ, Holaday JW. RESPONSE: re: antiangiogenic activity of prostate-specific antigen. J Natl Cancer Inst 2000; 92: 345A–346.

55. Gentile S. Clinical utilization of atypical antipsychotics in pregnancy and lactation. Ann Pharmacother 2004; 38: 1265–71.

56. Gerlach J, Rye T, Kristjansen P. Effect of baclofen on tardive dyskinesia. Psychopharmacology (Berl) 1978; 56: 145–51.

57. Gilbert PL, Harris MJ, McAdams LA, Jeste DV. Neuroleptic withdrawal in schizophrenic patients. A review of the literature. Arch Gen Psychiatry 1995; 52: 173–88.

58. Glassman AH, Bigger JT Jr. Antipsychotic drugs: prolonged QTc interval, torsade de pointes, and sudden death. Am J Psychiatry 2001; 158: 1774–82.

59. Glazer WM. Review of incidence studies of tardive dyskinesia associated with typical antipsychotics. J Clin Psychiatry 2000; 61(Suppl 4): 15–20.

60. Goetz CG, Klawans HL. Drug-induced extrapyramidal disorders—a neuropsychiatric interface. J Clin Psychopharmacol 1981; 1: 297–303.

61. Grebb JA. Medication induced movement disorders. In: Kaplan HI, Sadock BJ (eds) Comprehensive Textbook of Psychiatry. New York, Williams & Wilkins, 1995.

62. Green AI, Salomon MS, Brenner MJ, Rawlins K. Treatment of schizophrenia and comorbid substance use disorder. Curr Drug Targets CNS Neurol Disord 2002; 1: 129–39.

63. Gregorakos L, Thomaides T, Stratouli S, Sakayanni E. The use of clonidine in the management of autonomic overactivity in neuroleptic malignant syndrome. Clin Auton Res 2000; 10: 193–6.

64. Gupta S, Masand P. Aripiprazole: review of its pharmacology and therapeutic use in psychiatric disorders. Ann Clin Psychiatry 2004; 16: 155–66.
65. Haddad PM. Antipsychotics and diabetes: review of non-prospective data. Br J Psychiatry Suppl 2004; 47: S80–6.
66. Haddad PM, Anderson IM. Antipsychotic-related QTc prolongation, torsade de pointes and sudden death. Drugs 2002; 62: 1649–71.
67. Harvey PD, Keefe RS. Studies of cognitive change in patients with schizophrenia following novel antipsychotic treatment. Am J Psychiatry 2001; 158: 176–84.
68. Heimberg H, De Vos A, Pipeleers D, Thorens B, Schuit F. Differences in glucose transporter gene expression between rat pancreatic alpha- and beta-cells are correlated to differences in glucose transport but not in glucose utilization. J Biol Chem 1995; 270: 8971–5.
69. Hellewell JS. Oxcarbazepine (Trileptal) in the treatment of bipolar disorders: a review of efficacy and tolerability. J Affect Disord 2002; 72(Suppl 1): S23–34.
70. Jeste DV. Tardive dyskinesia in older patients. J Clin Psychiatry 2000; 61(Suppl 4): 27–32.
71. Kane JM, Woerner M, Sarantakos S. Depot neuroleptics: a comparative review of standard, intermediate, and low-dose regimens. J Clin Psychiatry 1986; 47: 30–3.
72. Kane JM, Woerner M, Weinhold P et al. Epidemiology of tardive dyskinesia. Clin Neuropharmacol 1983; 6: 109–15.
73. Kasper S. Do we need another atypical antipsychotic? Eur Neuropsychopharmacol 2008; 18: S146–S152.
74. Keefe RS, Silva SG, Perkins DO, Lieberman JA. The effects of atypical antipsychotic drugs on neurocognitive impairment in schizophrenia: a review and meta-analysis. Schizophr Bull 1999; 25: 201–22.
75. Killian JG, Kerr K, Lawrence C, Celermajer DS. Myocarditis and cardiomyopathy associated with clozapine. Lancet 1999; 354: 1841–5.
76. Kleinberg DL, Davis JM, de Coster R, Van Baelen B, Brecher M. Prolactin levels and adverse events in patients treated with risperidone. J Clin Psychopharmacol 1999; 19: 57–61.
77. Konitsiotis S, Pappa S, Mantas C, Mavreas V. Levetiracetam in tardive dyskinesia: an open label study. Mov Disord 2006; 21: 1219–21.
78. Koro CE, Fedder DO, L'Italien GJ et al. Assessment of independent effect of olanzapine and risperidone on risk of diabetes among patients with schizophrenia: population based nested case-control study. BMJ 2002; 325: 243.
79. Kutcher S, Williamson P, MacKenzie S, Marton P, Ehrlich M. Successful clonazepam treatment of neuroleptic-induced akathisia in older adolescents and young adults: a double-blind, placebo-controlled study. J Clin Psychopharmacol 1989; 9: 403–6.
80. La Grenade L, Graham D, Trontell A. Myocarditis and cardiomyopathy associated with clozapine use in the United States. N Engl J Med 2001; 345: 224–5.
81. Leucht S, Pitschel-Walz G, Abraham D, Kissling W. Efficacy and extrapyramidal side-effects of the new antipsychotics olanzapine, quetiapine, risperidone, and sertindole compared to conventional antipsychotics and placebo. A meta-analysis of randomized controlled trials. Schizophr Res 1999; 35: 51–68.
82. Lima AR, Weiser KV, Bacaltchuk J, Barnes TR. Anticholinergics for neuroleptic-induced acute akathisia. Cochrane Database Syst Rev 2004; 1: CD003727.
83. Linnoila M, Viukari M, Kietala O. Effect of sodium valproate on tardive dyskinesia. Br J Psychiatry 1976; 129: 114–9.
84. Littrell KH, Hilligoss NM, Kirshner CD, Petty RG, Johnson CG. The effects of an educational intervention on antipsychotic-induced weight gain. J Nurs Scholarsh 2003; 35: 237–41.
85. Lopez-Mato A, Rovner J, Illa G, Vieitez A, Boullosa O. [Randomized, open label study on the use of ranitidine at different doses for the management of weight gain associated with olanzapine administration]. Vertex 2003; 14: 85–96.
86. Lu ML, Lane HY, Lin SK, Chen KP, Chang WH. Adjunctive fluvoxamine inhibits clozapine-related weight gain and metabolic disturbances. J Clin Psychiatry 2004; 65: 766–71.

87. Marder SR, Essock SM, Miller AL et al. Physical health monitoring of patients with schizophrenia. Am J Psychiatry 2004; 161: 1334–49.

88. Marder SR, Fenton W. Measurement and treatment research to improve cognition in schizophrenia: NIMH MATRICS initiative to support the development of agents for improving cognition in schizophrenia. Schizophr Res 2004; 72: 5–9.

89. McCreadie RG, Padmavati R, Thara R, Srinivasan TN. Spontaneous dyskinesia and parkinsonism in never-medicated, chronically ill patients with schizophrenia: 18-month follow-up. Br J Psychiatry 2002; 181: 135–7.

90. McCreadie RG, Srinivasan TN, Padmavati R, Thara R. Extrapyramidal symptoms in unmedicated schizophrenia. J Psychiatr Res 2005; 39: 261–6.

91. McCreadie RG, Thara R, Kamath S et al. Abnormal movements in never-medicated Indian patients with schizophrenia. Br J Psychiatry 1996; 168: 221–6.

92. McGrath JJ, Soares-Weiser KVS. Neuroleptic reduction and/or cessation and neuroleptics as special treatments for tardive dyskinesia (Cochrane Review).The Cochrane Library, Issue 2. Chichester, UK, John Wiley & Sons, Ltd, 2004.

93. McKenna K, Koren G, Tetelbaum M et al. Pregnancy outcome of women using atypical antipsychotic drugs: a prospective comparative study. J Clin Psychiatry 2005; 66: 444–9.

94. Meco G, Fabrizio E, Epifanio A et al. Levetiracetam in tardive dyskinesia. Clin Neuropharmacol 2006; 29: 265–8.

95. Melamed E, Achiron A, Shapira A, Davidovicz S. Persistent and progressive parkinsonism after discontinuation of chronic neuroleptic therapy: an additional tardive syndrome? Clin Neuropharmacol 1991; 14: 273–8.

96. Meltzer HY, Bobo WV, Nuamah IF et al. Efficacy and tolerability of oral paliperidone extended-release tablets in the treatment of acute schizophrenia: pooled data from three 6-week, placebo-controlled studies. J Clin Psychiatry 2008; 69: 817–29.

97. Meltzer HY, McGurk SR. The effects of clozapine, risperidone, and olanzapine on cognitive function in schizophrenia. Schizophr Bull 1999; 25: 233–55.

98. Menza M, Vreeland B, Minsky S et al. Managing atypical antipsychotic-associated weight gain: 12-month data on a multimodal weight control program. J Clin Psychiatry 2004; 65: 471–7.

99. Messer T, Tiltscher C, Schmauss M. [Polypharmacy in the treatment of schizophrenia]. Fortschr Neurol Psychiatr 2006; 74: 377–91.

100. Miller DD. Review and management of clozapine side effects. J Clin Psychiatry 2000; 61(Suppl 8):14–7.

101. Möller HJ. Antidepressive effects of traditional and second generation antipsychotics: a review of the clinical data. Eur Arch Psychiatry Clin Neurosci 2005; 255: 83–93.

102. Möller HJ, Riedel M, Jager M et al. Short-term treatment with risperidone or haloperidol in first-episode schizophrenia: 8-week results of a randomized controlled trial within the German Research Network on Schizophrenia. Int J Neuropsychopharmacol 2008; 11(7): 985–97.

103. Möller HJ, von Zerssen D. Depression in schizophrenia 120. In: Burrows GD, Norman TR, Rubinstein G (eds) Handbook of studies on schizophrenia. Amsterdam Oxford New York, Elsevier, 1986: 183–91.

104. Morgenstern H, Glazer WM. Identifying risk factors for tardive dyskinesia among long-term outpatients maintained with neuroleptic medications. Results of the Yale Tardive Dyskinesia Study. Arch Gen Psychiatry 1993; 50: 723–33.

105. Morrison JA, Cottingham EM, Barton BA. Metformin for weight loss in pediatric patients taking psychotropic drugs. Am J Psychiatry 2002; 159: 655–7.

106. Mota M, Lichiardopol C, Mota E, Panus C, Panus A. Erectile dysfunction in diabetes mellitus. Rom J Intern Med 2003; 41: 163–77.

107. Naber D, Karow A. Good tolerability equals good results: the patient's perspective. Eur Neuropsychopharmacol 2001; 11(Suppl 4): S391–6.

108. Naber D, Lambert M. Aripiprazole: a new atypical antipsychotic with a different pharmacological mechanism. Prog Neuropsychopharmacol Biol Psychiatry 2004; 28: 1213–9.

109. Nair NP, Yassa R, Ruiz-Navarro J, Schwartz G. Baclofen in the treatment of tardive dyskinesia. Am J Psychiatry 1978; 135: 1562–3.

110. Nasrallah HA. Atypical antipsychotic-induced metabolic side effects: insights from receptor-binding profiles. Mol Psychiatry 2008; 13: 27–35.

111. Newcomer JW. Antipsychotic medications: metabolic and cardiovascular risk. J Clin Psychiatry 2007; 68: 8–13.

112. Nisijima K, Ishiguro T. Electroconvulsive therapy for the treatment of neuroleptic malignant syndrome with psychotic symptoms: a report of five cases. J ECT 1999; 15: 158–63.

113. Oehl M, Hummer M, Fleischhacker WW. Compliance with antipsychotic treatment. Acta Psychiatr Scand 2000; 102: 83–6.

114. Pelonero AL, Levenson JL, Pandurangi AK. Neuroleptic malignant syndrome: a review. Psychiatr Serv 1998; 49: 1163–72.

115. Poyurovsky M, Isaacs I, Fuchs C et al. Attenuation of olanzapine-induced weight gain with reboxetine in patients with schizophrenia: a double-blind, placebo-controlled study. Am J Psychiatry 2003; 160: 297–302.

116. Poyurovsky M, Pashinian A, Gil-Ad I et al. Olanzapine-induced weight gain in patients with first-episode schizophrenia: a double-blind, placebo-controlled study of fluoxetine addition. Am J Psychiatry 2002; 159: 1058–60.

117. Poyurovsky M, Tal V, Maayan R et al. The effect of famotidine addition on olanzapine-induced weight gain in first-episode schizophrenia patients: a double-blind placebo-controlled pilot study. Eur Neuropsychopharmacol 2004; 14: 332–6.

118. Pujalte D, Bottai T, Hue B et al. A double-blind comparison of clonazepam and placebo in the treatment of neuroleptic-induced akathisia. Clin Neuropharmacol 1994; 17: 236–42.

119. Purdon SE, Jones BD, Stip E et al. Neuropsychological change in early phase schizophrenia during 12 months of treatment with olanzapine, risperidone, or haloperidol. The Canadian Collaborative Group for research in schizophrenia. Arch Gen Psychiatry 2000; 57: 249–58.

120. Rabinowitz T, Frankenburg FR, Centorrino F, Kando J. The effect of clozapine on saliva flow rate: a pilot study. Biol Psychiatry 1996; 40: 1132–4.

121. Rohde A, Schaefer C. Psychopharmakotherapie in Schwangerschaft und Stilzeit. Möglichkeiten und Grenzen. 2. Aufl ed. Thieme, Stuttgart, 2006.

122. Rupniak NM, Jenner P, Marsden CD. Acute dystonia induced by neuroleptic drugs. Psychopharmacology (Berl) 1986; 88: 403–19.

123. Ryan DH, Espeland MA, Foster GD et al. Look AHEAD (Action for Health in Diabetes): design and methods for a clinical trial of weight loss for the prevention of cardiovascular disease in type 2 diabetes. Control Clin Trials 2003; 24: 610–28.

124. Sacchetti E, Guarneri L, Bravi D. H(2) antagonist nizatidine may control olanzapine-associated weight gain in schizophrenic patients. Biol Psychiatry 2000; 48: 167–8.

125. Sachse J, Koller J, Hartter S, Hiemke C. Automated analysis of quetiapine and other antipsychotic drugs in human blood by high performance-liquid chromatography with column-switching and spectrophotometric detection. J Chromatogr B Analyt Technol Biomed Life Sci 2006; 830: 342–8.

126. Sakkas P, Davis JM, Janicak PG, Wang ZY. Drug treatment of the neuroleptic malignant syndrome. Psychopharmacol Bull 1991; 27: 381–4.

127. Sentissi O, Epelbaum J, Olié JP, Poirier MF. Leptin and ghrelin levels in patients with schizophrenia during different antipsychotics treatment: a review. Schizophr Bull 2008; 34(6): 1189–99.

128. Sharpe JK, Hills AP. Atypical antipsychotic weight gain: a major clinical challenge. Aust N Z J Psychiatry 2003; 37: 705–9.

129. Shim JC, Shin J, Kelly DL et al. Adjunctive treatment with a dopamine partial agonist, aripiprazole, for antipsychotic-induced hyperprolactinemia: a placebo-controlled trial. Am J Psychiatry 2007; 164: 1404–10.

130. Sletten IW, Sundland D, Pichardo J, Viamontes G. Chlorphentermine and phenmetrazine compared: weight reduction, side effects and psychological change. Mo Med 1967; 64: 927–9.

131. Slone D, Siskind V, Heinonen OP et al. Antenatal exposure to the phenothiazines in relation to congenital malformations, perinatal mortality rate, birth weight, and intelligence quotient score. Am J Obstet Gynecol 1977; 128: 486–8.

132. Soares K, Rathbone J, Deeks J. Gamma-aminobutyric acid agonists for neuroleptic-induced tardive dyskinesia. Cochrane Database Syst Rev 2004; Issue 3: CD000203.

133. Soares KV, McGrath JJ. Vitamin E for neuroleptic-induced tardive dyskinesia (Cochrane Review).The Cochrane Library, Issue 2. Chichester, UK, John Wiley & Sons, Ltd, 2000.

134. Soares-Weiser K, Rathbone J. Calcium channel blockers for neuroleptic-induced tardive dyskinesia. Cochrane Database Syst Rev 2004; Issue 4: CD000206.

135. Susman VL. Clinical management of neuroleptic malignant syndrome. Psychiatr Q 2001; 72: 325–36.

136. Tammenmaa IA, Sailas E, McGrath JJ, Soares-Weiser K, Wahlbeck K. Systematic review of cholinergic drugs for neuroleptic-induced tardive dyskinesia: a meta-analysis of randomized controlled trials. Prog Neuropsychopharmacol Biol Psychiatry 2004; 28: 1099–07.

137. Tandon R, Belmaker RH, Gattaz WF et al. World Psychiatric Association Pharmacopsychiatry Section statement on comparative effectiveness of antipsychotics in the treatment of schizophrenia. Schizophr Res 2008; 100: 20–38.

138. Thaker GK, Tamminga CA, Alphs LD et al. Brain gamma-aminobutyric acid abnormality in tardive dyskinesia. Reduction in cerebrospinal fluid GABA levels and therapeutic response to GABA agonist treatment. Arch Gen Psychiatry 1987; 44: 522–9.

139. Trixler M, Gati A, Fekete S, Tenyi T. Use of antipsychotics in the management of schizophrenia during pregnancy. Drugs 2005; 65: 1193–06.

140. Tschoner A, Engl J, Laimer M et al. Metabolic side effects of antipsychotic medication. Int J Clin Pract 2007; 61: 1356–70.

141. Umbricht D, Flury H, Bridler R. Cognitive behavior therapy for weight gain. Am J Psychiatry 2001; 158: 971.

142. Velligan DI, Newcomer J, Pultz J et al. Does cognitive function improve with quetiapine in comparison to haloperidol? Schizophr Res 2002; 53: 239–48.

143. Walker P, Soares KVS. Benzodiazepines for neuroleptic-induced tardive dyskinesia (Cochrane Review).The Cochrane Library, Issue 2. Chichester, UK, John Wiley & Sons, 2004.

144. Wang HC, Hsieh Y. Treatment of neuroleptic malignant syndrome with subcutaneous apomorphine monotherapy. Mov Disord 2001; 16: 765–7.

145. Warner B, Alphs L, Schaedelin J, Koestler T. Clozapine and sudden death. Lancet 2000; 355: 842.

146. Weber SS, Dufresne RL, Becker RE, Mastrati P. Diazepam in tardive dyskinesia. Drug Intell Clin Pharm 1983; 17: 523–7.

147. Weiden PJ, Daniel DG, Simpson G, Romano SJ. Improvement in indices of health status in outpatients with schizophrenia switched to ziprasidone. J Clin Psychopharmacol 2003; 23: 595–600.

148. Werneke U, Taylor D, Sanders TA, Wessely S. Behavioural management of antipsychotic-induced weight gain: a review. Acta Psychiatr Scand 2003; 108: 252–9.

149. Wirshing DA, Boyd JA, Meng LR et al.. The effects of novel antipsychotics on glucose and lipid levels. J Clin Psychiatry 2002a; 63: 856–5.

150. Wirshing DA, Boyd JA, Pierre JM et al. Delusions associated with quetiapine-related weight redistribution. J Clin Psychiatry 2002b; 63: 247–8.

151. Wirshing DA, Wirshing WC, Kysar L et al. Novel antipsychotics: comparison of weight gain liabilities. J Clin Psychiatry 1999; 60: 358–63.

152. Woods SW, Saksa JR, Baker CB, Cohen SJ, Tek C. Effects of levetiracetam on tardive dyskinesia: a randomized, double-blind, placebo-controlled study. J Clin Psychiatry 2008; 69: 546–54.

153. Working group for the Canadian Psychiatric Association and the Canadian Alliance for Research on Schizophrenia. Canadian clinical practice guidelines for the treatment of schizophrenia. Can J Psychiatry 1998; 43(Suppl 2): 25–40.

154. Zimbroff DL, Kane JM, Tamminga CA et al. Controlled, dose-response study of sertindole and haloperidol in the treatment of schizophrenia. Sertindole Study Group. Am J Psychiatry 1997; 154: 782–91.

155. Zimmermann U, Kraus T, Himmerich H, Schuld A, Pollmacher T. Epidemiology, implications and mechanisms underlying drug-induced weight gain in psychiatric patients. J Psychiatr Res 2003; 37: 193-220.

20 Rehabilitation in schizophrenia: Social skills training and cognitive remediation

Joseph Ventura and Lisa H Guzik

SKILLS TRAINING AND COGNITIVE REMEDIATION INTERVENTIONS

In recent years, the conceptualization of schizophrenia has expanded beyond symptom control and relapse prevention. Current research shows that strides have been made in promoting recovery from schizophrenia. Newer skills training and cognitive rehabilitation treatment approaches are framed in a positive light that are grounded in a *recovery* rather than *deficit* model. This new emphasis is on the factors associated with improved quality of life, such as the ability to enjoy social and familial interactions, advance in educational endeavors, and/or perform well at work. This conceptual framework is fully consistent with the President's New Freedom Commission on Mental Health and is designed to instill both participants and clinicians with hope. The underlying theoretical framework comes from a developmental neuroscience perspective, which supports the idea that the brain is capable of change and development throughout the lifespan. Most cognitive interventions are based, in principle, on the large literature supporting the concept of brain plasticity and neurogenesis. Cognitive science purports that skill development can occur at any age and can help advance or restore the brain's capacity for improved cognitive or social performance. Learning in a properly stimulating environment can help the patient capitalize on brain malleability and improve functioning. There is wide acceptance that patients with schizophrenia are severely impaired in fundamental domains of neurocognitive functioning including executive control, attention, working memory, and declarative learning and memory. These deficits are severe, generally ranging from 1 to 2 standard deviations below healthy comparison groups, and are present even in first episode patients who are neuroleptic naive (1, 2). There has been increasing recognition that these core cognitive deficits have important implications for everyday functioning in schizophrenia and therefore are potentially appropriate targets for remediation (3, 4). Major initiatives are under way to find new nonpharmacological treatment interventions for cognitive impairment in schizophrenia that aim to improve functional outcomes. In recent years, theoretical frameworks to guide interventions, improved scientific methods for conducting research, and evidence supporting their effectiveness have emerged. These advances in the field have resulted in an increased optimism about the effectiveness of social skills training (SST) and cognitive remediation as interventions (5, 6).

SOCIAL SKILLS TRAINING (SST)

Individuals with schizophrenia exhibit uncommonly high rates of social skills impairments. These impairments are thought to be associated with poor premorbid learning history, limited environmental stimulation or isolation, psychiatric symptoms, and the loss of skill due to repeated hospitalizations. Over the past three decades, a variety of SST approaches have been developed for people with schizophrenia to address impairments in social skills. Accordingly, SST programs for schizophrenia patients have been developed based largely on behavioral therapy principles and techniques. Trainers use active teaching methods that include didactic instruction, modeling, behavior rehearsal, coaching of desired responses, corrective feedback, contingent social reinforcement, and homework assignments to facilitate the acquisition of the new skills. Performance reviews and positive reinforcements are an integral part of the lesson formatting. The term "skills" implies that social skills are largely based on learning experiences, as opposed to innate talent. Although skills training programs vary widely in content, duration, and the setting in which the training is delivered, they share a common set of strategies for teaching skills including goal setting, role modeling, role playing, behavioral rehearsal, positive reinforcement, corrective feedback, and homework assignments. SST aims to build social competence, conceived as the full range of human social behavior and performance including verbal and nonverbal behavior, as well as paralinguistic behavior, accurate social perception, proper understanding of social situations as to allow for appropriate responses that meet social expectations such as assertiveness, conversational skills, skills related to management of a mental condition, as well as the ability to show emotion that is contextually appropriate. A fundamental and common goal for skills training is to promote generalization to community functioning. Strengthening social skills and social competence has been viewed as a protective factor in the Vulnerability-Stress-Protective factors model of schizophrenia, because social skills and social competence can help minimize the "harmful" effects of cognitive deficits, neurobiological vulnerability, stressful life events, and social maladjustment (6–8).

Although the application of skills training to populations with deficits calls for various instructional methods, the core feature of all skills training remains the same. Patients are taught to perform component cognitive and behavioral responses sequentially, gradually combining simpler behaviors into more complex reactions. Repeated practice or overlearning is essential to ensure assimilation and duration of interpersonal use. A key principle is that observable behaviors are more accessible to therapeutic intervention, and are therefore more readily acquired than covert cognitions and emotions. Group therapy is the principal modality for the delivery of SST. Training patients in a group, as opposed to individually, is more cost effective, and has a greater chance of success because of the cohesion established among the participants, the ability of peers serve as models for change, the opportunity for self-help, and a context for real-life experiences and efforts at problem solving. Groups usually involve 4–12 patients and are typically led by 1–2 therapists. Patients who complete a skills training program can act as training aides, sharing their knowledge with the new trainees. Sessions are conducted for 45–90 minutes and meet 1–5 times per week. Training is typically presented in a nonstigmatizing fashion as education, so that the patients are able to tell their family and friends that they are attending a class in human relations or community life. In this way patients can list their training experiences on their resumes as an educational accomplishment with the academic or social agency listed as the sponsor. SST is often delivered over long periods of time to allow for patients to reach specific personal goals at their own pace (6–8).

The results from several studies indicate that the effect of SST is strongest on those outcomes such as the mastery of skills that are taught directly in SST groups. The next strongest effect has been observed on the skills measured by performance-based measures of social and independent living skill and psychosocial functioning, and then negative symptoms. Apparently, the impact of SST was the weakest on the domains that are furthest from the direct experience of the training, which is, psychotic relapse, followed by small effects on other symptoms. Considering all of these findings, there is evidence of generalization of SST interventions, from the training group setting to the more complex domains of daily functioning. In addition, there is some evidence to indicate SST helps patients with schizophrenia achieve personal goals through practicing effective behaviors, when combined with abundant social reinforcement that may bolster self-efficiency and the willingness or desire to use these skills at least in some patients (6–8).

Robert P. Liberman, MD, a psychiatrist and Professor, in the UCLA Department of Psychiatry, has come to be known as the "Grandfather" of psychiatric rehabilitation. Professor Liberman developed a modular approach to social and independent living skills with these goals in mind. Skills training modules have been developed in the areas of community re-entry, medication and symptom management, conversation skills, grooming, and recreation/leisure. The modular procedures designed to compensate for cognitive and learning disabilities by presenting information in a highly structured format, using frequent repetition of new material, auditory and visual presentation of the material, and verbal reinforcement for attention and participation. Trainers use a combination of techniques including focused instructions, video modeling of skills, and behavior rehearsal with immediate positive feedback, overlearning, cognitive restructuring, and generalization planning. These techniques are used to overcome patients' apathy, distractibility, poor memory, and deficient problem-solving ability. Training in a specific skill area continues until each patient achieves the mastery criterion of 80 percent of the knowledge and skill presented in the lesson, as determined by behavioral role-play tests. The modules come with a manual for the group trainer, videotapes, and patient workbooks. The SST modules have been successfully used by a broad array of professionals, and paraprofessionals in the United States and around the world with evidence of clinical efficacy. These methods have been applied in individual and group formats to improve schizophrenia patients' self-care, social, and independent living skills in hospital, clinic, and residential settings. In addition, the behavioral learning principles used in skills training, such as shaping modeling, behavioral rehearsal, prompting, reinforcement, and in vivo homework assignments have been effectively used in teaching communication and problem-solving skills to families of patients with schizophrenia (6–8).

The effectiveness of psychosocial skills training has been evaluated by assessing skill acquisition (learning and demonstration of skills), maintenance (ability to exhibit the skill continuously over time), and generalization (using the skill effectively across situations or environments), as well as through other outcome variables related to overall social functioning, symptom level, and quality of life. Studies have consistently shown the lack of a significant relationship between the effect of the treatment and characteristics such as patients' gender, number of psychiatric hospitalizations, and months of prior inpatient care. Other variables, such as patients' premorbid social competence, illness subtype, and comorbidity have not been sufficiently explored enough for any firm conclusions to be made (6–8).

The 1995 PORT review of randomized clinical trials evaluated the impact of psychosocial skills training methods on schizophrenia patients' social functioning, psychiatric symptoms, and resistance to relapse. Two subsequent analysis of this literature (one narrative, and one a meta-analysis) have appeared since the PORT findings, and have derived conclusions that are consistent and can be summarized as follows:

1. Patients with schizophrenia can be taught a wide range of social and instrumental skills, from simple behaviors such as gazing and reciprocity during conversations, to more complex and involved behaviors such as assertiveness, conversational skills, and medication self-management.

2. SST programs have a positive effect on patients' perceptions of themselves as more assertive and less socially anxious after treatment. Skills training has only a moderate impact on psychiatric symptoms, relapse, and rehospitalization.
3. Skills training appears to generalize well to measures and settings similar to training situations, but less consistently to more novel environments.
4. Despite some evidence that trained skills can be maintained over time few studies have addressed the question of long-term treatment question.

In response to these findings and the concern that skills training does not generalize, community supports have been explicitly designed to help participants transfer newly learned skills from a training environment to real world settings (6–8). One example known as "In Vivo Amplified Skills Training" (IVAST) utilizes specialized case managers who facilitate opportunities in the community for patients to use newly acquired skills. The community based informal interactions help them adapt their behaviors to their own environment, and practice and implement the skills they have adapted. The case manager acts to offer encouragement and reinforcement as well as softening the obstacles that might hinder a patient's ability to use the skill. Evaluations of IVAST have reported that participants with the extra support achieved higher levels of interpersonal problem-solving skills, significantly greater social adjustment, and better quality of life over a 2 year period than patients who only received the skills training (9).

In the last decade neurocognition in patients with schizophrenia has been extensively studied, and it has been found that certain cognitive impairments are considered to be traits in most individuals with schizophrenia. Accordingly it comes as little surprise that cognitive functioning has often been thought to impact how much a patient is capable of learning. However, there has been evidence showing that cognitive functioning and learning interact in complex ways. Learning is not just the result of intelligence, but motivation is also a factor. Skills training used to teach increasingly complex problem solving tasks has resulted in significant improvements in both success in solving problems and community functioning. Cognitive factors have been known to explain a moderate portion of the variance in the relationship between neurocognition with social functioning (10). However, the prediction of social or vocational performance by cognitive functioning cannot be fully explained by neurocognition. Social factors such as social cognition (as perception of emotion), social competence, and social support have been shown to mediate the relationship between neurocognition and functioning (11). These types of social cognitive factors are related concepts and skills taught in skills training for people with schizophrenia (6).

Although results from recent studies suggest that long periods of coordinated skills-based treatment are useful for subjects with chronic schizophrenia, many questions remain regarding the form and content of this treatment. Should treatment be delivered intensively followed by longer periods of less intensive therapy or should intensity remain constant? Should skills training be presented in a particular order, or can patients be assigned to intervention without regard to sequence? Here is what is known. Based on three decades of research the model patient is a young white man whose history of mental illness spans a decade or longer. Usually, the patient is a high school graduate, an armed services veteran, unemployed, and has no recent history of drug or alcohol problems. Usually such an individual achieves modest clinical gains while in the social skills program. Training programs with younger age individuals produced better effects. Beyond these general features, no patient characteristics other than cognitive processing impairments have been consistently associated with success or failure in skills training programs. In very different versions behavioral skills training have proven effective in acutely ill inpatients, persistent psychotic patients, individuals in the sub-acute phase of illness, and those with severe and persistent forms of schizophrenia. Most patients are able to learn to new skills if the content, form, and duration of training are adjusted to match their stress tolerance or information processing limits or both. Accordingly clinicians should consider how general skills training procedures could be adapted to match a particular patient's profile of symptoms, skills deficits, learning impairments, and motivational characteristics (6–8).

UNIQUE APPLICATIONS OF SKILLS TRAINING

Conducting skills training with family members present in the home can directly influence family communication and problem solving that can result in reductions in the stress inducing "emotional temperature" often found in families dealing with an ill family member. When family members understand the skills being learned by their mentally ill relative, they can encourage and reinforce those skills when they are used in the home setting. To this end one study examining Latino families trained patients on illness management skills. In addition, family members were taught how to provide opportunities and encouragement for their ill relatives to implement behavioral assignments related to the skills learned in the clinic. The leaders of the SST groups taught the family members' ways to encourage and reward generalization during home visits and multifamily sessions at the clinic. Participants learned the skills, transferred them to their living environments, and maintained their use for at least 6 months after training which was the duration of study follow-up. Moreover, there were fewer hospitalizations for individuals in the disease management program during the 9 months of the study, and 1 year later than for those receiving usual care alone (7).

Skills training for increasingly complex problem solving tasks have resulted in significant improvements in both success in solving problems and neurocognitive functioning. In addition, the predication of social or vocational performance by cognitive functioning is largely explained by the mediation of knowledge related to the social or vocational tasks and the patients. Along similar lines, treatment refractory patients with thought disorder and high levels of distractibility have been viewed as poor candidates for SST. Recent advances in training sustained attention have allowed this subset of patients to be considered as candidates for SST, and accordingly have been able to improve their conversational ability. In this approach basic attention skills were taught through repetition in discrete trials where behavioral learning responses were used to help elicit correct responses. Another approach used tokens and praise to reinforce gradually increasing durations of attention while the patients were learning the skills (8).

COGNITIVE REMEDIATION

Cognitive Remediation (CR) attempts to improve and/or restore cognitive functioning using a range of approaches. Recent cognitive remediation approaches that aim for improvements in cognitive performance are framed as educational and are grounded in a *recovery* rather than *deficit* model. Bottom-up approaches start by remediation of basic neurocognitive skills, such as attention, and advance to more complex skills, such as problem solving. In contrast, top-down approaches use more complex skills to improve individual components of neurocognition (12). In addition, there are two primary approaches to interventions for neuropsychological deficits, compensatory and restorative, each representing different theoretical orientations and cognitive remediation methods. Compensatory, as compared to restorative approaches, emphasize situational and environmental adaptations and are designed to circumvent residual neurocognitive deficits to improve community functioning. The underlying theoretical framework from restorative approaches comes from a developmental neuroscience perspective that is based on human cognitive development theory supporting the idea that the brain is capable of change and development throughout the lifespan (13, 14).

Cognitive Adaptive Training (CAT) has applied compensatory strategies to individuals with schizophrenia and was developed by Dawn Velligan and colleagues. CAT is delivered in an individualized training program that includes adjunctive supports, e.g., checklists, and adaptive equipment, for example signs, that are designed to cue and sequence adaptive behaviors. CAT is based on the idea that impairments in executive functioning lead to problems in initiating and/or inhibiting appropriate behaviors. Using behavioral principles such as antecedent control, environments are set-up to cue appropriated behaviors, discourage distraction and maintain goal directed activity. In addition, adaptations are customized for specific cognitive strategies or limitations in attention memory, and fine motor control, e.g., changing the color of a sign frequently to capture attention, using Velcro closures instead of buttons for a person with fine-motor problems. Examples of CAT interventions includes signs asking, "Did I take my medication today?" placed on the back of the front door, medication containers with alarms to cue taking medication at specific times, reorganization of closets to prevent soiled or inappropriate clothing from being worn, money management of job-hunting notebooks, and checklists reminding the individual to perform specific grooming or leisure task. CAT has been shown to improve adherence to medication, community functioning, and rate of relapse for individuals with schizophrenia. Large effect sizes have been found for improvements in functioning and medication adherence with CAT relative to control and treatment as usual conditions. Recent evidence suggests that environmental adaptations are highly likely to be used in a comprehensive program such as CAT in which supports are individualized and set-up in the patient's home environment. Supports are less likely to be used when they are generic and given to patients in the clinic rather than on home visits (14, 15).

Although several independent cognitive remediation programs have been developed, most cognitive remediation interventions are based in principle on the large literature supporting the concept of brain plasticity and neurogenesis. Cognitive remediation by nature purports that learning can occur at any age and can help improve or restore the brain's capacity for improved cognitive performance. These types of techniques have been used for years in the rehabilitation of individuals who have had physical injuries, such as head injuries, or those with developmental disability. One restorative approach that has been successful with schizophrenia patients involves the use of computer based software training delivered in a group setting. The Neuropsychological Educational Approach to Remediation (NEAR) was developed by Alice Medalia and is based on the educational software programs developed for training cognitive skills of children and adolescents in educational settings. The NEAR approach, promotes intrinsic motivation in patients by allowing task engagement and choice. The conceptual model emphases a top-down approach that develops higher-order, strategy-based methods of learning over drill-and-practice exercises as compared to learning of fundamental cognitive skills (bottom-up). Training involves participation in computer-based cognitive exercises (e.g., computer games such as "Where in the USA is Carmen San Diego?") that are designed to be enjoyable, engaging, and intrinsically motivating. These methods have been effective in the treatment of cognitive deficits because they combine computer-based technologies, the teaching of cognitive strategies, and learning principles from the field of education (16–18).

Another unique method of cognitive remediation, Neurocognitive Enhancement Therapy (NET), used by Morris Bell and colleagues subscribes to a restorative philosophy through the use of cognitive remediation programs developed for traumatic brain injured patients delivered thorough repeated drill-and-practice in the context of work rehabilitation (19). This program uses computerized software programs targeting attention, memory, including working memory, verbal memory, and executive skills. Training begins with relatively simple exercises and proceeds to more complex ones involving time delays (20).

Similarly, Cognitive Remediation Therapy (CRT) used by Til Wykes and colleagues focuses on teaching patients to develop their own individualized set of problem-solving strategies. The individually delivered training program targets deficits in executive process including cognitive flexibility, working memory, and planning. The program uses paper-and-pencil exercises for training, begins with simper tasks and proceeds to more difficult ones, and emphasizes teaching through procedural learning, scaffolding, and errorless learning (12).

Yet another cognitive remediation method, Cognitive Enhancement Therapy (CET) developed by Gerald Hogarty and colleagues, is a comprehensive rehabilitation program designed to enhance abstraction of social themes and alter cognitive schemas for individuals who have a recent onset of schizophrenia that suggests the disturbance in neurodevelopment results in delays in social cognition. Social cognitive milestones such as perspective taking are the focus of treatment. Computer-based cognitive exercises focus on attention, memory, and problem-solving abilities. In addition, participants attend a social-cognitive training group. Social interaction is emphasized through out the treatment and even the computer sessions are conducted in pairs of patients who assist one another by suggesting strategies and offering encouragement (21).

These cognitive remediation techniques are showing promise in remediation the core deficits in schizophrenia that are proposed to interfere with important aspects of community functioning, such as interacting with friends and family, attending school, or working. Effect sizes for improvements in specific training exercises generally have been large, with more moderate effect sizes for other cognitive outcomes and improvements in community functioning. A recent meta-analysis of 27 studies in the field reported that participation in clinic-based cognitive remediation was associated with a .41 effect size, indicating moderate improvement in cognition for patients with schizophrenia. This meta-analysis also found that cognitive remediation has a medium range effect of .35 on psychosocial functioning and small effect of size of .28 on symptoms (5). For six of seven cognitive domains the effect sizes ranged from 0.39 to 0.54, with verbal working memory, a potentially fundamental component of cognition, showing a moderate effect size of 0.52. Follow-up studies have shown that the effects, especially when combined with strategy coaching, appear to be durable (5, 20, 22). In addition, studies that involved follow-up of cognitive remediation patients indicate that the effects of remediation can be durable and can generalize to improvement in social and work outcomes in chronic schizophrenia patients (20, 22, 23). In fact, there is some evidence that even markedly severe cognitive deficits can be partially normalized by existing treatments (24). These studies conducted with chronic schizophrenia patients provide some evidence that the effects of cognitive remediation are robust, durable, and appear to have real world implications for improving the lives of the participants.

Although the mechanisms of action for successful cognitive remediation programs are not yet known, some investigators have suggested several critical components of effective cognitive remediation. Wykes and colleagues credit the use of procedural learning, principles of errorless learning, and targeted reinforcement in an individualized approach for improving memory and problem-solving skills (12). Medalia et al. believes that the key principle to facilitating both generalization and durability of patient gains from cognitive remediation is to incorporate proven educational learning principles that teach fundamental problem-solving strategies such as concept formation, reasoning, and planning. According to Medalia and colleagues, the computer-based tasks they used were designed to promote intrinsic rather than extrinsic motivation, proposing that the effectiveness of cognitive remediation procedures depends largely on patients' perception of the tasks as inherently interesting, engaging, and relevant to real-world functioning. Intrinsic motivation, active learning, and task engagement were all promoted through patient involvement in the nonessential aspects of the learning environment, the multisensory presentation of software programs, and personalizing the learning material. Strategy coaching involves helping the patient consolidate the cognitive strategies learned from working with the computer programs, e.g., chunking of information, organizing objects according to a category. In fact, strategy coaching was associated with increases in verbal memory. In addition, the effects appear to generalize to community functioning, even if only for patients who achieve a threshold of improved performance (20, 22, 23, 25).

SUMMARY AND FUTURE DIRECTIONS FOR SKILLS TRAINING AND COGNITIVE REMEDIATION

Advances in the field of psychiatric rehabilitation have resulted in greater effectiveness than in the past using behavioral treatments to promote the recovery of people with schizophrenia. Depending on the type of rehabilitation program, improvements have been found in a wide range of outcomes, including improved cognition, independent living skills, and social adjustment. Although there is no consensus regarding which approach at rehabilitation is best for particular patients, the importance of an adequate amount of training of therapists conducting rehabilitation and motivational factors are important factors for maximizing outcomes. Further improvements in implementing, understanding, and developing more comprehensive SST and cognitive remediation programs are needed so that an improved quality of life can be reached. Achieving goals in line with newer models of recovery from schizophrenia will require closer integration of SST and cognitive remediation with mainstream hospital and community programs. Recent research suggests that cognitive remediation programs are successful because they are embedded in comprehensive rehabilitation programs where the skills training or cognitive exercises are used in combination with psychosocial groups or work rehabilitation programs. As with other evidence-based treatments for schizophrenia, the greatest challenge to moving the field forward is the slow pace of dissemination and adoption by private clinicians and nonacademic systems of service. Increased success will likely be seen in the coming years for the diffusion of SST into customary, clinical settings for the treatment of schizophrenia. Charting future direction for SST and cognitive remediation is an absolute must for ensuring that these approaches remain vital and inseminated with new ideas.

REFERENCES

1. Bilder RM, Goldman RS, Robinson D et al. Neuropsychology of first-episode schizophrenia: initial characterization and clinical correlates. Am J Psychiatry 2000; 157: 549–59.
2. Keefe RS, Mohs RC, Bilder RM et al. Neurocognitive assessment in the Clinical Antipsychotic Trials of Intervention Effectiveness (CATIE) project schizophrenia trial: development, methodology, and rationale. Schizophr Bull 2003; 29(1): 45–55.
3. Carpenter WT. Clinical constructs and therapeutic discovery. Schizophr Res 2004; 72(1): 69–73.

4. Gold JM. Cognitive deficits as treatment targets in schizophrenia. Schizophr Res 2004; 72(1): 21–8.
5. McGurk SR, Twamley EW, Sitzer DI, McHugo GJ, Mueser KT. A meta-analysis of cognitive remediation in schizophrenia. Am J Psychiatry 2007; 164(12): 1791.
6. Kurtz MM, Mueser KT. A meta-analysis of controlled research on social skills training for schizophrenia. J Consult Clin Psychol 2008; 76(3): 491–504.
7. Kopelowicz A, Liberman RP, Zarate R. Recent advances in social skills training for schizophrenia. Schizophr Bull 2006; 32(Suppl 1): S12–23.
8. Silverstein SM, Spaulding WD, Menditto AA et al. Attention shaping: a reward-based learning method to enhance skills training outcomes in schizophrenia. Schizophr Bull 2009; 35(1): 222–32.
9. Glynn SM, Marder SR, Liberman RP et al. Supplementing clinic-based skills training with manual-based community support sessions: effects on social adjustment of patients with schizophrenia. Am J Psychiatry 2002; 159(5): 829–37.
10. Green MF, Kern RS, Braff DL, Mintz J. Neurocognitive deficits and functional outcome in schizophrenia: are we measuring the "right stuff"? Schizophr Bull 2000; 26(1): 119–36.
11. Brekke J, Kay DD, Lee KS, Green MF. Biosocial pathways to functional outcome in schizophrenia. Schizophr Res 2005; 80(2–3): 213–25.
12. Wykes T, Reeder C, Corner J, Williams C, Everitt B. The effects of neurocognitive remediation on executive processing in patients with schizophrenia. Schizophr Bull 1999; 25(2): 291–307.
13. Velligan DI, Bow-Thomas CC, Huntzinger C et al. Randomized controlled trial of the use of compensatory strategies to enhance adaptive functioning in outpatients with schizophrenia. Am J Psychiatry 2000; 157: 1317–23.
14. Velligan DI, Prihoda TJ, Ritch JL et al. A randomized single-blind pilot study of compensatory strategies in schizophrenia outpatients. Schizophr Bull 2002; 28(2): 283–92.
15. Velligan DI, Bow-Thomas CC, Mahurin RK, Miller AL, Halgunseth LC. Do specific neurocognitive deficits predict specific domains of community function in schizophrenia? J Nerv Ment Dis 2000; 188(8): 518–24.
16. Medalia A, Revheim N, Casey M. The remediation of problem-solving skills in schizophrenia. Schizophr Bull 2001; 27(2): 259–67.
17. Medalia A. Attention training procedures, in Encyclopedia of Psychotherapy, Herson M, Sledge W, eds. Academic Press: San Diego, CA, US, 2002: 131–37.
18. Medalia A, Revheim N, Casey M. Remediation of memory disorders in schizophrenia. Psychol Med 2000; 30: 1451–59.
19. Bell M, Bryson G, Wexler BE. Cognitive remediation of working memory deficits: durability of training effects in severely impaired and less severely impaired schizophrenia. Acta Psychiatr Scand 2003; 108: 101–09.
20. Bell M, Brsyon GJ, Fiszdon J, Greig TC, Wexler BE. Neurocognitive enhancement therapy and work therapy in schizophrenia: Work outcomes at 6 months and 12 month follow-up. Biol Psychiatry 2004; 55(8S): 1S–242S.
21. Hogarty GE, Flesher S, Ulrich R et al. Cognitive enhancement therapy for schizophrenia: Effects of a 2-year randomized trial on cognition and behavior. Arch Gen Psychiatry 2004; 61(9): 866–76.
22. Medalia A, Revheim N, Casey M. Remediation of problem-solving skills in schizophrenia: evidence of a persistent effect. Schizophr Res 2002; 57(2–3): 165–71.
23. Wykes T, Reeder C, Williams C et al. Are the effects of cognitive remediation therapy (CRT) durable? Results from an exploratory trial in schizophrenia. Schizophr Res 2003; 61: 163–74.
24. Fiszdon JM, McClough JF, Silverstein SM et al. Learning potential as a predictor of readiness for psychosocial rehabilitation in schizophrenia. Psychiatry Res 2006; 143(2–3): 159–66.
25. Wykes T, Reeder C, Landau S et al. Cognitive remediation therapy in schizophrenia: randomised controlled trial. Br J Psychiatry 2007; 190(5): 421–7.

21 Evidence-based psychosocial interventions for schizophrenia

Eric Granholm and Catherine Loh

INTRODUCTION

Historically, schizophrenia has been considered to be a chronic mental illness with little hope of remission or recovery. Whereas the treatment for schizophrenia has focused largely on symptom management, the psychosocial interventions for psychosis have largely been neglected. The recovery movement began as a response to social and political forces almost 40 years ago. Both consumers and providers of mental health services have expressed dissatisfaction with the singular focus on medication as *the* treatment for schizophrenia. Over the past two decades, there has been a definitive mainstream transformation in beliefs regarding the possibility of not just remission from symptoms but also recovery from schizophrenia and improvement in community functioning.

A recent consensus statement (1) prescribing standardized remission criteria defined remission not as an absence of symptoms but as a level of symptomatology that does not interfere with daily functioning. The consensus group was careful to note that remission is necessary but not sufficient to define the broader concept of recovery. There are no standardized criteria for recovery, and scientific definitions of recovery as an outcome differ in conceptualization from consumer-movement definitions of recovery as a process (2). Nonetheless, academic definitions of recovery generally involve remission of symptoms and a return to some level of role functioning, most typically occupational functioning, for a period of at least 1 year. Perhaps the most comprehensive definition of recovery is set forth by Liberman and his colleagues (3), which covers the following: requiring remission from symptoms, independent living, return to social functioning, and at least half-time occupational or school functioning sustained for a period of at least 2 years.

In the vision statement of *Achieving the Promise: Transforming Mental Health Care in America*, the President's New Freedom Commission on Mental Health (4), it states, " We envision a future when everyone with a mental illness will recover, a future when mental illnesses can be prevented or cured . . . ." But what are the chances of recovery for people with schizophrenia? It was previously assumed that the majority of people with schizophrenia experience continuing decline without a return to premorbid functioning during the course of illness (2). Several long-term outcome studies of schizophrenia, however, have demonstrated that recovery may be more commonplace than previously assumed. Indeed, recent trials of long-term outcome in schizophrenia indicate that about 50% of people diagnosed with schizophrenia have periods of recovery, as defined by remission of symptoms and resumed role functioning (i.e., occupational, social), maintained for at least 1 year (5, 6).

Within the current recovery atmosphere, a transformation in perspectives is taking place regarding service delivery, research, and expectations for people with severe mental illness and it focuses on treating not only symptoms but also *the* person him or herself by addressing his or her social, occupational, and relationship functioning.

The new recovery models emphasize increasing empowerment through consumer choice and active involvement in treatment. Consistent with the recovery model are current recommendations for the treatment of schizophrenia from academic, clinical, and institutional settings both in the United States and internationally, including the Schizophrenia Patient Outcomes Research Team (PORT: 7), Veterans Health Administration (8), the American Psychiatric Association (9), and the U.K. National Institute for Clinical Excellence (10). Universally, these recommendations advocate for the use of psychosocial interventions in addition to psychopharmacolgy for the treatment of schizophrenia. There are several evidence-based psychotherapeutic interventions for schizophrenia, effective for the wide range of difficulties associated with severe mental illness, including cognitive impairments, positive and negative symptoms, and social and occupational functioning.

RECOMMENDED PSYCHOSOCIAL INTERVENTIONS FOR SCHIZOPHRENIA

A number of national and international practice guidelines for the treatment of schizophrenia have been developed (for a review of recommendations, see Gaebel et al., 2005) (11). Practically all published treatment guidelines recommend the use of both psychotropic agents and adjunctive psychosocial treatment as best practice for treatment of schizophrenia. The most commonly recommended evidence-based practices (see Table 21.1) are consistent with the recovery model (2). One exception to this is token economy interventions, which are recommended by the Schizophrenia PORT (7) and the American Psychological Association (12) for the treatment of people with severe mental illness in long-term care or inpatient settings. Developed in the 1950s and based on principles of social learning and operant conditioning, token economies have been found to be effective for increasing adaptive behaviors for schizophrenia, although generalization of behavior to outpatient settings is questionable (13). With the growth of the recovery movement and consequent focus on least restrictive environments for people with schizophrenia, long-term inpatient care and token economies have largely fallen out of favor.

Family Interventions. Family intervention is perhaps the most well-studied psychotherapy for schizophrenia and typically involves elements of psychoeducation (14) regarding vulnerability–stress models, medication adherence, and treatment adherence. Behaviorally based family interventions may also include training in coping skills for the management of symptoms and social environments, using relapse prevention models, communication training, and problem-solving training.

There do not appear to be significant differences in outcome between types of family interventions (15). When compared to treatment as usual, family interventions have demonstrated efficacy for reducing relapse rates, reducing psychiatric hospitalizations, and increasing medication adherence in multiple, randomized clinical trials (15,16). The length of family interventions is important, with long-term interventions (greater than 9 months) being significantly more effective in reducing relapse and hospitalization than short-term interventions (7, 17, 18). Psychoeducation is an active element in family therapy for schizophrenia (14). One of the benefits of family psychoeducation is a greater understanding of the illness, as well as expectations for behavior, achievement, and motivation within the family system. There is some evidence to suggest that these changes in expectations may lead to increases in both family functioning (15) and client improvement in social functioning and symptom reduction (18).

Unfortunately, although family interventions for schizophrenia have been very successful in reducing hospitalization and relapse, people with schizophrenia and

TABLE 21.1 Evidence Based Psychosocial Interventions for Schizophrenia

	Elements	Format	Recommendations	Treatment Target(s)
Family Intervention[a,b,c,d]	Psychoeducation Crisis intervention/relapse prevention Communication training Coping skills for symptoms Problem-solving training	Single family Multifamily Outpatient	Length: >6 mos	Reduce relapse rates Reduce hospitalization Improve medication adherence Reduce stress/expressed emotion
Supported Employment (SE)[a,b,c,d]	Individualized job development Rapid placement Ongoing job support Integrated services	Individual Group Outpatient	Should be offered to anyone who expresses an interest in working	Acquire competitive employment
Assertive Community Treatment (ACT)[a,b,c,d]	Multidisciplinary team Shared caseload Direct service provision High frequency contact Low patient-to-staff ratio Outreach/services in community	Individual Outpatient	For high utilizers of crisis and emergency care Must have a psychiatrist on the ACT team (NOT as consultant)	Reduce length of hospitalizations Improve living conditions
Social Skills Training (SST)[a,b,c,d]	Behavioral instruction Modeling Corrective feedback Contingent social reinforcement In vivo practice	Individual Group Inpatient Outpatient	Length: 6 mos – 2 years Small groups (<6) Repeated practice of skills	Improve social/communication skills Improve community functioning Reduce symptom severity Reduce relapse rates
Cognitive Behavioral Therapy (CBT)[a,b,d,e]	Relationship between thoughts, feelings and behaviors Shared understanding of illness Belief modification Coping skills	Individual Group Outpatient	Length: ≥6 mos Recommended for treatment resistant symptoms	Reduce positive symptom distress and dysfunction Reduce depression and negative symptoms Reduce social anxiety and improve functioning
Token Economies[a,d]	Contingent positive reinforcement Individualized treatment Avoid punishing consequences	Inpatient Mileu/Day Treatment	Inpatient care Long term care	Increase adaptive behaviors

NOTES: [a]Schizophrenia PORT recommendation; [b]American Psychiatric Association recommendation; [c]Veterans Health Administration recommendation; [d]American Psychological Association recommendation; [e]UK National Institute for Clinical Excellence recommendation their families do not routinely receive referrals for family care. Possibly in response to the growing need for family services, the newest development in family therapies for schizophrenia is service delivery by other family members (i.e., family to family) rather than trained clinical staff. Consumer-oriented resources, such as NAMI, have developed protocols for training family members to provide psychoeducation and support for other families who are interested in learning more about schizophrenia.

Supported Employment (SE). Employment confers benefits other than financial for people with schizophrenia, including daily structure, sense of value, and social responsibility; opportunities to use skills; opportunities for socialization; and increased self-esteem (19). SE programs are not the same as traditional, sheltered work programs or vocational rehabilitation programs. In traditional programs, people with disabilities participate in a series of available training opportunities, and after they achieve mastery of the task, they are placed in sheltered work environment with other people who have disabilities. Participants typically work part time for less-than-minimum wage, and once they are placed, support from the vocational rehabilitation staff is discontinued. In SE, client interest and choice are a key component, and the SE counselor provides assistance in finding preferred competitive employment in an integrated environment (i.e., coworkers may or may not have disabilities) where salaries are minimum wage or more. Job-related training occurs on the job, and perhaps most important, support from SE staff continues after job placement (19).

People in SE programs are more likely to obtain employment when compared to people in traditional vocational rehabilitation programs (19) or those in general psychosocial rehabilitation programs (20). Participants in SE programs also earn more money than those in other work-related programs (20). While participants in SE programs are able to obtain employment, employment retention is an issue that remains to be addressed by SE interventions. Not surprisingly, negative symptoms, persistent positive symptoms, cognitive impairments, and recent hospitalization negatively influence successful employment retention (21, 22). Enhancements of SE interventions using cognitive-behavioral and cognitive-remediation techniques are promising, as these additional interventions may be helpful in reducing the effects of both symptoms and cognitive impairments on employment retention.

Assertive Community Treatment (ACT). ACT models were developed approximately 30 years ago to address the needs of people with severe mental illness who had difficulty accessing services in the community after discharge from inpatient psychiatric treatment. Lack of access to readily available services can result in frequent crises necessitating costly emergency psychiatric treatment in emergency rooms or inpatient units. Clients who are referred to ACT are typically frequent users of emergency psychiatric services, are difficult to engage, and have severe impairment in psychosocial functioning.

ACT services are characterized by flexibility and multidisciplinary collaboration in outpatient treatment (23). Unlike traditional mental health and social services, all possible treatment is provided by the ACT team, rather than having multiple providers in different locations. ACT teams typically consist of psychiatrists, nurses, mental health professionals, employment specialists, and substance abuse specialists. In situations where specialty treatment is required, the ACT team will make the appointment, transport the client to the appointment, and ensure attendance at future appointments if necessary. ACT case managers share small caseloads (usually a 1:10 ratio of case managers to clients) and are available 24/7 for crisis intervention. ACT treatment is also provided *in vivo* (rather than in a clinic) and services are typically time unlimited. The goal of ACT intervention is rehabilitation and return to role functioning through skills training and therapy to reach individualized goals chosen by the client.

ACT is the most well-studied form of case management. One major benefit of ACT teams for clients is continuous contact with the same providers over time, ensuring collective understanding of each client's goals and current level of success at each goal. In general, ACT produces better outcomes than treatment as usual for decreasing the length of hospital stays and improving housing situations (24, 25). In addition, client satisfaction rating for ACT services is consistently greater than satisfaction ratings for treatment as usual (25). Unfortunately, many clients who may be appropriate for ACT services are often not referred for treatment with ACT teams (26).

Social Skills Training (SST). Poor social functioning is common in schizophrenia. With the increase in duration of illness, teenagers and young adults who develop schizophrenia become progressively distanced from their peer groups socially, occupationally, and recreationally, resulting in increased segregation from mainstream society. Social skills training is based on the social skills model of social competence, which involves *social perception* (the ability to accurately identify social cues), *social cognition* (the ability to integrate current and past information to plan an effective response), and *behavioral response* (ability to respond verbally and physically) (27).

The primary goal of SST is to teach skills related to each element of social competence to improve interpersonal communication and effectiveness. These skills are necessary for a number of functional outcomes, including social (meeting new people and making friends), occupational (obtaining and maintaining employment), independent living (communications, including negotiating rent and paying bills), and substance abuse treatment (asking for help and assertiveness skills for declining substances when offered). Skills are typically taught in small group format, with extensive role-play practice, but may be tailored for each client according to his or her goals in individual sessions. Groups begin with establishing the rationale for each new skill, and then skills are taught over time by parsing complex skills into simple tasks and emphasizing practice both in and out of sessions. Both facilitators and other group members engage in role plays with corrective feedback to improve skills for subsequent practices. Both verbal (i.e., feeling statements) and nonverbal (i.e., eye contact, body posture) aspects of communication are addressed. Facilitators demonstrate (e.g., model) the desired behavior, reinforce progressive approximations to the modeled behavior (e.g., shaping), and attempt to have clients generalize new skills learned in group to real-world situations through homework assignments.

SST is consistently effective in increasing behavioral skills for people with schizophrenia (e.g., improving eye contact, attending to voice volume, asking questions) (27–29). Having the requisite skills to operate effectively in social environments is also related to improved general psychological adjustment (30), reduced negative symptoms (29), as well as reduced self-reported social anxiety (28). In addition to improved functioning in the community (29), participants also report satisfaction with social skills interventions (31), greater self-efficacy in social situations (32), and greater self-reported assertiveness skills (28).

Cognitive-Behavioral Therapy (CBT). Clinical trials of CBT for psychosis (CBTp) have primarily focused on treatment-resistant schizophrenia. CBT has been traditionally used to treat depression and anxiety. The premise of CBT is that thoughts (or cognition—the process of acquiring knowledge and forming beliefs) can influence feelings and behaviors. CBT techniques are used to help people challenge and modify unhelpful thoughts that generate negative feelings and maladaptive behaviors. As applied to schizophrenia, CBT can be used to address and challenge beliefs about psychotic symptoms ("Voices can harm me"), as well as social aversion attitudes and defeatist performance beliefs that interfere with adaptive behaviors, including expectancies ("It won't be fun"), self-efficacy beliefs ("I always fail"), and anomalous beliefs ("Spirits will harm me") that interfere with community functioning. It is important to stress that CBTp typically does not directly focus on symptoms (e.g., hallucinations, delusions) but on the thoughts about psychotic symptoms or other beliefs that lead to distress or dysfunction.

CBTp is recommended in numerous national and international best-practice guidelines for schizophrenia (11) because clinical trials demonstrated beneficial effects for positive and negative symptoms, anxiety and depression, as well as improved community functioning (33–38). In addition, CBTp has been associated with low dropout rates (16), which has led some to speculate that CBT may improve adherence to other forms of treatment, like medication (39).

PROMISING PSYCHOSOCIAL INTERVENTIONS FOR SCHIZOPHRENIA
In addition to these most commonly recommended evidence-based practices, there are several noteworthy interventions that warrant discussion and consideration (see Table 21.2).

Integrated Dual Diagnosis Treatment (IDDT). Approximately 40%–60% of people with a severe mental illness also meet criteria for substance abuse or dependence (40). Psychiatric services and substance abuse services are typically delivered in separate settings (e.g., parallel treatment). Integration of these services may be hindered by systemic conflict between different care providers who have different treatment philosophies and funding sources. The recommendation to integrate mental health and substance abuse treatment began approximately three decades ago, as a response to poor patient outcomes in the existing system of parallel or sequential treatment models. In comparison, IDDT programs provide services for both psychiatric and substance abuse disorders in the same setting (e.g., in the same therapy groups), by the same providers, using integrated content from a unified conceptual framework (30, 41). The focus of IDDT is to ensure that the responsibility for congruent care of both issues is a burden on the health care system rather than the client.

Much of the evidence for IDDT is based on clinical trials focused on severe mental illness (i.e., schizophrenia, mood disorders with psychotic features, and post-traumatic stress disorder [PTSD]) rather than specifically on people with schizophrenia. These clinical trials have generally found that longer-term interventions (greater than 6 months) yield better outcomes (42). Research on the efficacy and effectiveness of IDDT specific to schizophrenia has been limited by lack of methodological standardization, small samples, and frequent use of quasi-experimental designs (42–44). Methodologically rigorous studies of IDDT specific to schizophrenia have found that integrated treatment is superior to routine care at end of treatment for symptoms and abstinence and for functioning at follow-up (45, 46). More research is necessary to determine the active elements of IDDT specific to people with schizophrenia.

Cognitive Remediation/Rehabilitation. Most people with schizophrenia manifest some level of cognitive impairment, most commonly in the areas of attention, memory, or executive functioning. Psychosocial interventions designed to address these deficits have been in development for the past 40 years, and NIMH has recently initiated projects focused on development of pharmacologic treatments for cognition in schizophrenia (MATRICS & CNTRICS). Also known as cognitive training and cognitive rehabilitation in the literature, the early psychosocial interventions focused on drill and practice methods using paper and pencil methods; however, they have evolved to include the use of computers as well as strategized coaching to improve performance (47). In addition, outcomes have expanded to include memory training, problem

TABLE 21.2 Promising Psychosocial Interventions for Schizophrenia

	Treatment Target(s)	Elements/Formats	Issues
Integrated Dual Diagnosis	Substance use Psychiatric symptoms Mental health services utilization Independent living	Group (CBT, education, peer support) Long term residential treatment (>1 yr) Contingency management Individual therapy (MI, CBT) Family (psychoeducation) Intensive case management Intensive outpatient treatment	Long-term maintenance of abstinence
Cognitive Remediation	Attention Memory Executive functioning Psychosocial functioning	Attention Process Training (APT) Integrated Psychological Therapy (IPT) Cognitive Enhancement Therapy(CET) Neurocognitive Enhancement Therapy (NET) Cognitive Remediation Therapy (CRT) Neuropsychological Educational Approach to Remediation (NEAR) Errorless Learning Approaches	Generalization of skills Maintenance of gains Best combined with other psychiatric rehabilitation (e.g., supported employment)
Compensatory Support	Psychiatric symptoms Mental health services utilization Independent living	Cognitive Adaptation Therapy (CAT)	Generalization of skills Maintenance of gains

solving, visual learning, processing speed, and working memory. Cognitive remediation does appear to improve the cognitive performance of people with schizophrenia and has shown some limited benefit for more general psychosocial functioning outcomes (17, 18, 48). At present, there is insufficient evidence to identify active elements or ideal conditions (e.g., length of treatment, frequency of sessions, etc.) for delivery of cognitive remediation interventions. Despite few long-term outcome studies and concerns about generalization of skills to real-world situations, cognitive remediation continues to be a very promising future intervention for schizophrenia.

Compensatory/Environmental Support. Compensatory strategies provide environmental supports in an effort to attempt to circumvent the negative outcomes of cognitive deficits. Although these interventions have been used in rehabilitation efforts with mental retardation, head injury, and memory loss, the approach has only recently been adapted for people with schizophrenia. Cognitive adaptation training (CAT) for schizophrenia involves individualizing cues in the environment to prompt adaptive behaviors (49–51). For example, a CAT intervention may involve alarms on medication bottles; arranging clothes so that outfits each day are appropriate and clean; checklists that remind clients to perform daily activities, such as grooming; and signs that cue specific behaviors, such as taking medications. CAT is also a personalized rehabilitation approach, as the nature of community support provided depends upon the patients' pattern of neurocognitive impairments (e.g., differential severity of executive memory deficits). CAT is a promising community support intervention and has been found to be effective for medication adherence, community functioning, and decreasing relapse (49–51). Long-term studies are necessary to examine maintenance of adaptive behaviors following discontinuation of CAT provider contact.

UTILITY VERSUS IMPLEMENTATION

The combination of psychopharmacology and psychosocial interventions is recommended by practically all best-practice guidelines for schizophrenia and does result in improved psychiatric and psychosocial outcomes. Despite these recommendations, the vast majority of patients with schizophrenia do not receive these evidence-based psychosocial interventions (52). Barriers to implementation of psychosocial interventions include larger societal and systems issues, such as health care policies, as well as more specific issues such as clinician education and training.

Successful implementation of evidence-based psychosocial interventions for schizophrenia requires navigating through barriers in the larger policy environment. The shift in focus from paternalistic care to the consumer empowerment/recovery model involves a number of policy changes, including billing, service delivery, and reimbursement (2). At present, psychosocial interventions are typically inadequately reimbursed, hindering development of additional psychosocial services. In addition, the limited number of therapists with specialized training required for some therapeutic services, such as CBTp, do not accept Medicare or Medicaid. People with schizophrenia who have been ill and unemployed for more than a decade also typically do not have private insurance or the means to pay for therapy, and Medicare and Medicaid do not emphasize reimbursement for evidence-based over other forms of psychosocial practices. These factors can lead to pessimism among provider organization administrators, who are often not willing to take the risk of implementing a new program, due to fears about financial sustainability.

Clinician education and training are also vital to the implementation of these interventions. Perhaps the most important concern involves the perception of schizophrenia as an illness characterized by continued deterioration over time and an inability to return to premorbid functioning. Provider hopelessness can be an impediment to successful psychiatric rehabilitation. The belief that people with schizophrenia cannot improve beyond a certain point may be a byproduct of the "clinician's illusion" (53), which asserts that clinicians are more likely to treat people who have persistent symptoms, because people who are able to manage symptoms on their own are less likely to continue in treatment. A surprising minority (one-third) of people who have a severe mental illness seek care in a specialty mental health clinic (53). Stigma associated with severe mental illness ensures that people who are able to self-manage their illness do not present to emergency clinics, outpatient psychiatry, or as participants in research protocols. These stereotypes affect the implementation of psychosocial interventions for schizophrenia at every level, from referral to direct delivery of services. Education about referral opportunities (see Appendix A) needs to emphasize the importance of providing psychosocial services to all people with schizophrenia, without making judgments beforehand regarding probability of success or failure of treatment. To meet the gap in service delivery and have sufficient placements for referrals, it is also essential that graduate training programs address these interventions for schizophrenia and train practitioners in appropriate service delivery and service methodologies.

CONCLUSIONS

Conventional wisdom and recent longitudinal studies have established that, at a minimum, periods of recovery from schizophrenia are commonplace (2, 54). Evidence-based psychosocial treatments for schizophrenia are effective in helping people achieve recovery goals. It should be cautioned that no individual could engage in all the recommended treatment options at once. Ideally, each person with schizophrenia would have the option to choose from all the treatments available, based on individual needs, strengths, and goals. Many of the treatments listed may be combined appropriately to address complementary issues. For example, the combination of social skills training with cognitive-behavioral interventions addresses both self-defeating beliefs that interfere with skill performance and skill capacity and improves the likelihood that people will engage in functional behaviors and use the skills acquired by them. Indeed, it has been recommended that social skills training is best conceptualized as a targeted treatment in conjunction with other psychosocial interventions (27). Psychoeducation, as an intervention, is also almost routinely used as part of all the discussed psychosocial treatments for schizophrenia.

The effectiveness of any of the interventions is largely dependent on nonspecific factors, perhaps most importantly, therapeutic alliance. Building trust and establishing rapport are critical for ensuring treatment adherence. Provider and client hopelessness regarding prognosis for schizophrenia is a major stumbling block for the widespread implementation and effectiveness of these services. Consequently, the most important element may be changing expectations and increasing hope in recovery for individuals with schizophrenia (55).

REFERENCES

1. Andreasen NC, Carpenter WT Jr, Kane JM et al. Remission in schizophrenia: proposed criteria and rationale for consensus. Am J Psychiatry 2005; 162(3): 441–9.
2. Bellack AS. Scientific and consumer models of recovery in schizophrenia: concordance, contrasts, and implications. Schizophr Bull 2006; 32(3): 432–42.

3. Liberman RP, Kopelowicz A, Ventura J, Gutkind D. Operational criteria and factors related to recovery from schizophrenia. International Rev Psychiatry 2002; 14: 256–72.

4. New Freedom Commission on Mental Health. Achieving the Promise: Transforming Mental Health Care in America. Executive Summary, editor. 2003. Rockville, MD. DHHS Pub No. SMA-03-3831.

5. Harrison G, Hopper K, Craig T et al. Recovery from psychotic illness: a 15- and 25-year international follow-up study. Br J Psychiatry 2001; 178: 506–17.

6. Harrow M, Grossman LS, Jobe TH, Herbener ES. Do patients with schizophrenia ever show periods of recovery? A 15-year multi-follow-up study. Schizophr Bull 2005; 31(3): 723–34.

7. Lehman AF, Kreyenbuhl J, Buchanan RW et al. The Schizophrenia Patient Outcomes Research Team (PORT): Updated treatment recommendations 2003. Schizophr Bull 2004; 30: 193–217.

8. U.S.Department of Veterans Affairs. Achieving the promise: Transforming mental health care in the VA. 2003. Washington, D.C.

9. American Psychiatric Association. Practice Guidelines for the Treatment of Patients with Schizophrenia. American Psychiatric Association [Second]. 2004. 6-25-2008. http://www.psychiatryonline.com/pracGuide/pracGuideTopic_6.aspx.

10. National Institute for Clinical Excellence. Core interventions in the treatment and management of schizophrenia in primary and secondary care: Clinical guideline 1. 2002. London, UK.

11. Gaebel W, Weinmann S, Sartorius N, Rutz W, McIntyre JS. Schizophrenia practice guidelines: international survey and comparison. Br J Psychiatry 2005; 187: 248–55.

12. American Psychological Association. Training Grid Outlining Best Practices for Recovery and Improved Outcomes for People with Serious Mental Illness. American Psychological Association . 2005. http://www.apa.org/practice/smi_grid2.pdf.

13. Dickerson FB, Tenhula WN, Green-Paden LD. The token economy for schizophrenia: review of the literature and recommendations for future research. Schizophr Res 2005; 75(2–3): 405–16.

14. Pitschel-Walz G, Leucht S, Bauml J, Kissling W, Engel RR. The effect of family interventions on relapse and rehospitalization in schizophrenia–a meta-analysis. Schizophr Bull 2001; 27(1): 73–92.

15. Pharoah F, Mari J, Rathbone J, Wong W. Family intervention for schizophrenia. Cochrane Database Syst Rev 2006; (4) CD000088.

16. Pilling S, Bebbington P, Kuipers E et al. Psychological treatments in schizophrenia: II. Meta-analyses of randomized controlled trials of social skills training and cognitive remediation. Psychol Med 2002; 32: 783–91.

17. Velligan DI, Gonzalez JM. Rehabilitation and recovery in schizophrenia. Psychiatr Clin North Am 2007; 30(3): 535–48.

18. Pfammatter M, Junghan UM, Brenner HD. Efficacy of psychological therapy in schizophrenia: conclusions from meta-analyses. Schizophr Bull 2006; 32(Suppl 1): S64–S80.

19. Twamley EW, Jeste DV, Lehman AF. Vocational rehabilitation in schizophrenia and other psychotic disorders: A literature review and meta-analysis of randomized controlled trials. J Nerv Ment Dis 2003; 191: 515–23.

20. Lehman AF, Goldberg R, Dixon LB et al. Improving employment outcomes for persons with severe mental illnesses. Arch Gen Psychiatry 2002; 59: 165–72.

21. McGurk SR, Mueser KT. Cognitive functioning, symptoms, and work in supported employment: a review and heuristic model. Schizophr Res 2004; 70(2–3): 147–73.

22. Razzano LA, Cook JA, Burke-Miller JK et al. Clinical factors associated with employment among people with severe mental illness: findings from the employment intervention demonstration program. J Nerv Ment Dis 2005; 193(11): 705–13.

23. Mueser KT, Bond GR, Drake RE, Resnick SG. Models of community care for severe mental illness: a review of research on case management. Schizophr Bull 1998; 24(1): 37–74.

24. Rosen A, Mueser KT, Teesson M. Assertive community treatment-Issues from scientific and clinical literature with implications for practice. J Rehabil Res Dev 2007; 44(6): 813–26.

25. Marshall M, Lockwood A. Assertive community treatment for people with severe mental disorders. Cochrane Database Syst Rev 2000; (2): CD001089.
26. Lehman AF, Steinwachs DM. Patterns of usual care for schizophrenia: Initial results from the Schizophrenia Patient Outcomes Research Team (PORT) Client Survey. Schizophr Bull 1998; 24: 11–20.
27. Bellack AS. Skills training for people with severe mental illness. Psychiatr Rehabil J 2004; 27(4): 375–91.
28. Benton MK, Schroeder HE. Social skills training with schizophrenics: A meta-analytic evaluation. J Consult Clin Psychiatr 1990; 58: 741–7.
29. Kurtz MM, Mueser KT. A meta-analysis of controlled research on social skills training for schizophrenia. J Consult Clin Psychol 2008; 76(3): 491–504.
30. Mueser KT, Bellack AS, Blanchard JJ. Comorbidity of schizophrenia and substance abuse: Implications for treatment. J Consult Clin Psychol 1992; 60: 845–56.
31. Prince JD. Determinants of care satisfaction among inpatients with schizophrenia. Community Ment Health J 2006; 42(2): 189–96.
32. Kopelowicz A, Liberman RP, Zarate R. Recent Advances in Social Skills Training for Schizophrenia. Schizophr Bull 2006; 32(1): 12–23.
33. Gould RA, Mueser KT, Bolton E, Mays V, Goff D. Cognitive therapy for psychosis in schizophrenia: An effect size analysis. Schizophr Res 2001; 48: 335–42.
34. Dickerson FB. Cognitive behavioral psychotherapy for schizophrenia: A review of recent empirical studies. Schizophr Res 2000; 43: 71–90.
35. Rector NA, Beck AT. Cognitive behavioral therapy for schizophrenia: An empirical review. J Nerv Ment Dis 2001; 189: 278–87.
36. Turkington D, Kingdon D, Weiden PJ. Cognitive behavior therapy for schizophrenia. Am J Psychiatry 2006; 163(3): 365–73.
37. Wykes T, Steel C, Everitt B, Tarrier N. Cognitive behavior therapy for schizophrenia: effect sizes, clinical models, and methodological rigor. Schizophr Bull 2008; 34(3): 523–37.
38. Zimmermann G, Favrod J, Trieu VH, Pomini V. The effect size of cognitive behavioral treatment on the positive symptoms of schizophrenia spectrum disorders: A meta-analysis. Schizophr Res 2005; 77: 1–9.
39. Turkington D, Dudley R, Warman DM, Beck AT. Cognitive-behavioral therapy for schizophrenia: a review. J Psychiatr Pract 2004; 10(1): 5–16.
40. Regier DA, Farmer ME, Rae DS et al. Comorbidity of mental disorders with alcohol and other drug abuse. Results from the Epidemiologic Catchment Area (ECA) Study. JAMA 1990; 264(19): 2511–18.
41. Ries R. Clinical treatment matching models for dually diagnosed patients. Psychiatr Clin North Am 1993; 16(1): 167–75.
42. Drake RE, O'Neal EL, Wallach MA. A systematic review of psychosocial research on psychosocial interventions for people with co-occurring severe mental and substance use disorders. J Subst Abuse Treat 2008; 34(1): 123–38.
43. McHugo GJ, Drake RE, Brunette MF et al. Enhancing validity in co-occurring disorders treatment research. Schizophr Bull 2006; 32(4): 655–65.
44. Cleary M, Hunt GE, Matheson S, Siegfried N, Walter G. Psychosocial treatment programs for people with both severe mental illness and substance misuse. Schizophr Bull 2008; 34(2): 226–8.
45. Barrowclough C, Haddock G, Tarrier N et al. Randomized controlled trial of motivational interviewing, cognitive behavior therapy, and family intervention for patients with comorbid schizophrenia and substance use disorders. Am J Psychiatry 2001; 158: 1706–13.
46. Haddock G, Barrowclough C, Tarrier N et al. Cognitive-behavioural therapy and motivational intervention for schizophrenia and substance misuse. 18-month outcomes of a randomised controlled trial. Br J Psychiatry 2003; 183: 418–26.
47. Twamley EW, Jeste DV, Bellack AS. A review of cognitive training in schizophrenia. Schizophr Bull 2003; 29: 359–82.

48. McGurk SR, Twamley EW, Sitzer DI, McHugo GJ, Mueser KT. A meta-analysis of cognitive remediation in schizophrenia. Am J Psychiatry 2007; 164(12): 1791–802.
49. Velligan DI, Bow-Thomas CC. Two case studies of cognitive adaptation training for outpatients with schizophrenia. Psychiatr Serv 2000; 51(1): 25–9.
50. Velligan DI, Prihoda TJ, Ritch JL et al. A randomized single-blind pilot study of compensatory strategies in schizophrenia outpatients. Schizophr Bull 2002; 28(2): 283–92.
51. Velligan DI, Mueller J, Wang M et al. Use of environmental supports among patients with schizophrenia. Psychiatr Serv 2006; 57(2): 219–24.
52. Lehman AF, Steinwachs DM. Patterns of usual care for schizophrenia: initial results from the Schizophrenia Patient Outcomes Research Team (PORT) Client Survey. Schizophr Bull 1998; 24: 11–20.
53. Cohen P, Cohen J. The clinician's illusion. Arch Gen Psychiatry 1984; 41(12): 1178–82.
54. Davidson L, Schmutte T, Dinzeo T, Andres-Hyman R. Remission and recovery in schizophrenia: practitioner and patient perspectives. Schizophr Bull 2008; 34(1): 5–8.
55. Substance Abuse and Mental Health Services Administration (SAMHSA). National consensus conference on mental health recovery and systems transformation. 2005. Rockville, MD. DHHS Pub No. SMA 05-4129.

APPENDIX A Psychosocial Interventions for Schizophrenia: Online Resources

General Resources	American Psychological Association	http://www.apa.org/practice/smi_grid2.pdf
	National Alliance for Mental Illness (NAMI)	http://www.nami.org/
	SAMHSA Evidence Based Toolkits	http://mentalhealth.samhsa.gov/cmhs/communitysupport/toolkits/
	National Institute for Clinical Excellence (UK)	http://www.nice.org.uk/nicemedia/pdf/CG1publicinfo.pdf
Family Interventions	NAMI Family to Family	http://www.nami.org/template.cfm?section=Family-to-Family
	SAMHSA: Family Psychoeducation Toolkit	http://mentalhealth.samhsa.gov/cmhs/communitysupport/toolkits/family/
	Support and Family Education (SAFE) Program	http://w3.ouhsc.edu/Safeprogram/
Supported Employment	SAMHSA: Supported Employment Toolkit	http://mentalhealth.samhsa.gov/cmhs/communitysupport/toolkits/employment/
Assertive Community Treatment	Assertive Community Treatment Association	www.actassociation.com
	National Alliance for the Mentally Ill	www.nami.org/about/PACT.htm
	SAMHSA: ACT Toolkit	http://mentalhealth.samhsa.gov/cmhs/communitysupport/toolkits/community/
Social Skills Training	UCLA Social and Independent Living Skills Modules	http://psychrehab.com/
Cognitive Behavioral Therapy	Massachusetts General Hospital	http://www.massgeneral.org/schizophrenia/scz_care_treatment-cogbeh.html
	Cognitive Behavioral Social Skills Training	http://www.nrepp.samhsa.gov/programfulldetails.asp?PROGRAM_ID=94
Integrated Dual Diagnosis	SAMHSA: Integrated Dual Diagnosis Toolkit	http://mentalhealth.samhsa.gov/cmhs/communitysupport/toolkits/cooccurring/
	Dual Recovery Anonymous	http://draonline.org/

22

Transcultural psychiatry and schizophrenia

Thomas Stompe

INTRODUCTION

In current anthropology, culture is a complex system formed by values, beliefs, customs, and practices (1). The construct of culture offers a way to conceptualize differences in psychopathology, allowing to bring together race, ethnicity, and ways of life (2). Schizophrenia has a special place in the field of cultural psychiatry. After his journey to Java, Kraepelin concluded already in 1903 that the basic forms of dementia praecox and manic-depressive insanity in the Javanese were generally the same as those in Europe. But he also conceded that "racial characteristics, religion and customs" might modify their clinical manifestations (3, 4).

CULTURE AND THE FREQUENCY OF SCHIZOPHRENIA

During the decades after the two basic transcultural-psychiatric papers of Emil Kraepelin, the sources of the epidemiology of schizophrenia in non-European countries mainly based on mental health hospital statistics or sporadic field surveys. Most of these studies pointed out the rarity of *true* schizophrenia in traditional cultures (5). The first epidemiological surveys that generated incidence and prevalence data on psychoses in traditional cultures were carried out by Rin and Lin (6) in Taiwan and Leighton et al. in Nigeria (7). Starting in the 1970s, two studies of the World Health Organization—the International Pilot Study of Schizophrenia (8) and Determinants of Outcome of Severe Mental Disorders (9)—set a benchmark for comparing this illness across cultures.

The most influential study of the incidence of schizophrenia was the 10-Nation International Pilot Study of Schizophrenia organized by the World Health Organization, employing standardized measures of course and outcome (10). When narrow criteria (CATEGO S+) were used, the incidence ranged from 7 to 14 per 100,000. Applying ICD-9 (International Classification of Diseases) criteria, the incidence ranged from 16 to 42 per 100,000. Although the difference between the highest and the lowest margin for the broad definition was statistically significant, this finding for many authors has underpinned the belief that schizophrenia is an egalitarian disorder. However, criticism has risen from many sides during the past two decades (11). Many anthropologists and social scientists claimed that these studies looked at commonalities and ignored the differences. However, meta-analyses yielded a slightly different "epidemiological landscape" of the disease. During their meta-analysis of 161 studies on the incidence of schizophrenia from 33 countries, McGrath et al (12) found a median value of 15.2 (7.7–43.0) new cases per 100,000 population. Another meta-analysis of 188 studies from 46 countries found that the calculated median value for lifetime prevalence was 4.0 (1.6–12.1) per 1,000 population (13). Regardless of the type of prevalence estimate (point, period, lifetime, lifetime morbid risk), these distributions show prominent variations (five- to six-fold differences based on conservative criteria) (11). The prevalence estimates for "least developed" countries (median = 2.62) were significantly lower (p = 0.02) than those from "emerging" (median = 4.69) and from developed sites (median = 3.30). A meta-analysis based on 353 incidence rates from 68 studies additionally showed that the prevalence and incidence of schizophrenia varies with latitude(14). Prevalence estimated from sites in the high-latitude band were significantly higher when compared with lower bands for both sexes, and incidence rates were positively associated with absolute latitude only for males. These findings are in line with the results of field studies in Papua New Guinea conducted by Torrey et al. (15). The prevalence rate among tribal population in the mountain districts was between 0.03 and 0.19 per 1.000 population, whereas the prevalence rate was significantly higher in the case of people living in the coastal districts and having closer contacts with Australians and Europeans (0.38 and 0.77 per 1,000).

CULTURE AND THE OUTCOME OF SCHIZOPHRENIA

One of the most striking findings of the World Health Organization (WHO) International Pilot Study of Schizophrenia (IPSS) conducted in the 1960s and 1970s was the more favorable outcome for patients in the developing world (16–19). The original IPSS consisted of 1,202 patients with a PSE (Present State Examination) diagnosis of schizophrenia drawn from China, Columbia, Czechoslovakia, Denmark, India, Nigeria, the United Kingdom, the United States, and the Union of Soviet Socialist Republics. The 5-year follow-up showed a broad heterogeneity and a more favorable outcome of the disorder in the developing countries (Table 22.1).

This result was confirmed by the following cross-cultural studies organized and performed by the WHO: the Determinants of Outcome of Severe Mental Disorder (DOSMeD, 20 and the International Study of Schizophrenia (ISoS; e.g., 21). The aim of the DOSMeD project was to identify all persons suffering from the first onset of schizophrenia in 13 catchment areas located in 10 different countries over a period of 2 years. Like with the IPSS, the most important finding of this research was the existence of consistent and marked differences in the prognosis of schizophrenia between the centers of developed countries and the centers of developing countries (9, 10, 20). A series of further studies in India continued the program of the IPSS. In a multicenter study in Lucknow, Vellore, and Madras of 323 early-course schizophrenic patients, the authors found a 66% remission rate at 2-year follow up (22). Comparable with a similar study conducted in Columbia (23), there was only a 2% suicide rate, and 40% of patients were employed at 2 years. In a second Indian survey, the Madras Longitudinal Study, both positive and negative symptoms showed a significant decline at the end of 10 years. About 67% of the sample showed a good favourable course leading to partial or complete recovery (24,25). In a 7-year follow-up study conducted in Nigeria, 7-years follow up study 50.7% of the patients, most of them with an acute onset followed by an episodic course with rapid remission in response to treatment, achieved a good outcome and 23.9% a moderate outcome (26). Similarly, Bhugra found in a 1-year follow-up of 56 patients with schizophrenia from Trinidad poor outcome rates in only 19% (27). The better outcome in low-income cultures has been attributed to acute onset, being married, and stable personal social networks. Jablensky noted that the factors underlying this better outcome are likely to be the result of interactions between genetic variations and specific aspects of environment (28). In contrast, Patel et al. (29) pointed at methodological limitations of the three WHO cross-national studies, but they also mentioned the lack of evidence on the sociocultural factors that apparently contribute to the better outcome. While a substantial gap between the health and mortality between people with schizophrenia and the general population exists, there were no

TABLE 22.1 Two-year course and outcome in the International Pilot Study of Schizophrenia

Course and outcome measures	% patients in developing countries	% patients in developed countries
Remitting, complete remissions	62.7	36.8%
Continuous or episodic, no complete remissions	35.7	60.9%
Psychotic < 5% of follow-up	18.4	18.7%
Psychotic > 75% of follow-up	15.1	20.2%
No complete remissions during follow-up	24.1	57.2%
Complete remission for > 75% of follow-up	38.3	22.3%
On antipsychotic medication > 75% during follow-up	15.9	60.8%
No antipsychotic medication during follow-up	5.9	2.5%
Hospitalized for > 75% during follow-up	0.3	2.3%
Never hospitalized	55.5	8.1%
Impaired social functioning throughout follow-up	15.7	41.6%
Unimpaired social functioning > 75% during follow-up	42.9	31.6%

Source: Jablensky (28)

differences found, however, in the standardized mortality rates between developing and developed countries (30).

CULTURE AND SCHIZOPHRENIA PHENOTYPES

Kraepelin performed the first study on schizophrenia in traditional cultures by investigating psychotic patients in Java (3,4). He found all classical clinical features of dementia praecox with different accentuations and frequencies: Initial depression was rare, however, and the psychosis usually started with confusion and agitation. Auditory hallucinations, thought influence, and hypochondriac delusions played a minor role; delusions were seldom systematized; and negativistic stupor was rare (31). The first systematic investigation on schizophrenia subtypes in different cultures was carried out by Murphy in the 1960s (32). He found that the catatonic subtypes were rare among Euro-Americans, hebephrenic subtypes occurred more often in Japanese and Okinawan, and that there were only simple subtypes in Asian patients. The IPSS was a milestone for our knowledge of the cultural distribution of schizophrenic subtypes (8). Schizophrenic patients from 10 sites were subclassified according to the ICD-9 criteria of schizophrenia subtypes. Acute onset characterized 40.3% of all the cases in developing countries, compared to 10.9% in the developed countries. The largest diagnostic subgroup in the total sample was paranoid schizophrenia with 39.8%. It accounted for 75% of all patients in London, 53% in Aarhus and Washington, and 40% or more in Ibadan and Taipei. The hebephrenic subtype was assigned in 10.6% of all patients, with the highest rates in Cali and Taipei. In this group, 10.6% were classified as catatonic schizophrenia, with the highest rates in the centers of the developing countries (Agra, Cali, Ibadan). Another cross-sectional study on schizophrenia showed that paranoid subtype was more prevalent in developed European countries compared to the West African states and Pakistan (33).

In contrast to the findings of studies on schizophrenic subtypes conducted in Africa during the last century (32), the rate of catatonic subtypes was very similar in

TABLE 22.2   Culture and DSM-IV schizophrenia subtypes (*N* = 1080)

	Austria (*N* = 350)	East-Europe (*N* = 227)	Pakistan (*N* = 103)	West-Africa (*N* = 400)
Disorganized	13 (3.7%)	13 (5.7%)	24 (23.3%)	25 (6.6%)
Catatonic	26 (7.4%)	12 (5.3%)	3 (2.9%)	25 (6.6%)
Paranoid	248 (70.9%)	174 (76.6%)	45 (43.7%)	92 (24.2%)
Residual	36 (10.3%)	13 (5.7%)	14 (13.6%)	10 (0.3%)
Indifferent	11 (3.1%)	–	–	34 (8.9%)
Schizoaffective	16 (4.6%)	10 (4.4%)	–	122 (32.1%)
Schizophreniform	–	5 (2.2%)	–	92 (24.2%)

Source: Stompe & Friedmann (33)

all sites (Table 22.2). In line with the results of the IPSS, West African countries are characterized by higher rates of acute schizoaffective and schizophreniform disorders. Confirming the results of Murphy (32), the prevalence of paranoid subtype was significantly lower in the non-European countries.

CULTURE, DELUSIONS, AND HALLUCINATIONS IN SCHIZOPHRENIA
The shape of psychotic symptoms is influenced to a high extent by personal and cultural values. For example, delusions of grandeur are usually not prevalent in traditional collectivistic societies (34, 35). Religious delusions and delusional guilt are prevalent in societies with a Christian tradition, but infrequent in Islamic, Hindu, or Buddhist societies (35–42).

The first large cross-cultural investigation on the frequency of different kinds of hallucinations yielded a high prevalence of visual and tactile hallucinations in patients from Africa and the Near East (43), a result which was confirmed 20 years later by Ndetei and Vadher (44). Suhail and Cochrane compared a sample of patients from Pakistan living in their home country, with a sample of Pakistanis, who immigrated to Great Britain, and with White patients of British origin (45). Patients living in Pakistan reported statistically significantly more often visual hallucinations and also visualizations of spirits or ghosts compared with the two British groups, a result that underlines the importance of the immediate environment.

MIGRATION AND SCHIZOPHRENIA
The effects of migration on the incidence and prevalence of schizophrenia and related psychoses have been studied extensively since the 1930s (46).

Studies of migrants provide compelling support for the notion that social factors contribute to the development of schizophrenia. Meta-analyses found an increased risk for schizophrenia not only among first-generation immigrants but also among second-generation migrants (47). The mean weighted risk (RR) among first-generation migrants was 2.7 (95% CI: 2.3–3.2); among second generation migrants, the risk to develop schizophrenia was even higher, however, with a broader range (RR: 4.5; 95% CI: 1.5–13.1). The meta-analysis of subgroups yielded a RR of 3.3 (95% CI: 2.8–3.9) for migrants from developing countries, compared to a RR of 2.3 (95% CI: 1.7–3.1) of those from developed countries. The greatest effect size was found in migrants from areas with a Black majority (RR = 4.8; 95% CI: 3.7–6.2). This result was confirmed by a

Swedish 3-year incidence study (48). Here too, the highest risk to develop a psychotic disorder was found in first-generation Black immigrants (RR = 5.8; 95% CI: 2.8–13.4).

In a prevalence study among 10,000 people in the United Kingdom, Brugha et al. (49) found an increased risk of psychotic disorder in the immigrant groups of African Caribbeans and Africans (odds ratio = 4.5) but not in the South Asian ethnical groups. It is important for the interpretation of these data that epidemiological studies in the countries of origin found incidence rates in the Caribbean, similar to those for White Europeans in Europe (27, 50, 51).

Hutchinson et al. (52) found an increased rate of schizophrenia in the siblings of second-generation African Caribbean index cases, as compared to the incidence of schizophrenia in the siblings of White index cases with schizophrenia, a result suggesting a lower threshold for the expression of the disorder in carriers of susceptibility alleles that might be induced by environmental stress. This environmental stress comprises a lack of supportive community structure, acculturation stress, demoralization resulting from racial discrimination, and blocked opportunity for upward social mobility (53). Migrants are exposed to higher levels of competition. Those migrant groups that are the least successful in their host society (like the Moroccan males in the Netherlands or the African Caribbeans in Great Britain) have the highest risk to develop schizophrenia. Therefore Selten and Cantor-Graae suggested that the chronic experience of social defeat might lead to sensitization of the mesolimbic dopamine system (54).

CULTURE, PSYCHOPHARMACOLOGY, AND SCHIZOPHRENIA

Ethnic and cultural issues are becoming more and more important in the field of psychopharmacology (55). Both genetic and environmental factors need to be considered in the use of antipsychotic medication. Variations among ethnic groups in the use of medications, dosages, and therapeutic and side effects may be influenced by genetic and biological in pharmacokinetics (i.e., protein-binding absorption, distribution, metabolism, and excretion) and pharmacodynamics (i.e., receptor-coupled response or tissue sensitivity). The plasma concentration of α_1-acid glycoproteins are significantly lower among Asians than among African Americans and Whites (56). The activities of transferases involved in the metabolism of most psychotropic medications are known as genetically determined. The CYP system has been found to demonstrate genetic polymorphism. Especially the CYP2D6 is an important metabolizing enzyme for many antipsychotics like ariprazole, clozapine, flupentixol, haloperidol, levomepromazine, olanzapine, perazine, perphenazine, pimozide, risperidone, thioridazine, and zuclopenthixol (57). Caused by genotyping variations, four different levels of activity of CYP2D4 have been distinguished: ultrarapid metabolizers, extensive metabolizers, intermediate metabolizers, and poor metabolizers. In White populations, the frequency of poor metabolizers is 5%–10%, in Black Africans 0%–8%, in African Americans 3.7%, and in Chinese 1%. In Asians the CYP2D6*10 allele causes a decreased enzyme activity, with an allele frequency of about 50%, in contrast to Caucasians with an allele frequency about 0.05% (56). Increased enzyme activity is due to a gene duplication of CYP2D6*2xn allele, which is prevalent in Ethiopians and Saudi Arabians (10%–29%). These and other results imply that Asians should receive lower dosages of antipsychotic medication.

But also psychosocial and cultural factors such as diet, health beliefs, patients' compliance, patients' and family members' attitudes toward medication, societal demands and tolerance of psychotic symptoms, physicians' diagnostic and therapeutic skills, the availability of medication, and folk treatment must be considered when trying to explain the differences in the use of antipsychotics.

CONCLUSION

Culture has a major impact on prevalence and outcome, shape, and treatment of schizophrenic disorders. Despite the fact that many facets of the way culture influences mental disorders are still unknown, it is an established notion in the meantime that in the era of globalization cultural knowledge and sensitivity are essential qualities of professionals treating foreign as well as native-born patients with mental illness.

REFERENCES

1. Kuper A. Culture. The Anthropologists' Account. Cambridge: Havard University Press; 1999.
2. Kirmayer LJ. Culture Psychiatry in Historical Perspective. In: Bhugra D, Bhui K, eds. Textbook of Cultural Psychiatry. Cambridge: Cambridge University Press; 2007: 3–19.
3. Kraepelin E. Vergleichende Psychiatrie. Zentralbl Nervenhlk Psychiatr 1904; 27: 433–7.
4. Kraepelin E. Psychiatrisches aus Java. Zentralbl Nervenhlk Psychiatr 1904; 27: 468–9.
5. Carothers JC. The African Mind in Health and Disease. A Study of Ethnopsychiatry. Geneva: World Health Organization; 1953.
6. Rin H, Lin TY. Mental illness among Formosan aborigines compared with the Chinese in Taiwan. J Ment Science 1962; 198: 134–46.
7. Leighton AH, Lambo TA, Hughes HH et al. Psychiatric disorders among the Yoruba. Ithaka NY: Cornell University Press; 1963.
8. World Health Organisation Report of the International Pilot Study of Schizophrenia. Vol 1. Geneva: World Health Organisation; 1973.
9. Craig TJ, Siegel C, Hopper K et al. Outcome in schizophrenia and related disorders compared between developing and developed countries. A recursive partitioning re-analysis of the WHO DOSMeD data. Br J Psychiatry 1997; 70: 229–33.
10. Jablensky A, Sartorius N, Ernberg G et al. Schizophrenia: manifestations, incidence and course in different cultures. A World Health Organization ten-country study. Psychol Med Monograph Supplement 1992; 20: 1–97.
11. McGrath J. Variations in the incidence of schizophrenia: data versus dogma. Schizophr Bull 2006; 32: 195–7.
12. McGrath J, Saha S, Welham J et al. A systematic review of the incidence of schizophrenia: the distribution of rates and the influence of sex, urbanicity, migrant status and methodology. BMC Med 2004; 28: 13.
13. Saha S, Chant D, Welhalm J et al. A systematic review of the prevalence of schizophrenia. PLoS Med 2005; 2: 413–33.
14. Saha S, Chant D, Welhalm J et al. The incidence and prevalence of schizophrenia by latitude. Acta Psychiatr Scand 2006; 114: 36–9.
15. Torrey EF, Torrey B, Burton-Bradley BG. The epidemiology of schizophrenia in Papua New Guinea. Am J Psychiatry 1974; 131: 567–73.
16. Jablensky A. Multicultural studies and the nature schizophrenia: a review. J Royal Soc Med 1987; 80: 162–7.
17. Jablensky A. Epidemiology of schizophrenia: the global burden of disease and disability. Eur Arch Psych Clin Neurosci 2000; 250: 274–85.
18. Leff J, Sartorius N, Jablensky A et al. The International Pilot Study of Schizophrenia: five-year follow-up findings. Psychol Med 1992; 22: 131–45.
19. Sartorius N, Jablensky A, Korten A et al. Early manifestations and first-contact incidence of schizophrenia in different cultures. A preliminary report on the initial evaluation phase

of the WHO Collaborative Study on determinants of outcome of severe mental disorders. Psychol Med 1986; 16: 909–28.

20. Edgerton RB, Cohen A. Culture and schizophrenia: the DOSMeD challenge. Br J Psychiatry 1994; 164: 222–31.

21. Hopper K, Wanderling J. Revisiting the developed versus developing country distinction in course and outcome in schizophrenia: results from ISoS, the WHO collaborative follow-up project. International Study of Schizophrenia. Schizophr Bull 2000; 26: 835–46.

22. Verghese A, John JK, Rajkumer S et al. Factors associated with the course and outcome of schizophrenia in India: results of a two-year multicentre follow-up study. Br J Psychiatry 1993; 163: 535–41.

23. Leon CA. Clinical course and outcome of schizophrenia in Cali, Columbia: a 10-year follow-up study. J Nerv Ment Dis 1989; 177: 593–606.

24. Thara R, Henrietta M, Joseph A et al. Ten-year course of schizophrenia: the Madras Longitudinal Study. Acta Psychiatr Scand 1994; 90: 329–36.

25. Thara R. Twenty-year course of schizophrenia: the Madras Longitudinal Study. Can J Psychiatry 2004; 49: 564–9.

26. Ohaeri JU. Long-term outcome of treated schizophrenia in a Nigerian cohort. Retrospective analysis of 7-year follow-ups. J Nerv Ment Dis 1993; 181: 514–6.

27. Bhugra D, Hilwig M, Hossein B et al. First-contact incidence rates of schizophrenia in Trinidad and one-year follow-up. Br J Psychiatry 1997; 169: 587–92.

28. Jablensky A. Schizophrenia and Related Psychoses. In: Bhugra D, Bhui K, eds. Textbook of Cultural Psychiatry. Cambridge: Cambridge University Press, 2007: 207–23.

29. Patel V, Cohen A, Thara R et al. Is the outcome of schizophrenia really better in developing countries? Rev Bras Psichiatr 2006; 28: 149–52.

30. Saha S, Chant D, McGrath J. A systematic review of mortality in schizophrenia. Arch Gen Psychiatry 2007; 64: 1123–31.

31. Jilek WG. Emil Kraepelin and comparative sociocultural psychiatry. Eur Arch Psych Clin Neurosci 1995; 245: 231–38.

32. Murphy HBM. Comparative Psychiatry. Berlin, Heidelberg, New York: Springer; 1982.

33. Stompe T, Friedmann A. Culture and Schizophrenia. In: Bhugra D, Bhui K, eds. Textbook of Cultural Psychiatry. Cambridge: Cambridge University Press, 2007: 314–23.

34. Pfeiffer WM. Transkulturelle Psychiatrie, 2nd ed. Stuttgart, New York: Thieme; 1994.

35. Stompe T, Friedmann A, Ortwein G et al. Comparison of delusions among schizophrenics in Austria and in Pakistan. Psychopathology 1999; 32: 225–34.

36. Murphy HBM. Cultural aspects of the delusion. Studium Generale 1967; 11: 684–92.

37. Kala AK, Wig NN. Delusions across cultures. Int J Soc Psychiatry 1982; 28: 185–93.

38. Ndetei DM, Vadher A. Frequency and clinical significance of delusions across cultures. Acta Psychiatr Scand 1984; 70: 73–6.

39. Tateyama M, Masahiro A, Kamisada M et al. Transcultural study of schizophrenic delusions. Tokyo versus Vienna and Tübingen. Psychopathology 1998; 31: 59–68.

40. Kim K, Hwu H, Zhang LD et al. Schizophrenic delusions in Seoul, Shanghai and Taipei: a transcultural study. J Kor Med Science 2001; 16: 88–94.

41. Stompe T, Bauer S, Ortwein-Swoboda G et al. Delusions of guilt: The attitude of Christian and Islamic confessions towards Good and Evil and the responsibility of men. J Muslim Ment Health 2006; 1: 43–56.

42. Tateyama M, Asai M, Hashimoto M, Bartels M, Kasper S. Transcultural study of s chizophrenic delusions: Tokyo vs. Vienna and Tübingen (Germany). Psychopathology 1998; 31: 59–68.

43. Murphy HBM, Wittkower ED, Fried J et al. Cross-cultural survey of schizophrenic symptomatology. Int J Soc Psychiatry 1963; 10: 237–49.

44. Ndetei DM, Vadher A. A comparative cross-cultural study of the frequencies of hallucinations in schizophrenia. Acta Psychiatr Scand 1984; 70: 545–9.

45. Suhail LK, Cochrane R. Effect of culture and environment on the phenomenology of delusions and hallucinations. Int J Soc Psychiatry 2002; 48: 126–38.

46. Ødegaard Ø. Emigration and insanity: a study of mental disease among Norwegian born population in Minnesota. Acta Psychiatr Neurol Scand 1932; 7(Suppl. 4): 1–206.

47. Selten JP, Cantor-Graae E, Kahn RS. Migration and schizophrenia. Curr Opin Psychiatry 2007; 20: 111–5.

48. Cantor-Graae E, Zolkowska K, McNeil TF. Increased risk of psychotic disorder among immigrants in Malmö: a 3-years first-contact study. Psychol Med 2005; 35: 1155–63.

49. Brugha T, Jenkins R, Bebbington P et al. Risk factors and the prevalence of neurosis and psychosis in ethnic groups in Great Britain. Soc Psychiatry Psychiatr Epidemiol 2004; 39: 939–46.

50. Hickling F, Rodgers-Johnson P. The incidence of first contact schizophrenia in Jamaica. Br J Psychiatry 1995; 167: 193–6.

51. Mahy GE, Mallet R, Leff J et al. First-contact incidence rates of schizophrenia on Barbados. Br J Psychiatry 1999; 175: 28–33.

52. Hutchinson G, Takei N, Bhugra D. Morbid risk of schizophrenia in first-degree relatives of White and African-Caribbean patients with psychosis. Br J Psychiatry 1996: 776–80.

53. Bhugra D, Mallett R, Leff J. Schizophrenia and the African-Caribbeans: a conceptual model of aetiology. Int Rev Psychiatry 1999; 11: 145–52.

54. Selten JP, Cantor-Graae E. Social defeat: risk factor for schizophrenia? Br J Psychiatry 2005; 187: 101–2.

55. Pi EH, Simpson GM. Cross-cultural psychopharmacology: a current clinical perspective. Psychopharmacology 2005; 56: 31–3.

56. Zhou HH, Adedoyin A, Wilkinson GB. Differences in plasma binding of drugs between Caucasian and Chinese subjects. Clin Pharm Therap 1990; 48: 10–7.

57. Yu S-H, Liu S-K, Lin K-M. Psychopharmacology across Cultures. In: Bhugra D, Bhui K, eds. Textbook of Cultural Psychiatry. Cambridge: Cambridge University Press, 2007: 402–13.

23

Electroconvulsive therapy in schizophrenia

Georgios Petrides and Raphael J Braga

BACKGROUND

Electroconvulsive therapy (ECT) is the oldest surviving biological treatment in modern psychiatry. It is now more than 70 years old and its efficacy in treating severe mental illness remains unsurpassed. Convulsive therapy was initially introduced in 1934 in Hungary by Ladislaus von Meduna as a treatment for schizophrenia. It was thought at the time that epilepsy and schizophrenia were "antagonistic" illnesses (1). This concept was based on the interpretation of neuropathological studies showing a robust growth of glial cells in brains of epileptic patients and lack of glial growth in brains of schizophrenic patients, as well as the observation that epileptic patients diagnosed with schizophrenia had better overall prognosis (2).

Meduna decided to follow this line of research by investigating the possibility that epileptic seizures have a therapeutic effect on schizophrenic patients. The first patient treated with an injection of camphor oil was a patient diagnosed with schizophrenia in a catatonic stupor, bedridden, and tube fed for 4 years. He recovered completely after 11 treatments (3). Convulsive therapy was born and heralded as a major step toward the cure of schizophrenia. Camphor oil was quickly replaced by metrazol, a more soluble and easier to administer compound. However, inducing seizures by chemical means was unreliable and often very unpleasant for the patients. Researchers sought to replace chemicals with more efficient methods. Ugo Cerletti and his assistant Lucio Bini in Rome experimented with electricity. After a series of studies in animals, they applied their technique to a human for the first time in April of 1938 (4). As in Meduna's case, the first patient that they attempted to treat was a patient diagnosed with schizophrenia exhibiting agitation, disorganized speech replete with neologisms, and delusional ideas that his thoughts were controlled by others and broadcasted to strangers. The induction of generalized grand-mal seizures was successful and the patient recovered completely after 11 treatments. It is fortuitous that both of these patients presented, as will be discussed later, with conditions highly responsive to convulsive therapy. ECT became very popular for the management of severe mental illness, and during this period of limited treatment options, hundreds of thousands of patients around the world received the treatment. ECT was tried on patients with a variety of mental problems, and for the first time in history, large numbers of severely mentally ill patients found a treatment that was effective, improving the quality of their lives and allowing them to rejoin the community. However, the initial enthusiasm was tempered as the indiscriminate use of ECT for the management of any psychiatric condition, maladaptive behaviour, or even homosexuality, failed to become a panacea. As might be expected, in hindsight, in many cases the results were very poor and even counterproductive. On the other hand, it became quite clear that certain conditions responded quite dramatically to ECT. Most strikingly, patients with depressive symptoms received maximal benefit from the treatment. Other conditions for which ECT was shown to be effective were mania, epilepsy, motor syndromes such as catatonia, and Parkinson's disease. In some cases, the effects of ECT were not only dramatic and life altering, but they were also truly life saving.

It is a very difficult task to evaluate the studies regarding the efficacy of ECT in various psychiatric disorders that were performed during the "premedication psychiatry" period due to the differences in diagnosing psychiatric disorders between then and now. Many of the patients who would likely be diagnosed as having bipolar illness or major depressive disorder by modern diagnostic criteria were considered schizophrenics. Research methodology was also different, resulting in reports that are difficult to interpret or even accept today. However, the efficacy of ECT in the treatment of affective disorders has been established beyond a doubt in numerous studies over the years (5) and the review of those studies is beyond the scope of this chapter. Ironically, the role of ECT in the treatment of schizophrenia, the disorder for which it was first introduced, remains unclear.

With the introduction of antipsychotic medications in the 1950s, the use of ECT in schizophrenia sharply declined along with the overall use of ECT. The ease of administration of medications, lower cost compared to ECT, acceptable efficacy, and the well-promoted interests of the pharmaceutical industry were some of the reasons for the quick displacement of ECT. In addition, the strong antipsychiatry movement that swept Western Europe and North America in the 1960s and 1970s offered the fertile ground for unjustifiably labeling ECT as barbaric and obsolete, bundling it together with the already scientifically discredited biological treatments of that era, namely, insulin coma and lobotomy (6). However, despite the remarkable scientific progress in understanding schizophrenia and the introduction of medications that control many symptoms, a high percentage of patients do not respond or respond only partially. Others cannot tolerate medications or experience severe side effects. For those patients, ECT remained the last resort. Many practitioners continued to recommend ECT for their patients, albeit in smaller numbers (7).

ECT has undergone an unprecedented revival the past 30 years mainly due to its superior effectiveness in treating affective illnesses. The technique of the administration has been substantially improved and refined, resulting in better outcomes and fewer side effects. As ECT has become again less stigmatized and more easily accessible, the interest in its use for the management of schizophrenia has been renewed (8, 9). The evolution of our diagnostic classification systems and research methodologies allows us to study the role of ECT in schizophrenia more systematically. It is not surprising that after an essential paucity of publications for many years, several new reports on ECT and schizophrenia have appeared in the literature since 1980, the year when *DSM-III* was introduced. Thus, in this chapter, we will focus primarily on studies pertaining to the use of ECT in schizophrenia published after 1980.

STUDIES ON EFFICACY

Initial studies regarding the efficacy of ECT as compared to antipsychotic medications indicate no superiority of the former (10–12). Unfortunately, due to the limitations already mentioned in the early literature, its conclusions should be viewed with caution.

Since 1980, all studies on ECT in schizophrenia focused on the efficacy of ECT as an augmentation to antipsychotics. Details of these studies are found in an earlier publication where we reviewed the use of ECT in combination with antipsychotic medications (13). It became clear to us that ECT in schizophrenia has been poorly studied even after 1980. Besides the general ambivalence of the medical and research community toward its use and the lack of financial support, (14) ECT research also suffers from innate methodological challenges such as the lack of an adequate control group. The "optimal" control is the simulated or sham ECT that consists of the induction of general anesthesia without the electrical stimulus and the seizure. Due to the ethical challenges of exposing subjects to the procedure's risks without getting any benefit, the use of the sham strategy in modern protocols is avoided in most countries. However, there were eight double-blind studies with sham conducted since 1980. Most of them suffer from methodological problems and report conflicting results.

Three of the studies using simulated ECT suggested that real ECT plus antipsychotic therapy is more effective than sham treatment plus medications. Taylor and Fleminger randomly assigned 20 patients who failed 2 weeks of 300 mg of chlorpromazine to receive up to 12 real ECT or sham treatments as an adjunct to chlorpromazine (15). Nine patients in the ECT group and one in the sham group showed improvement. The two groups differed significantly in rating scores for psychopathology after the sixth treatment and at the end of the course at 4 weeks. However, the differences were not significant at 1 and 3 months after the end of treatment. Brandon et al. randomly assigned 19 schizophrenic patients to receive eight ECT or eight sham sessions in addition to the antipsychotic medications they were already receiving (16). At the end of the treatment phase, the ECT group fared significantly better than the sham group. There was no difference between the groups at Week 12 and Week 28 naturalistic follow-up. In a study by Abraham and Kulhara, 22 patients were randomly assigned to receive 8 ECT or sham treatments in addition to 20 mg/day of trifluoperazine(17). The ECT group showed significantly greater and more rapid improvement than the simulated ECT at the end of 4 weeks. Again, there were no differences between the groups at Week 16, 20, and 26.

Four other studies fail to show differences between ECT plus medication versus sham plus medication. Agarwal and Winny randomized 30 patients to receive 8 ECT or sham plus 1200 mg of chlorpromazine(18). Both groups improved, and there were no differences in BPRS reductions at the end of ECT course. Sarkar et al. tested the two strategies using 6 ECT or sham sessions in 30 subjects receiving 15 mg of haloperidol. Again, both groups improved, and there was no difference between them after six treatments(19). Upkong and collaborators randomized 16 subjects to 6 sessions of ECT plus chlorpromazine or sham plus chlorpromazine (20). After six treatments they failed to show any differences between the groups. Sarita et al. compared bitemporal, right unilateral, and sham ECT in groups of 12 patients receiving >10 mg/day of haloperidol(21). All three groups improved after 4 weeks, and there were no statistically significant differences among them.

It is difficult to ignore that the above studies suffered from significant methodological flaws and had small samples of 30 subjects or less, raising the question of lack of power to detect differences. Furthermore, with few exceptions, the studies used a small number of ECT sessions, on account of the ethical challenges of submitting patients to a prolonged use of sham ECT. The inclusion of patients in various stages of their illness, including patients with schizophreniform disorder and patients free of medication, is also problematic, as many of these patients are particularly responsive to medications and may artificially inflate response rates in both groups. Finally, Small et al. reported that they conducted a randomized controlled trial where the blind applied not to the ECT condition but to the medication (22). They included 75 patients and used thiothixene and right unilateral ECT. The presented details of the study are very limited, with no data on medication dosages, number of patients in each group, treatment parameters, and statistical analyses. Nevertheless, they concluded that medication alone and medication plus ECT were equally effective.

We identified two studies using a single-blind design with masked raters. Janakiramaiah et al. compared 4 groups of 15 patients who were administered 300 or

500 mg of chlorpromazine with or without ECT (23). None of these patients were on medications at baseline. Those who received ECT had an average of 10 treatments. Despite a faster response noted at Week 1, with the combination of 500 mg and ECT, analysis at the end of Week 4, 5, and 6 indicated that 500 mg of chlorpromazine alone was better than 300 mg of chlorpromazine alone or 300 mg + ECT, while the addition of ECT did not result in further improvement.

These results are in contrast to a more recent and well-designed study by Chanpattana and colleagues (24). This was a multicenter study, divided into acute and continuation phases. Patients had a diagnosis of schizophrenia in acute exacerbation and were defined as treatment resistant, according to modified Kane and Miller criteria (25, 26) requiring at least 2 failed medication trials. In the acute phase, subjects were started on flupenthixol up to 24 mg/day, and bilateral ECT was given 3 times per week. Response was defined as a BPRS score of 25 or less and sustaining it at this level throughout a stabilization period. This period was comprised of the following schedule: 3 ECT treatments in the first week, then once a week for the Weeks 2 and 3. A minimum of 20 treatments was necessary for a patient to be considered a nonresponder. In all, 101 patients completed the acute phase, and 57% of the subjects were considered responders. Responders were eligible to go on to the continuation phase. In this second phase, patients were randomly assigned to either continuation-ECT (C-ECT) alone, C-ECT combined with flupenthixol, or flupenthixol alone. C-ECT was given weekly for 1 month (4 treatments) and then biweekly for 5 months (10 treatments). As many 51 patients were enrolled and 45 completed the second phase of the study. Among the completers, 60% maintained remission after 6 months in the combined C-ECT+ flupenthixol group, while 93% relapsed in both the C-ECT-alone and the flupenthixol-alone groups, which represented a significant difference between groups. This study is significant not only due to its sound design and relatively large sample size but also because it employed longer courses of ECT. In the acute phase, they required 20 treatments before declaring someone as nonresponder. They also showed that a substantial percentage of responders (60%) may maintain their improvement if treated with the combination of maintenance ECT and medications. This is particularly important when someone takes into consideration that these patients had been already declared nonresponders to medication.

These auspicious results seem to be in concordance with a large number of open studies and chart reviews of more than 850 patients, which indicates that the combination of ECT and antipsychotic medications is a safe and more effective strategy for schizophrenia, especially for those patients who failed previous treatments with medications (27–46).

CLOZAPINE AND ECT

A particular case could be made for the use of ECT in individuals with schizophrenia refractory to clozapine. Clozapine is the only drug shown to be effective in the treatment of the medication-resistant patients. Still, as many as 70% of those who are able to receive an adequate trial of clozapine fail to receive any benefit from this drug (25). Hence, a possible next step for these patients would be the combination of ECT and clozapine. It is, therefore, surprising that very few researchers have tried to evaluate such a treatment strategy.

Case reports and retrospective studies attest to the safety of combination ECT and clozapine and generally report positive outcomes (47–53). Three small prospective studies provide promising data on the combination of clozapine and ECT. James et al.

studied individuals with schizophrenia who were refractory to conventional antipsychotic treatment (not clozapine) and who had refused the blood tests necessary for clozapine introduction (54). All six subjects included were inpatients in secure facilities. Clozapine treatment was only started after the sixth ECT session. After 12 treatments, all patients were out of seclusion and offered no resistance to clozapine treatment. Mean BPRS improvement was 32%. No prolonged seizures or other side effects were noted. Kho and collaborators selected patients who were nonresponsive to clozapine treatment, with a diagnosis of schizophrenia according to the Mini International Psychiatric Interview (55). Eleven patients received right-unilateral ECT, twice a week. If by the sixth session there was insufficient clinical response, the placement was switched to bitemporal. If the patient was still not responding (defined as a reduction of the PANSS scores greater than 30%) after the sixth bitemporal ECT session, the treatment was discontinued. Two of the patients discontinued ECT prematurely, one of them due to lack of efficacy after the sixth session. Of the 9 completing patients, 8 were considered responders. Interestingly, a comparable improvement was seen in both positive and negative symptoms. Finally, Masoudzadeh and Khalilian randomized 18 treatment-resistant schizophrenic patients into 3 groups: clozapine alone, ECT alone, and clozapine plus ECT(56). They reported a reduction in the PANSS ratings by 46%, 40%, and 70%, respectively. They also reported improvement both in positive and negative symptoms.

The association of clozapine use with EEG abnormalities and increased risk of seizures has raised concerns about the safety of its combination with ECT. The above mentioned reports do not support such concerns and encourage further study of the combination of clozapine and ECT for the treatment of treatment-resistant schizophrenia.

CATATONIA AND NEUROLEPTIC MALIGNANT SYNDROME

Among different presentation of schizophrenia, catatonia merits special attention in discussions of ECT. Catatonia is a motor syndrome that presents itself with a variety of symptoms, including muscle rigidity, mutism, staring, negativism, posturing, psychomotor retardation, and autonomic instability. It also presents in a range of severity with the most severe form being the malignant or lethal catatonia with high mortality rates. Traditionally catatonia is considered to be a part of the schizophrenic presentation and a subtype of the illness according to *DSM* and ICD classifications. Although it is now known that the condition is more commonly associated with affective illness and medical conditions (57, 58) and classification systems allow for the use of a modifier for catatonia in affective and medical conditions, many patients with schizophrenia also present with catatonic symptoms. Nevertheless, many reports testify to the effectiveness of ECT in treating the catatonic syndrome regardless of its underlying psychopathology and severity. In the case of malignant catatonia, ECT can be life saving (59).

Due to the relatively low incidence of the syndrome, it is very difficult to perform prospective randomized studies with ECT in catatonia. Nevertheless, there are several case reports and open studies attesting to the marked effectiveness of ECT for this syndrome. It is evident from these reports that more favorable results and reduced morbidity are obtained when ECT is initiated during the early stages of catatonia (59–61).

One particularity of the ECT technique in treating catatonia is that in severe forms daily treatments for up to 5 days are preferred with continuation at more conventional frequencies when the acute symptoms are resolved. Furthermore, catatonia is the only situation for which the concomitant use of benzodiazepines and ECT is considered to be synergistic (62).

Several lines of data suggest that neuroleptic malignant syndrome (NMS)—a syndrome characterized by fever, rigidity, altered mental state, mutism, autonomic instability, and elevated serum CPK—can be conceptualized as a more severe condition in a catatonia spectrum, resembling lethal catatonia (59, 60, 63). Therefore, it is not surprising that several case reports indicated that ECT is effective, often dramatically so, for the treatment of NMS. For instance, in a review of 734 cases of NMS, Davis and colleagues found that ECT was used in 48 cases. The results suggest that ECT is at least as effective as specific drug treatments (i.e., amantadine, bromocriptine, L-dopa, and dantrolene), reducing mortality by about 50% (64).

However, it should be stressed that ECT for NMS is not without risks, as subjects diagnosed with NMS are frequently in a compromised medical condition. Reports of thrombophlebitis and cardiac events are potential complications of the procedure in NMS, and clinicians should weigh the risks and benefits of ECT in individual cases (64–66).

ECT TECHNIQUE AND SAFETY

The vast majority of the papers found in the literature used the traditional bitemporal placement. Two controlled studies compared different electrode placements for ECT in subjects with schizophrenia (21, 67). Both studies suggest that bilateral and right-unilateral placements have comparable efficacy and that the latter might offer a better side-effect profile. However, these studies have serious methodologic shortcomings, leaving the question of which is the optimal placement for ECT in schizophrenia unanswered. At least one controlled study suggests that higher stimulus intensities can have some benefits in bilateral ECT for schizophrenia. Chanpattana et al. randomized 62 patients to 3 ECT different dosage strategies at just above seizure threshold (1xST), twofold (2xST), and fourfold threshold (4xST) (68). At the end of the study, all groups exhibited similar response rates, but patients in the twofold (2xST) group required fewer treatments, with no additional side-effect burden.

Despite being an important issue regarding ECT technique, very few studies have presented extensive data on safety measures or side effects. Only two controlled studies reported the effects of ECT on cognition and their results are conflicting. Taylor and Fleminger (15) indicated that subjects treated with ECT combined with antipsychotics exhibited memory performance comparable to patients treated with antipsychotic and sham ECT, while Sarita et al. (21). concluded that patients treated with sham ECT performed significantly better in cognitive evaluations than patients treated with unilateral or bilateral ECT. Two other longitudinal studies failed to detect any deleterious impact of ECT on cognitive function, although this finding should be viewed with caution because these studies had extremely small samples (69) and/or used coarse cognitive measures (27, 31, 32).

Overall, most reports regard the combination of antipsychotics and ECT as a safe strategy. No life-threatening side effects or deaths have been reported. Memory effects and muscle aches (44, 67) are described in some of the studies, but they do not seem to differ from those typically associated with ECT.

CONCLUSION

The review of the current literature points to the fact that the body of data available regarding the role of ECT in schizophrenia is still far from adequate. Large studies with careful, blinded, controlled research designs; operationalized criteria; and comprehensive assessments of treatment response and safety are needed. However, the available data indicate that ECT can be a very useful strategy, particularly for individuals with affective or pharmacological treatment-resistant symptoms. There is good evidence that ECT in combination with antipsychotics can be more effective than ECT or medications alone for these conditions. In addition, descriptions of a dramatic improvement in life-threatening conditions, such as neuroleptic malignant syndrome and malignant catatonia, strongly point to the importance of ECT as a treatment option.

REFERENCES
1. Gazdag G, Bitter I, Ungvari GS, Baran B, Fink M. Laszlo Meduna's Pilot Studies With Camphor Inductions of Seizures: The First 11 Patients. J ECT 2009 (e-pub ahead of print).
2. Abrams R. Electroconvulsive Therapy. Fourth ed. New York: Oxford University Press; 2002.
3. Fink M. Meduna and the origins of convulsive therapy. Am J Psychiatry 1984; 141(9): 1034–41.
4. Cerletti U, Binni L. Un Nuevo Metodo de Shocktherapie "L'elettroshock". Bolletino Accademia Medica Roma 1938; 64; 136–8.
5. Pagnin D, de QV, Pini S, Cassano GB. Efficacy of ECT in depression: a meta-analytic review. J ECT 2004; 20(1): 13–20.
6. Fink M. Impact of the antipsychiatry movement on the revival of electroconvulsive therapy in the United States. Psychiatr Clin North Am 1991; 14(4): 793–801.
7. Thompson JW, Weiner RD, Myers CP. Use of ECT in the United States in 1975, 1980, and 1986. Am J Psychiatry 1994; 151(11): 1657–61.
8. Chanpattana W, Kunigiri G, Kramer BA, Gangadhar BN. Survey of the practice of electroconvulsive therapy in teaching hospitals in India. J ECT 2005; 21(2): 100–4.
9. Gazdag G, Sebestyen G, Zsargo E, Tolna J, Ungvari GS. Survey of referrals to electroconvulsive therapy in Hungary. World J Biol Psychiatry 2008 Jul 25; 1–5.
10. Bagadia VN, Abhyankar RR, Doshi J , Pradhan PV, Shah LP. A double blind controlled study of ECT vs chlorpromazine in schizophrenia. J Assoc Physicians India 1983; 31(10): 637–40.
11. Childers RT, Therrien R. A comparison of the effectiveness of trifluoperazine and chlormpromazine in schizophrenia. Am J Psychiatry 1961; 118: 552–4.
12. Langsley DG, Enterline JD, HICKERSON GX Jr. A comparison of chlorpromazine and EST in treatment of acute schizophrenic and manic reactions. AMA Arch Neurol Psychiatry 1959; 81(3): 384–91.
13. Braga RJ, Petrides G. The Combined Use of Electroconvulsive Therapy and Antipsychotics in Patients With Schizophrenia. J ECT 2005; 21(2): 75–83.
14. Salzman C. ECT, research, and professional ambivalence. Am J Psychiatry 1998; 155(1): 1–2.
15. Taylor P, Fleminger JJ. ECT for schizophrenia. Lancet 1980; 1(8183); 1380–2.
16. Brandon S, Cowley P, McDonald C et al. Leicester ECT trial: results in schizophrenia. Br J Psychiatry 1985; 146: 177–83.
17. Abraham KR, Kulhara P. The efficacy of electroconvulsive therapy in the treatment of schizophrenia. A comparative study. Br J Psychiatry 1987; 151: 152–5.
18. Agarwal AK, Winny GC. Role of ECT Phenotiazine Combination in Schizophrenia. Indian J Psychiatry 1985; 27(3): 233–6.
19. Sarkar P, Andrade C, Kapur B et al. An exploratory evaluation of ECT in haloperidol-treated DSM-IIIR schizophreniform disorder. Convuls Ther 1994; 10(4): 271–8.
20. Ukpong DI, Makanjuola RO, Morakinyo O. A controlled trial of modified electroconvulsive therapy in schizophrenia in a Nigerian teaching hospital. West Afr J Med 2002; 21(3): 237–40.
21. Sarita EP, Janakiramaiah N, Gangadhar BN, Subbakrishna DK, Jyoti Rao KM. Efficacy of Combined ECT after Two Weeks of Neuroleptics in Schizophrenia: A Double Blind Controlled Study. NIMHANS Journal 1998; 16(4): 243–51.
22. Small JG, Milstein V, Klapper M, Kellams JJ, Small IF. ECT combined with Neuroleptics in the Treatment of Schizophrenia. Psychopharmacol Bull 1982; 18(1): 34–5.

23. Janakiramaiah N, Channabasavanna SM, Murthy NS. ECT/chlorpromazine combination versus chlorpromazine alone in acutely schizophrenic patients. Acta Psychiatr Scand 1982; 66(6): 464–70.

24. Chanpattana W, Chakrabhand ML, Sackeim HA et al. Continuation ECT in treatment-resistant schizophrenia: a controlled study. J ECT 1999; 15(3): 178–92.

25. Kane J, Honigfeld G, Singer J, Meltzer H. Clozapine for the treatment-resistant schizophrenic. A double-blind comparison with chlorpromazine. Arch Gen Psychiatry 1988; 45(9): 789–96.

26. Miller DD, Perry PJ, Cadoret RJ, Andreasen NC. Clozapine's effect on negative symptoms in treatment-refractory schizophrenics. Compr Psychiatry 1994; 35(1): 8–15.

27. Chanpattana W, Chakrabhand ML, Kongsakon R, Techakasem P, Buppanharun W. Short-term effect of combined ECT and neuroleptic therapy in treatment-resistant schizophrenia. J ECT 1999; 15(2): 129–39.

28. Chanpattana W, Buppanharun W, Raksakietisak S, Vaughn MW, Somchai Chakrabhand ML. Seizure threshold rise during electroconvulsive therapy in schizophrenic patients. Psychiatry Res 2000; 96(1): 31–40.

29. Chanpattana W. Maintenance ECT in treatment-resistant schizophrenia. J Med Assoc Thai 2000; 83(6): 657–62.

30. Chanpattana W, Chakrabhand ML. Combined ECT and neuroleptic therapy in treatment-refractory schizophrenia: prediction of outcome. Psychiatry Res 2001; 105(1–2): 107–15.

31. Chanpattana W, Chakrabhand ML. Factors influencing treatment frequency of continuation ECT in schizophrenia. J ECT 2001; 17(3): 190–4.

32. Chanpattana W, Kramer BA. Acute and maintenance ECT with flupenthixol in refractory schizophrenia: sustained improvements in psychopathology, quality of life, and social outcomes. Schizophr Res 2003; 63(1–2): 189–93.

33. Das PS, Saxena S, Mohan D, Sundaram KR. Adjunctive Electroconvulsive Therapy for Schizophrenia. Natl Med J India 1991; 4(4): 183–4.

34. Dodwell D Goldberg D. A study of factors associated with response to electroconvulsive therapy in patients with schizophrenic symptoms. Br J Psychiatry 1989; 154: 635–9.

35. Friedel RO. The combined use of neuroleptics and ECT in drug resistant schizophrenic patients. Psychopharmacol Bull 1986; 22(3): 928–30.

36. Gujavarty K, Greenberg LB, Fink M. Electroconvulsive Therapy and Neuroleptic Medication in Therapy-Resistant Positive-Symptom Psychosis. Convuls Ther 1987; 3(3): 185–95.

37. Hirose S, Ashby CR Jr, Mills MJ. Effectiveness of ECT combined with risperidone against aggression in schizophrenia. J ECT 2001; 17(1): 22–6.

38. Konig P, Glatter-Gotz U. Combined electroconvulsive and neuroleptic therapy in schizophrenia refractory to neuroleptics. Schizophr Res 1990; 3(5–6): 351–4.

39. Kramer BA. ECT in elderly patients with schizophrenia. Am J Geriatr Psychiatry 1999; 7(2): 171–4.

40. Milstein V, Small JG, Miller MJ, Sharpley PH, Small IF. Mechanisms of action of ECT: schizophrenia and schizoaffective disorder. Biol Psychiatry 1990; 27(12): 1282–92.

41. Nahshoni E, Manor N, Bar et al. Alterations in QT dispersion in medicated schizophrenia patients following electroconvulsive therapy. Eur Neuropsychopharmacol 2004; 14(2): 121–5.

42. Natani GD, Gautam S, Gehlot PS. Comparison of Three Treatment Regimes in Schizophrenia. Indian J Psychiatry 1983; 25(4): 306–11.

43. Sajatovic M, Meltzer HY. The Effect of Short-Term Electroconvulsive Treatment Plus Neuroleptics in Treatment-Resistant Schizophrenia and Schizoaffective Disorder. Convuls Ther 1993; 9(3): 167–75.

44. Tang WK, Ungvari GS. Efficacy of electroconvulsive therapy combined with antipsychotic medication in treatment-resistant schizophrenia: a prospective, open trial. J ECT 2002; 18(2): 90–4.

45. Suzuki K, Awata S, Takano T et al. Improvement of psychiatric symptoms after electroconvulsive therapy in young adults with intractable first-episode schizophrenia and schizophreniform disorder. Tohoku J Exp Med 2006; 210(3): 213–20.

46. Ucok A, Cakr S. Electroconvulsive therapy in first-episode schizophrenia. J ECT 2006; 22(1): 38–42.
47. Benatov R, Sirota P, Megged S. Neuroleptic-resistant schizophrenia treated with clozapine and ECT. Convuls Ther 1996; 12(2): 117–21.
48. Bhatia SC, Bhatia SK, Gupta S. Concurrent administration of clozapine and ECT: a successful therapeutic strategy for a patient with treatment-resistant schizophrenia. J ECT 1998; 14(4): 280–3.
49. Dean CE. Severe self-injurious behavior associated with treatment-resistant schizophrenia: treatment with maintenance electroconvulsive therapy. J ECT 2000; 16(3): 302–8.
50. Husni M, Haggarty J, Peat C. Clozapine does not increase ECT-seizure duration. Can J Psychiatry 1999; 44(2): 190–1.
51. Safferman AZ, Munne R. Combining Clozapine with ECT. Convuls Ther 1992; 8(2): 141–3.
52. Frankenburg FR, Suppes T, McLean PE. Combined Clozapine and Electroconvulsive Therapy. Convuls Ther 1993; 9(3): 176–80.
53. Cardwell BA, Nakai B. Seizure activity in combined clozapine and ECT: a retrospective view. Convuls Ther 1995; 11(2): 110–3.
54. James DV, Gray NS. Elective combined electroconvulsive and clozapine therapy. Int Clin Psychopharmacol 1999; 14(2): 69–72.
55. Kho KH, Blansjaar BA, De Vries S et al. Electroconvulsive therapy for the treatment of clozapine nonresponders suffering from schizophrenia. An open label study. Eur Arch Psychiatry Clin Neurosci 2004; 254(6): 372–9.
56. Masoudzadeh A, Khalilian AR. Comparative study of clozapine, electroshock and the combination of ECT with clozapine in treatment-resistant schizophrenic patients. Pak J Biol Sci 2007; 10(23): 4287–90.
57. Rosebush PI, Hildebrand AM, Furlong BG, Mazurek MF. Catatonic syndrome in a general psychiatric inpatient population: frequency, clinical presentation, and response to lorazepam. J Clin Psychiatry 1990; 51(9): 357–62.
58. Bush G, Fink M, Petrides G et al. Rating scale and standardized examination. Acta Psychiatr Scand 1996; 93(2): 129–36.
59. Petrides G, Malur C, Fink M. Convulsive Therapy. In: Caroff SN, Mann SC, Francis A, Fricchione GL, editors. Catatonia: from psychopathology to neurobiology. 1st ed. Washington, DC: American Psychiatric Publishing, 2004: 151–60.
60. Philbrick KL, Rummans TA. Malignant catatonia. J Neuropsychiatry Clin Neurosci 1994; 6(1): 1–13.
61. Hawkins JM, Archer KJ, Strakowski SM, Keck PE. Somatic treatment of catatonia. Int J Psychiatry Med 1995; 25(4): 345–69.
62. Petrides G, Divadeenam KM, Bush G, Francis A. Synergism of lorazepam and electroconvulsive therapy in the treatment of catatonia. Biol Psychiatry 1997; 42(5): 375–81.
63. Koch M, Chandragiri S, Rizvi S, Petrides G, Francis A. Catatonic signs in neuroleptic malignant syndrome. Compr Psychiatry 2000; 41(1): 73–5.
64. Davis JM, Janicak PG, Sakkas P, Gilmore C, Wang Z. Electroconvulsive Therapy in the Treatment of the Neuroleptic Malignant Syndrome. Convuls Ther 1991; 7(2): 111–20.
65. Hughes JR. ECT during and after the neuroleptic malignant syndrome: case report. J Clin Psychiatry 1986; 47(1): 42–3.
66. Regestein QR, Kahn CB, Siegel AJ, Blacklow RS, Genack A. A case of catatcnia occurring simultaneously with severe urinary retention. J Nerv Ment Dis 1971; 152(6): 432–5.
67. Bagadia VN, Abhyankar R, Pradhan PV, Shah LP. Reevaluation of ECT in Schizophrenia: Right Temporoparietal versus Bitemporal Electrode Placement. Convuls Ther 1988; 4(3): 215–20.
68. Chanpattana W, Chakrabhand ML, Buppanharun W, Sackeim HA. Effects of stimulus intensity on the efficacy of bilateral ECT in schizophrenia: a preliminary study. Biol Psychiatry 2000; 48(3): 222–8.
69. Rami L, Bernardo M, Valdes M et al. Absence of additional cognitive impairment in schizophrenia patients during maintenance electroconvulsive therapy. Schizophr Bull 2004; 30(1): 185–9.

24 Schizophrenia and stigma: Old problems, new challenges

Marina P Economou, Nick C Stefanis, and
George N Papadimitriou

STIGMA THROUGH HISTORY

The word *stigma* originates from the Greek language, στίμα, and specifically from the verb στίω, which means "to prick, to puncture." It connotes a mark and its use can be traced back to ancient years. In the Genesis of the Bible, God stigmatized Cain in order to identify him as the first murderer in the history of mankind. In ancient Greece, stigma was a sign, placed on slaves in order to acknowledge and indicate their inferiority within the social structure. In a similar vein, in the *Anatomy of Melancholy*, Burton (1) described the stigmatization of a criminal with hot iron to induce his public humiliation. Consistent with these two examples, and especially throughout Middle Ages, stigma took on the meaning of branding and publicly discrediting a criminal. In sharp contrast to the aforementioned negative meanings, the word *stigma* has also been used in a positive light. In the tradition of Christianity, stigmata (i.e. the plural of stigma) constituted wounds equivalent to those of Jesus Christ and thus manifested a life of extraordinary holiness. Nevertheless, with the passage of time, the negative meaning of the word has prevailed over the positive.

Modern thinking about stigma is heavily influenced by Erving Goffman's seminal publication of "Stigma—Notes on the Management of Spoiled Identity" (2). According to him, stigma is the "situation of the individual who is disqualified from full social acceptance." Consistent with this, nowadays, the term is restricted to denote a distinct mark, which induces the devaluation of the person who bears it within the society. In medicine, this mark or characteristic is indicative of a history of a disease or abnormality. Thus, medical conditions such as leprosy and tuberculosis in the past, AIDS in the contemporary society, and mental illness throughout history are all surrounded by stigma and discrimination against people suffering from them. The stigma attached to mental illness and specifically to schizophrenia is undoubtedly the most serious form of stigma (3, 4).

CONCEPTUAL ASPECTS

Since the early work of Goffman, many definitions of stigma have been put forward. The conceptualization of the stigma attached to mental illness is based on two leading conceptual frameworks, that of Corrigan (5) and that of Link and Phelan (6).

Corrigan (5) focuses on the cognitive, emotional, and behavioral core features of the mental-illness stigma and identify three components: *stereotypes*, defined as cognitive knowledge structures that are learned by most members of a social group; *prejudice*, which is the cognitive and emotional response to stereotypes; and *discrimination*, which is a negative behavioral consequence of prejudice. Furthermore, he divides stigma in two genres: *public stigma*, which is the general population's reaction to people with mental illness, and *self-stigma*, which is the prejudice people with mental illness turn against themselves.

Link and Phelan (6) have developed a model whereby they argue that when the five interrelated components of labeling, stereotyping, separation, status loss, and discrimination co-occur in a power situation and get unfolded, stigma is the outcome. Specifically, the "labeled" person is viewed as an outcast, as "them" and not "us." Furthermore, they (7) have identified three major forms of discrimination: *direct*, which involves overt rejection; *structural*, which is more subtle; and *insidious*, which occurs when stigmatized individuals realize that they are viewed as less trustworthy and intelligent and more dangerous and incompetent.

Another conceptual model of stigma and its consequences is that of Sartorius (8), which focuses on schizophrenia and has provided the foundation on which the antistigma initiatives taken by the World Psychiatric Association (WPA) are based. According to his formulation, a marker that allows the identification of a person can be loaded with negative contents by association with previous knowledge. Once the marker is loaded, it becomes stigma and the person who bears it gets stigmatized. Stigmatization then yields negative discrimination that in turn leads to numerous disadvantages in terms of access to care, poor health service, setbacks that impinge on self-esteem, and additional stress. As a result, the condition of the consumer might get exacerbated; the marker might get amplified; and a vicious circle is then established, as it is more likely for the person to be identified and stigmatized.

PUBLIC BELIEFS AND ATTITUDES

There is now a voluminous literature on stigma largely based on attitudinal surveys. The first studies exploring lay attitudes toward mental illness were conducted in the United States throughout the 1950s (9,10) by employing research techniques, such as vignettes and open-ended interviews, which determined to a large extent the subsequent methodology of the field. At the same period, Whatley (11) developed a social-distance scale by refining an existing one by Bogardus (12), with the purpose of measuring the degree of social proximity people would be willing to have to a person with mental illness. Social distance is still considered a fundamental measure of stigma (13,14,15) and current attitudes' surveys conducted by centers participating in the WPA program against stigma and discrimination due to schizophrenia (16, 17, 18) use a more developed instrument (19) incorporating the Social Distance Scale (12).

Many studies exploring community beliefs and attitudes have shown that stigmatizing opinions about psychiatric disorders are widely held in the population (14, 20, 21, 22, 23, 24) with schizophrenia being the disorder that is associated with the highest amount of stigma (4, 25, 26). Patients with schizophrenia are perceived primarily as unpredictable and dangerous, stereotypes that elicit feelings of uneasiness, uncertainty, and fear as well as rejective behaviors against them (25, 26, 27, 28).

For this reason, WPA embarked a program to fight the stigma and discrimination due to schizophrenia and placed only schizophrenia on the forefront of attention. Under this international program, several studies were conducted and revealed various similarities and differences between subgroups. Regarding the knowledge of schizophrenia, a Canadian sample (16) was found to be relatively well informed and progressive, whereas a Greek one (29) appeared to be poorly informed. Social distance was found to be strikingly higher in the Greek population (18) in comparison to the Canadian (16) and German samples (17). Interestingly, in spite of following a slightly different methodology, an Austrian study (30) on a representative sample of the general population found that the Austrian public reported a more negative view of schizophrenia and a greater extent of social distance in comparison to results of studies conducted in neighboring Germany (24, 31).

Negative attitudes and social distance toward individuals with mental illness are not only endorsed by the general public but also by other population groups, even health or mental health professionals (32, 33, 34). Psychiatrists in particular have been documented to hold more positive attitudes toward people with mental illness, especially schizophrenia, in comparison to the general population (35); however, no differences have been found in terms of the levels of social distance to mentally ill people (36). Studies focusing on medical students have revealed stigmatizing attitudes mainly based on fear and insufficient knowledge, which get improved, though, as medical education progresses, or after specific educational interventions (37, 38).

FACTORS INFLUENCING BELIEFS AND ATTITUDES

A line of research on stigma has concentrated on the factors that shape the beliefs toward mental illness and the attitudes toward people who suffer from it. Some of these factors are pertinent to the lay respondent, some to the person with mental illness and others to the interaction between the two.

From the perspective of the respondent, sociodemographic factors have been found to play a prominent role. Cultural background, older age, and male gender are all predictors of social distance toward people with mental illness (27,39). Converging evidence from Canada, Germany, and Greece have supported that old age of the respondent (16, 17, 18), especially over 60 years; low social class (18); low educational level (18); and being resident in semiurban or rural areas (16, 18) are all associated with greater social distance. By contrast, better-educated people and residents of urban areas have demonstrated better knowledge of mental illness and consequently more favorable attitudes (29, 30), whereas families with young children independently of their educational and sociodemographic background endorse negative attitudes (40).

From the same perspective, lay people who explain psychiatric disorders from a biological point of view (41) endorse negative attitudes. In addition, people who regard people with mental illness, especially with schizophrenia, as violent and dangerous (perceived dangerousness) tend to be less tolerant, to hold more negative attitudes, and to discriminate against them (42, 43). This association between perceived dangerousness, fear, and increased social distance has been validated in different countries, such as Germany (43), Russia (25), and the United States (44), indicating that one of the most significant dimensions of stigma is the assumed potential of patients for violent and dangerous behavior. Strengthening the importance of perceived dangerousness, a Greek study (18) comparing attitudes toward people with schizophrenia to other vulnerable-to-stigmatization groups revealed that the general public stigmatized people with schizophrenia the most, even more than serious law offenders. This finding might suggest that the public's perception about schizophrenia is associated with criminality rather than with other social taboos.

From the patient's perceptive, research has shown that several patient and illness factors predict social distance like the severity of mental illness (31), negative outcome (15), disturbances in patient's affective expression in social interaction (45), as well as actual violent and dangerous behaviors (25, 30). Violent and dangerous behaviors along with labeling one with a psychiatric diagnosis (28, 42) are considered the most prominent factors influencing attitudes. The impact of the label "schizophrenia" seems to be very powerful. In psychiatric day care, it was found that most clients were extremely anxious about being labeled as "mad", while "schizophrenia" was their most feared label (46). This is not surprising, as the term *schizophrenia* is negatively perceived in all cultures (47), especially in the Greek culture, as the word itself is of Greek origin and literally means a split mind, giving in this way a misleading connotation of split personality (e.g., Jekyll and Hyde) (18). In addition, in Japan the stigmatizing effect of the label *schizophrenia* on lay attitudes led the Japanese professionals to argue for changing the name (48). However, other studies have argued for the relative importance of the diagnostic label versus the person's behavior in determining public attitudes. Specifically, these have found that the effect of labeling was significant but that the person's behavior was more potent (49). Similarly, Penn and colleagues argued that knowledge of the symptoms of a person's acute schizophrenic episode created more stigma than the label *schizophrenia* itself (50).

The characteristics of the interaction between the lay person and the one with mental illness have also been indicated to have an impact on public beliefs, attitudes, and behavior. Prior contact with someone who suffers from mental illness decreases fear of dangerousness and stigma, while people who have never met or spoken to a psychiatric patient have more negative attitudes and feelings about mental illness (25, 41, 44, 51). It is noteworthy that when consistent and closer contact between the lay person and the individual with mental illness is necessitated, lay attitudes are more wary and conservative. Various studies have provided evidence for this relationship between closeness and social distance, where social distance has been found to increase with the level of intimacy required in the relationship (16, 17, 29).

STIGMA EXPERIENCED BY PATIENTS AND RELATIVES

While many studies on the field have explored the beliefs and attitudes of individuals who do not face stigmatization personally, little research has been conducted on the subjective stigma experiences of the affected individuals and their families. Only recently, studies employing primarily qualitative techniques have begun to enquire this subjective perspective (52, 53, 54, 55). Focus group studies on patients with schizophrenia and their relatives have revealed the following four dimensions of stigma to be affecting their lives: *interpersonal interaction*, *access to social roles* (e.g., work, partnership), *public image of mental illness*, and *structural discrimination* (i.e., imbalances and injustices observed in social structures, political decisions, and legislations) (52, 53). In addition to the aforementioned dimensions, in a recent study (55), patients and their relatives reported negative experiences regarding the availability and quality of mental health services as a manifestation of structural discrimination; while internalization of stigma emerged as a fifth dimension leading to self-induced discrimination.

The internalization of stigma is considered a further complication, as some individuals with mental illness agree with the stereotypical public conceptions, apply them to themselves, and consequently their self-confidence and self-esteem are diminished; a process known as self-stigmatization (56). In a proposed model of self-stigma; stereotype awareness (being aware of the stereotypes pertinent to mental illness), stereotype agreement (endorsing them), stereotype self-concurrence (applying them to the self-concept), group identification (identifying oneself with the mentally ill group), and perceived legitimacy (perceiving the stereotypes as accurate) have been found to influence either directly or indirectly the self-esteem and self-efficacy of individuals with mental illness (56, 57). Moreover, many studies have found a negative relationship between stereotype awareness and self-esteem (58, 59), while feelings of responsibility for one's illness lead to greater levels of self-blame and diminished self-worth (60).

Overall, both patients and their relatives have described a variety of stigmatizing experiences in all areas of life; feelings of self-blame, shame, and guilt, and they have reacted to these experiences with concealment of mental illness, avoidance, and isolation (54, 61).

MEDIA AND STIGMA

It is unanimously accepted that the mass media constitute a primary source of information on mental illness, influencing public opinion and shaping the public image of people with mental disorders (62, 63). In line with this, the media have been criticized/accused/blamed for contributing to psychiatric stigma via the images of characters with mental illness they portray, the misinformation communicated, and the inaccurate use of psychiatric terms (64). The studies that have endeavored to address this relationship between the media and the stigma attached to mental illness have approached the issue from different perspectives: how people with mental illness are portrayed in the various forms of media; how these images affect lay beliefs, attitudes, and behaviors pertinent to mental illness; and how the media can be used to combat psychiatric stigma.

With regard to the first perspective, people with mental illness are negatively portrayed in the various types of media, with violence being the most highlighted characteristic. As far as the print media are concerned, several studies from different countries (65, 66, 67, 68) have shown that the representations of people with mental illness are frequent, negatively biased toward the severe forms of illness, and disproportionately covering bizarre or criminal behavior rather than achievements of patients. In a recent trend analysis between 1989 and 1999, Wahl et al. (69) found that while the number of references to dangerousness in articles discussing mental illness had decreased, dangerousness was still the most common theme. Relevant studies on TV coverage of mental illness have yielded similar results (70, 71), a finding of special importance, as television has been argued to be the primary contributor of mental health information (62). Specifically, characters with mental illness in prime-time televisions are depicted physically violent and their representations have been found to be "outstandingly negative" (70), a finding that also emerges in children's television programs (71). It is noteworthy that people with mental illness are not the only ones with a distorted image in the media. Mental health professionals are also portrayed in one of the following negative ways: as being incompetent, controlling, neurotic, manipulative, stupid, drug or alcohol dependent, uncaring or mentally ill themselves (72, 73).

It is, therefore, clear that the images of people with mental illness in the media are negative, and consequently, various studies have sought to explore how these images influence stigma endorsement (74, 75, 76). Survey research has shown that people who watch television regularly are less likely to live next to someone diagnosed with mental illness (75), while more time spent in television viewing is associated with expressing greater intolerance toward mental illness (76) and with strongly believing that mental health services in a residential neighborhood would jeopardize the safety of the residents (75).

Another line of research has endeavored to find ways to use the media in order to combat psychiatric stigma. Based on the rationale that if the mass media can influence public perception of mental illness in such a negative way, they can also affect it in a positive way; many have seen into the media a potential ally to counteract stigma (72, 74). Indeed, the media can play a prominent role in educating the public, raising its awareness, and improving its attitudes toward mental illness, provided sophisticated techniques and well-organized interventions will be used. This was exactly the finding of some recent studies that examined the effect of an educational film material about schizophrenia and a computer-based antistigma intervention (77, 78) as well as of an educational intervention targeting journalists (79).

STRATEGIES AGAINST STIGMA

It has been argued, primarily by Corrigan and Penn (80), that the most effective approaches to diminish the stigma attached to mental illness can be grouped into three processes: protest, education, and contact.

Protest is a reactive strategy; often applied against stigmatizing public statements, media reports, and advertisements, it views stigma as a moral injustice. Consistent with this, protest strategies encompass public rallies and boycotts targeting business behaviors that are stigmatizing. An example of a protest effort is the StigmaBusters, a group developed in the United States with the purpose of challenging stigmatizing images presented in the media. With regard to the effectiveness of the protest approach, Wahl (62) has contended that citizens are encountering far fewer sanctioned examples of stigma and stereotypes because of protest initiatives. However, it is noteworthy that while protest efforts are helpful in diminishing negative attitudes, there is no compelling evidence to suggest that they can promote favorable attitudes, indicating in this way an important direction for future research.

Education attempts to diminish stigma by providing accurate information, so that the public can make more informed decisions about mental illness. Research has suggested that persons who evince a better understanding of mental illness are less likely to endorse stigma and discrimination (21, 51); therefore, the strategic provision of information about mental illness seems capable of lessening negative stereotypes. Education programs have been shown to be effective for a wide variety of participants; such as police officers, students, and journalists (81) as well as mental health professionals (32).

It merits discussion that the content of education programs is of paramount significance. Because neurobiological models of mental illness are predominant in current Western psychiatry, biological causes of schizophrenia, for example, constitute an integral part of the message relayed in educational programs. The rationale underlying this approach is that by emphasizing on the biochemical and hereditary components of mental illness, the shame and blame associated with it will be reduced. However, for some patients and their families, the knowledge of carrying a "genetic deficit" evokes strong negative feelings and impinges on their self-esteem (82). In addition, Mehta and Farina (83) found that describing mental illness in medical instead of psychosocial terms actually led to harsher behavior toward people with mental illness. A recent international study found similar results by showing that the view of schizophrenia being of biological origin led to a greater desire for social distance from the patients (84). Given these findings and the complexities of interactions between genes and the environment, the message of mental illness as being "genetic" or "neurological" may not only be overly simplistic but also of little use to educational interventions aiming at reducing stigma (85).

Contact with persons with mental illness may help to augment the effects of education on reducing stigma. Research has shown that contact challenges stereotypes and improves positive attitudes (86), and it is, therefore, regarded as an important strategy to fight stigma. In a number of interventions on secondary school students, where education and contact were combined, contact emerged as the most efficacious part of the intervention (81, 87). Particularly interesting in this respect is an Austrian study, which compared an educational intervention without contact to that of a combination of both education and contact, and found a positive change of students' attitudes only when a consumer was also involved in the intervention (contact and education condition) (88).

ANTISTIGMA INITIATIVES

Even today, the stigma of mental illness is one of the main obstacles to better mental health care and quality of life for patients, their families, and their communities. Stigma is pernicious and in spite of advances in psychiatry and medicine, it continuous to grow and to have terrible consequences for patients and their families. As such, it was recognized in the 2001 World Health Report of the World Health Organization (89) and in the Conference of EU Ministers of Health, which resulted in political commitment to fight stigma across the European Union (90).

Stigma constitutes a challenge for modern society, making it imperative to take specific steps with the aim of dispelling it. Various antistigma programs and campaigns have been initiated in many countries by governmental, professional, or consumer groups in order to target the stigma attached to mental illness in general. In 1996, the World Psychiatric Association (WPA) launched an international program to fight stigma and discrimination associated with schizophrenia, named "Schizophrenia: Open the Doors" (4, 8). Schizophrenia was chosen as the focus of this program because it is considered to be a typical example of mental illness in the public's mind. Specifically, when lay people were asked to describe a person with mental illness, they invariably listed symptoms such as delusions and hallucinations—hallmarks of schizophrenia—as the defining features of a "madman." Furthermore, rehabilitation of people with schizophrenia is often hampered by stigma-associated difficulties (91), and the stigma related to it is more pronounced than the stigma attached to other psychiatric conditions. Consequently, a success in the prevention or removal of the stigma related to schizophrenia may show the way to those fighting to remove the stigma of other mental disorders and of other stigmatizing illnesses. The main objectives of the WPA program are as follows: to raise awareness and improve knowledge about schizophrenia, to shape public attitudes toward individuals with schizophrenia and their families, and to generate actions against prejudice and discrimination. A characteristic of the program is the participation not only of psychiatrists but also of all parties concerned with schizophrenia, varying from those responsible for the administration to the users and their families. Up to now, the WPA program has been implemented in more than 20 countries around the world, resulting in numerous antistigma interventions.

Research on antistigma interventions has made considerable progress (92, 93). Nonetheless, there is still a pressing need for further studies that will incorporate sophisticated methodology, such as the testing of theory-based models and the implementation of cross-cultural comparisons on representative samples, which will cast light on the relationship between beliefs, attitudes, and behaviours; show ways of dealing with the nagging issue of discrimination; and, finally, provide the foundation for the creation of evidence-based antistigma programs. While the research community has made remarkable progress, there is still a long road ahead with many issues to be addressed.

REFERENCES

1. Burton R. The anatomy of melancholy. Oxford: Clarendon; 1989.
2. Goffman E. Stigma: Notes on the Management of Spoiled Identity. Harmondsworth: Penguin; 1970.
3. Lopez-Ibor JJ. The WPA and the fight against stigma because of mental diseases. World Psychiatry 2002; 1(1): 16–20.
4. Sartorius N, Schulze H. Reducing the stigma of mental illness: A report from a global programme of the World Psychiatric Association. New York: Cambridge University Press; 2005.
5. Corrigan PW. Mental health stigma as social attribution: Implications for research methods and attitude change. Clin Psychol Sci Pract 2000; 7: 48–67.
6. Link BG, Phelan JC. Conceptualizing stigma. Annu Rev Sociol. 2001; 27: 363–85.
7. Link BG, Phelan JC. Stigma and its public health implications. Lancet 2006; 367: 528–29.
8. Sartorius N. Breaking the vicious circle. Ment Health Learn Disabil Care 2000; 4(3): 80.
9. Star S. The publics' ideas about mental illness. Annual Meeting of the National Association for Mental Health, Indianapolis; Nov 5 1955.
10. Cumming E, Cumming G. Closed ranks: an experiment in mental health education. Cambridge: Harvard University Press; 1957.
11. Whatley C. Social attitudes towards discharged patients. Soc Problems 1958–1959; 6: 313–20.
12. Bogardus EM. Measuring social distance. J Appl Sociol 1925; 9: 299–308.
13. Owen CA, Eisner HC, McFaul TR. A half century of social distance research: National replication of the Bogardus' studies. Sociol Soc Res 1981; 66: 80–98.
14. Angermeyer MC, Matschinger H. Social distance towards the mentally ill: results of representative survey in the Federal Republic of Germany. Psychol Med 1997; 27: 131–41.
15. Angermeyer MC, Beck M, Matschinger H. Determinants of the public's preference for social distance from people with schizophrenia. Can J Psychiatry 2003; 48(10): 663–8.
16. Stuart H, Arboleda-Florez J. Community attitudes towards people with schizophrenia. Can J Psychiatry 2001; 46: 245–52.
17. Gaebel W, Baumann A, Witte AM et al. Public attitudes towards people with mental illness in two German cities. Results of a public survey under special considerations of schizophrenia. Eur Arch Psychiatry Clin Neurosci 2002; 252: 278–87.
18. Economou M, Gramandani C, Richardson C et al. Public attitudes towards people with schizophrenia in Greece. World Psychiatry 2005; 4(Supplement 1): 40–44.
19. Thompson A, Stuart H, Bland RC et al. Attitudes about schizophrenia from the pilot site of the WPA worldwide campaign against the stigma of schizophrenia. Soc Psychiatry Psychiatr Epidemiol 2002; 37: 475–82.
20. Crocetti G, Spiro JR, Siassi I. Are the ranks closed? Attitudinal social distance and mental illness. Am J Psychiatry 1971; 127: 1121–7.
21. Brockington I, Hall P, Levings J et al. The community's tolerance of the mentally ill. Br J Psychiatry 1993; 162: 93–9.
22. Madianos M, Economou M, Hatjiandreou M et al. Changes in public attitudes towards mental illness in the Athens area (1979/1980-1994). Acta Psychiatr Scand 1999; 99: 73–8.
23. Eker D. Attitudes toward mental illness: recognition, desired social distance, expected burden and negative influence on mental health among Turkish freshmen. Soc Psychiatry Psychiatr Epidemiol 1989; 24: 146–50.
24. Angermeyer MC, Dietrich S. Public beliefs about and attitudes towards people with mental illness: a review of population studies. Acta Psychiatr Scand 2006; 113: 163–79.
25. Angermeyer MC, Matschinger H, Corrigan P. Familiarity with mental illness and social distance from people with schizophrenia and major depression: Testing a model using data from a representative population survey. Schizophr Res 2004; 69: 175–82.
26. Magliano L, Fiorillo A, de Rosa C et al. Beliefs about schizophrenia in Italy: a comparative nationwide survey of the general public, mental health professionals, and patients' relatives. Can J Psychiatry 2004; 49: 322–30.

27. Lauber C, Nordt C, Falcato L et al. Factors influencing social distance toward people with mental illness. Community Ment Health J 2004; 40: 265–74.
28. Martin JK, Pescosolido BA, Tuch SA. Of fear and loathing: The role of "disturbing behavior", labels and causal attributions in shaping public attitudes toward people with mental illness. J Health Soc Behav 2000; 41: 208–23.
29. Economou M, Richardson C, Gramandani C et al. Knowledge about schizophrenia and attitudes towards people with schizophrenia in Greece. Int J Soc Psychiatry 2008; in press.
30. Grausgruber A, Meise U, Katsching H et al. Patterns of social distance towards people suffering from schizophrenia in Austria: a comparison between the general public, relatives and mental health staff. Acta Psychiatr Scan 2007; 115: 310–9.
31. Gaebel W, Zäske H, Bauman AE. The relationship between mental illness severity and stigma. Acta Psychiatr Scand Suppl 2006; 429: 41–5.
32. Lopez-Ibor JJ, Cuenca O, Reneses B. Stigma and health care staff. In Okasha A, Stefanis C Eds. Perspectives on the stigma of Mental illness. World Psychiatric Association; 2005: 21–9.
33. Ucok A, Polat A, Sartorius N et al. Attitudes of psychiatrists towards schizophrenia. Psychiatry Clin. Neurosci 2004; 58: 89–91.
34. Ozmen E, OgelK, Aker T et al. Public attitudes to depression in urban-Turkey - the influence of perceptions and causal attributions on social distance towards individuals suffering from depression. Soc Psychiatry Psychiatr Epidemiol 2004; 39(12): 1010–6.
35. Kingdon D, Sharma T, Hart D et al. What attitudes do psychiatrists hold towards people with mental illness? Psychiatr Bull 2004; 28: 401–6.
36. Lauber C, Anthony M, Ajdacic-Gross Y et al. What about psychiatrists' attitudes to mentally ill people? Eur Psychiatry 2004; 19(7): 423–7.
37. Altindag A, Yanik M, Ucok A et al. Effects of an antistigma program on medical students' attitudes towards people with schizophrenia. Psychiatry Clin Neurosci 2006; 60: 283–8.
38. Kerby J, Calton T, Dimambro B et al. Anti-stigma films and medical students' attitudes towards mental illness and psychiatry: randomised controlled trial. Psychiatr Bull 2008; 32: 345–9.
39. Corrigan PW, Watson AC. The stigma of psychiatric disorders and the gender, ethnicity, and education of the perceiver. Community Ment Health J 2007; 43: 439–58.
40. Wolff G, Pathare S, Craig T et al. Public education for community care: a new approach. Br J Psychiatry 1996; 168: 441–7.
41. Read J, Law A. The relationship of causal beliefs and contact with users of mental health services to attitudes to the 'mentally ill'. Int J Soc Psychiatry 1999; 45 (3): 216–29.
42. Link BG, Cullen FT, Frank J et al. The social rejection of former mental patients: Understanding why labels matter. Am J Soc 1987; 92: 1461–500.
43. Angermeyer MC, Matschinger H. The stigma of mental illness: effects of labelling on public attitudes towards people with mental disorders. Acta Psychiatr Scand 2003; 108: 304–9.
44. Corrigan PW, Edwards AB, Green A et al. Prejudice, social distance and familiarity with mental illness. Schizophr Bull 2001; 27(2): 219–25.
45. Baumann AE, Craig E, Zäske H et al. Interpersonal factors contributing to the desire for social distance. The XIIIth World Congress of Psychiatry, Cairo, Egypt, 2005.
46. Teasdale K. Stigma and psychiatric day care. J Adv Nurs 1987; 12: 339–46.
47. Haghighat R. A unitary theory of stigmatization: pursuit of self-interest and routes to destigmatisation. Br J Psychiatry 2001; 178: 207–15.
48. Sugiura T, Sakamoto S, Tanaka E et al. Labeling effect of Seishin-bunretsu-byou, the Japanese translation for schizophrenia: an argument for relabeling. Int J Soc Psychiatry 2001; 47(2): 43–51.
49. Link BG, Phelan JC, Bresnahan M et al. Public conceptions of mental illness: Labels causes, dangerousness and social distance. Am J Publ Health 1999; 89: 1328–33.
50. Penn D, Guynan K, Daily T et al. Dispelling the stigma of schizophrenia: what sort of information is best? Schizophr Bull 1994; 20: 567–78.

51. Link BG, Cullen FT. Contact with the mentally ill and perceptions of how dangerous they are. J Health Soc Behav 1986; 27: 289–302.

52. Schulze B, Angermeyer MC. Subjective experiences of stigma. A focus group study of schizophrenic patients, their relatives and mental health professionals. Soc Sci Med 2003; 56: 299–312.

53. Angermeyer MC, Schulze B, Dietrich S. Courtesy stigma. A focus group study of relatives of schizophrenic patients. Soc Psychiatry Psychiatr Epidemiol 2002; 38: 593–602.

54. Gonzales-Torres M, Oraa R, Aristegui M et al. Stigma and discrimination towards people with schizophrenia and their family members – A qualitative study with focus groups. Soc Psychiatry Psychiatr Epidemiol 2007; 42: 14–23.

55. Buizza C, Schulze B, Bertocci E et al. The stigma of schizophrenia from patients' and relatives' view: A pilot study in an Italian rehabilitation residential care unit. Clin Pract Epidemiol Ment Health 2007; 3: 23.

56. Corrigan PW, Watson AC. The paradox of self-stigma and mental illness. Clin Psychol Sci Pract 2002; 9: 35–53.

57. Watson AC, Corrigan PW, Larson JE et al. Self-stigma in people with mental illness. Schiz Bull 2007; 33: 1312–8.

58. Link BG, Struening EL, Neese-Todd S et al. The consequences of stigma on the self esteem of people with mental illness. Psychiatr Serv 2001; 52: 1621–6.

59. Lysaker PH, Roe D, Yanos P et al. Toward understanding the insight paradox : internalised stigma moderates the association between insight and social functioning, hope and self-esteem among people with schizophrenia spectrum disorders. Schiz Bull 2007; 33: 192–9.

60. Winnie WS, Crystal FM. Cognitive insight and causal attribution in the development of self-stigma among individuals with schizophrenia. Psych Serv 2006; 57: 1800–2.

61. Madianos M, Economou M, Dafni O et al. Family disruption, economic hardship and psychological distress in schizophrenia: can they be measured? Eur Psychiatry 2004; 19: 408–14.

62. Wahl OF. Mass media images of mental illness: a review of the literature. J Community Psychol 1992; 20: 343–52.

63. Philo G. Media and Mental Distress. London: Longman; 1996.

64. Wahl OF. Media madness: Public images of mental illness. New Brunswick, NJ: Rutgers University Press; 1995.

65. Economou M, Kourea A, Gramandani Ch et al. Mental disorder and mental health representations in Greek newspapers and magazines. World Psychiatry 2005; 4: 45–9.

66. Coverdale J, Nairn R, Claasen D. Depictions of mental illness in print media: a prospective national sample. Aust N Z J Psychiatry 2002; 36: 697–700.

67. Angermeyer MC, Schulze B. Reinforcing stereotypes: How the focus on forensic cases in news reporting may influence public attitudes toward the mentally ill. Int J Law Psychiatry 2001; 24: 469–86.

68. Capriniello B, Girau R, Orru MG. Mass-media, violence and mental illness. Evidence from some Italian newspapers. Epidemiol Psichiatr Soc 2007; 16: 251–5.

69. Wahl OF, Wood A, Richards R. Newspaper coverage of mental illness: Is it changing? Psychiatr Rehabil Skills 2002; 6: 9–31.

70. Wilson C, Nairn R, Coverdale J et al. Mental illness depictions in prime-time drama: Identifying the discursive resources. Aust N Z J Psychiatry 1999; 33: 232–9.

71. Wahl OF. Depictions of mental illnesses in children's media. J Ment Health 2003; 12: 249–58.

72. Stout PA, Villegas J, Jennings NA. Images of mental illness in the media: Identifying gaps in the research. Schiz Bull 2004; 30: 543–61.

73. Schulze B. Stigma and mental health professionals: a review of the evidence on an intricate relationship. Int Rev Psychiatry 2007; 19: 137–55.

74. Stuart H. Media portrayal of mental illness and its treatments: what effect does it have on people with mental illness? CNS Drugs 2006; 20: 99–106.

75. Diefenbach D, West M. Television and attitudes towards mental health issues: Cultivation analysis and the third-person effect. J Community Psychol 2007; 35(2): 181–95.
76. Granello DH, Pauley PS. Television viewing habits and their relationship to tolerance toward people with mental illness. J Ment Health Counsel 2000; 22: 162–75.
77. Ritterfeld U, Jin S. Addressing media stigma for people experiencing mental illness using an entertainment - education strategy. J Health Psychology 2006; 11(2): 247–67.
78. Finkelstein J, Lapshin O, Wasserman E. Randomised study of different anti-stigma media. Patient Educ Couns 2008; 71(2): 204–14.
79. Nairn R. Media portrayal of mental illness, or is it madness? A review. Austr Psychol 2007; 42(2): 138–46.
80. Corrigan PW, Penn DL. Lessons from social psychology on discrediting psychiatric stigma. Am Psychol 1999; 54: 756–76.
81. Baumann AE, Gaebel W et al. "Fighting stigma and discrimination because of schizophrenia-Open the Doors": a collaborative review of the experience from the German project centres. In Arboleda-Florez J, Sartorius N, Eds. Understanding the stigma of mental illness: Theory and interventions. Wiley & Sons 2008: 49–67.
82. Papadimitriou GN, Dikeos DG. How does recent knowledge on the heredity of schizophrenia affect genetic counselling? Curr Psychiatry Rep 2003; 5: 239–40.
83. Mehta S, Farina A. Is being "sick" really better? Effect of the disease view of mental disorder on stigma. J Soc Clin Psychol 1997; 16: 405–19.
84. Dietrich S, Beck M, Bujantugs B et al. The relationship between public causal beliefs and social distance toward mentally ill people. Aust N Z J Psychiatry 2004; 38: 348–54.
85. Phelan JC. Genetic bases of mental illness – a cure for stigma? Trends Neurosci 2002; 25: 430–1.
86. Kolodziej ME, Johnson BT. Interpersonal contact and acceptance of persons with psychiatric disorders: a research synthesis. J Consult Clin Psychol 1996; 64: 387–96.
87. Schulze B, Richter-Werling M, Matschinger H et al. Crazy? So what? Effects of a school project on students' attitudes towards people with schizophrenia. Acta Psychiatr Scand 2003; 107: 142–50.
88. Meise U, Sulzenbracher H, Kemmier G et al. «...nicht gefahlich, aber doch furchterregend». Ein Programm gegen Stigmatisierung von Schizophrenie in Schulen. Psychiatr Prax 2000; 27: 340–6.
89. World Psychiatric Association. The Madrid Declaration. Curr Opin Psychiatry 1998; 1.
90. Stefanis CN, Economou M. The unprecedented initiative of European Ministers of Health. In Okasha A, Stefanis CN, eds. Perspectives of the Sigma of Mental Illness. World Psychiatric Association, 2005: 7–20.
91. Sartorius N. Stigma: what can psychiatrists do about it? Lancet 1998; 352: 1058–9.
92. Pitre N, Stewart S, Adams S et al. The use of puppets with elementary school children in reducing stigmatizing attitudes towards mental illness. J Ment Health 2007; 16(3): 415–29.
93. Warner R. Implementing local projects to reduce the stigma of mental illness. Epidemiol Psychiatr Soc 2008; 17(1): 20–5.

25 Patient rights: Ethics and the clinical care of patients with schizophrenia

Evan G DeRenzo, Steve Peterson, Jack Schwartz,
Alexis Jeannotte, and Steve Selinger

INTRODUCTION

Much has been written on the subject of patient rights. Even a cursory search of the literature reveals many documents—both published in print and on Web sites. And, although these documents, some generic and some specific to mental health, have been produced by diverse professional organizations, they reflect a consistent identification of patient needs and benefits. They define patient rights in terms of providing patients with the following:

- respectful and nondiscriminatory care
- a safe and secure environment
- protection of privacy and confidentiality
- provision of information, and involvement of surrogates where appropriate, for sound medical decision making
- access to, and insurance coverage of, appropriate services

We agree that everything on this list is essential to moral medical and psychiatric care, to which all patients have a right. We believe, also, that emphasis needs to be placed on the quality of *how* such rights are fulfilled. That is, the right to "be cared for" implies that patients' health care needs are to be met not only with technical skill but also with empathy and compassion.

Excellence in medical care, thus defined, is the right of every patient, regardless of whether the patient has schizophrenia alone, schizophrenia and a somatic illness, or schizophrenia and psychiatric or behavioral comorbidities. The ways in which excellence in care manifests itself in any particular medical encounter are unique. Addressing comprehensively the panoply of patient rights issues associated with the clinical care of patients with schizophrenia would be impossible. Rather, we have selected the following three, contemporary ethical issues, all related in one way or another to the collection and use of medical information relevant to meeting the clinical needs of patients with schizophrenia and to protecting the rights of such patients.

1. psychiatric consultation in the critical care setting
2. criteria for and approach to capacity assessment
3. appropriate use of genetic and neurophysiological data

These issues, which illustrate the ethical complexities of upholding the rights of patients with schizophrenia in the clinical care setting, all involve important patient information. Specifically, this chapter addresses barriers to acquiring patient information, sophistication in applying patient information to well-accepted ethical (and legal) criteria, and caution in relying on data produced by cutting-edge technology.

NOTES ON OUR APPROACH

Setting the Context

Although we acknowledge the significance of international issues and cultural diversity, the issues discussed in this chapter are seen through the ethical lens of the authors' immersion in the secular bioethics that predominates in affluent Western nations, especially the United States. This view incorporates a default bias toward individual, autonomously driven decision making.

The Importance of Language

We use the term "patients with schizophrenia," not "schizophrenic patient," because the latter term tends to label rather than describe, entrenching stigma (1, 2). By contrast, the term "patients with schizophrenia" can be a salutary reminder that at times schizophrenia may be better thought of as merely a part of the patient's history rather than as a description of the patient's primary condition.

Along the same lines, we use the term "patient" and not any other, such as "consumer" or "client." We believe that a person with a serious disease or condition who seeks out the help of a health care professional, particularly one licensed to prescribe drugs, is in a special status best captured by the word "patient." Furthermore, we believe that the status of patient results in a power differential in favor of the health care professional that the patient can never totally equalize. Although we respect the position of advocacy groups that take offense at the use of the term "patient" on the basis that it is disempowering, we believe that terminology such as "consumer" or "client," derived from economic transactions, tends to obfuscate the true nature of the medical encounter. That is, when an individual goes to or is brought to a clinician, that individual is suffering and in need of care. That need creates obligations for the clinician to act in certain ways, here summarized as the core ethical obligation to act, first and foremost, in the best interest of the patient. Clearly, professionals' obligations do not change when they enter into a relationship of caring for a suffering person, no matter whether that person is called patient or client or consumer, nor does the power differential change with the label applied. But, the nuanced differences in emotional response these different terms evoke can be expected to color the ways in which the clinician reacts to the needs and vulnerabilities of a patient. Because we believe the term "patient" most fully defines those needs and vulnerabilities, we believe its use sets the most appropriate tone and points clinicians in directions that promise excellence in care.

A Patient's Moral Right to Excellent Care

We take as our starting point that it is the moral—as distinct from legal—right of every patient to receive excellent clinical care. While we take note of the complex relationship between moral claim and legal right, acknowledging that this relationship is a fraught problem (3), this chapter focuses on the ethical, not the legal, aspects of patient rights. Insofar as law establishes rules of conduct for actors in society, here it rests on a moral substratum. Thus, for example, a competent patient's legal right to give informed consent is a manifestation of the ethical principle of autonomy. Law, however, is significantly shaped by process, whether in the political sphere (enactments of legislatures) or the limited-party adversarial arena (court decisions). Consequently, in scope and detail laws usually depart from what might be seen as the logic of a moral position. For example, a patient may have a moral right to excellent clinical care, but the patient's legal rights are violated only if care is negligent (4). While a fuller account of these legal and moral distinctions is beyond the scope of this chapter, we underscore that future references to "rights" should be understood as meaning moral rights, not necessarily legal rights.

Important Distinctions between Psychiatric Illness and Somatic Disease

We make the claim that psychiatric illness is qualitatively different from somatic disease and that this difference is relevant to the protection of the rights of patients with schizophrenia. We accept that, as research about the brain and brain disease continues to break new ground, we will understand much more about the healthy mind and psychiatric illness. We also believe that certain social, political, and interpersonal phenomena so frequently associated with psychiatric illness (and so infrequently part of the care of patients without psychiatric illness) render psychiatric illness, at least for the foreseeable future, as qualitatively different from somatic disease. And, although we accept the possibility that these differences may melt away in the face of advanced knowledge about how the brain works, we believe that such refined understanding, which depends upon both future scientific advances and social acceptance, is not immediately relevant for protecting the rights of patients with schizophrenia.

Competence Is Not Enough

Finally, we advance the view that, although scientifically and technically competent practice is a necessary condition for excellence in medical care, it is not sufficient. What is both necessary and sufficient for excellent medical care is the ability to provide technically competent care while aspiring to ensure that every patient's rights are honored. While this may be understood as the art of medicine, the practice of such ideals is no longer a matter of intuitively adhering to standards of professionalism. Working through the ethical complexities presented by contemporary, high-tech medicine—in a context of multicultural values, interconnecting but often disjointed medical delivery systems, and socioeconomic constraints—requires specialized training in ethics for skilled clinical practice (5–7). As such, it is important that each clinician take the time to become familiar with the basic scholarship of contemporary bioethics.

In sum, we recognize that honoring patient rights while meeting the medical needs of patients with schizophrenia is complex and ethically challenging. We write this chapter with that humbling appreciation and with the goal of helping those who provide such care.

IMPROVING UTILIZATION OF PSYCHIATRIC CONSULTATION FOR THE SERIOUSLY SOMATICALLY ILL PATIENT WITH SCHIZOPHRENIA

When people become seriously ill, especially in the United States, they often are hospitalized. Once hospitalized, patients often have multiple subspecialty consultations, especially if the patient is admitted to an intensive care unit (ICU). Calling for a psychiatric consultation, however, is not quite the same as calling for a consultation for other subspecialties, even when the somatically seriously ill patient also has schizophrenia. Although exact data are unavailable, observers of routine hospital practices recognize that the question of whether to call for a psychiatric consultation is seen as more difficult than calling for other consultations, which often deters clinicians from calling the consultation. This disinclination to call for a psychiatric consultation may be attributable in part to the patient's concurrent diagnosis of schizophrenia. In the general medical literature, much has been written about stigma and discrimination in the diagnosis and treatment of schizophrenia (8, 9), including data presenting consistent findings of stigma and discrimination cross-culturally (10–13). Also, data are plentiful about the increased morbidity and mortality of patients with schizophrenia in the general medical population compared with those without schizophrenia (14, 15), but this finding is not universal (16). The scant literature about patients with schizophrenia in the critical care setting (17–20), focuses primarily on suicidal patients (21, 22). Here we consider ethical barriers to calling for a psychiatric consultation and why such barriers might contribute to poor outcomes for somatically seriously ill patients with schizophrenia.

Although the well understood sources of stigma and discrimination can discourage psychiatric consultation, we speculate here that the sources of the problem are far more complex, including deeply embedded biases that go well beyond simple psychological discomfort posed by diagnosis of schizophrenia. Rather, important aspects potentially accounting for the seemingly chronic disinclination to call a psychiatric consultation for somatically ill patients who also have serious psychiatric disease may be the differences in purpose, structure, and format of psychiatric consultation compared with consultations by other medical subspecialties.

Seriously ill patients with schizophrenia can be expected to present complexities beyond those presented by the nonpsychiatrically ill acute care hospital patient. For example, delays in treatment may result from aspects inherent in the psychiatric disease itself. Somatic delusions and hallucinations, psychotic denial, and thought disorder may result in having physical symptoms misperceived or ignored by patients or clinicians. If a patient with schizophrenia is taking drugs for his or her psychiatric disease, the potential for drug-to-drug interactions is increased. In addition, advanced patient age can further complicate diagnosis and treatment of a patient with schizophrenia and critical somatic illness. For instance, there is evidence that older patients with schizophrenia may have a higher risk for late-onset depression (23), a well-known predictor of poor somatic outcome. These examples of the complexities inherent in the care of the seriously somatically ill patient who also has schizophrenia may require clinicians to have highly specialized expertise in the physiology and psychopharmacology of psychiatric illness (24).

To provide acute care hospital patients with schizophrenia subspecialty attention comparable with the subspecialty attention given to patients without schizophrenia, clinicians must adopt a fundamental change in the way psychiatric consultation is ordered, delivered, and understood. Central to this change is to encourage clinicians to call for the psychiatric consultant early on—as is ordinary practice for cardiology, neurology, and other subspecialty consultations—*before* the situation deteriorates, so that the psychiatrist has time to do the required work.

Despite the fact that a psychiatric consultation would help the attending physician manage the comorbidity and polypharmacy issues that may arise when a patient with schizophrenia is admitted to a general medicine or surgical unit, or especially to a critical care unit, this logic often does not prevail. As mentioned earlier, the problem is that calling for a psychiatric consultation has a different "feel" to it than calling a consultation in other subspecialties. In general, "requests for a psychiatric consultation are notoriously vague and imprecise…" (25). In part, this is due to the confusing and wide array of symptoms and issues for the patient with behavioral problems, especially those with psychotic presentations. In the face of these complexities, it is of first concern to determine a proper diagnosis, because psychotic symptoms may be due to an underlying medical illness.

In addition, unlike calling for a cardiology or oncology consult, a somatically ill patient who also has schizophrenia may present qualitative characteristics that discourage clinicians from providing the consultative attention related to his or her psychiatric disease. This qualitative difference in "feel" of calling for a psychiatric consultation may derive from an insidious mixture of stigma and discrimination about psychiatric patients and a discriminatory response to psychiatry itself (26). The difference in feel, however, also may derive from the differences between somatic and psychiatric disease. For instance, patients with schizophrenia, due to their paranoia, negativism, lack of insight, and oppositional behavior, often have great difficulty cooperating with complex medical care. As a result, such patients may produce powerful feelings of frustration and elicit a variety of problematic responses in health care staff, including negative counter-transference reactions.

Furthermore, an attending physician may be disinclined to call for a psychiatric consultation because of differences in the purpose, structure and format of a psychiatric consultation as compared with other medical consultations. Typically, the purpose of the psychiatric consultation is not simply to evaluate one symptom, such as when a nephrologist is called for renal insufficiency. Rather, the psychiatrist must ascertain the patient's world view and make a comprehensive assessment of the patient's coping mechanisms, levels of trust, cognitive functions, awareness of illness, and ability to understand and make judgments. Furthermore, the psychiatrist must identify any disturbances in these areas and initiate appropriate treatments. Thus, a psychiatric consultation often is far more complex and time-consuming than other subspecialty consultations. In an era when intense focus is on reducing length of inappropriate stay for hospital patients, especially ICU patients, attending physicians might be loath to start a consultation process that may extend an in-patient stay.

Nonetheless, appreciating the profound and complex purposes of a psychiatric consultation can improve utilization of the psychiatric consultation in hospital settings. The psychiatrist's duty is to help the patient—through interpersonal and pharmacological interventions—to foster coping, improve trust and cooperation, reduce false perceptions of the world (and of the treatment team), and help restore the patient's decisional capacity. All this takes time but is essential in helping a patient with schizophrenia to survive a serious somatic illness and successfully convalesce. Too often, medical attending physicians are impatient with what can be a several-day process. Nevertheless, patients with complex conditions need more time, because they need more complex help.

The literature supports our theory that a revised view of the role of psychiatric consultation in the medical setting may better ensure the rights of patients with schizophrenia. The affinities between a psychiatric consultation and ethics have long been noted (27–36). And, recent literature has shown an increased appreciation for the prevalence and under-diagnosis of psychiatric illnesses, such as delirium (37–39) and post-traumatic stress disorder (40), among the general population of critically ill patients. Intellectually connecting the ethics of patient rights to a greater understanding and utilization of psychiatric consultation in the care of seriously somatically ill patients with schizophrenia can be expected to lead to a substantial improvement in quality of care.

THE PROBLEM OF CAPACITY ASSESSMENT IN A SOMATICALLY ILL PATIENT WITH SCHIZOPHRENIA

One of the most important, studied, and discussed issues in the medical ethics literature about patients with schizophrenia is the degree to which such individuals have the capacity to provide ethically and legally valid informed-consent. Much of the existing literature focuses on capacity to give consent to research participation, with recent literature looking toward refining and standardizing methods for assessing research capacity (41–45). The literature addressing capacity to provide consent to treatment often is focused on the issue of consent to psychiatric treatment (46, 47). Many articles combine attention to capacity assessment in both research and clinical care venues (48, 49).

One can also find growing numbers of articles about capacity in the related literatures on neuropsychological deficits (50) and advance directives in psychiatry (51, 52). In addition, the issue of capacity is discussed in court cases (53) and legislation (54, 55). The generally accepted criteria for capacity assessment in the clinical setting, however, are often considered too narrowly, without adequate attention to two factors already well articulated in the research ethics literature: vulnerability and voluntariness.

The indicia of capacity to provide valid consent, generally accepted by commentators and applied by some courts (56), include all of the following abilities

1. to express a choice
2. to understand the information provided
3. to appreciate the implications of the consequences of one's decisions, and
4. to reason in a way that is consistent with what the individual considers to be in his or her own best interest

These criteria are applied to potential subjects and study participants in clinical research and to patients in the clinical care setting (57). It is generally recognized that patients in a research setting must be able to give consent *voluntarily* in addition to showing the cognitive ability to provide meaningful consent (58). In addition, it is generally accepted that in research settings clinicians also must pay attention to the degree of vulnerability of the prospective or participating research subject. In the clinical care setting, however, the importance of considering the factors of voluntariness and vulnerability in assessing a patient's capacity has not been well articulated.

Worse still, it is common experience in the clinical care setting that capacity assessment of seriously ill patients often is poorly executed. In fact, somatic physicians often are unable to identify the well-established criteria against which capacity is to be assessed. And, it is rare to find any documentation in a patient's chart that such an assessment was performed. Because self-reflective somatic physicians are aware of their own shortcomings in managing psychiatric issues, such as decisional capacity, they may call for a psychiatric consultation to have a patient's decisional capacity assessed. Indeed, this may be the most frequent reason for a psychiatric consultation. Yet, a psychiatric consultation for capacity assessment in the in-patient setting often does not result in better attention to the ethically relevant issues (59).

An error in capacity assessment by a somatic physician may be in one direction or the other; that is, the error may be that a capacitated patient is assessed as lacking decisional capacity or that a not-capacitated patient is assessed as capable. On the other hand, a psychiatrist may be *a priori* biased toward assessing a patient as capacitated given the gravity of assessing a psychiatrically ill patient as decisionally incapable in light of the implications for future competency hearings and the subsequent potential loss of liberty.

In any case, the consulting psychiatrist can be expected to assess for the patient's cognitive capacities indicated by the standard criteria for capacity. If, however, the patient does not meet diagnostic criteria and is not so blatantly cognitively impaired as to be obviously unable to process information, then the consulting psychiatrist can be expected to deem the patient capable, when the patient in fact may not be capable. Furthermore, this result can leave the somatic physician in a worse position than if the consultation had not been called in the first place. Because it takes thoughtfulness and moral courage to override the recommendation of a subspecialist, the patient's capacity may be inaccurately assessed, sending treatment decisions in an unhelpful or ethically ill-analyzed direction.

Our Western ethical bias toward assuming persons to be autonomous unless proven otherwise may be the appropriate default position. However, for the somatically ill patient, with or without schizophrenia, assessment of cognitive function is not sufficient to determine whether or not a patient should be permitted to make his or her own decisions. Such a decision ought not to be made merely on the basis of cognitive capacity considered in isolation, but rather on the basis of cognitive capacity within a context of morally acceptable additional considerations. These additional considerations include whether or not the patient is made vulnerable in some other way that limits the patient's ability to be self-determining—one of those limitations is lack of voluntariness.

When, for example, a seriously or chronically somatically ill patient refuses treatments that make sense to a multidisciplinary team of clinicians, concern should be high that such a patient's refusal may be the product of exhaustion, withdrawal from addiction, pain, or other distress. Serious illness or chronic disease renders patients vulnerable in ways other than cognitive impairment of decisional capacity. Such vulnerabilities are morally relevant to ensuring that patient rights are upheld, specifically related to matters of informed consent and the involvement of surrogates. For example, it is ethically wrong to accept as valid, without further assessment, a refusal of life-extending technology in a patient whose cognitive capacity is seemingly intact but whose vulnerabilities nevertheless compromise autonomous decision making.

Consideration of voluntariness is rarely given in the process of capacity assessment, whether by a somatic or psychiatric physician, but virtually all seriously somatically ill patients, have constraints on their voluntary actions. These constraints may be as minimal as simply depending on their physician to renew their medication prescriptions or as all-encompassing as being sedated and ventilated in an ICU. Under both conditions, and in virtually all situations in between, there are constraints on patients' voluntary choices.

It is the patient's right, when decision making is constrained, to be provided with protections in the medical encounter. Such protections can range from merely including a family member or friend the patient wants present, to having a hospital's patient advocate included, to having a guardian appointed. Such protections in the nonpsychiatrically ill patient may be less complicated than in the case of a somatically ill patient who also has schizophrenia. For example, for a patient with schizophrenia who has paranoid features as characteristics of his or her disease, the choice of who that patient might accept to help make decisions may be quite complicated. Thus, it is important that performance of capacity assessment be improved, including applying the now standard four-part criteria with careful attention to a patient's state of vulnerability and voluntariness.

APPROPRIATE USE OF GENETIC AND NEUROPHYSIOLOGICAL DATA IN DIAGNOSIS AND TREATMENT OF SCHIZOPHRENIA

While the previous two sections considered patient rights related to information gathering and assessment for the already ill patient, this last section contemplates patient rights' implications of medical information gathering and utilization more upstream. Here we focus on the rights of individuals thought to have, or having risk factors for, schizophrenia, on the basis of data produced by the cutting-edge technologies of genetic screening and neural imaging.

Historically, a diagnosis of schizophrenia has been based primarily on behavioral assessment. And, although these traditional diagnostic methods continue to be used, much current research seeks to develop new ways to better understand, diagnose, and treat schizophrenia. Two of the most promising of these new lines of research use genetic screening and brain imaging in combination with the classical battery of exams. These new tools attempt to address the complex epigenetic nature of schizophrenia.

There are, however, ethical concerns raised by the use of data produced by these technologies, the implications of which have the potential to infringe on patient rights. Indeed, inappropriate reliance on these technologies risks premature or inaccurate diagnoses, which in turn can lead to unnecessary treatment, psychological burden, social stigma, and possible discrimination in access to health care, insurance, and employment.

The effects of psychiatric illness, including its assaults on personhood and potentially severe social isolation (60), create an acute need to improve the treatment of schizophrenia. Adding to this urgency is our relative lack of understanding of brain function, which creates an urgent need to improve our means of diagnosing schizophrenia. In the face of these urgent needs, the natural impulse of the clinician is to grab onto innovations that appear to provide useful insights. It is important, however, to keep such impulses in check when presented with data from promising new technologies. Clinicians must exercise the appropriate wise restraint needed to integrate these innovations into practice soundly, not prematurely.

Genetic screening and improvements in neural scanning are two such promising and ethically challenging technologies, and both have been advancing rapidly in clinical utility (61, 62). For example, genetic screening has been quite useful in advancing the treatment of such relatively rare genetic diseases as Alpha-1 antitrypsin deficiency (63). And, newer generations of scanning technologies have produced improvements in the diagnosis and treatment of coronary disease, resulting in widespread use of the technology (64, 65) even though there is still much to be learned about the outcomes associated with applying these innovations broadly (66, 67). Thus, especially in psychiatry, where information about the brain has implications beyond and qualitatively different from information about lung or cardiac function, unbridled enthusiasm about the utility of such data can lead psychiatrists and somatic physicians astray diagnostically and therapeutically and, thus, ethically.

There are many reasons clinicians should exercise caution in the use of genetic or neurophysiological data for the diagnosis of schizophrenia. The rate of false positives in clinical genetics studies of at-risk populations has been as high as 60% to 90% (68–70). In light of studies finding a disease concordance rate in monozygotic twins of up to 48%, it would be dangerous for clinicians to rely too heavily on genetic information without learning the role of environmental factors in schizophrenia susceptibility (71). Although genetic screening is being touted as a predictive tool (72, 73), especially by those eager to be "early adopters" of an exciting and promising technology (74, 75), we still do not have sound scientific evidence as to how these genes are expressed and how they affect an individual's physical and mental well-being in relation to other influencing factors.

To be sure, classical behavioral tests can be used in combination with both well-established techniques, such as electroencephalography (EEG) and the recently developed functional magnetic resonance imaging (fMRI). Yet, even an approach that includes data from these varied sources may not be sufficient to develop a definitive diagnosis. For example, it has been shown that patients with schizophrenia *and* their healthy siblings (who share a mutation associated with increased risk for schizophrenia) have similarly poor performance on working memory tasks and abnormal activation in the prefrontal cortex. Such disease indicators, however, provide only statistical risk, not correct and absolute diagnosis (62).

Inaccurate interpretation and use of data from genetic screening or imaging may lead to inaccurate diagnosis in specific individuals who might never have gone on to develop a full-blown case of schizophrenia. Such misinterpretation can then produce a harmful cascade of events, resulting in unnecessary treatment, with all its attendant negative outcomes for patients and society (76).

Even if the predictive data turn out to be accurate, serious privacy and confidentiality concerns arise. Inappropriate disclosure of such information about a patient, or an at-risk sibling, can produce the harms identified previously in this chapter. When such data are generated about minor children, an additional problem is the potential for pejorative influencing of family and school expectations.

These cautionary notes, however, are not to suggest that genetic or neurophysiological imaging data will not be, or perhaps in certain circumstances are not already, helpful. Until these technologies are fully and carefully integrated into practice, clinicians must be vigilant about protecting the rights of patients and others from the potentially serious negative outcomes associated with the application of unvalidated data from such technologies.

CONCLUSION: PROGRESS TOWARD EXCELLENCE IN THE SOMATIC CARE OF PATIENTS WITH SCHIZOPHRENIA

There are myriad opportunities that must be taken and challenges that must be overcome in protecting the rights of somatically ill patients with schizophrenia. For the somatically ill patient with schizophrenia and for the individual for whom a diagnosis is being sought, clinicians must provide both care that is comparable to that of the patient without psychiatric overlay *and* care that takes into account the additional complexities posed by psychiatric disease. In the chapter we have presented examples related to information gathering, assessment, and utilization because today's clinicians face information overload, with so much information to gather, evaluate, and use or discard. And, although information management has always been part of mastering the *art* of medicine, information gathering and management today requires exceptional effort.

In the end, it is attention to the unique and ubiquitous ethical aspects of care of somatically ill patients with schizophrenia that presents the greatest chance for protecting their rights and, thus, provides the best chance for providing excellent medical care. We hope the issues we raised in this chapter will encourage improvement in these areas and others.

REFERENCES

1. Reynaert CC, Gelman SA. The influence of language form and conventional wording on judgments of illness. J Psycholinguist Res 2007; 36(4): 273–95.
2. Cain DM, Detsky AS. Everyone's a little bit biased (Even physicians). JAMA 2008; 299(24): 2893–5.
3. Dickson J. Evaluation and Legal Theory. Oxford: Hart Publishing; 2001.
4. Weiler PC, Hiatt HH, Newhouse JP et al. A measure of malpractice: Medical injury, malpractice litigation, and patient compensation. Cambridge, Mass: Harvard University Press; 1993.

5. Have H. UNESCO's ethics education programme. J Med Ethics 2008; 34(1): 57–9.
6. Andorno R. Global bioethics at UNESCO: in defence of the Universal Declaration on Bioethics and Human Rights. J Med Ethics 2007; 33(3): 150–4.
7. Fox E, Myers S, Pearlman RA. Ethics consultation in United States Hospitals: a national survey. Am J Bioeth 2007; 7(2): 13–25.
8. Corrigan PW, Watson AC. The stigma of psychiatric disorders and the gender, ethnicity, and education of the perceiver. Community Ment Health J 2007; 43(5): 439–58.
9. Sajatovic M, Jenkins JH. Is antipsychotic medication stigmatizing for people with mental illness? Int Rev Psychiatry 2007; 19(2): 107–12.
10. Buizza C, Schulze B, Bertocchi E et al. The stigma of schizophrenia from patients' and relatives' view: a pilot study in an Italian rehabilitation residential care unit. Clin Pract Epidemol Ment Health 2007; 3: 23.
11. Charles H, Manoranjitham SD, Jacob KS. Stigma and explanatory models among people with schizophrenia and their relatives in Vellore, South India. Int J Soc Psychiatry 2007; 53(4): 325–32.
12. Yang LH. Application of mental illness stigma theory to Chinese societies; synthesis and new directions. Singapore Med J 2007; 48(11): 977–85.
13. Yang LH, Kleinman A, Link BG et al. Culture and stigma: adding moral experience to stigma theory. Soc Sci Med 2007; 64(7): 1524–35.
14. Goff DC, Newcomer JW. Integrating general health care in private community psychiatric practice. J Clin Psychiatry 2007; 68(7): e19.
15. Leucht S, Burkard T, Henderson J et al. Physical illness and schizophrenia: A review of the literature. Acta Psychiatr Scand 2007; 116(5): 317–33.
16. Rasanen S, Mayer-Rochow VB, Moring J et al. Hospital-treated physical illness and mortality: an 11-year follow-up study of long-stay psychiatric patients. Eur Psychiatry 2007; 22(4): 211–8.
17. Salomon JB, Armstrong RF, Cohen SL et al. Schizophrenic patients requiring intensive care. BMJ 1993; 307(6902): 508.
18. Jones C, Griffiths RD, Humphris G. A case of Capgras delusion following critical illness. Intensive Care Med 1999; 25(10): 1183–4.
19. Daumit GL, Pronovost PJ, Antthony CB et al. Adverse events during medical and surgical hospitalizations for persons with schizophrenia. Arch Gen Psychiatry 2006; 63(3): 267–72.
20. Hoyer D, Frank B, Gotze C et al. Complex autonomic dysfunction in cardiovascular, intensive care, and schizophrenic patients assessed by autonomic information flow. Biomed Tech (Berl) 2006; 51(4): 182–5.
21. Juarez-Aragon G, Castanon-Gonzalez JA, Perez-Morales AJ et al. [Clinical and epidemiological characteristics of severe poisoning in an adult population admitted to an intensive care unit] [Article in Spanish] Gac Med Mex 1999; 135(6): 669–75.
22. Pajonk FG, Ruchholtz S, Waydhas C et al. Long-term follow-up after severe suicide attempt by multiple blunt trauma. Eur Psychiatry 2005; 20(2): 115–20.
23. Diwan S, Cohen CI, Bankole AO et al. Depression in older adults with schizophrenia spectrum disorders: prevalence and associated factors. Am J Geriatr Psychiatry 2007; 15(12): 991–8.
24. Misra S, Ganzini L. Delirium, depression, and anxiety. Crit Care Clin 2003; 19(4): 771–87.
25. Levenson JL (ed). Textbook of Psychosomatic Medicine. Washington, DC: American Psychiatric Publishing, Inc, 2005: 243.
26. Schulze B. Stigma and mental health professionals: a review of the evidence on an intricate relationship. In Rev Psychiatry 2007; 19(2): 137–55.
27. Youngner SJ. Consultation-liaison psychiatry and clinical ethics. Historical parallels and diversions. Psychosomatics 1997; 38(4): 309–12.
28. Steinberg MD. Psychiatry and bioethics. An exploration of the relationship. Psychosomatics 1997; 38(4): 313–20.
29. Powell T. Consultation-liason psychiatry and clinical ethics. Representative cases. Psychosomatics 1997; 38(4): 321–6.

30. Morris J, McFadd A. The mental health team on a burn unit: a multidisciplinary approach. J Trauma 1978; 18(9): 658–63.
31. Leeman CP. Psychiatric consultations and ethics consultations. Similarities and differences. Gen Hosp Psychiatry 2000; 22(4): 270–5.
32. Leeman CP, Blum J, Lederberg MS. A combined ethics and psychiatric consultation. Gen Hosp Psychiatry 2001; 23(2): 73–6.
33. Desan PH, Powsner S. Assessment and management of patients with psychiatric disorders. Crit Care Med 2004; 32(4 Suppl): S166–S173.
34. Bourgeois JA, Cohen MA, Geppert CM. The role of psychosomatic-medicine psychiatrists in bioethics: a survey study of members of the academy of psychosomatic medicine. Psychosomatics 2006; 47(6): 520–6.
35. Geppert CM, Cohen MA. Consultation-liason psychiatrists on bioethics committees: opportunities for academic leadership. Acad Psychiatry 2006; 30(5): 416–21.
36. Schneider PL, Bramstedt KA. When psychiatry and bioethics disagree about patient decision making capacity (DMC). J Med. Ethics 2006; 32(2): 90–3.
37. Ely EW, Inouye SK, Bernard GR et al. Delirium in mechanically ventilated patients: Validity and reliability of the confusion assessment method for the intensive care unit (CAM-ICU). JAMA 2001; 286(21): 2703–10.
38. Gunther ML, Jackson JC, Ely EW. The cognitive consequences of critical illness: practical recommendations for screening and assessment. Critical Care Clinics 2007; 23(3): 491–506.
39. Larson C, Axell AG, Ersson A. Confusion assessment method for the intensive care unit (CAM-ICU): translation, retranslation and validation into Swedish intensive care settings. Acta Anaesthesiol Scand 2007; 51(7): 888–92.
40. Schelling G. Post-traumatic stress disorder in somatic disease: Lessons from Critically Ill Patients. In: de Kloet ER, Oizi MS, Vermetten E, eds. Progress in Brain Research, 2008: 229–37.
41. Palmer BW, Dunn LB, Appelbaum PS et al. Assessment of capacity to consent to research among older persons with schizophrenia, Alzheimer disease, or diabetes mellitus: comparison of a 3-item questionnaire with a comprehensive standardized capacity instrument. Arch Gen Psychiatry 2005; 62(7): 726–33.
42. Appelbaum PS. Decisional capacity of patients with schizophrenia to consent to research: Taking stock. Schizophr Bull 2006; 32(1): 22–5.
43. Dunn LB, Palmer BW, Appelbaum PS et al. Prevalence and correlates of adequate performance on a measure of abilities related to decisional capacity: differences among three standards for the MacCat_CR in patients with schizophrenia. Schizophr Res 2007; 89(1–3): 110–8.
44. Nokes KM, Nwakeze PC. Assessing cognitive capacity for participation in a research study. Clin Nurs Res 2007; 16(4): 336–49.
45. Jeste DV, Palmer BW, Appelbaum PS et al. A new brief instrument for assessing decisional capacity for clinical research. Arch Gen Psychiatry 2007; 64(8): 966–74.
46. Cairns R, Maddock C, Buchanan A et al. Reliability of mental capacity assessments in psychiatric in-patients. Br J Psychiatry 2005; 187: 372–8.
47. Okai D, Owen G, McGuire H et al. Mental capacity in psychiatric patients: Systematic review. Br J Psychiatry 2007; 191: 291–7.
48. Dunn LB, Nowrangi MA, Palmer BW et al. Assessing decisional capacity for clinical research or treatment: A review of instruments. Am J Psychiatry 2006; 163(8): 1323–34.
49. Eyler LT, Jeste DV. Enhancing the informed consent process: a conceptual overview. Behav Sci Law 2006; 24(40): 553–68.
50. Palmer BW, Savia GN. The association of specific neuropsychological deficits with capacity to consent to research or treatment. J Int Neuropsychol Soc 2007; 139: 1047–59.
51. Srebnik DS, Kim SY Competency for creation, use, and recovation of psychiatric advance directives. J Am Acad Psychiatry Law 2006; 34(4): 501–10.
52. Davis JK. How to justify enforcing a Ulysses contract when Ulysses is competent to refuse. Kennedy Inst Ethics J 2008; 18(1): 87–106.

53. Sklar R. Starson v Swayze: the Supreme Court speaks out (not all that clearly) on the question of "capacity" Can J Psychiatry 2007; 52(6): 390–6.
54. Carney T. Mental health legislation in the commonwealth. Curr Opin Psychiatry 2007; 20(5): 482–5.
55. Dimond B. Mental capacity and decision making: defining capacity. Br J Nurs 2007; 16(18): 1138–9.
56. In re Farrell, 529 A.2d 404 (N.J. 1987).
57. Appelbaum PS. Clinical practice: assessment of patients' competence to consent to treatment. N Engl J Med 2007; 357(18): 1834–0.
58. The National Commission for the Protection of Human Subjects of Biomedical and Behavioral Research. The Belmont Report: Ethical Principles and Guidelines for the Protection of Human Subjects of Research. Washington, DC: U.S. Department of Health, Education, and Welfare; 1979.
59. Geppert CM, Abbott C. Voluntarism in consultation psychiatry: the forgotten capacity. Am J Psychiatry 2007; 164(3): 409–13.
60. Nilsson LL, Logdberg B. Dead and forgotten—Postmortem time before discovery as indicator of social isolation and inadequate mental healthcare in schizophrenia. Schizophr Res 2008; 102(1–3): 337–9.
61. Caspi A, Moffitt TE. Opinion: Gene–environment interactions in psychiatry: joining forces with neuroscience. Nat Rev Neurosci 2006; 7: 583–90.
62. Meyer-Lindenberg A, Weinberger DR. Intermediate phenotypes and genetic mechanisms of psychiatric disorders. Nat Rev Neurosci 2006; 7: 818–27.
63. American Thoracic Society/European Respiratory Society Statement. Standards for the diagnosis and management of individuals with Alpha-1 antitrypsin deficiency. Am J Respir Crit Care Med 2003; 168: 818–900.
64. Gani F, Jain D, Lahiri A. The role of cardiovascular imaging techniques in the assessment of patients with acute chest pain. Nucl Med Commun 2007; 28(6): 441–9.
65. Wu HD, Kwong RY. Cardiac magnetic resonance imaging in patients with coronary disease. Curr Treat Options Cardiovasc Med 2008; 10(1): 83–92.
66. Mieres, JH, Shaw LJ, Arai A et al. Role of noninvasive testing in the clinical evaluation of women with suspected coronary artery disease: Consensus statement from the Cardiac Imaging Committee, Council on Clinical Cardiology, and the Cardiovascular Imaging and Intervention Committee, Council on Cardiovascular Radiology and Intervention, American Heart Association. Circulation 2005; 111(5): 682–9.
67. Beller GA. Assessment of new technologies: surrogate endpoints versus outcomes, and the cost of health care. J Nucl Cardiol 2008; 15(3): 299–300.
68. Klosterkotter J, Hellmich M, Steinmeyer EM et al. Diagnosing schizophrenia in the initial prodromal phase. Arch Gen Psychiatry 2001; 58: 323–4.
69. Yung AR, Phillips LJ, Yuen HP et al. Psychosis prediction: 12-month follow up of a high risk ("prodromal") group. Schizophr Res 2003; 60: 21–32.
70. Yung AR, Phillips LJ, Yuen HP et al. Risk factors for psychosis in an ultra high-risk group: Psychopathology and clinical features. Schizophr Res 2004; 67: 131–42.
71. Gottesman II. Schizophrenia genesis: The origins of madness. New York: W.H. Freeman; 1991.
72. Peltonen L, McKusick VA. Dissecting human disease in the postgenomic era. Science 2001; 291: 1224–9.
73. Subramanian G, Adams MD, Venter JC et al. Implications of the human genome for understanding human biology and medicine. JAMA 2001; 286(18): 2296–07.
74. Blow N. Genomics: The personal side of genomics. Nature 2007; 449: 627–30.
75. Weinshilboum R, Wang L. Pharmacogenomics: bench to bedside. Nat Rev Drug Discov 2004; 3(9): 739–48.
76. Corcoran C, Malaspina D, Hercher L. Prodromal interventions for schizophrenia vulnerability: The risks of being "at risk" Schizophr Res 2005; 73(2–3): 173–84.

26 Genetic counseling in schizophrenia

Dimitris G Dikeos, Evangelos Vassos, and
George N Papadimitriou

INTRODUCTION

The fact that major psychiatric disorders tend to cluster in families has raised the question about the role of heredity in their manifestation. This question is not new, as since Kraepelin's separation of major psychiatric disorders into schizophrenia and affective disorder empirical observations have shown that these disorders were frequently expressed in the families of affected persons (1).

Genetic epidemiology studies show unequivocally that schizophrenia is predominantly a genetic disorder with estimates of heritability of around 80% (2, 3). In family studies, the rates for schizophrenia and schizophrenia spectrum disorders have been found to be significantly higher among the relatives of affected individuals than among the relatives of normal subjects (4, 5). Twin and adoption studies have demonstrated that the reason for this familial aggregation of schizophrenia is mainly common genetic factors shared by family members, rather than common environment (2, 6). In fact, having a family history of the disorder is currently the best predictor for the development of severe mental disorders, like schizophrenia (7).

In the past decades, the dramatic advance of molecular biology allowed the identification of numerous DNA markers associated with schizophrenia, spanning the whole human genome (e.g., 8–11). Following a long period of failure to demonstrate the universality of any finding, however, it is believed that no single major causative gene exists and that the etiology of schizophrenia should be complex, with hereditary factors involving a multitude of genes of small effect and possibly rare variants of large effect (12–14). Environmental factors conferring an increased risk for the development of schizophrenia include cannabis use; prenatal infection or malnutrition; perinatal complications; and a history of winter birth, migration, and childhood trauma (15, 16).

The recent progress in the field of genetic research and its wide publicity have created an ever-rising demand for genetic counseling regarding many disorders, and, among them schizophrenia. Clinicians are increasingly confronted with questions from patients and families regarding risks for themselves and their children, but currently only few individuals are offered psychiatric genetic counseling services. In a recent survey, over 40% of patients with schizophrenia and their relatives indicated that their family-planning decisions were influenced by the presence of schizophrenia in the family and over 70% of either group thought that genetic counseling would be useful; however, only 6% of all respondents had been offered genetic counseling (17).

Traditionally, genetic counseling has concentrated on conditions with well-known patterns of inheritance, such as Huntington's disease. The practice of genetic counseling in psychiatry is relatively new and underdeveloped, mainly due to the inability to individualize risks, which is a consequence of the absence of genetic testing for psychiatric disorders. However, contemporary research using larger samples, more accurate diagnoses, modern molecular genetics techniques, and more sophisticated statistical methods is anticipated to improve risk prediction. The coming years

TABLE 26.1 Usual questions posed in genetic counseling

What is the risk of disease to the relatives of a patient?
Is prenatal diagnosis/selective abortion possible?
What are the risks from marrying someone who has a close relative with this illness?
Should we adopt a child from a family with individuals with this illness?
Is it safe to have children if a prospective parent is affected with this illness?
What are the consequences of pregnancy on illness and what are those of medication during
   pregnancy (if needed)?

will likely see significant advances in the clinical application of this knowledge in psychiatric practice (18).

DEFINITION OF GENETIC COUNSELING

According to the U.S. "National Society of Genetic Counselors" (NSGC), genetic counseling is defined as "the process of helping people understand and adapt to the medical, psychological and familial implications of genetic contributions to disease. This process integrates the following: a) Interpretation of family and medical histories to assess the chance of disease occurrence or recurrence, b) Education about inheritance, testing, management, prevention, resources and research and c) Counseling to promote informed choices and adaptation to the risk or condition" (19).

PEOPLE INVOLVED IN GENETIC COUNSELING

1. Client

Usually the demand for genetic counseling comes from individuals who have reasons to be afraid for the development of a mental illness by themselves or other members of their family. The more common questions asked are about (Table 26.1) the risk of possible future illness in a relative of an individual with schizophrenia, the decision to marry with someone who has the disease or family loading for schizophrenia, the decision whether to have or not to have children, the possibility of prenatal diagnosis and performance of selective abortion, the adoption of a child from a family with individuals affected with this illness, and the use of psychiatric medication during pregnancy (18). It is important to remark that the individuals who request genetic counseling have different interests and opinions. The patients, relatives, or potential partners, and their relatives, have dissimilar approaches to the illness and different anxieties and queries. This has to be taken into account before offering genetic counseling (20).

Who has the right to an answer? In this very critical question, it is commonly accepted that people thinking of becoming parents are entitled to having access to valid information, in order to make their choice. If genetic counseling is requested only by one spouse (especially the one who does not have the illness) or by individuals who are thinking of marrying someone with a diagnosis or genetic loading for schizophrenia, the common practice is to advise them to include in the process their partner and return for counseling together. If this is not feasible, the counselor can disclose information only if they do not breach medical confidentiality for the person in question, always explaining that this is general information on the subject, not personalized on the specific patient. The indirect conveyance of information is discouraged, to avoid misinterpretations. In addition, as the counseling process has to be handled with sensitivity to the personal opinions, attitudes to the disease, and ability to understand of each individual, the counselor can only assess these attitudes and decide on how much information to convey, by direct contact.

In general, the demand for genetic counseling should never be rejected immediately (even when the counselor believes that the client is not entitled to receive information) because the person may be led to other sources of information, which are less reliable. An understanding/supportive approach should be adopted, and the limitations of the counseling process should be explained. It also needs to be stated that the counseling center is at the disposition of the family, if they want to proceed with the patient or other family members for further information.

2. Counselor
Family doctors, treating psychiatrists, or other specialists trusted by the individual are usually approached initially to provide information. The family doctors may be appropriate to give genetic counseling because they are aware of the family and its dynamics, but may not be adequately informed on the recent developments in the area of psychiatric genetics. The same applies for the treating psychiatrist who is not up to date with the progress in genetics. A recent survey of psychiatrists demonstrated gaps in genetic knowledge and a directive approach in response to questions about the continuation or termination of a pregnancy (21).

The counselor must possess the current knowledge concerning the role of genetic factors in the pathogenesis of mental illness and needs to have a good, scientific understanding of the source of relevant risk figures and the potentials, as well as the limitations, of current clinical and molecular strategies in risk prediction. He or she also should base counseling on the ethical standards of medical genetics (22, 23). In addition he or she needs to have experience in psychiatric disorders because part of his or her duty is to investigate the opinion and the attitude of the family toward schizophrenia and to correct misconceptions. The counselor should also examine if possible the family members who are labeled "psychiatrically ill." For all these reasons, genetic counseling requires a competent psychiatrist with well-established knowledge of genetics, as well as with certain abilities in communicating with patients and assessing personality traits, social interests, psychological motivation, and attitudes (23, 24). The genetic counselor must use flexible, interactive, skill-based counseling. This approach must be respectful, not only of the counselee's values and ultimate decisions but also of his or her need for direction, guidance, and emotional engagement (25).

When available, it is appropriate to refer the family to centers of psychiatric genetic counseling, where the counselors have clinical experience with schizophrenia and are informed on the developments in the research of genetic predisposition to the disorder, and where a multidisciplinary, collaborative approach between psychiatrists and geneticists may provide the best outcome for patients and their families (18).

GENETIC COUNSELING PROCESS

The process of genetic counseling should follow a number of steps (Table 26.2).

1. Gathering Information: Family History
Before offering genetic counseling, it is important to collect and verify information on mental and medical conditions of the family members and to draw the family tree.

TABLE 26.2 Steps of genetic counseling

Gathering information/taking a detailed family history
Estimating the morbidity risk
Assisting clients to understand the notion of morbidity risk and its limitations, and to deal with genetic information
Assisting clients to make their choices

This will allow an overview of mental and physical illness to be quickly recorded and visually displayed (18, 26). In addition, it can be used to process information that may indicate the presence of a genetic syndrome underlying the psychotic illness; the most important (but probably not the only one) is the velo–cardio–facial syndrome (VCFS), which is due to a 22q11.2 deletion (27, 28). VCFS is found among about 1% of patients with schizophrenia and represents the highest known genetic risk factor for the development of the disorder with up to 30% of patients manifesting psychotic symptoms (29, 30). Diagnoses are preferably made with personal interview, where the interviewer applies valid diagnostic criteria to establish a rigorous diagnosis. If one of the patients cannot be examined with personal interview, the assessment should be based on the interview of as many relatives as possible, medical records, and telephonic interview with the patient, if necessary. Various structured instruments are available for research purposes (31). Best-estimate diagnoses should be reached when information is not conclusive.

The importance of accurate diagnosis needs to be emphasized because one of the greatest limitations in estimating morbidity risks is the potential for misdiagnosis of relatives (32). For every affected member of the family, it is also useful to establish the severity of the disease (26). Factors that indicate more severe disease are (a) early age of onset; (b) severe symptomatology; (c) frequent relapses; (d) lengthy admissions to hospital; (e) personal, professional, and social decline; and (f) violent and self-destructive acts. In addition, it is essential to assess the capacity of the patient to fulfill parental role (33).

The systematic exploration of the family history is important because, sometimes, distant relatives are considered "healthy," either because their condition is hidden by themselves and their close relatives or because they have milder forms of the disorder or its spectrum. Occasionally, other concomitant conditions (e.g., alcohol or substance abuse) modify the clinical picture and may conceal the correct diagnosis. The counselor needs to take into account these limitations in the family history before estimating the morbidity risk, which is to some degree diagnosis depended (20).

2. Estimation of Morbidity Risk

In order to assist individuals in formulating personal plans, an effort is made for the estimation of the risk of occurrence in an unaffected individual, the risk of possible recurrence in one who has already manifested the disease, the genetic risk of children to be born, and the potential consequences of a spouse's illness with regard to the person's ability to function as a parent. Because (unlike Mendelian disorders like Huntington's disease) no definite genetic factors that predict the development of schizophrenia have been established so far, there is no way to ascertain a prenatal or presymptomatic diagnosis. Consequently, the morbidity risk remains an empirical estimation based on the morbidity of other members of the family and the closeness of the relationship.

TABLE 26.3   Risk of schizophrenia in relatives of patients
and the general population (approximate values)

MZ twins	49%
Children of affected (both) parents	46%
DZ twins	15%
Children of an affected parent	13%
Siblings	10%
Half siblings, grandchildren, nephews	3%
First cousins	1.5%
General population	0.8%

In schizophrenia, while the morbidity risk is about 0.8% for the general population, it is significantly higher for the first-degree relatives of schizophrenic probands
(Table 26.3): about 6% for parents, 10% for siblings (17% if one parent is also affected),
49% for monozygotic and 15% for dizygotic twins (34), 13% for children, and 46% if
both parents are affected. For second-degree relatives (half-siblings, grandchildren,
grandparents, nephews, uncles, aunts) the risk is about 3%, while for third-degree relatives (first cousins) the risk is about 1.5% (4). These estimations, however, are empiric
calculations based on averaging several studies, and they do not reflect the true probability of a given individual to become ill. The morbidity risk for a particular family
may be larger or smaller than the average; thus calculations must be based on the number of affected family members and their symptomatology, as greater familial risk has
been associated with earlier age of onset, poor premorbid adjustment, disorganized or
negative symptomatology (35, 36). A dimensional approach of psychotic symptoms, if
possible, may be superior to the categorical approach in predicting course, outcome,
and treatment response (37). In addition, the counselor needs to explore variations
in severity based on need of hospitalizations or history of suicide attempts; course,
prognosis, and recurrence rate; response to available treatments; social functioning,
presence of impairment, or incapacitation; and the role of possible environmental factors. Also, genetic factors such as rare cases of heavy familial aggregation or specific
modes of transmission in the given family, implying an underlying genetic syndrome
and assortative mating (marriage between individuals with similar symptomatology
or predisposition to mental disorders) should be taken into consideration (33).

According to the multifactorial inheritance model, the greater the number of
affected individuals, the more severe their symptomatology and the higher the risk
of developing the disease. A limitation for a more accurate calculation of morbidity
risks is that because several relatives may have not exceeded the age range at risk for
schizophrenia, not all cases in the family are identified. To overcome this problem in
research, the Weinberg method for age correction of morbidity risks has been used
(4). An additional complexity in estimating morbidity risks is the evidence for a continuum of psychosis. The presence of relative with schizophrenia spectrum disorders
probably conveys risk for schizophrenia in family members. The counselor should
take into account studies that estimate the risk of schizophrenia when family members
have conditions of the broader spectrum (38).

3. Family Education About Genetic Risks
The procedure of genetic counseling for schizophrenia should start with the identification of the exact needs of the person(s) seeking counseling and exploration of

all the dimensions of the problem should be made, including the ability of patients and their families to participate in decision making. Before providing estimates of risk, the counselor must carefully examine whether the clients want to know morbidity risks, assess their intellectual and emotional capacity, and explore their perception of risk (20).

The report must not be a simple reference to the calculated morbidity risks but should also contain the information that these are estimates at best and that genes are not necessarily destiny, as the influence of environmental factors may have a deleterious or protective effect for the manifestation of the disorder. Despite the fact that the estimate of morbidity risk is essential information for genetic counseling, the understanding of probabilities varies from person to person (39). Thus, it is advisable to discuss how risks are derived and to provide information on the distinction between classic single-gene and complex, multifactorial inheritance. It should be made clear that genes may confer risk for a disorder but that the expression of the phenotype and the probability of the disorder's occurring may be difficult to predict (18).

The counselor should explain in lay language current knowledge about pathogenesis, ongoing research, issues around the potential for genetic testing for psychiatric disorders, and why testing for schizophrenia is not currently clinically available. Understanding that in a majority of cases both genetic and environmental factors contribute to disease pathogenesis may help relieve the fatalistic attitude of the individual and provide a source of hope, empowerment, and an increased sense of personal control, which may ultimately improve self-esteem (20).

Genetic counseling also offers an opportunity to reduce damaging misattributions of etiology and reduce the guilt, shame, and stigma for affected individuals and their families (40). This part of the discussion can also alleviate some common misconceptions (e.g., "if a disorder is genetic, it inevitably occurs in those carrying the harmful gene or it is untreatable") (41). For some patients and their families the knowledge that they carry a "genetic defect" creates strong negative feelings, fear, and affects self-esteem. In these cases, it should be explained that, despite the genetic predisposition, the probability of developing the illness by the children is not 100%, but much smaller. On the other hand, this knowledge may reduce the family's self-blame, as the disorder can be attributed to biological rather than social factors. Furthermore, understanding that the illness is mainly due to a biological aberration helps the individual and the family to accept the necessity of pharmacotherapy and other treatments (42). A letter to the family, summarizing the consultation is advisable and, when possible, follow-up sessions to ensure continued assessment of the client's understanding of pertinent information and follow-up of life events (43).

4. Promotion of Informed Choices
A general principle of genetic counseling is that the advice should be nondirective.

In other words, the counselor's values should not be forced on the family. The role of the genetic counselor, according to Sheldon Reed, the geneticist who coined the expression "genetic counseling" in 1947, is "to explain thoroughly what the genetic situation is, but the decision must be a personal one between the husband and wife, and theirs alone" (44). Thus, families must be assisted to make their own informed decisions by weighing the consequences of either choice. The counselor should remain neutral in the process of decision making, informing and supporting the family where needed. If the clients have erroneous ideas about the disease, the counselor should portray the usual clinical characteristics, including symptoms, age of onset, course, impact on personal and social functioning, and existing treatment options.

The nondirective approach respects the autonomy, consent, voluntary attendance, and confidentiality, which are the central principles of medical practice. This approach differentiates genetic counseling from the methodology of eugenics, which has raised increased social sensitivity (45). Given the existing knowledge on genetics of schizophrenia, it cannot be advocated that advice against childbearing in families with genetic loading can eliminate the disorder. The benefits of having children vary with each individual's culture, values, religion, and personality; these benefits should be explored and discussed against the burden of disease. Only in the case of particularly severe hereditary loading and/or a prospective parent suffering from clinically unmanageable illness, which diminishes considerably the ability to make decisions or the responsibility required for the parental role, the families may be advised against having children. Even then, advice should be nondirective and must protect the patients' and their spouses' choices in reproduction because nondirectiveness is a generally professed standard for genetic counseling (46).

In cases where the couple decides to bear a child, the only prenatal advice that can be given to prospective parents who have schizophrenia is to inform the obstetrician, in order to avoid perinatal complications. Caesarian section is advisable in cases at high risk for perinatal complications, as they are major environmental risk factor for the development of schizophrenia-like disorders. Prospective parents or other relatives of susceptible individuals should also be informed about the need for a protective social environment at home as well as at school, and about the premorbid symptoms of the disease, so that medical advice is sought without delay if they appear, in order to minimize the detrimental effects of the illness through early implementation of treatment. In addition, genetic counseling may promote adherence to prescribed treatment and decrease risk behaviors, such as illicit drug use (47).

LIMITATIONS—FUTURE DIRECTIONS

The limitations of psychiatric genetic counseling are that mental disorders, such as schizophrenia, are complex behavioral diseases that are genetically heterogeneous, caused by interactions of genes, and environmental factors operating over a lifespan. Because no robust genetic marker has been identified for the psychiatric disorders and there is lack of knowledge about their etiology and exact mode(s) of transmission, the subject is inappropriate for accurate risk prediction. Even if susceptibility genes for schizophrenia are finally identified, it will not be possible to predict the development of the disorder with certainty until the nature of the complex interactions between genes and environmental factors are understood (48). In the meanwhile, risk estimates from family studies constitute the best available knowledge on which to predict the risk of the development of mental disorders. These risk estimates, however, represent mean values from many families and cannot be considered as reflecting the real morbidity risk for any particular case.

On the other hand, recent technological advances, including DNA genotyping microarrays, permit the analysis of hundreds of thousands of genetic markers. At least seven genomewide association studies of schizophrenia and bipolar disorder, each in excess of 1,000 cases and controls, are ongoing (49). The first published results indicate that rare de novo copy number variants may have a large effect on schizophrenia risk, which could potentially be clinically useful in a minority of cases (50,51). It is conceivable that in the coming years, the ability to simultaneously assay multiple susceptibility genes could substantially improve the predictive value of genetic testing (52). Gaining understanding of the significance of genetic risk factors and learning proper interpretation of their meaning for patients and their families will ultimately become part of clinical practice, and clinicians will be involved more than ever in helping patients to comprehend the meaning and potential impact of genetic risk (7). Before any predictive or diagnostic genetics tests are introduced to clinical practice, studies need to be conducted measuring the benefits and adverse effects of this practice (17).

ETHICAL CONSIDERATIONS

Even at this early stage, and much more in the future when prenatal diagnosis will also be applied to multifactorial disorders, the implementation of genetic counseling raises very serious ethical and clinical questions, as recent developments in genetics are likely to exacerbate the ethical issues in clinical practice, especially with regard to privacy and disclosure of genetic information (53). It must be ensured that the diagnostic and therapeutic technologies do more than open a Pandora's box of dangerous or uncontrollable technology. The problem of the availability of genetic data to third parties such as relatives, employers, or insurance companies is central and difficult to be tackled. The difficulty lies in finding the balance between the interests of individuals and those of relatives or the community (54).

Questions of ethics in genetic testing most commonly center on whether there is a clear clinical benefit to be gained from learning one's genetic status. This question is particularly important because the onset of schizophrenia commonly occurs during adolescence or early adulthood, and the appropriateness of genetic testing of children must be considered (41). Another controversial ethical issue is the question of assisted versus surrogate decision making in pregnant women with schizophrenia. The management of pregnancy in these cases poses particularly difficult clinical ethical challenges to the obstetrician. These challenges center mainly on the patient's capacity for decision making, which can be adversely affected by psychosis (55).

Despite the limitations in risk prediction from the current knowledge on the genetics of mental illnesses, private companies have already introduced genetic testing for psychiatric disorders. They are advertised in the Internet and provide "direct-to-consumer" genetic testing. In most cases, the DNA sample is sent by post and no face-to-face contact, let alone genetic counseling, is provided (56). In addition to the controversial use of genetics tests, there is enormous potential for misinterpretation of information by the clients, with potentially very damaging consequences. Furthermore, based on the current state of knowledge, there is no evidence that genetic testing should be used to alter risk, diagnosis, or treatment of psychiatric disorders (57,58), and it has been even supported that "the premature marketing of insensitive and confusing genetic tests is misleading to consumers and may cause human suffering" (57). The American College of Neuropsychopharmacology has released a statement in May 2008 (http://www.acnp.org/asset.axd?id=b6808602-acf9-4fa5-8edb-bee40e09164e) declaring that genetic testing in psychiatric illness is "scientifically unsupportable for general clinical use and certainly inappropriate in the direct-to-consumer arena." In spite of the strong opposition of individualized psychiatric genetic testing by the scientific community, the industry is currently poorly regulated (20). Regulatory bodies, scientists, and service users, and families, arguably need to examine the ethics of such practice and develop relevant legislation and codes of practice, but it must be anticipated that as tests for the genes involved become more easily available, pressures will arise to use them for prenatal testing, screening of children and adults, selection of potential adoptees, and premarital screening (59). Thus, the scientific community, as well as the society, are faced with the problems of (a) the development of ethical and legal principles for medical genetics, and (b) the control over their proper use. The main challenge is to establish an interaction between the aims of molecular genetics and the interests and rights of the individual, family members, and society at large (45).

CONCLUSIONS

Despite the lack of a presymptomatic or prenatal test for schizophrenia, genetic counseling for this disorder is available, based on the understanding that the disease has a strong hereditary component and that genetic factors are in interplay with environmental ones. Even with the anticipated improvement in risk prediction, considerable uncertainty will probably remain, and the clinical utility of this information and its ethical consequences may remain unknown (48,60). Nevertheless, genetic counseling for schizophrenia should be part of the routine clinical practice, as it can offer help to patients and their relatives regarding family planning, correct many of the misconceptions about the disease, enhance treatment compliance, assist patients achieving their parenting goals, and reduce morbidity through preventive measures. Last but not least, ethical guidelines concerning genetic information should be always kept in mind, following the Hippocratic principle of "primum non nocere."

REFERENCES

1. Slater E, Cowie V. The genetics of mental disorders. London: Oxford University Press; 1971.
2. Sullivan PF, Kendler KS, Neale MC. Schizophrenia as a complex trait: evidence from a meta-analysis of twin studies. Arch Gen Psychiatry 2003; 60: 1187–92.
3. Harrison PJ, Weinberger DR. Schizophrenia genes, gene expression, and neuropathology: on the matter of their convergence. Mol Psychiatry 2005; 10: 40–68.
4. Gottesman I. Schizophrenia genesis: The origins of madness. New York: Freeman; 1991.
5. Kendler KS. Schizophrenia genetics. In: Sadock B, Sadock V editors. Kaplan and Sadock's comprehensive textbook of psychiatry: 7th ed, Vol 1. Philadelphia: Lippincott, Williams and Wilkins, 2000: 1147–59.
6. Kety SS, Wender PH, Jacobsen B et al. Mental illness in the biological and adoptive relatives of schizophrenic adoptees. Replication of the Copenhagen Study in the rest of Denmark. Arch Gen Psychiatry 1994; 51: 442–55.
7. Merikangas KR, Risch N. Will the genomics revolution revolutionize psychiatry? Am J Psychiatry 2003; 160: 625–35.
8. Antonarakis SE, Blouin JL, Pulver AE et al. Schizophrenia susceptibility and chromosome 6p24-22. Nat Genet 1995;11: 235–6.
9. Blouin JL, Dombroski BA, Nath SK et al. Schizophrenia susceptibility loci on chromosomes 13q32 and 8p21. Nat Genet 1998; 20: 70–3.
10. Pulver AE, Mulle J, Nestadt G et al. Genetic heterogeneity in schizophrenia: stratification of genome scan data using co-segregating related phenotypes. Mol Psychiatry 2000; 5: 650–3.
11. O'Donovan MC, Craddock N, Norton N et al. Identification of loci associated with schizophrenia by genome-wide association and follow-up. Nat Genet 2008 Sep; 40: 1042–4.
12. Pulver A, Pearlson G, McGrath J et al. Schizophrenia. In: King R, Rotter J, Motulsky A editors. Genetic Basis of Common Diseases. New York: Oxford University Press, 2002: 850–75.
13. Karayiorgou M, Gogos JA. Schizophrenia genetics: uncovering positional candidate genes. Eur J Hum Genet 2006; 14: 512–9.
14. Craddock N, O'Donovan MC, Owen MJ. Phenotypic and genetic complexity of psychosis. Invited commentary on ... Schizophrenia: a common disease caused by multiple rare alleles. Br J Psychiatry 2007; 190: 200–3.

15. Murray RM, Morrison PD, Henquet C, Di Forti M. Cannabis, the mind and society: the hash realities. Nat Rev Neurosci 2007; 8: 885–95.
16. Tandon R, Keshavan MS, Nasrallah HA. Schizophrenia, "just the facts" what we know in 2008. 2. Epidemiology and etiology. Schizophr Res 2008; 102: 1–18.
17. Lyus VL. The importance of genetic counseling for individuals with schizophrenia and their relatives: potential clients' opinions and experiences. Am J Med Genet B Neuropsychiatr Genet 2007; 144B: 1014–21.
18. Finn CT, Smoller JW. Genetic counseling in psychiatry. Harv Rev Psychiatry 2006; 14: 109–21.
19. Resta R, Biesecker BB, Bennett RL et al. A new definition of Genetic Counseling: National Society of Genetic Counselors' Task Force report. J Genet Couns 2006; 15: 77–83.
20. Austin JC, Honer WG. The genomic era and serious mental illness: a potential application for psychiatric genetic counseling. Psychiatr Serv 2007; 58: 254–61.
21. Finn CT, Wilcox MA, Korf BR et al. Psychiatric genetics: a survey of psychiatrists' knowledge, opinions, and practice patterns. J Clin Psychiatry 2005; 66: 821–30.
22. Pardes H, Kaufmann CA, Pincus HA, West A. Genetics and psychiatry: past discoveries, current dilemmas, and future directions. Am J Psychiatry 1989; 146: 435–43.
23. Rainer J. Genetic counseling and ethical dilemmas in neuropsychiatric disorders. In: Papadimitriou G, Mendlewicz J editors. Genetics of Mental Disorders Part II: Clinical Issues. Bailliere Tindall, 1996: 153–9.
24. Papadimitriou GN. Genetic counseling for major psychiatric disorders. In: Christodoulou GN, Kontaxakis VP editors. Topics in Preventive Psychiatry. Basel: Karger, 1994: 8–13.
25. Weil J, Ormond K, Peters J et al. The relationship of nondirectiveness to genetic counseling: report of a workshop at the 2003 NSGC Annual Education Conference. J Genet Couns 2006; 15: 85–93.
26. Peay HL, Sheidley BR. Principles of Genetic Counseling. In: Smoller JW, Sheidley BR, Tsuang MT editors. Psychiatric Genetics: Applications in Clinical Practice. Washington, DC: American Psychiatric Publishing, Inc, 2008: 27–46.
27. Pulver AE, Nestadt G, Goldberg R et al. Psychotic illness in patients diagnosed with velo-cardio-facial syndrome and their relatives. J Nerv Ment Dis 1994; 182: 476–8.
28. Bassett AS, Chow EW, Husted J et al. Clinical features of 78 adults with 22q11 Deletion Syndrome. Am J Med Genet A 2005; 138: 307–13.
29. Murphy KC. Schizophrenia and velo-cardio-facial syndrome. Lancet 2002; 359: 426–30.
30. Bassett AS, Chow EW. Schizophrenia and 22q11.2 deletion syndrome. Curr Psychiatry Rep 2008; 10: 148–57.
31. Nurnberger JI Jr, Blehar MC, Kaufmann CA. Diagnostic interview for genetic studies. Rationale, unique features, and training. NIMH Genetics Initiative. Arch Gen Psychiatry 1994; 51: 849–59; discussion 863–44.
32. Stefanis CN, Dikeos DG, Papadimitriou GN. Clinical strategies in genetic research. In: Mendlewicz J, Papadimitriou GN editors. Genetics of Mental Disorders Part I: Theoretical Aspects: Bailliere Tindall, 1995: 1–18.
33. Papadimitriou GN, Dikeos DG. The Role of Genetics in the Prevention of Psychiatric Disorders In: Christodoulou GN, Lecic-Tosevski D, Kontaxakis VP editors. Issues in Preventive Psychiatry. Basel: Karger, 1999: 7–16.
34. Kringlen E. Twin studies in mental disorders. In: Mendlewicz J, Papadimitriou GN editors. Genetics of Mental Disorders Part I: Theoretical Aspects: Bailliere Tindall, 1995: 47–62.
35. Cardno AG, Holmans PA, Harvey I et al. Factor-derived subsyndromes of schizophrenia and familial morbid risks. Schizophr Res 1997; 23: 231–8.
36. Ritsner M, Ratner Y, Gibel A, Weizman R. Familiality in a five-factor model of schizophrenia psychopathology: findings from a 16-month follow-up study. Psychiatry Res 2005; 136: 173–9.
37. Dikeos DG, Wickham H, McDonald C et al. Distribution of symptom dimensions across Kraepelinian divisions. Br J Psychiatry 2006; 189: 346–53.

38. Kendler KS, McGuire M, Gruenberg AM et al. The Roscommon Family Study. I. Methods, diagnosis of probands, and risk of schizophrenia in relatives. Arch Gen Psychiatry 1993; 50: 527–40.

39. Marteau TM. Communicating genetic risk information. Br Med Bull 1999; 55: 414–28.

40. Austin JC, Honer WG. The potential impact of genetic counseling for mental illness. Clin Genet 2005; 67: 134–42.

41. Arehart-Treichel J. Psychiatric Genetic Counseling: Don't Expect Easy Answers. Psychiatr News 2008; 43: 20.

42. Hill MK, Sahhar M. Genetic counselling for psychiatric disorders. Med J Aust 2006; 185: 507–10.

43. Tsuang MT. Genetic counseling for psychiatric patients and their families. Am J Psychiatry 1978; 135: 1465–75.

44. Reed S. Counseling in Medical Genetics. Philadelphia: W.B. Saunders Co; 1955.

45. Hoge SK, Appelbaum PS. Ethical, Legal, and Social implications of psychiatric genetics and genetic counseling. In: Smoller JW, Sheidley BR, Tsuang MT editors. Psychiatric Genetics: Applications in Clinical Practice. Washington, DC: American Psychiatric Publishing, Inc, 2008: 27–46.

46. Andrews L, Fullarton J, Holzman N, Motulsky A. Assessing genetic risks; Implications for health and social policy. Washington: National Academy Press; 1994.

47. Papadimitriou GN, Dikeos DG. How does recent knowledge on the heredity of schizophrenia affect genetic counseling? Curr Psychiatry Rep 2003; 5: 239–40.

48. Scourfield J, Owen M. Genetic Counselling. In: McGuffin P, Owen M, Gottesman I editors. Psychiatric Genetics & Genomics. Oxford: Oxford University Press, 2002: 419–27.

49. Sullivan PF. Schizophrenia genetics: the search for a hard lead. Curr Opin Psychiatry 2008; 21: 157–60.

50. International Schizophrenia Consortium. Rare chromosomal deletions and duplications increase risk of schizophrenia. Nature 2008; 455: 237–41.

51. Stefansson H, Rujescu D, Cichon S et al. Large recurrent microdeletions associated with schizophrenia. Nature 2008; 455: 232–6.

52. Yang Q, Khoury MJ, Botto L et al. Improving the prediction of complex diseases by testing for multiple disease-susceptibility genes. Am J Hum Genet 2003; 72: 636–49.

53. Meslin EM, Thomson EJ, Boyer JT. The Ethical, Legal, and Social Implications Research Program at the National Human Genome Research Institute. Kennedy Inst Ethics J 1997; 7: 291–8.

54. Nuffield Council on Bioethics. Genetic Screening: Ethical Issues. London: Nuffield Counsil on Bioethics; 1993.

55. McCullough LB, Coverdale JH, Chervenak FA. Ethical challenges of decision making with pregnant patients who have schizophrenia. Am J Obstet Gynecol 2002; 187: 696–702.

56. Couzin J. Science and commerce. Gene tests for psychiatric risk polarize researchers. Science 2008; 319: 274–7.

57. Braff DL, Freedman R. Clinically responsible genetic testing in neuropsychiatric patients: a bridge too far and too soon. Am J Psychiatry 2008; 165: 952–5.

58. de Leon J. The future (or lack of future) of personalized prescription in psychiatry. Pharmacol Res 2008 Oct 17. [Epub ahead of print]

59. Appelbaum PS. Ethical issues in psychiatric genetics. J Psychiatr Pract 2004; 10: 343–51.

60. DeLisi LE, Bertisch H. A preliminary comparison of the hopes of researchers, clinicians, and families for the future ethical use of genetic findings on schizophrenia. Am J Med Genet B Neuropsychiatr Genet 2006; 141B: 110–5.

Violence in schizophrenia: Risk factors and assessment

John Rabun and Susan Boyer

VIOLENCE IN SCHIZOPHRENIA: RISK FACTORS AND ASSESSMENT

Clinicians routinely interview and treat individuals with schizophrenia. At certain times, those practitioners must decide whether a particular individual under their care is at imminent risk for violence and then take steps to reduce that risk. It is now recognized in the literature that individuals with schizophrenia are at an increased risk for violence compared to the general public (1–4). Violence in schizophrenia, therefore, must be addressed, but in a thoughtful manner guided by the scientific evidence, not by speculation or fear.

To actually predict violence in a specific individual is difficult. Monahan has noted that predictions of violence in those suffering from a mental disorder are accurate only one-third of the time (5). Some authorities on this subject suggest that psychiatrists overpredict violence by 40% to 90% (6). Given those odds, a psychiatrist would be better served by flipping a coin when asked to state whether a particular person will act violently in the near future. Despite a growing body of evidence pointing to key factors that increase risk for violence, the actual commission of violence is infrequent. Because violent behavior is infrequent and the overall prevalence is low, even small errors in sensitivity and specificity result in significant errors in outcome when a psychiatrist tries to predict that a particular person will act violently. Much like the meteorologist trying to predict where lightening will strike, the psychiatrist's attempt to predict whether a patient will commit violence is hampered by the infrequency of this event.

Although it is widely acknowledged that individuals with schizophrenia are at an increased risk for violence, the specific factors offered as causal links continue to be debated in the literature. To compound the problem, researchers have changed their opinions regarding various mental disorders and the risk for violence, initially opining that there was no link, then offering that certain diagnoses were associated with violence, then shifting to investigating symptom categories such as hallucinations, then turning to specific, narrow symptoms such as threat/control-override delusions, and most recently focusing on static versus dynamic factors in risk assessments (7, 8). This means that many methods of studying violence have been used, leading to conflicting outcomes.

Despite the differences in opinion about what symptoms cause violence in schizophrenia, and the level of risk posed by those symptoms, it is common for psychiatrists to assess their patients' level of risk for harm. Furthermore, society expects that psychiatrists will take appropriate action when an individual poses a risk to the public. In line with societal expectations, the legal community seemingly defined the standard of care for psychiatry in this area. The seminal legal case is the Tarasoff decision handed down by the California Supreme Court in 1976. This legal action was filed after Tatiana Tarasoff, a college student, was murdered by a male student. Several months before the homicide, the male student revealed his homicidal thoughts to his therapist, who did not alert Tarasoff. After hearing the case twice, the California Supreme Court articulated the following standard: When "a therapist determines, or according to the standard of his profession, should determine that his patient presents a serious danger of violence to another, he incurs an obligation to use reasonable care to protect the intended victim from danger" (9). This specific standard, with its variations, has been adopted by multiple higher courts hearing similar cases of patient violence. This means that mental health professionals are expected to know the risk factors for potential violence. It also means that if a patient is determined to be at an elevated risk for violence, mental health professionals are expected to take reasonable steps to protect the intended target, such as by increasing medications, seeking hospitalization, contacting the intended victim, or notifying the police.

It is important to note that the Tarasoff decision does not state that psychiatrists must predict which patient will act violently. Instead, the language of the Tarasoff decision suggests that psychiatrists should assess violence risk potential and if a patient is judged to be at an elevated risk, institute appropriate measures to minimize that risk. In other words, assessing risk for violence is not the same as actually predicting violence. As numerous studies point out, psychiatrists have no special ability to predict who will be violent. Given the difficulties in predicting violence, it would be a misrepresentation of expertise for a psychiatrist to offer in court that an individual will act violently. Despite all the inherent problems identifying who will act violently, society views psychiatrists as barometers of violence potential for individuals with a mental disorder.

Due to Tarasoff and its progeny, psychiatrists must assess risk for violence on an ongoing basis in their patient populations. Furthermore, civil commitment laws frequently require psychiatric opinions about risk for violence before a court can order involuntary hospitalization. Like it or not, throughout their clinical careers, psychiatrists will be faced with questions about "future dangerousness." When faced with such a question, psychiatrists should not overreach their expertise and predict that a patient will act violently. Instead, psychiatrists should offer a risk assessment, using known factors that are associated with potential violence. In fact, psychiatrists should familiarize themselves with known risk factors and then use these factors as an anchor for clinical judgment in this area. In other words, psychiatrists can meet their clinical duties by conducting a thorough risk assessment, while avoiding the slippery slope of actual prediction.

The actual violence risk assessment should be similar to assessing suicide potential. When assessing suicide potential, psychiatrists probe for known, general risk factors and then adjust the level of risk based on information unique to the patient. For instance, the literature on suicide suggests that a middle-aged, divorced White male, who has access to weapons, lives alone, and suffers from depression and alcohol dependence is similar to a population of individuals who have completed suicide. The terse, general risk factors in this case could represent a psychiatric emergency. The psychiatrist's duty in this case, however, has not been fully discharged because information unique to this patient must be elicited to further guide the final risk calculus. Consider then, that the psychiatrist gathers important additional information, including that this patient would not consider suicide for familial and religious reasons. What was at first look an elevated risk for suicide has now become an acceptable risk in the final analysis.

The violence risk assessment should be approached in a similar manner. During an interview with a patient, the psychiatrist should elicit recognized, general risk factors and then move to information distinct to the patient. Furthermore, the psychiatrist should repeatedly assess patients for violence potential because some risk factors, particularly those termed *dynamic*, can change over time, much like blood glucose measurements can fluctuate throughout the day in diabetes. Using the diabetes example, it would not meet the standard of practice for a clinician to merely check blood glucose once a day in a hospitalized patient suffering from brittle, insulin-dependent diabetes. This would also be true in assessing violence potential. The psychiatrist should elicit general risk factors, or those viewed as static in nature, and then over the course of treatment, hone the assessment by uncovering and then monitoring factors unique to the patient, or those viewed as dynamic.

Performing risk assessments in this manner means that every time a psychiatrist interviews a patient, whether for the first time or in follow-up, information should be gathered that will aid in assessing that patient's current violence potential. Psychiatrists who view their duty in this area as ongoing, and therefore, monitor for changing risk factors are best able to insulate themselves from a successful claim of malpractice, even if a patient acts violently. It is important to understand that in malpractice, professionals are more easily faulted for failing to gather relevant information, so called errors of omission, than for making an incorrect final judgment on an issue (10). It is also important to be mindful of the fact that judging a patient to be at an increased risk for violence is not the same as stating that the patient will actually commit violence. Rather, such a judgment indicates that the patient currently poses an unacceptable risk for imminent violence.

THE ASSOCIATION BETWEEN SCHIZOPHRENIA AND VIOLENCE

Research findings now suggest that schizophrenia is associated with an increased risk for violence (11). One study in the United States noted that the prevalence for violence in schizophrenia was 8%, but in those without a mental illness it was 2% (12, 13). A more recent study found that 19.1% of individuals with schizophrenia acted violently over a 6-month period and that 3.6% of that same study group was involved in serious violent acts (14). Furthermore, in a national survey of homicides that occurred over a 3-year period in England and Wales, researchers found that 5% of the offenders had schizophrenia (15, 16). This does not mean that the diagnosis of schizophrenia per se increases the afflicted individual's potential for violence. In fact, the majority of individuals with schizophrenia do not engage in violent behavior (17, 18). Rather, only during symptomatic periods, and in certain subgroups, does the individual with schizophrenia pose an elevated risk for violence. This means that similar to the individual with alcohol dependence who while sober poses no increased risk driving a vehicle, the individual with schizophrenia who is in remission poses no increased risk of violence due to this illness.

Therefore, when a patient is acutely psychotic, a clinician should be most vigilant for signs of potential violence and maintain a low threshold for hospitalization. Despite continued debates over the degree of threat posed by particular delusions and hallucinations, it is clear that during acute psychotic episodes certain subgroups of individuals with schizophrenia are at increased risk for violence. It becomes the clinician's task to recognize the symptoms and look for the signs in schizophrenia that distinguish the violence-prone patient from all others in treatment. In order to do this, the clinician must know the risk factors for violence in the general population and then utilize that information while probing the patient for factors unique to schizophrenia.

GENERAL RISK FACTORS

The following general factors are important for assessing risk for violence whether someone is or is not afflicted by a mental disorder. Despite being labeled as "general," these factors need to be considered in all patients because it is likely that multiple factors result in a synergistic effect.

Demographics

It is well known that violence peaks in late adolescence and early adulthood, typically between the ages of 15 and 24 (19). All other factors being equal, psychiatric patients tend to peak in violence potential at a slightly later age, around the mid-20s (13, 20). Gender is of course an important issue, with males being more likely to commit violence in the general population (21). This factor is so well known that unfortunately it can foster mistakes when assessing risk in psychiatric patients. Contrary to the general population, among individuals with a mental disorder, males and females do not significantly differ in risk for violence (19). Therefore, a psychiatrist should be mindful of this finding while interviewing a female patient. Another factor to consider is socioeconomic status because violence is 3 times more likely in the lowest socioeconomic class compared to the highest (19). In addition, the lower a person's intellectual capacity, the higher the risk of violence, to a degree (22). Obviously, individuals who are severely and profoundly mentally retarded are incapacitated to such an extent that the likelihood of engaging in serious violence is hampered by their mental and physical situation. Violence is also more likely if the person is unemployed and has a limited education (6). In regards to living circumstances, homeless mentally ill individuals commit 35 times more crimes than those in a stable situation (23).

Personality Traits

The literature suggests that particular personality traits are associated with violent behavior (17). One study on this issue suggested that these traits include impulsivity, low frustration tolerance, inability to tolerate criticism, reckless driving, entitlement, antisocial behavior, superficial relationships, and dehumanizing others (24). These individuals may display glibness and projection of internal difficulties on the world around them. Another study suggested that violent behavior is the defining characteristic of two specific personality disorders, borderline and antisocial (25). Furthermore, the individual with antisocial personality disorder is often seeking revenge when planning and executing a violent act. Such an individual may also act violently after a period of alcohol consumption, a substance known to enhance impulsivity. The resulting violent act often lacks the emotionality found among those who do not have antisocial personality disorder (26). Additional personality traits that contribute to violence are lack of empathy, shallow affect, lack of remorse, and denial of responsibility (25).

Recently, research has focused on separating criminal offenders with schizophrenia into two groups, those who start offending at an early age, typically before their illness emerges, and those who start offending in adulthood, usually after the onset of their illness. This concept has also been used to distinguish early-onset criminal offenders from those who started offending in adulthood (27). It is hypothesized that the causes of criminality in the so called early-start offenders with schizophrenia has less to do with their mental disorder and more to do with their life pattern of offending (11). One study found that homicides committed by early-start offenders with schizophrenia were more frequently preceded by arguments, with one possible interpretation for this finding being that early starters come from environments that foster more criminal behavior compared to late-start offenders (11). It was noted that the majority of early starters had committed a prior violent offense, suggesting that they had been exposed to situations where violence was used to resolve conflicts (11). An additional interpretation of these findings could be that early-start offenders are more comfortable with using violent force due to their history of misconduct and persistent antisocial behavior. It was further discovered that 70% of the early starters were intoxicated at the time of the violent act, compared to 43% of the late starters (11). More important, this line of research suggests that the likelihood of violence is enhanced by several factors working synergistically, including an underlying personality disorder, in particular, antisocial personality (28).

Childhood Factors
Children who have been physically abused by a caregiver are more likely to become violent as adults (29). In general, abused boys identify with the aggressor and become aggressive, whereas abused girls appear to replicate their victimization in relationships as an adult (30). Additional general factors associated with violence include truancy, low educational levels, and impoverished socioeconomic status (6, 17). The literature on violence assessment also suggests that a person has an increased risk for aggression if that person suffered from childhood hyperactivity (31); has prior arrests for violent behavior (32); was psychiatrically hospitalized before the age of 18 (33); and has a history of enuresis, setting fires, and abusing animals (34, 35).

Substance Use
One of the most robust findings in the literature is that substance use increases the potential for violence. This factor was well documented by the Epidemiological Catchment Area study in 1990 in which thousands of people in the community were questioned about violence over the previous year. This study discovered that 25% of those who met criteria for alcohol abuse or dependence were violent within the previous year and that 35% of those who met criteria for illicit substance use or dependence were violent within the previous year (13). This study also noted that the combination of substance use with mental disorder was more volatile than either finding alone. The data from the Epidemiological Catchment Area study revealed that mental disorder alone caused less violence than substance use, with substance use being about twice as prevalent in the violent subgroup (13, 36). The finding that substance use is strongly correlated with risk for violence has been replicated in other studies. In an article that reviewed risk for violence in schizophrenia, it was noted that schizophrenia alone increased an individual's risk of committing a homicide by a factor of 10, and by adding a comorbid substance use disorder the risk jumped by a factor of 17 (18). It is now accepted that substance abuse or dependence alone are significant risk factors for violence, and it is further accepted that the combination of substance abuse or dependence and mental disorder increases the risk to a considerable degree, likely higher than any one mental disorder standing alone (37–39).

Behavior History
One of the strongest indicators for future violence is a past history of violent behavior (1, 15, 33). Therefore, if someone has been violent in the past, it is important to not

only consider this fact but to also inquire further about the incident, what led to it, and whether it could have been avoided. Furthermore, it is important to inquire about the patient's perceptions of the victim's intentions because such perceptions can sometimes uncover psychotic beliefs.

RISK FACTORS IN SCHIZOPHRENIA

Particular Subtype
The literature suggests that the paranoid subtype of schizophrenia is at greater risk for violent behavior when compared to other diagnostic groups (40). Another study found that a significant majority of individuals with schizophrenia who had acted violently were diagnosed with the paranoid subtype of this disorder (17). It has been postulated that the paranoid subtype of schizophrenia is at increased risk for violence when acutely ill because this subtype retains the cognitive ability to formulate a plan and act while avoiding outside detection (12). Furthermore, clinical experience invites the conclusion that an individual suffering from structured delusions, a common finding in paranoid schizophrenia, would be more likely to act on those beliefs than the person with disorganized delusions. Clearly, the patient who firmly believes that his family is plotting to harm him is more of a concern than the patient who contends that he is able to communicate with animals.

Particular Delusions
Individuals suffering from paranoid schizophrenia are likely a greater potential for violence because their illness is characterized by persecutory delusions. In support of this assumption, the literature suggests that persecutory delusions in particular increase the risk for violence (17, 28, 41–43). Furthermore, individuals afflicted by psychosis are more likely to act on persecutory delusions than any other type of delusion (40, 44–46). One study at a forensic hospital found that the frequency of committing murder was highest in those individuals harboring persecutory delusions (47). Although persecutory delusions are associated with violence, it may not be the delusion standing alone that causes this association. Rather, it appears to be the co-occurrence of persecutory delusions with specific emotional states that increases the overall risk. The literature reports that there is an increased risk for violence when patients experience negative emotions of anxiety, anger, sadness, and fright flowing from their delusions (28, 41, 42, 48–50). What this important finding means is that when a patient is distressed or frightened by their delusion, the patient has adopted the delusion as reality and is no longer able to consider alternative explanations. With this in mind, it becomes obvious that if a patient believes that a particular individual is trying to cause harm, then he or she may devise a plan for a preemptive strike.

As an example, one of the authors evaluated an individual who believed that his father was having him followed and this was a part of a plot to harm him. The individual purchased a weapon, laid in wait, and subsequently shot and killed his father. This individual had never divulged his persecutory delusions or intentions to anyone before the incident. This example highlights several findings noted in the literature, including that paranoid individuals frequently plan their actions, hide their intentions, act in a manner consistent with their delusion, and often target family members (12, 40, 51).

As a part of the risk assessment, it is essential to consider potential victims. A growing body of literature suggests that individuals with schizophrenia often target family members and friends (3, 18, 37). One study noted that between 50% and 60% of victims were family members of the patient, adding that only 12% to 16% of victims were unknown (17). Furthermore, most of the violence occurred in a residence, not a public area (17). If a patient is living with his or her mother, that parent is at particular risk (3, 37). It appears that if a patient is financially dependent, this increases the risk that family members will be targeted (3). The literature also suggests that persons with schizophrenia who start to commit offenses after their illness emerges are more likely to target family members than persons with schizophrenia who begin offending before the onset of their psychosis (11).

Another type of delusion associated with violence is the misidentification syndrome. Capgras is the most common misidentification delusion (52). The patient with Capgras delusion believes that the appearance of an individual remains the same but the identity is altered (53). Patients suffering from Capgras delusion are often paranoid and hostile toward the perceived psychological stranger (52). The literature suggests that such patients are at an increased risk of acting violently toward the perceived stranger (52, 54). One study suggested that the most important finding in judging the patient's response to the Capgras delusion was the degree of threat perceived from the object of the delusion (55). The authors have been involved in several cases of violence stemming from the misidentification delusion syndrome. One case involved a patient who believed that his mother had been replaced by an imposter. He contacted authorities and told them of his suspicions. He later lamented that authorities did nothing to help him. He subsequently armed himself and shot the object of his delusions, though fortunately she was only wounded. He afterwards described the belief that his actual mother was held hostage by the imposter and her life was in peril. This example highlights not only the dangerousness of misidentification delusion syndrome but also that family members are often the victim of persons with a psychotic illness.

Research in this area has uncovered another set of delusions called threat/control-override delusions that can, in certain situations, increase the risk of violence (56). Threat/control-override delusions cause the individual to lose internal control and this enhances the probability of violent behavior. These delusions are well known in psychiatry and include thought insertion and thought control. The seminal research on this issue discovered that a specific set of delusions designated as threat/control-override delusions contributed to an increased rate of violent behavior and illegal acts in those individuals who had been or who were in psychiatric treatment, compared to community residents who had never been in treatment (56, 57). Later studies have also found an association between threat/control-override delusions and potential for violence (41,45). Although some researchers have recently challenged this association, these same researchers caution clinicians not to conclude that delusions never lead to violence (58). This study pointed out that this new data should not replace the long-held opinion that if a patient has acted on delusions in the past, it is likely that a similar course of behavior will take place in the future. What appears to be important in assessing the risk potential of any delusion is whether and to what degree the patient has surrendered to the psychotic belief (50, 56). This means that the psychiatrist should test the tenacity of the patient's delusions, not just the content.

We have some additional insights in this area stemming from our own experience in forensic psychiatry. Even though our insights are anecdotal, some of these insights are supported by the literature. We opine that individuals with schizophrenia are more likely to act on delusions than any other psychotic symptom (59). The literature supports our opinion, and in fact, one study suggested that males with schizophrenia were more likely to engage in violence if their illness followed an exclusively delusional course (17, 60–62). Furthermore, our experience has led us to the opinion that persecutory delusions combined with either delusions of grandiosity or jealousy often significantly increase the risk for violence over any one of these delusions (59). One study that addressed this issue found that the mixture of delusions of persecution and jealousy could spark violent behavior (63). Finally, we have noted that patients with a history of noncompliance with treatment and repeated hospitalizations are at increased risk for violence. Noncompliance with treatment as a risk factor for violence is supported by the literature, in particular if the patient is also using substances (17).

Particular Hallucinations

Clinical wisdom and the literature both support the opinion that certain hallucinations are associated with violent behavior. Similar to delusions, hallucinations that generate negative emotions such as anger, irritability, and sadness, are more likely to cause violent behavior (42). The risk for violence is further increased when hallucinations are related to a delusion (41, 64–66). Another important feature to consider when questioning a patient is whether any command hallucinations are present. Data exist which suggest that certain command hallucinations are followed but apparently only in specific situations and when other factors are present. Research in this area has found that if the command hallucination is recognized, or familiar, and is consistent with the patient's delusions, the risk for complying with the command is increased (7, 65, 66). In addition, research has noted that compliance with hallucinations is higher if the command is harmless and the voice is identifiable (67). Violent commands to harm others are less frequently obeyed than harmless commands and commands to harm self (68). This means that patients who report commands to harm themselves are at greater risk for acting on those commands than directives to harm others. In summary, the data suggest that the risk for acting on a command hallucination to harm others is increased when several factors exist, including delusions consistent with the theme of the hallucination, a familiar voice, and if the voice generates negative emotions.

USING THE RISK FACTORS IN THE RISK ASSESSMENT

Research has demonstrated that actuarial instruments are useful in assessing the risk for recidivism, in particular with sex offenders (69). The actuarial approach utilizes information from the research literature that suggests certain factors are associated with sexual recidivism (8). These instruments are useful as guides to assessing risk in sexual offenders because such instruments force the expert to consider key factors that are correlated with sexual offending. In other words, the instruments serve as an anchor in the risk assessment, which is then further honed by uncovering factors unique to the individual. The final risk assessment is, therefore, an appraisal of both actuarial data and distinct information gathered from the interview. The authors are of the opinion that clinicians should use a similar approach when interviewing a patient with schizophrenia. The clinician should weigh those general factors associated with an increased risk for violence and then develop facts unique to the patient, using those facts to guide the final judgment in this area. By conducting an assessment in this manner, the clinician avoids making judgments based solely on anecdotal experience or "gut" instinct. The final opinion should be presented as a risk assessment, not as a prediction of violence in a particular patient.

To summarize, the authors offer the following factors for consideration in judging risk for violence.

General Factors Associated with an Increased Potential for Violence

Gender:	male, but if the assessment involves a psychiatric patient, be mindful of the finding that males and females may not differ in risk
Age:	late adolescent to early 20s
Substance Use:	current abuse or dependence
Weapons:	owning a weapon
Training:	military, paramilitary, or police experience
Personality:	cluster B features, *DSM-IV-TR* definition (70)
Employment:	unemployed or unstable employment
Education:	high school or less
Family dynamics:	estranged from or complete lack of family support
Housing:	homeless or living alone
Marital:	single
Legal:	criminal record, violent acts in particular
Intelligence:	below average
Organic status:	history of head injuries or present cognitive deficits
Childhood history:	conduct disorder or attention-deficit disorder
Abuse:	history of physical or sexual abuse
Family history:	unstable parenting and/or poor role models
Thoughts:	documented history of violent thoughts from statements or records

Factors in Schizophrenia Associated with an Increased Potential for Violence

Diagnostic subtype:	paranoid schizophrenia
State of illness:	acutely psychotic
Delusions:	persecutory, threat/control-override, and misidentification
Delusional enhancement:	persecutory delusions associated with grandiose and jealous delusions
Target linked to delusions:	risk-enhancing delusions that target a specific person who is readily accessible
Delusional conviction:	risk-enhancing delusions that are accepted without question
Primary symptom:	psychotic illness characterized primarily by risk-enhancing delusions
History of reacting to delusions:	patient has a history of acting on risk-enhancing delusions
Negative emotions and delusions:	delusions that cause fear, sadness, or anxiety
History of illness:	repeated hospitalizations beginning at an early age
Insight:	lack of insight and noncompliance with treatment
Psychotic enhancement:	hallucinations that buttress risk-enhancing delusions
Type of hallucinations:	command hallucinations to harm self or others
Type of voice associated with the hallucination:	familiar voice
History of reacting to hallucinations:	patient has a history of acting on hallucinations

Hallucinatory conviction:	hallucinations that are firmly accepted as real and the content is generally believed
Negative emotions and hallucinations:	hallucinations that cause fear, sadness, or anxiety
Target linked to hallucinations	Hallucinations that target a specific person who is readily accessible
Living circumstances and financial dependency:	Living with family, in particular mother, and dependent

CASE STUDY

The following vignette highlights many of the risk factors that have been discussed. In a murder case, one of the authors was retained to evaluate an individual's mental state at the time of the charged offense. The individual had a history of psychosis and was already diagnosed with paranoid schizophrenia. The police report indicated that the individual was charged with killing a family member with a weapon at that family member's residence. The evaluation revealed that the individual was genetically loaded for schizophrenia in that a parent suffered from that disorder. Furthermore, despite above-average intelligence, the individual did not complete high school. The individual had used illicit substances but had ceased drug use many years before the offense. The individual's childhood did not uncover evidence of problems with behavior or attention. In addition, the individual's legal history as an adult found one prior arrest for a minor offense. The individual was primarily living with family around the time of the allegations due to psychiatric issues and unemployment. The individual claimed a history of sexual abuse, but the description of this abuse suggested it was delusional. The individual was single, having gone through a divorce as a young adult. The individual had developed paranoid schizophrenia several years before the charged offense, requiring hospitalizations for bizarre behavior. Interestingly, one of the individual's treatment providers documented that the patient had become adept at hiding his symptoms from mental health professionals and family. Months prior to the offense, the individual was noncompliant with treatment.

The facts that led up to the homicide included that the individual had secured a weapon for protection. Furthermore, the individual had developed persecutory and religious delusions about the victim, believing that the victim was endowed with supernatural powers. The individual had argued with the victim before the murder, demanding a religious cure from the victim. The individual was experiencing hallucinations, some of which he blamed on the victim, asserting that the victim had this ability because of the victim's religious powers. In the days leading up to the incident, the individual was increasingly fearful of the victim, a fear that flowed from the individual's persecutory delusions about the victim. Furthermore, just prior to the homicide, the individual told a witness about a command hallucination to kill. On the night of the offense, the individual confronted the victim at the victim's residence and then shot and killed the victim. The individual later explained that the victim was using supernatural powers of a religious nature to cause harm so a preemptive strike was necessary. The individual was evaluated after the incident by multiple experts, all of whom agreed that the homicide flowed from delusions caused by paranoid schizophrenia. The individual was subsequently found not guilty by reason of mental disease.

Final Thought

The authors have been involved in evaluating or treating many individuals who have committed serious acts because of their mental disorder. The authors have repeatedly noted that in the majority of these cases there were clear, at times stark, warning signs of a growing threat of violence. All too often, these warning signs were ignored or explained away. It is a shocking truth that if the same individual had complained of chest pain, or blood in their urine, or any other serious physical symptom, no one would have allowed that individual to forego an initial exam. We, therefore, recommend that psychiatrists educate family members about the factors that suggest an increased risk for violence, stress the seriousness of such factors, and provide information about available community resources in psychiatric emergencies.

REFERENCES

1. Walsh E, Buchanan A, Fahy T. Violence and schizophrenia: examining the evidence. Br J Psychiatry 2001; 180: 490–5.
2. Silver H, Goodman C, Knoll G et al. Schizophrenia Patients with a History of Severe Violence Differ From Nonviolent Schizophrenia Patients in Perception of Emotions but Not Cognitive Function. J Clin Psychiatry 2005; 66(3): 300–8.
3. Nordstrom A, Kullgren G. Do Violent Offenders With Schizophrenia Who Attack Family Members Differ From Those With Other Victims? Int J Forensic Ment Health 2003; 2(2): 195–200.
4. Soyka M, Graz C, Bottlender P et al. Clinical correlates of later violence and criminal offences in schizophrenia. Schizophr Res 2007; 94: 89–98.
5. Monahan J. The prediction of violent behavior: toward a second generation of theory and policy. Am J Psychiatry 1984; 141(1): 10–5.
6. Resnick P. Violence Risk Assessment. Forensic Psychiatry Review Course, American Academy of Psychiatry and the Law, New Orleans, LA, Oct 1998: 19–21.
7. Bjorkly S. Psychotic symptoms and violence toward others – a literature review of some preliminary findings, Part 2 Hallucinations. Aggression and Violent Behavior 2002; 7: 605–15.
8. Hanson R, Bussiere M. Predicting relapse: a meta-analysis of sexual offender recidivism studies. J Consult Clin Psychol 1998; 66(2): 348–62.
9. Tarasoff vs. Regents of the University of California. 551 P.2d 334, 1976.
10. Keeton W, Dobbs D, Keeton R et al. Negligence: Standard of Conduct. In: Prosser and Keeton on the Law of Torts, 5th ed., Keeton W, ed. Hornbook Series, Westlaw, the West Publishing Co., St. Paul, MN, 1984: 235–62.
11. Laajasalo T, Hakkanen H. Offence and offender characteristics among two groups of Finnish homicide offenders with schizophrenia: Comparison of early- and late-start offenders. J Forensic Psychiatry and Psychol 2005; 16(1): 41–59.
12. Pontius A. Violence in schizophrenia versus limbic psychotic trigger reaction: Prefrontal aspects of volitional action. Aggress Violent Behav 2004; 9: 503–21.
13. Swanson J, Holzer C, Ganju V et al. Violence and psychiatric disorder in the community: evidence from the epidemiological catchment area surveys. Hosp Community Psychiatry 1990; 41: 761–70.
14. Swanson J, Swartz M, Van Dorn R et al. A national study of violent behavior in persons with schizophrenia. Arch of Gen Psychiatry 2006; 63: 490–9.
15. Meehan J, Flynn S, Hunt I et al. Perpetrators of Homicide with Schizophrenia: A National Clinical Survey in England and Wales. Psychiatr Serv 2006; 57(11): 1648–51.
16. Shaw J, Hunt I, Flynn S et al. Rates of mental disorder in people convicted of homicide. Br J Psychiatry 2006; 188: 143–7.
17. Joyal C, Putkonen A, Paavola P et al. Characteristics and circumstances of homicidal acts committed by offenders with schizophrenia. Psychol Med 2004; 34: 433–42.

18. McNamara N, Findling R. Guns, Adolescents, and Mental Illness. Am J Psychiatry 2008; 165(2): 190–4.
19. Borum R, Swartz M, Swanson J. Assessing and managing violence risk in clinical practice. J Pract Psychiatry Behav Health 1996; 2(4): 205–15.
20. Pearson M, Wilmot E, Padi M. A study of violent behavior among inpatients in psychiatric hospitals. Br J Psychiatry 1986; 149: 232–5.
21. Tardiff K, Sweillman A. Assault, suicide, and mental illness. Arch Gen Psychiatry 1980; 37: 164–9.
22. Quinsey V, MacGuire A. Maximum security psychiatric patients: actuarial and clinical prediction of dangerousness. J Interpersonal Violence 1986; 1: 143–71.
23. Martell D, Rosner R, Harman R. Base-rate estimates of criminal behavior by homeless mentally ill persons in New York City. Psychiatr Serv 1994; 46(6): 596–601.
24. Reid W, Balis G. Evaluation of the violent patient. In: Hales R, Frances A, eds. American Psychiatric Association Annual Review, 1987: 491–509.
25. Widiger T, Trull T. Personality Disorders and Violence. In: Monahan J, Steadman H, eds. Violence and Mental Disorder: Developments in Risk Assessment. Chicago: University of Chicago Press, 1994: 203–26.
26. Williamson S, Hare R, Wong S. Violence: criminal psychopaths and their victims. Can J Behav Sci 1987; 19: 454–62.
27. Moffit T. Adolescence limited and life-course persistent antisocial behavior: A developmental taxonomy. Psychol Rev 1993; 100: 674–701.
28. Vandamme M, Nandrino J. Temperament and Character Inventory in Homicidal, Nonaddicted Paranoid Schizophrenic Patients: A Preliminary Study. Psycholo Rep 2004; 95: 393–406.
29. Yesavage J, Brizer D. Clinical and historical correlates of dangerous inpatient behavior. In: Brizer D, Crowner M, eds. Current Approaches to the Prediction of Violence. Washington, DC: American Psychiatric Press, 1989.
30. Carmen E, Reiker P, Mills T. Victims of violence and psychiatric illness. Am J Psychiatry 1984; 141: 378–9.
31. Manuzza S, Klein R, Konig P et al. Hyperactive boys almost grown up. IV. Criminality and its relationship to psychiatric status. Arch Gen Psychiatry 1989; 46: 1073–9.
32. Convit A, Jaeger J, Lin S et al. Predicting assaultiveness in psychiatric inpatients: a pilot study. Hosp Commun Psychiatry 1988; 39: 429–34.
33. Klassen D, O'Connor W. A prospective study of predictors of violence in adult male mental health admissions. Law Hum Behav 1988; 12: 143–58.
34. Hellman D, Blackman N. Enuresis, firesetting, and cruelty to animals: a triad predictive of adult crime. Am J Psychiatry 1966; 122: 1431–5.
35. Felthous A, Kellert S. Childhood cruelty to animals and later aggression against people: a review. Am J Psychiatry 1987; 144: 710–7.
36. Swanson J. Mental disorder, substance abuse, and community violence: an epidemiological approach. In: Monahan J, Steadman H, eds. Violence and Mental Disorder: Developments in Risk Assessment. Chicago: University of Chicago Press, 1994: 101–36.
37. Nordstrom A, Dahlgren L, Kullgren G. Victim relations and factors triggering homicides committed by offenders with schizophrenia. J Forensic Psychiatr and Psychol 2006; 17(2): 192–203.
38. Schwartz R, Reynolds C, Austin J et al. Homicidality in Schizophrenia: A Replication Study. Am J Orthopsychiatry 2003; 73(1): 74–7.
39. Pulay A, Dawson D, Hasin D et al. Violent Behavior and DSM-IV Psychiatric Disorders: Results from the National Epidemiologic Survey on Alcohol and Related Conditions. J Clin Psychiatry 2008; 69(1): 12–22.
40. Krawkowski M, Volavaka J, Brizer D. Psychopathology and violence: a review of the literature. Compr Psychiatry 1985; 27(2): 131–48.
41. Bjorkly S. Psychotic symptoms and violence toward others – a literature review of some preliminary findings, Part 1 Delusions. Aggress Violent Behav 2002; 7: 617–31.

42. Cheung P, Schweitzer I, Crowley K et al. Violence in schizophrenia: role of hallucinations and delusions. Schizophr Res 1997; 26: 181–90.
43. Swanson J, Swartz M, Van Dorn R et al. A National Study of Violent Behavior in Persons With Schizophrenia. Arch Gen Psychiatry 2006; 63: 490–9.
44. Junginger J. Psychosis and violence: the case for a content analysis of psychotic experience. Schizophr Bull 1996; 22(1): 91–03.
45. Link B, Stueve A, Phelan J. Psychotic symptoms and violent behaviors: probing the components of "threat/control override" symptoms. Soc Psychiatry Psychiatr Epidemiol 1998; 33: S55–S60.
46. Wessely S, Buchanan A, Reed A et al. Acting on Delusions. I. Prevalence. Br J Psychiatry 1993; 163: 69–76.
47. Benezech M, Bourgeois M, Yesavage J. Violence in the mentally ill: a study of 547 patients at a French hospital for the criminally insane. J Nerv Ment Dis 1980; 168: 698–700.
48. Appelbaum P, Robbins P, Roth L. Dimensional approach to delusions: comparison across types and diagnoses. Am J Psychiatry 1999; 156(12): 1938–43.
49. Buchanan A, Reed A, Wessely S et al. Acting on Delusions. II. The phenomenological correlates of acting on delusions. Br J Psychiatry 1993; 163: 77–81.
50. Taylor P, Garety P, Buchanan A et al. Delusions and violence. In: Monahan J, Steadman H, eds. Violence and Mental Disorder: Developments in Risk Assessment. Chicago: University of Chicago Press, 1994: 161–82.
51. Addad M, Benezech M, Bourgeois M et al. Criminal acts among schizophrenics in French mental hospitals. J Nerv Ment Dis 1981; 169: 289–93.
52. Silva J, Leong G, Weinstock R. The dangerousness of persons with misidentification syndromes. Bull Am Acad Psychiatry Law 1992; 20(1): 77–86.
53. Silva J, Leong G, Shaner A. A classification system for misidentification syndromes. Psychopathol 1990; 23: 27–32.
54. Nestor P, Haycock J, Doiron S et al. Lethal violence and psychosis. A clinical profile. Bull Am Acad Psychiatry Law 1995; 23(3): 331–41.
55. Aziz M, Razik G, Donn J. Dangerousness and Management of Delusional Misidentification Syndrome. Psychopathol 2005; 38: 97–102.
56. Link B, Stueve A. Psychotic symptoms and the violent/illegal behavior of mental patients compared to community controls. In: Monahan J, Steadman H, eds. Violence and Mental Disorder: Developments in Risk Assessment. Chicago: University of Chicago Press, 1994: 137–59.
57. Link B, Andrews H, Cullen F. The violent and illegal behavior of mental patients reconsidered. Am Sociol Rev 1992; 57: 275–92.
58. Appelbaum P, Robbins P, Monahan J. Violence and delusions. Data from the MacArthur Violence Risk Assessment Study. Am J Psychiatry 2000; 157(4): 566–72.
59. Rabun J, Boyer S. Violence and Forensic Issues in Schizophrenia. In: Csernansky J, ed. Schizophrenia, A New Guide for Clinicians. New York: Marcel Dekker, Inc., 2002: 247–65.
60. Taylor P. Motives for offending among violent and psychotic men. Br J Psychiatry 1985; 147: 491–8.
61. Martell D, Dietz P. Mentally disordered offenders who push or attempt to push victims onto subway tracks in New York City. Arch Gen Psychiatry 1992; 49: 472–5.
62. Robertson G, Taylor P. The presence of delusions and violence among remanded male prisoners with schizophrenia. In: Gunn J, Taylor P, eds. Forensic Psychiatry: Clinical, Ethical and Legal Issues. Oxford: Heinemann-Butterworth, 1993: 338–9.
63. Silva J, Ferrari M, Leong G et al. The dangerousness of persons with delusional jealousy. J Am Acad Psychiatry Law 1998; 26(4): 607–23.
64. Junginger J. Predicting compliance with command hallucinations. Am J Psychiatry 1990; 147: 245–7.
65. Braham L, Trower P, Birchwood M. Acting on command hallucinations and dangerous behavior: A critique of the major findings in the last decade. Clin Psychol Rev 2004; 24: 513–28.

66. McNiel D, Eisner J, Binder R. The Relationship Between Command Hallucinations and Violence.Psychiatr Serv 2000; 51(10): 1288–92.
67. Junginger J. Command hallucinations and the prediction of dangerousness. Psychiatr Serv 1995; 46(9): 911–4.
68. Kasper M, Rogers R, Adams P. Dangerousness and command hallucinations: an investigation of psychotic inpatients. Bull Am Acad Psychiatry Law 1996; 24: 219–24.
69. Hanson R, Thornton D. Improving risk assessments for sex offenders: a comparison of three actuarial scales. Law Hum Behav 2000; 24(1): 57–66.
70. American Psychiatric Association. The Diagnostic and Statistical Manual of Mental Disorders. 4th edition, text revision. Washington, DC: American Psychiatric Press; 2000.

28 Economic evaluation and schizophrenia

Martin Knapp and Denise Razzouk

1. THE RELEVANCE OF ECONOMICS

The underlying challenge that stimulates a need for economic insights is scarcity: there are not enough resources to meet all needs, and there never will be. Scarcity is the reason why difficult choices have to be made between alternative uses of a skilled professional's time, in-patient beds in a hospital, or the pharmacy budget for medications. Economic evaluation aims to provide evidence that can inform decisions about how to allocate these scarce resources. It does so by building on a theoretically sound platform to provide a comprehensive measure of the resources employed (usually measured by their costs) in comparison to what those resources achieve (usually measured in terms of better health, functioning and quality of life) for two or more treatment or policy options.

The primary aim of a health system is to alleviate symptoms and so improve personal and social functioning, and quality of life. But pursuit of such a laudable, widely accepted objective cannot proceed without regard for the economic consequences of the therapies, support arrangements or broad policy strategies put in place. Consequently, money is never far from the surface in policy and practice discussions. For example, the psychiatrist prescribing a course of antipsychotic medications might not have to be concerned about the associated costs at the point of taking the treatment decision (although increasingly in many health systems they *will* be aware of them). However, there will always be someone further along the management chain who *does* have to watch expenditure levels and to balance the annual budget.

In other words, decision-makers in mental health systems have to be aware of not just effectiveness in responding to needs but also cost-effectiveness in the use of resources. This awareness generates demands for economic evidence, including: information on the overall cost of an illness such as schizophrenia; the association between what is spent on (say) a new treatment and what is saved later because patients use fewer health care or other resources (the *cost-offset* association); and the link between what is spent and what is achieved (*cost-effectiveness*). The last of these is the most important, and is the focus of this chapter.

Section 2 describes the costs of schizophrenia and its treatment, and provides an example of cost-offset arguments, illustrated by early intervention services for psychosis. Section 3 sets out how cost-effectiveness analyses are undertaken, identifying the different approaches to outcome measurement employed by health economists in order to address various policy and practice questions. Section 4 illustrates the application of these approaches in some recent evaluations, and Section 5 outlines the main challenges in carrying out cost-effectiveness studies. A final concluding section brings the chapter to a close.

2. COSTS
2.1 Cost range
A chronic, debilitating condition such as schizophrenia will have wide-ranging economic impacts, most obviously sizable health care costs. The impact of schizophrenia is typically estimated to be 1.5% to 3% of total national spending on health care (1). But there can also be high costs elsewhere, particularly to social care, housing, and criminal justice agencies. On top of these service-related impacts are various 'indirect' costs to patients, families and the wider society, including out-of-pocket payments by patients and families for medications, treatment services or transport, as well as lost income (for the individual) and lost productivity (for the economy) resulting from unemployment and disrupted employment. The employment impact is especially important: only around one-fifth of people with schizophrenia can find paid work (2). Lack of social support, low educational attainment, limited availability of jobs, employers' negative attitudes about people with mental health problems, and self-stigmatising behaviour can each contribute to employment difficulties. A recent UK study illustrates the overall impact: total societal cost of schizophrenia of £6.7 billion in 2004/05, spread widely (3).

Decision-makers need to be aware of this breadth of cost impacts, spreading well beyond the health system as conventionally defined. Because a mental illness such as schizophrenia can have consequences across a number of life domains and for so many years, the quality of life and economic impacts should usually be seen in this broader and longer-term context. For certain purposes it makes sense to focus on particular costs (such as the acquisition cost for medications or the total health spend on schizophrenia), but these elements are likely to be just a small part of the overall picture. Indeed, there could well be strong justification for higher spending on treatment and other health care support because of savings and outcomes elsewhere. Similarly, decision making will inevitably focus on the immediate impacts of an illness and its treatment, but the longer-term impacts do need to be borne in mind when taking decisions that affect the life course. We come back to these issues later in the chapter.

2.2 Cost drivers
Some events in the lives of people with schizophrenia and the responses they stimulate from health and other systems are particularly influential in driving the costs. These include: relapse; inpatient services; specialist community accommodation; medication; mortality; lost employment; family impact; public safety and concern (4). The most important of these when thinking about treatment planning is relapse, while the largest of these in terms of spending is inpatient care.

Relapse is enormously distressing to patients and their families. The exacerbation or onset of debilitating symptoms requires urgent responses from specialist professionals and services. Across most health care systems, the most common response to relapse—just as it is to an initial episode of psychosis—is admission to an inpatient setting. The subsequent length of stay will obviously depend on the course taken by the illness, and personal circumstances will also have a considerable influence. Almond et al. (5) compared costs, clinical outcomes and quality of life for a group of schizophrenia patients in England who experienced relapse with another group of patient who did not. Over a 6-month period, costs for the patients who relapsed were more than four times greater than costs for the nonrelapse group.

2.3 Cost-offset comparisons: early intervention

A question that governments, insurance funds, and strategic decision-makers usually want answered is whether expenditure on a treatment or policy initiative will partly or wholly 'pay for itself' by reducing future expenditure. For example, would the use of a new medication, which costs more to purchase than medications currently in use, improve patient health sufficiently to reduce inpatient admissions and hence costs?

Unidentified or untreated psychosis can have a number of adverse consequences, including poor educational attainment, school difficulties more generally, employment problems, deliberate self-harm and suicide, violent behaviour and homicide (6–10). In principle, therefore, it might be expected that early detection and treatment of psychosis would help avoid many of these negative impacts. There could be economic benefits as a result, for example from reduced use of inpatient services.

Ten years ago, Mihalopoulos et al. (11) addressed the question of whether the initial investment in an early detection or early intervention service would generate savings that would outweigh the set-up costs. They reported evidence on the costs and effectiveness of the phase-specific community-orientated treatment of early onset psychosis (EPPIC) approach in Melbourne, Australia. EPPIC consisted of an early psychosis assessment team, inpatient unit, outpatient case management, day programme and smaller therapeutic programmes. A simple before-after design compared 51 EPPIC patients treated between 1993 and 1994 with 51 matched retrospective controls who received the pre-EPPIC treatment model between 1989 and 1992. Costs were measured so as to cover inpatient stays, outpatient appointments, medication, community mental health team contacts, general practitioner contacts and private therapy and psychiatry. These costs were lower for the EPPIC patients than the pre-EPPIC patients: in particular, reductions in inpatient costs outweighed increases in community services.

3. COST-EFFECTIVENESS METHODS
3.1 The key questions

Knowing the costs associated with treating and supporting people with schizophrenia helps decision-makers to gauge the overall societal impact. Knowing whether financial savings might flow from current treatment expenditure could also help those same decision-makers if they are considering whether to invest in a preventive or early intervention programme. But these bodies of evidence only look at costs, and so are not providing the decision-maker with information about how to make *better* or *best* use of available resources. Costs need to be examined alongside outcomes for this purpose.

Consider what happens following the introduction of a new treatment (say a new medication). Decision-makers first want an answer to the *clinical* question: is the medication effective in alleviating psychotic symptoms and generally improving health and quality of life, while avoiding unpleasant side-effects? Looking at two or more different drugs, which has the better outcomes and/or the less harmful side-effects? If the answer to the clinical question is that the new medication is no better than treatments currently in use, then there is usually no need to ponder its use any further, since neither psychiatrists nor patients will be attracted to such a treatment. But if the new medication looks clinically effective, the decision-maker will then want an answer to the cost-effectiveness question. Does the new medication achieve the improved clinical and other outcomes at a cost that is worth paying? Cost-effectiveness analysis therefore does what it says: it looks at *both* costs and effectiveness (outcomes).

It asks whether improved outcomes are *worth* the extra cost. Deciding what outcome is or is not 'worth' the cost is far from straightforward, as discussed below, but is the very crux of an economic evaluation.

There are different variants of cost-effectiveness analysis. They share a common approach to the conceptualisation, definition and measurement of costs, but they differ in the approaches employed to measure outcomes. The principal reason for looking at different outcomes is in order to address slightly different questions (see below). However, although the choice of evaluation question influences the type of analysis needed, the choices are operationally not mutually exclusive in that a single study could support more than one type of analysis. A body of evidence which is well located within the clinical domain will be exactly what the treating professional or the local formulary committee needs but may not be sufficient for a higher level decision-making body, such as a health ministry. The broader the research question, the more demanding are the data needs.

3.2 Cost measurement

Before costs can be calculated in an economic evaluation, all relevant services used by patients must be identified. Once a list of likely services has been drawn up, there are a number of methods available to record each patient's use of them, including questionnaires, diaries or case files. The first of these—employing a service-use questionnaire—is the most common in trials, with information gathered from patients, relatives and/or treatment staff through face-to-face or telephone interviews, or (sometimes) through postal survey. One example of a service-use questionnaire is the Client Service Receipt Inventory (CSRI), which includes sections on accommodation, employment, income, service receipt, informal support and satisfaction with services (12). The CSRI has been adapted for use in many studies across many countries (13).

The accuracy of questionnaire-based information is dependent on the accuracy of recall of interviewees. Service-use diaries could potentially improve recall: patients or family members record service use prospectively over the period of a study. However, they place a greater burden on patients, and often are not completed or returned (14). Another option is to draw information directly from case notes, but this can be time-consuming unless full data are recorded electronically, and has the additional disadvantage that the data will usually be limited to the services provided by the agency keeping the case files. Given that many people with schizophrenia have multiple needs and hence service contacts across a number of agencies, it would be necessary to look at potentially many agencies' case files. These data on service use then need to be multiplied by unit costs (e.g., cost per in-patient day or per therapy hour), calculated from expenditure and workload data (15), or drawn from previous research. In England, an annual compendium of previous unit cost calculations is widely used (16).

3.3 Opportunity costs

Costs are not exactly synonymous with money expended, for they should also cover opportunities lost. The best example is time given up by family members in supporting a relative with schizophrenia. No money may change hands, but the family member has given up time that could have been spent in employment or leisure activities which generally will have some value. Evaluations should therefore be cognisant of the opportunities lost by individuals in providing care and support, and include these in the evaluation. When set alongside other (expenditure) costs, the opportunity costs of unpaid care can often be substantial.

3.4 Evaluation perspective

An early decision has to be taken on study perspective. Is the evaluation needed to help resource allocation within a particular agency (such as a psychiatric clinic), or a particular service system (such as the health care system), or across the whole of government, or for society as a whole? The breadth of perspective will determine the breadth of cost and outcome measurement. Thus, a study undertaken from a health system perspective would only look at health system costs and would measure outcomes in perhaps quite narrow health terms. (An even narrower perspective would look only at medication acquisition costs and psychotic symptoms. These acquisition costs are clearly important to a chief pharmacist having to keep within their budget, but in fact the relative prices of medications can be misleading. We return to this in section 4.4 when describing the appraisal by the National Institute for Health and Clinical Excellence in England.) In contrast, a study undertaken from a societal perspective would include costs to all service-providing agencies as well the opportunity costs to family carers and of lost productivity.

3.5 Effectiveness measurement

The choice between different types of health economic evaluation depends on the treatment or policy question being addressed (17). If the question is essentially clinical—what is the most appropriate treatment for someone with schizophrenia in particular circumstances, and whether to opt for one therapeutic strategy over another—then information is needed on the comparative costs of the different therapies and the comparative outcomes measured in terms relevant to the clinical decision (probably relapse rate, symptom alleviation, personal and social functioning, and quality of life). A standard *cost-effectiveness analysis* would then be appropriate and sufficient. Cost-effectiveness analysis (CEA) is the most intuitive mode of economic evaluation, and aims to help decision makers choose between alternative interventions for a *specific* patient group, such as people with a particular pattern of symptoms.

A CEA would look at a single outcome dimension—such as change in symptoms—and would then compute and compare the ratio of the difference in costs between two treatments to the difference in (primary) outcome (called the incremental cost-effectiveness ratio). For example, the CATIE (Clinical Antipsychotic Trials of Intervention Effectiveness) study looked (in turn) at improvements in positive and negative syndrome scale (PANSS) scores and neurocognitive performance, and at total health care costs (18; see below).

An obvious weakness with the strict cost-effectiveness methodology is the focus on a single outcome dimension (in order to compute ratios) when many people with schizophrenia often have multiple needs and when most psychiatrists would be aiming to achieve improvements in a number of them. Cost-effectiveness ratios are therefore sometimes computed for each of a number of outcome measures in turn (as in CATIE). This has the advantage of breadth but poses a challenge if two or more ratios point to different interventions as the more cost-effective: i.e. using one outcomes measure, treatment A might look more cost-effective than treatment B, but using another outcome the ranking of treatments could be the other way around (B looks more cost-effective than A).

3.6 Utility measurement

If, to take a broader stance, the question addressed in an evaluation is whether to invest available resources to treat either schizophrenia or asthma, then decision makers again need to know the relative costs of the alternatives, but they now need a different measure of effectiveness. They need something that has relevance and validity for both schizophrenia and asthma. The most commonly such employed measure is 'utility', generated from health-related quality of life scales.

A *cost-utility analysis* (CUA), as this form of evaluation is sometimes called, measures the impact of an intervention in terms of improvements in a unidimensional, preference-weighted, health-related quality of life measure. This utility measure is usually calculated from the combination of mortality and quality of life effects; societal weightings of different health states are generally recommended. The best known utility index is the Quality-Adjusted Life Year (QALY). One problem is that the utility measure may be seen as too reductionist (19). In particular, there are worries that the available generic utility-generating instruments, the best known being the EQ-5D or EuroQol (20), are insufficiently sensitive to the typical changes in symptoms and functioning observed for people with schizophrenia. A better measure has been developed from the widely used PANSS (21).

3.7 Benefit measurement
The broadest kind of question addressed by an economic evaluation asks whether it is better to invest more money in the health system or more money in (say) improving transport. The evaluation thus needs data that allow comparison of costs and outcomes across these broad investment options, and 'outcome' now needs to be measured so as to be broadly relevant. The usual choice of broad 'outcome' measure is monetary. A *cost-benefit analysis* (CBA) has the merit of examining whether the benefits of a treatment or policy exceed the costs. With two or more alternative treatments or policies, the one with the greatest excess of benefits over costs would be seen as the more efficient. Comparing costs incurred with costs saved later is not a cost-benefit analysis, but a cost-offset comparison of the kind described earlier. A cost-benefit analysis *must* measure outcomes (in terms of improved health or improved quality of life, for example) and convert them to monetary values.

The practical challenge of conducting a CBA is that it is hard to compute the monetary value of something as nebulous as a health improvement. Approaches have been developed for this purpose—seeking to obtain direct valuations of health outcomes by patients, relatives or the general public (called 'willingness-to-pay' estimates) or using discrete choice experiments to get indirect valuations (17)—but they are difficult to do well.

3.8 Making trade-offs
Many evaluations of new interventions find them to be both more effective (the outcome profiles are better than for old or current interventions) but simultaneously more expensive. The approach employed to reveal the trade-off between the better outcomes and the higher expenditure necessary to achieve them is to plot a cost-effectiveness acceptability curve (CEAC) (22). This curve shows the likelihood of one treatment being seen as cost-effective relative to another given different (implicit, prespecified monetary) values placed on incremental outcome improvements.

4. COST-EFFECTIVENESS EVIDENCE
There are now quite a number of completed economic evaluations of treatments for schizophrenia, although many have some limitations in terms of the methods

employed or the ways that they were implemented. This is not the place to attempt a comprehensive review of the literature (see, for example (23–25)). Instead we focus on three recent economic evaluations.

4.1 The CATIE study

The government-funded, North American multicentre CATIE study examined the comparative effectiveness and cost-effectiveness of four second-generation antipsychotics (olanzapine, risperidone, quetiapine, ziprasidone) and one first-generation (perphenazine) antipsychotic (18, 26). In this trial, 1,493 schizophrenia patients recruited from many sites across the US were randomly assigned to a medication and assessed over an 18-month follow-up. The main outcome measures were: discontinuation of treatment (primary outcome), overall symptoms, side-effects, quality of life, psychosocial functioning, neurocognitive performance. QALYs were the main outcome for the cost-effectiveness analysis, built on PANSS scores (21). The study perspective was the health system, and so only health care costs were measured.

There was an improvement on PANSS scores, neurocognitive performance and QALYs for all medication groups over the 18-month period, but no significant differences between them. Average health care costs were 20–30% lower for the perphenazine group than for patients given second-generation antipsychotics, due entirely to lower drug costs. This led to the conclusion that perphenazine was more cost-effective than second-generation antipsychotics (18).

Given its importance and scale, and indeed its conclusions, the CATIE trial has attracted much attention (27–30). The trial team themselves caution against generalisation to excluded patient groups (those who are first episode, elderly, learning disabled, refractory, long-term institutionalised, noncompliant and some others) and beyond 18 months. They also noted the high sample attrition rate. However, in a later paper they argued that their results were robust to a number of limitations (31). Attention has particularly focused on three areas. The exclusion of patients with existing tardive dyskinesia from receiving perphenazine may have biased the effectiveness and hence cost-effectiveness findings in favour of the first-generation medication. The 18-month follow-up may have been too short to observe the effects of any long-term differential development of side-effects, although this duration is longer than most trials. Third, high rates of discontinuation and the intent-to-treat design complicate the interpretation of medication effects and their economic consequences. The CATIE study was also not powered to be able to detect meaningful differences in costs, something that occurs quite often when cost-effectiveness evaluations are 'piggy-backed' onto clinical trials.

4.2 The CUtLASS study

The Cost Utility of the Latest Antipsychotic Drugs in Schizophrenia Study (CUtLASS) was designed to verify whether second-generation antipsychotics are more cost-effective than first-generation antipsychotics for treating patients with schizophrenia, schizoaffective or delusion disorders in the UK. A pragmatic randomised trial assessed quality of life as primary outcome over 12 months, having recruited 227 patients. A wide range of medications were used to treat these patients. No differences in quality of life were observed between them, and health service costs were similar (32). The cost-effectiveness analysis concluded that first-generation medications may be cost-saving and generate better QALY gains than second-generation medications (33).

Concerns about CUtLASS have focussed on the small sample and limited statistical power (particularly in relation to the economic hypotheses), the measurement of only health care costs (although this is a very common limitation across all schizophrenia trials), and the aggregation of medications into 'classes' when there are likely to be marked differences in response and cost *within* each such group.

4.3 The SOHO study

The European Schizophrenia Outpatient Health Outcomes (SOHO) study sought to determine the effectiveness and cost-effectiveness of treating schizophrenia patients with olanzapine (manufactured by Lilly, which funded the study) compared with other antipsychotics (34–36). Using a 3-year, prospective, outpatient, observational design, 10,972 patients were enrolled at baseline study across ten European countries; 80% of these individuals were eligible for analyses at 12 months (the time period for the economic evaluation). Outcome measures included functioning, clinical global impression of symptoms, tolerability of medication, and health-related quality of life. Health care resource use (covering only the main services) and QALYs generated from the EQ-5D data generated the cost-effectiveness results, based on data collected at baseline, 3, 6 and 12 months. Multivariate regression analyses were used to estimate the incremental cost and utility gains, after adjusting for patients' baseline characteristics. If a funding threshold of £30,000 per QALY gained is assumed—which is used by the National Institute for Health and Clinical Excellence in England for the purposes of making trade-offs—olanzapine was found to have a high probability of being the most cost-effective treatment compared with other antipsychotic treatments.

The observational design was both strength and limitation. RCTs (randomised controlled trials) have high internal validity and remain the 'design of choice' for addressing many clinical questions. But they often abstract too much from everyday practice and do not easily allow generalisation. The SOHO design permitted much more flexibility in drug dosage, switching and combinations, and the careful statistical analyses revealed interesting associations between a range of patient characteristics, outcomes and costs. The analyses also allowed examination of the outcome and cost consequences of switching medications. On the other hand, costs were more narrowly measured than in either CATIE or CUtLASS, and outcomes measured less comprehensively.

4.4 NICE clinical guidelines

The National Institute for Health and Clinical Excellence in England (NICE) is, as its website explains, 'an independent organization responsible for providing national guidance on promoting good health and preventing and treating ill health'. Its most recent clinical guidelines for schizophrenia were issued in 2009 (38), based on probably the most thorough health technology appraisal ever undertaken of the various therapeutic options in this clinical area. The full report is an encyclopaedic source of summary evidence.

In order to pull together evidence from a wide range of trials and other sources, the schizophrenia appraisal used meta-analytic techniques and decision analytic modelling. This latter is an approach that aims to simulate the treatment pathways and associated 'events' (such as relapse and treatment discontinuation) and their consequences for costs and outcomes. Each of a number of different treatments can be simulated in this way, and comparisons made between them. The perspective for the cost-effectiveness modelling was the health and social care system in England, although patients' (modest) out-of-pocket costs were also included. The model took explicit account of relapse (which, as noted earlier, is such an important cost driver in schizophrenia), discontinuation of treatment, side effects, complications related to diabetes and mortality.

The central finding of this extensive analysis was that the antipsychotics did not clearly separate from each other in terms of their cost-effectiveness, mainly because of the high level of uncertainty in the available clinical data. Zotepine appeared to be the most cost-effective in the English and Welsh context, followed by olanzapine and paliperidone ER. Relapse prevention was particularly influential in determining cost-effectiveness; side-effects were not. Nor did drug acquisition costs exert much influence. Another finding was that the choice of time horizon for the analysis—over what period were costs and outcomes measured and compared—did make a difference to the result.

As with any study, the technology appraisal commissioned by NICE has its limitations. It adopts a relatively narrow perspective, and uses modelling to pool data from a range of studies and countries. Only randomised controlled trial evidence was used, which begs questions about external validity (see above). Lack of data meant that quetiapine was excluded from the analysis. On the other hand, the comprehensive, very thorough and independent reviewing and analyses of data by the NICE appraisal team ensure that their conclusions warrant considerable attention.

5. CHALLENGES WITH COST-EFFECTIVENESS STUDIES

Compared to a decade ago, there is now not only considerably more but also better cost-effectiveness on treatments for schizophrenia. But the completed studies have some limitations, similar to the challenges that face most economic evaluations in the mental health field.

5.1 Purpose and target

Evaluations are undertaken for a variety of purposes: to inform treatment decisions, support purchasing decisions by formulary committees, for policy monitoring, or for marketing. An evaluation carried out for one purpose may not provide useful evidence for other purposes. Consequently, evidence generated (say) by a pharmaceutical company in support of their marketing might not be very helpful for a national body considering whether to put that treatment on to its formulary, or it might need supplementation before it can be used. This common problem is perhaps exacerbated by the tension between requirements for registration and for reimbursement.

A linked issue is that the choice of comparator in a trial—such as the choice of medication to be taken by the control group, while the new group try a newly licensed antipsychotic—is driven by a range of motives. A pharmaceutical company may want to choose a comparator which demonstrates to best effect the positive qualities of their own product (say haloperidol), whereas a health ministry would be more interested in how the new medication compared to the most commonly used drug or group of drugs. Of course, different medications within such a group will usually have different profiles of action, and presumably therefore different costs, as illustrated by the results of the SOHO study (36). The target audience for the findings will therefore usually influence choice of research design and how it is implemented, and evidence may not carry over easily from one context to another.

5.2 Location
The majority of completed schizophrenia treatment trials (including those looking at cost-effectiveness) have been undertaken in North America, but it is increasingly common for studies to be carried out elsewhere and using multicountry designs. Unfortunately, the results of economic evaluations generally do not readily transfer easily from one health system to another because of the structure of health systems, financing arrangements, incentive structures and hence relative costs (17, 37). There might also be differences in the appropriate choice of comparator: a new medication or psychological therapy might look attractive compared to current treatment arrangements in one country but not in comparison to what is the norm elsewhere. The problem is that it is infeasible (and actually unnecessary) to carry out a new, local evaluation every time a new policy or clinical decision needs to be taken, but using the results from a study carried out in one country to inform decisions in another requires careful adaptation to local context, perhaps through some kind of simulation modelling.

5.3 Patient characteristics
Ideally, an evaluation will include every 'patient type' that could potentially benefit from the treatments under consideration in real-world contexts. In contrast, of course, many trials have strict exclusion criteria: commonly excluded groups include patients with comorbid substance misuse, those who are involuntarily detained, those without competence in the dominant language of the country, children, adolescents and older people. There may be understandable practical or ethical reasons for such exclusions, but the upshot is that the evidence is based on data for a relatively narrow subset of the overall population of people with schizophrenia, even if generalisations are nevertheless later made to the whole such population.

The particular challenge for economic evaluations is that many of the excluded patients are likely to have quite high costs (such as those with comorbid substance misuse), or to have different personal contexts (such as the lesser importance of paid employment for older people), or different attitudes to treatment, resulting in different patterns of compliance (and hence different outcomes and downstream costs). These exclusions therefore make generalisation of economic evidence from trials to the wider 'real world' quite problematic.

An associated consideration is patient heterogeneity, with wide outcomes and cost variations between patients. Some events in people's lives tend to be associated with higher costs (e.g., admission to hospital, symptomatic relapse), while there are also behaviours linked to higher costs (e.g., poor adherence with medication and poor engagement with community services). Some personal characteristics and needs can influence costs too, including age, gender, ethnicity, duration and severity of symptoms, and personal and social functioning. Many of these cost-influencing events, behaviours and characteristics are interconnected: for example, medication side-effects could exacerbate nonadherence, in turn raising the risk of relapse, to which the most common response is in-patient admission.

5.4 Perspective
The choice of perspective for a study is usually the result of negotiation between researcher, funding body and decision maker. Economic theory would recommend a societal perspective, covering all costs and outcomes within a well-defined 'society'

(usually a country). But the research funding body might want a narrower perspective, perhaps looking only at the health system. A well-designed study does not have to rule out multiple perspectives, but good science would dictate that a decision is taken on the primary perspective before a trial commences. As noted earlier, the choice of perspective determines the costs and outcomes that are measured, and hence quite possibly influences the results.

5.5 Cost and outcome measurement

Most completed schizophrenia trials have measured only health care costs and not looked wider at costs associated with criminal justice contacts, social care services, uncompensated family support, lost employment/productivity or premature mortality. These omissions could be significant. Even when a study purports to measure health care costs, it is common to find that data are actually collected on only a few health services.

Similarly, most completed economic evaluations—and the clinical trials with which most of them are closely associated—have measured a relatively narrow range of outcomes. Good schizophrenia care is not just symptom alleviation, but also about improving a patient's personal and social functioning (perhaps including ability to work) and their quality of life. Of course, respondent fatigue should be a consideration when designing a study, which would caution against employing too many measures, but the neglect of the outcomes experienced by families is less defensible. There is also the perennial challenge of trying to draw inferences from across a number of studies that employ different primary or secondary outcome measures. These omissions mean that cost-effectiveness conclusions are reached on the basis of just a partial view of what is happening. The neglect of family costs and effects in particular could lead decision makers to choose treatment and support options that are suboptimal.

A related question is whether it makes sense conceptually and strategically to seek to measure QALYs, and if so whether the tools currently available are up to the task. A generic outcome measure such as the QALY, when combined with cost estimates, can point to ways of achieving better value for money, but few studies have included a QALY-generating tool that is valid, reliable and sensitive to change for schizophrenia patients.

5.6 Time frames

Over what periods are interventions delivered to patients, and how do these periods compare with the time frame chosen for an evaluation? Most mental health problems are chronic and require long-term treatment, whereas most studies are short in duration. Decisions therefore need to be taken on the basis of often seriously incomplete evidence. Health economists conduct modelling studies to project future (posttrial) costs and outcomes, but these are less reliable than observational evidence. The analyses that underpin the NICE guidance (38)—themselves based on the modelling of trial data—demonstrate how significant the time horizon of analysis can be.

The longer a trial the greater the risk of sample attrition, the greater the challenge of maintaining a fixed external environment, the higher the research cost, and the longer the delay in feeding back results. But short follow-up periods can be problematic for an economic evaluation because some of the potential economic benefits of an intervention might not manifest themselves immediately. The most obvious example would be the impact of symptom alleviation on ability to work, which might not lead to any observed change in employment rates until some months have elapsed, yet which could be one of the most important longer-term benefits of successful treatment for patients and families.

5.7 Evaluation design

RCTs are rightly seen as providing the most robust and internally valid data for assessing efficacy and safety issues. Economic evaluations can conveniently be built onto an RCT design too. However, the low external validity of an RCT restricts the relevance and generalisability of findings to everyday clinical settings, particularly with tightly drawn patient selection criteria. This is a particular issue when evaluating socially complex interventions (such as combinations of pharmacotherapy, psychotherapy and medication management) because of a low signal-to-noise ratio. Pragmatism in the design of trials should be encouraged, and other designs should be explored, if good economic evidence is to be generated. Observational studies generally enrol less narrowly restrictive samples of patients, have fewer problems with longer follow-ups, impose fewer limitations on drug dosage or concomitant medication, and therefore can better represent the complexities of clinical practice. They cannot replace RCT-generated evidence, but observational and modelling studies can improve understanding of real world effectiveness and cost-effectiveness.

5.8 Sample size

Sample size is always a key consideration in designing a study, but is especially challenging for economic evaluations, since the sample required to detect a significant difference in costs is often larger than that needed for outcomes (39, 40). The reason is the commonly right-skewed distribution of costs—a large number of people with very low costs, and a small number with very high costs because of long periods of inpatient stay. Most schizophrenia trials also experience high drop-out rates, and not all have adequately tested for bias or adjusted for discontinuation. Studies that are powered on the primary clinical outcome alone will usually be underpowered in relation to costs. Rarely has the larger sample needed for an economic evaluation been chosen; budgetary, logistical and sometimes ethical reasons are cited. Given this widespread underpowering, studies that report no significant difference in costs between experimental and control interventions may not be reaching the correct conclusions regarding cost-effectiveness.

In fact, the issue is more complicated. What is the criterion? In principle, it should be a prespecified difference in cost-effectiveness, but is usually specified in terms of a difference in *cost*. Unfortunately, mathematical calculations based upon a ratio measure (such as cost-effectiveness) are far from straightforward. A related difficulty is that there is no consensus on what constitutes an economically important difference.

In the last decade or so, health economists have explored different statistical methodologies and alternative decision-making criteria, not based on conventional 'frequentist' tests of the statistical significance of cost and outcome differences between interventions, but on a decision-making approach embodying Bayesian principles (41). The cost-effectiveness acceptability curve described earlier is one such approach.

5.9 Funding body

Funding source can determine a study's choice of comparator treatment, patient groups to be included, outcome and cost dimensions to be measured (and the tools for their measurement), study duration, and how, where and when findings are disseminated. Conflicts of interest are potentially an issue. Ideally, decision makers would be able to call upon a multiplicity of studies, funded by a multiplicity of sponsors.

6. CONCLUSIONS

The starting point for an interest in the economics of schizophrenia treatment is scarcity: there will never be enough resources to meet population health or other needs. Difficult choices therefore have to be made about how to use available resources, and economic evaluation offers evidence to inform or support those choices by looking at the cost-effectiveness of different treatment options. If it is found that a new intervention (such as a new medication) can generate better clinical and other outcomes than an existing intervention, but at a higher cost, then economic evaluation seeks to clarify the trade-off to be made: Are the better outcomes *worth* the higher cost?

These approaches and methods were illustrated by describing recent economic evaluations of antipsychotics. No evaluation has ever been described as perfect, and while these recent studies of schizophrenia treatment were well designed and competently conducted, they nevertheless illustrate some of the difficulties encountered in analysing cost-effectiveness. Three aspects of economic evaluation stand out as especially challenging, and in need of more attention as new studies are designed. One is the question of whether to include 'utility' among the outcome measures, and particularly whether a robust QALY measure can be found that is sensitive to change for people with schizophrenia. Another design feature that continues to generate problems is sample size, with a great many economic evaluations being underpowered. Third is the perennial question of patient selection, with the narrow recruitment strategies of most major trials excluding people who are among the most expensive to support and treat. Health system decision-makers need to be aware of these limitations, although it would be inadvisable to ignore the findings of the best cost-effectiveness studies.

REFERENCES

1. Knapp M, Mangalore R, Simon J. The global costs of schizophrenia. Schizophr Bull 2004; 30: 279–93.
2. Marwaha S, Johnson S, Bebbington P et al. Rates and correlates of employment in people with schizophrenia in the UK, France and Germany. Br J Psychiatry 2007; 191: 30–7.
3. Mangalore R, Knapp M. Cost of schizophrenia in England. J Ment Health Policy Econ 2007; 109: 23–41.
4. Knapp M, Simon J, Percudani M, Almond S. Economics of schizophrenia: a review, in M Maj and N Sartorius eds. WPA Series in Evidence-Based Psychiatry: Schizophrenia, John Wiley and Sons, Chichester, substantially revised second edition, 2002: 413–60.
5. Almond S, Knapp M, Clement Francois C et al. Relapse in schizophrenia: costs, clinical outcomes and quality of life. Br J Psychiatry 2004; 184: 346–51.
6. Ang YG, Tan HY. Academic deterioration prior to first episode schizophrenia in young Singaporean males. Psych Research 2004; 121: 303–7.
7. Cannon C, Jones P, Huttunen M et al. School performance in Finnish children and later development of schizophrenia. Arch Gen Psychiatry 1999; 56: 457–63.
8. Foley S, Kelly B, Clarke M et al. Incidence and clinical correlates of aggression and violence at presentation in patients with first episode psychosis. Schizophr Res 2005; 72: 161–68.
9. Hollis C. Adult outcomes of a child and adolescent onset schizophrenia. Am J Psychiatry 2000; 157: 1652–59.

10. Nielssen O, Westmore B, Large M et al. Homicide during psychotic illness in New South Wales between 1993 and 2002. Med J Australia 2007; 186: 301–4.

11. Mihalopoulos C, McGorry PD, Carter EC. Is phase-specific, community-orientated treatment of early psychosis an economically viable method of improving outcome? Acta Psychiatr Scand 1999; 100: 47–55.

12. Beecham JK, Knapp MRJ. Costing psychiatric interventions. In: Thornicroft G, ed. Measuring Mental Health Needs, 2nd ed. London: Gaskell, 2001: 200–24.

13. Chisholm D, Knapp M, Knudsen HC et al. Client Socio-demographic and Service Receipt Inventory—EU version: development of an instrument for international research. EPSILON Study. Br J Psychiatry 2000; 177: 28–33.

14. Stone AA, Shiffman S, Shwartz JE et al. Patient non-compliance with paper diaries. BMJ 2002; 324: 1193–4.

15. Brouwer W, Rutten F, Koopmanschap M. Costing in economic evaluations. In: Drummond M, McGuire A, eds. Economic Evaluation in Health Care: Merging Theory with Practice. New York: Oxford University Press, 2001.

16. Curtis L. Unit Costs of Health and Social Care 2008. University of Kent: PSSRU; 2008.

17. Drummond M, Sculpher M, Torrance G et al. Methods for the Economic Evaluation of Health Care Programmes. Oxford: Oxford University Press; 2005.

18. Rosenheck R, Leslie D, Sindelar J et al. Cost-effectiveness of second-generation antipsychotics and perphenazine in a randomized trial of treatment for chronic schizophrenia. Am J Psychiatry 2006; 63: 2080–9.

19. Knapp M, Mangalore R. The trouble with QALYs—Epidemiologia e Psichiatria Sociale 2007; 16: 289–93.

20. EuroQol Group. EuroQol—a new facility for the measurement of health-related quality of life. Health Policy 1990; 16: 199–208.

21. Lenert L, Sturly A, Rapaport M et al. Public preferences for health states with schizophrenia and a mapping function to estimate utilities from positive and negative syndrome scale scores. Schizophr Res 2004; 71: 155–65.

22. Fenwick E, O'Brien B, Briggs A. Cost-effectiveness acceptability curves—facts, fallacies and frequently asked questions. Health Econ 2004; 13: 405–15.

23. Bagnall AM, Jones L, Ginnelly L et al. A systematic review of atypical antipsychotic drugs in schizophrenia. Health Technol Assess 2003; 7(13): 131–214.

24. Basu A. Cost-effectiveness-analysis of pharmacological treatments in schizophrenia: critical review of results and methodological issues. Schizophr Res 2004; 71: 445–62.

25. Rosenheck R, Leslie D, Doshi J. Second-generation antipsychotics: cost-effectiveness, policy options, and political decision making. Psychiatr Serv 2008, 59, 515–520.

26. Lieberman JA, Stroup TS, McEvoy JP et al. Effectiveness of antipsychotic drugs in patients with chronic schizophrenia. N Engl J Med 2005; 12: 1209–23.

27. Manschreck TC. The CATIE schizophrenia trial: results, impact, controversy. Harv Rev Psychiatry 2007; 15: 245–8.

28. Frank R. Policy towards second-generation antipsychotic drugs: a cautionary note. Psychiatr Serv 2008; 59: 521–2.

29. Rosenheck R, Leslie D, Doshi J. Policy implications of CATIE (letter). Psychiatric Services 2008; 59: 695.

30. Ohlsen R, Taylor D, Tandon K et al. Returning to the issue of the cost-effectiveness of antipsychotics in the treatment of schizophrenia. Clin Neuropsychiatry 2008; 5: 184–94.

31. Rosenheck R, Swartz R, McEvoy J et al. Second-generation antipsychotics: reviewing the cost-effectiveness component of the CATIE trial. Expert Rev Pharmacoecon Outcomes Res 2007; 7: 103–11.

32. Jones P, Barnes T, Davies L et al. Randomised controlled trial of the effect on quality of life of second- vs. first-generation antipsychotic drugs in schizophrenia. Arch Gen Psychiatr 2006; 63: 1079–87.

33. Davies LM, Lewis PB, Barnes RE et al. Cost-effectiveness of first v. second-generation antipsychotic drugs: results from a randomised controlled trial in schizophrenia responding poorly to previous therapy. Br J Psychiatry 2007; 191: 14–22.

34. Haro JM, Edgell ET, Jones PB et al. The European Schizophrenia Outpatient Health Outcomes (SOHO) study: rationale, methods and recruitment. Acta Psychiatr Scand 2003; 107: 222–32.

35. Haro JM, Edgell ET, Novick D et al. Effectiveness of antipsychotic treatment for schizophrenia: 6-month results of the Pan-European Schizophrenia Outpatient Health Outcomes (SOHO) study. Acta Psychiatr Scand 2005; 111: 220–31.

36. Knapp M, Windmeijer F, Brown J et al. Cost-utility analysis of treatment with olanzapine compared with other antipsychotic treatments in patients with schizophrenia in pan-European SOHO study. Pharmacoeconomics 2008; 26: 341–58.

37. Knapp M, Chisholm D, Leese M et al. Comparing patterns and costs of schizophrenia care in five European countries: the EPSILON study. Acta Psychiatr Scand 2002; 105(1): 42–54.

38. National Institute for Health and Clinical Excellence. Core interventions in the treatment and management of schizophrenia in primary and secondary care (update). National Clinical Practice Guideline 82, NICE, London.

39. Sturm R, Unützer J, Katon W. Effectiveness research and implications for study design: sample size and statistical power. Gen Hosp Psychiatry 1999; 21: 274–83.

40. Briggs A. Economic evaluation and clinical trials: size matters. BMJ 2000; 321: 1362–3.

41. Claxton K. The irrelevance of inference: a decision making approach to the stochastic evaluation of health care technologies. J Health Econ 1999; 18: 341–64.

Transcultural aspects of schizophrenia and old-age schizophrenia

Tarek Okasha and Ahmed Okasha

INTRODUCTION

Schizophrenia is a chronic disease that afflicts approximately 1% of the population worldwide. It usually afflicts people at a young age and is among the seven most disabling diseases in the age group between 20 and 45 according to the World Health Organization (1), surpassing diabetes, cardiovascular disease, and HIV-AIDS.

The economic cost of schizophrenia has been estimated to be 6 times the cost of myocardial infarction.

The onset of schizophrenia generally occurs at the end of adolescence or beginning of adulthood and, in many cases, the symptoms continue for a lifetime, there being different forms of evolution. Both the positive symptoms as well as negative ones are generally seen; however, cognitive and mood symptoms may be overlooked, but the detection of the disorder is not generally excessively delayed. A study by Melle et al. (2), found a median duration to treatment of a first psychotic episode of 5 weeks in an area with an early detection program and 16 weeks in an area without such a program. However, the wide range in both cases (up to 1,196 weeks, which is equal to more than 22 years) indicates that there are patients who remain without treatment for very long periods.

FIRST-EPISODE SCHIZOPHRENIA

The issue of first-episode schizophrenia has been discussed earlier in the book in details; however, an extensive clinical and research effort is directed internationally toward patients in very early stages of their illness and especially during their first psychotic breakdown with a focus on early and effective intervention. First episode provides a unique opportunity to intervene early and effectively and possibly change the course of the illness. It is known that there is usually an average delay of 1 to 2 years between the onset of psychosis and the start of treatment. The concept of duration of untreated psychosis is an independent predictor of likelihood and extent of recovery from a first episode of psychosis and as a prognostic factor.

Long-term studies suggest that negative symptoms tend to be less common and less severe in the early stages of the illness but increase in prevalence and severity in the later stages. Following the onset of the illness, patients experience substantial decline in cognitive functions from their premorbid levels. Patients with first-episode psychosis usually have a very good response to antipsychotic treatment early in the course of their illness compared to chronic multiepisode patients (3, 4).

According to Emsley et al. (5) the most important factor by far in management of first-episode patients is non- and partial-adherence to medication. Poor adherence is greatest, early in the illness. Relapses and partial response result in accruing morbidity and enduring deficits in cognition and psychosocial function.

PHENOMENOLOGY

Schizophrenia appears relatively similar across a range of cultures; however, variability has been noted in symptom presentation and development (6). The WHO international study of schizophrenia found that schizophrenia was a fairly ubiquitous disorder with an almost similar picture over many cultures. However, the way in which the particular types of symptoms appear may vary from individual to individual and culture to culture (7). Furthermore, owing to differences in social customs and expectations, cultures differ in their assessment of the importance of different symptoms (8, 9).

Manifestations of Schizophrenia

Historically, there are a number of studies comparing the manifestations of schizophrenia across cultures (10). The phenomenology and evaluation of symptomatology in schizophrenia have been discussed before; however, some light should be shed on the differences in the symptomatology of schizophrenia in the Arab cultures that have been a subject of investigation and research with interesting results (11). While Taleb et al. (12) found few clinical differences in their comparative study between schizophrenic patients from Morocco and France, Gawad et al. (13) showed a number of important differences in the diagnosis of schizophrenia in Egypt compared to the United States and the United Kingdom. Gawad et al. studied the cross-national differences in symptom importance in the diagnosis of schizophrenia between the three countries. They found that restriction and incongruity of affect ranked first in the Egyptian study compared to the British and American ones. Their results are in agreement with other studies who stated that what is normal emotional expression in an Anglo-Saxon culture may suggest a schizoid reduction of emotional response in a Mediterranean culture (14). The top ten symptoms in the Egyptian hierarchy for diagnosis of schizophrenia were incongruity and restricted affect, formal thought disorder, thought block, thought withdrawal, incoherence, passivity feeling, neologisms, hallucination, delusions and ideas of reference. In the British study, formal thought disorder ranked first, followed by incongruity of affect, neologism, thought block, passivity of feeling, paranoid delusions, stereotype of other delusions, thought withdrawal and ideas of references (15). The Americans ranked symptoms of importance for diagnosis of schizophrenia as follows: formal thought disorder, delusions, paranoid delusions, incongruity of affect, hallucinations, ideas of reference, neologism, depersonalization, and thought block (16).

There was a striking difference in ranking neologism, though it is the third in the Anglo-American study, it was the seventh in Egyptian study because neologism is perhaps among the commonest symptom in hysterical dissociation, particularly occurring in religious pseudomystic ceremonies (17). The same finding was reported in Libya (18). The cultural and religious heritage absorbs many features that would otherwise be considered symptomatic of a psychiatric disorder (19, 20).

Clinical Presentations

Clinical analyses have shown differences in the clinical presentations of schizophrenia as a result of cultural pathoplastic influences (11). Findings highlighting these influences are summarized in the following sections.

Delusions

The themes of delusions are affected by the individual characteristics of the patients in relation to their culture. The most frequent themes of delusions in Egypt are religious, political, and social, and delusions related to health, while autistic delusions are less common (21). Religious delusions are more common among Muslims and Christians (22). Religious delusions are frequent due to highly religious standards in Egypt. Sexual delusions are commoner in groups in whom sexual behavior is severely suppressed, for example, delusions of sin are frequent in the masturbators in the younger, single, and the student group (23). Political delusions are positively correlated to the level of political sanctions and pressure. Fear of political persecution is a reality of life for people living under totalitarian regimens. Such fears may contribute to a higher prevalence of paranoid delusions (24).

The content of the patient's delusions varies directly in relation to his social class and education. For most of the lower-class men and women, the delusional symptoms are fantasized in terms of the cultural religious institutions. Middle- and upper-class patients, however, far more frequently "secularized" their restitutive narcissistic and self-esteem delusions in terms of science and class conception of power (25) .

Hallucinations
A study from a cultural angle suggests that the theory and treatment of hallucinations requires a broad biopsychosocial approach that is not limited to the consideration of biological and psychological factors only, but takes into account the sociocultural context (26).There are cultural variations in the frequency of different kinds of hallucinations within and between cultures (27).

A study of schizophrenic symptoms in selected regions in the world found that whereas visual hallucinations are the least frequently reported in urban Euro-Americans, they are the most frequently reported in Africa and the Near East (28).

Many investigators in the Arab countries studied the phenomenology and frequency of visual, kinesthetic, and haptic hallucinations. It is concluded that these types of hallucinations in schizophrenia are of common occurrence in these countries. However, the part played by cultural and other factors needs further investigations (29).

The cross-cultural study of the content of auditory hallucinations in schizophrenics living in Saudi Arabia compared to those living in the United Kingdom showed striking differences. Much of the content of the hallucinations of Saudi Arabian schizophrenics were religious and superstitious in nature, whereas instructional themes and running commentary were common among schizophrenic patients in the United Kingdom (30). Patients from both cultures had several coping mechanisms with auditory hallucinations, but these varied between cultures. The majority of Saudi patients used strategies associated with their religion, whereas UK patients were more likely to use distraction or physiologically based approaches. This study suggests that clinicians, when they attempt to facilitate the use of coping strategies, may find greater patient acceptance and efficacy if they are familiar with cultural-specific factors (31).

Attitudes toward hallucinations tend to affect the emotional reaction to and the degree of control of these experiences. Awareness of these attitudes may help the diagnostician to distinguish between pathological and culturally sanctioned hallucinations. It is important that therapists consider the functional significance and meaning of hallucinations as well as the social context and the stimuli associated with them.The cross-cultural differences in the attitudes of mental health professionals toward auditory hallucinations were studied by Wahass and Kent (32), and their results suggest that the cultural view of the causes and treatment of auditory hallucinations could affect attitudes.

Behavior
Behavioral problems in schizophrenia are traditionally attributed to acts of possession by spirits (jinn), sorcery, or envy by the evil eye. Families who entertain these beliefs

take their patients to native healers who are endowed with powers of exorcising evil spirits, undoing sorcery, or ending the harm of envy (33). When efforts along these lines are judged to have failed, and this may take months or years, the patient is finally brought under medical care.

Positive and Negative Symptoms

Studies to evaluate the pathoplastic influences of ethnicity and culture on the symptom of schizophrenia revealed that the core symptoms remained basically the same between different cultures. In the meanwhile, the content of positive symptoms was found to be more influenced by culture than negative symptoms (34).

Clinical assessment of schizophrenia in Egypt denoted that negative symptoms had a greater diagnostic and prognostic value than positive symptoms (35).

Okasha (36) stated that regretably the assessment of the quality of life of patients in religious families according to their adherence to religious rituals regardless of symptomatology, so negative symptoms are interpreted as deeper contemplation about God that makes this person virtuous. Also, positive symptoms are interpreted as being gifted from God by extraordinary perception that makes this person a blessed person. Similarly, personality disorders can be percieved in the same way as schizotypal personality as being close to God, schizoid personality as a kind person, paranoid personality as careful, avoidant personality as religious, and anankastic (obsessive) personality as meticulous in following religious rituals. This may delay treatment as the symptoms may be viewed as a desierable social trait (37).

Affective Phenomena in Schizophrenia

The importance of affective phenomenon in schizophrenia has been recognized since the early evolutionary stages of psychiatry. Fear is the most prominent affect followed by tension, anger, and hostility in Egyptian patients with schizophrenia (38).

Elevated mood, in general, is considered to be uncommon in schizophrenia, while symptoms of depression were found to be an integral part of the schizophrenic process whether patients are maintained on treatment or not (39)

Expressed Emotion and Schizophrenia

Family climate plays an important role in the prognosis of schizophrenic patients. In this respect, the concept of expressed emotion (EE) has gained respectable ground in the field of psychiatry. It includes five components: criticism, hostility, emotional overinvolvement, warmth, and positive remarks. A series of studies have demonstrated that family EE predicts a patient's symptomatic relapse, both in Anglo and American settings (40,41,42), and surprisingly reported that there is no association between emotional overinvolvement and relapse in Egyptian schizophrenic patients. Moreover, they proved that family-expressed emotions, mainly criticism and hostility, seem to be an independent risk factor for relapse of their patients. Their results seem to be similar to those found by Maosheng (43) in Chinese culture.

The presence of high warmth appeared to be associated with lower admission rate and better psychosocial adjustment. Leff (44) has suggested that high values of warmth may have an opposite effect to that of high EE, enhancing patient's psychosocial adjustment.

OLD-AGE SCHIZOPHRENIA

Patients with schizophrenia of later life include those with early-onset schizophrenia (EOS) who have grown older and those who develop the illness in later adult life late-onset schizophrenia (LOS).

There has also been much debate about what age range constitutes late onset in schizophrenia. Manfred Bleuler in 1943 described late-onset schizophrenia with a cutoff of 40 years; Roth and Morrisey in 1952 used the term *late paraphrenia* to describe patients with onset of schizophrenia after age 55. ICD-9 included late paraphrenia, and *DSM-III-R* provided a category for patients with onset of schizophrenia after age 45. These different classifications added to the confusion about LOS. Neither ICD-10 nor *DSM-IV* includes a separate diagnostic category for LOS, both requiring that all cases that fulfill the criteria for schizophrenia be classed accordingly, regardless of age of onset.

A recent consensus statement of the International Late Onset Schizophrenia Group stated that there is sufficient evidence to justify recognition of the two illness classifications; late-onset schizophrenia, with onset after age 40 and very late-onset schizophrenia-like psychosis, with onset after the age of 60 years (45).

All of these factors make caring for older adults with schizophrenia particularly challenging. Members of the interdisciplinary team—physicians, nurses, pharmacists, and other long-term care providers—must be knowledgeable about the most appropriate treatments for schizophrenia as well as the other conditions these patients may be likely to develop.

Epidemiology

Prevalence estimates for schizophrenia in individuals over the age of 65 ranges from 0.1% to 0.5%. The prevalence in some studies has been estimated at 0.3%. However, this figure is probably underestimated (46).

The proportion of patients with schizophrenia whose illness first emerges after the age of 40 has been estimated to be 23.5%, and after age 60, it is around 1.5%.

Risk factors

Later onset of schizophrenia among women and overrepresentation of women among late-onset cases are both robust findings. Patients with very late-onset schizophrenia have a high prevalence of nearly 40% of sensory deficits, especially conductive deafness, compared to normal and depressed elderly patients. The association is less strong in those who develop schizophrenia after the age of 40 years. Some reports suggest an improvement in the psychotic symptoms after the fitting of hearing aid (47). The diagnosis of LOS has also been associated with visual impairment. Premorbid educational, occupational, and psychosocial functioning is less impaired in LOS than EOS, although many LOS patients are reported to have premorbid schizoid or paranoid personality traits not reaching a threshold for the diagnostic criteria for personality disorders in either the ICD 10 or *DSM IV*.

Family history

There is evidence that the relatives of very late-onset schizophrenia patients have lower morbid risk for schizophrenia than the relatives of EOS patients. A controlled family study of late-onset, nonaffective psychosis, in which most cases fulfilled ICD-10 criteria for schizophrenia, found no differences in the lifetime risk of schizophrenia in relatives of cases compared to controls. However, it found that a history of depression was significantly more common among relatives of cases than among controls (48).

This familial link with depression has led to the suggestion that LOS has more in common aetiologically with affective disorders, especially in female patients.

Clinical features

Changes in the symptoms of schizophrenia over the life course need to be considered in association with normal aging. Usually, there is a trend toward a reduction in positive symptoms, with negative and depressive symptoms dominating the clinical picture. Negative symptoms may be difficult to identify in elderly patients because of depression, medication, and the effects of institutionalization.

Cognitive deficits are a recognized feature of all subtypes of schizophrenia. Several cross-sectional studies of poor outcome and chronically institutionalized EOS patients have reported profound cognitive impairment. Longitudinal studies of 30 months or longer have demonstrated cognitive and functional decline in such patients. Risk factors for this decline include more severe positive symptoms and lower educational attainment. These impairments have been shown to be different from normal age-related changes and from the changes associated with Alzheimer's disease.

Poor-outcome schizophrenia patients are more impaired in most domains of cognitive assessment than patients with mild Alzheimer's disease, except on tests of delayed recall and other automatic memory tests where Alzheimer patients underperform.

Studies of patients with EOS who have had a relatively good lifetime outcome find little evidence of decline in cognitive functioning. In a comparative study of elderly patients with schizophrenia, acutely psychotic patients who previously had a good lifetime functional outcome significantly outperformed institutionalized patients on cognitive assessment and both groups underperformed normative standards (49).

In both good- and poor-outcome EOS patients, there is little evidence of progressive cognitive decline over short follow-up periods, which argues against a degenerative dementia being the cause of cognitive decline in this group.

Cross-sectional studies have generally reported that patients with late-onset schizophrenia have cognitive deficits that are similar to those seen in age-matched patients with EOS (49). Comparisons of cross-sectional studies of LOS patients with Alzheimer's disease patients report significant differences in the cognitive profiles of the two patient groups (50). Longitudinal studies have not always been consistent with this. A 5-year follow-up study of 27 patients who developed schizophrenia at age 50 years or over and 34 healthy controls reported that 9 of the LOS groups and none of the control group were found to have a clinical diagnosis of dementia, mainly Alzheimer's disease at 5 years (51).

Postmortem studies of patients with chronic schizophrenia do not reveal an excess of cases that fulfil neuropathologic criteria for Alzheimer's disease, when compared to the general population (52). A link between LOS and dementia would have major implications for the treatment and prognosis of such conditions and may even need further studies using antidementia drugs.

Differences between EOS and LOS

There are a number of significant differences between EOS and LOS. LOS patients are more likely to complain of the following:

1. Visual, tactile, and olfactory hallucinations
2. Persecutory delusions
3. Third-person auditory hallucinations
4. Running commentary
5. Abusive auditory hallucinations.

LOS patients are less likely to display formal thought disorder, affective flattening, or blunting. Formal thought disorder and negative symptoms are even rarer in cases with onset after age 60. The coexistence of affective symptoms, particularly depression, is well recognized clinically.

Differential Diagnosis and overall assessment:
The differential diagnosis of LOS includes the following:

1. Organic psychotic disorders such as delirium, dementia, and focal psychosis
2. Alcohol and substance-induced psychosis
3. Mood disorders with psychotic symptoms
4. Delusional disorder
5. Schizoaffective disorder
6. Psychosis not otherwise specified

A full psychiatric and medical history and examination, including neuroimaging, should always be performed. The presence of any sensory impairment should be addressed in the treatment.

Treatment of schizophrenia in later life requires a biopsychosocial approach, involving multiple disciplines. The role of psychosocial and behavioural approaches, including cognitive–behavioural therapy and social skills training, are important adjuncts to pharmacotherapy for patients with schizophrenia. Like in the case of patients with dementia and Alzheimer, treatment should also focus and address the caregivers and the burden they face caring for such patients.

COMORBIDITIES

Physical comorbidities
Several reviews have shown that there is an excess mortality in people suffering from schizophrenia, being twice as high as the general population (53,54), leading schizophrenia to be termed and categorized as a "life-shortening disease" (55). Despite the excess mortality, people with schizophrenia suffer from many physical disorders that are usually neglected and even when detected are, unfortunately, not attended to or treated properly. Some experts theorize that patients with schizophrenia are more likely to miss the warning signs of cancer and other physical illnesses. What is known is that these people are less likely to receive appropriate medical care for medical illnesses. This could be because patients with schizophrenia are inattentive to or unable to act upon physical problems. However, it may also be due to health care providers incorrectly assuming that the physical complaints of such patients are "delusional". Thus, as patients with schizophrenia grow older, they are more likely than others to experience poor general medical health and have a lower-than-average life expectancy.

In a recent study by Leucht et al. (56) they searched MEDLINE from 1996 to May 2006 combining the term *schizophrenia* with 23 terms of general physical disease categories to identify relevant epidemiological studies during that time.

It was found that regarding infectious diseases, patients with schizophrenia had a higher incidence of tuberculosis than the general population, as well as a higher prevalence of HIV positivity ranging from 1.3% to 22.9% compared to the general population at 0.6% that may be related to sexual risk behavior and substance abuse (57). Several studies also showed an increased prevalence of hepatitis in patients with schizophrenia (58). Several studies found osteoporosis (decreased bone mineral density) in patients with schizophrenia compared to the general population (59,60). Similarly, several studies found that people with schizophrenia die more frequently from cardiovascular disease and experience sudden death than control populations (61). A study carried out in Australia found that patients with schizophrenia received revascularization procedures more rarely than the general population (62).

Psychiatrists must be aware of the frequent medical comorbidities in patients with schizophrenia and play an active role in the prevention, diagnosis, and treatment of such disorders as well as education of patients, families, and colleagues in the different specialties in medicine about patients with schizophrenia and these medical disorders.

Psychiatric comorbidities

1) Substance abuse: Patients with schizophrenia have high rates of substance abuse, more than 50% in some samples. Thus, the development of cardiovascular and hepatic diseases associated with the abuse of these substances, especially alcohol, is very common (63).

2) Dementing diseases: Although patients with schizophrenia are not more likely than the general population to develop dementia (including Alzheimer's disease), the cognitive deficits intrinsic to schizophrenia may become more severe as some patients grow older. Uncommon, though, this culminates in chronic disability.

The most important prerequisite for treating people of all ages with schizophrenia is a complete and comprehensive diagnosis. This should also include consideration of other illnesses, both psychiatric and physical. Providing proper treatment for the patient's physical conditions will often have a dramatically positive effect on his or her capacity to cooperate with and respond to psychiatric treatment.

3) Anxiety and Depression: Comorbidity of anxiety and affective disorders in people with schizophrenia is common. A study carried out by Karatzias et al. (64) investigated the hypothesis that greater negative beliefs about illness and lower self-esteem will be significantly associated with the presence of anxiety or affective comorbidity. In a sample of young patients with schizophrenia, they found that 44.9% had a comorbid anxiety or affective disorder. Those with comorbid anxiety or affective disorder had significantly lower levels of functioning, more negative appraisals of entrapment in psychosis, and lower levels of self-esteem. We can assume that patients with schizophrenia with a late onset and a long history of schizophrenia will have the same result if not higher comorbidity with anxiety and affective disorders.

TREATMENT OPTIONS IN OLD AGE

The existence of psychiatric patients who do not receive treatment is frequent. Several studies have found percentages between 35% and 54% of schizophrenia patients who have not received treatment in the last 12 months. A study by Kessler et al. (65) showed that the most frequent reason for not receiving treatment is lack of disease awareness, as reported by 51% of the study participants. Several studies have found out an association between the duration of psychosis until the onset of treatment and clinical evolution, with worse prognosis based on the greater time without treatment (66). The mechanism of this association have not been explained; thus, a long period without treatment could represent an epiphenomenon or a marker of preexisting factors that would contribute to worse prognosis (67,68).

A Cochrane review carried out in 2003 by Arunpongpasil et al. (69) concluded that there was no trial-based evidence upon which to produce guidelines for the treatment of LOS. Despite this, clinical experience and efficacy of antipsychotics in EOS justify their use in the treatment of schizophrenia and other psychoses in older adults.

The response rate is lower in LOS patients compared to EOS patients. Around 45%-60% of patients show remission of psychotic symptoms in LOS cases, although compliance may render treatment in the community less successful. LOS cases may respond to dose amounts that are about 50% of those given to EOS cases.

Elderly patients are more sensitive to the side effects of both typical and atypical antipsychotic agents. The effects of ageing on hepatic and renal function generally lengthen the half-life of these medications, increasing the susceptibility to adverse effects even at recommended therapeutic doses. Also, physical illness and the excessive use in some cases of polypharmacy, nutritional deficiencies, and dehydration, all predispose to the development of adverse events. Therefore, lower doses and lower dose increments are advised in those older than 65 years of age. Older patients who have been clinically stable while receiving antipsychotic should be regularly reviewed with a view to dose reduction to reduce side effects, while monitoring closely for signs of psychotic relapse. The goal should be to minimize the risk of adverse events.

The National Institute for Clinical Excellence (NICE) in 2005 (70) recommends second-generation antipsychotics for patients with first-episode psychosis and those at high risk of developing extra pyramidal side effects. This would include many elderly patients with both EOS and LOS. First-generation antipsychotics carry a considerable side-effect burden; therefore, second-generation antipsychotics are often chosen as first-line agents in the elderly. They have a more favorable side-effect profile, causing fewer extrapyramidal and anticholinergic side effects. The reported improvements not only in positive symptoms but also in negative and cognitive symptoms are an added advantage in this age group.

In the elderly population, extrapyramidal side effects not only occur more commonly and at lower doses than in younger patients but they are also more troublesome, leading to increased risk of falls. The annual incidence of tardive dyskinesia is reported to be 5 to 6 times greater in older patients (26%) than in younger patients with schizophrenia on first-generation antipsychotics (4%-5%) (71). Autonomic side effects of neuroleptics such as postural hypotension and anticholinergic effects of constipation, urinary hesitancy, and tachycardia can cause considerable morbidity in the elderly.

Currently recognized side effects of second-generation antipsychotics may pose significant risk to elderly patients, known as the "metabolic syndrome," including hyperglycaemia and development or exacerbation of diabetes, hyperlipidemia (especially with olanzapine and clozapine), possible increased risk of cerebrovascular adverse events (reported in patients with dementia on olanzapine and risperidone), and QTc prolongation (reported with ziprasidone) (72).

Clinicians must be vigilant when prescribing antipsychotics in this age group. The clinician must ensure accurate diagnosis; consideration of medical history; discussion of side effects with patient and carer; and the use of minimum effective dose and regular review, as well as regular evaluation of the patient's blood sugar, lipid profile, ECG, and so on.

Table 29.1 Differences between Traditional and Nontraditional Societies regarding relationships and medical treatment

Traditional Societies	Nontraditional Societies
Family and group oriented	Individually oriented
Extended family (less geographical than previously, but conceptual)	Nuclear family
Status determined by age, position in family, and care of elderly	Status achieved by own efforts
Relationship between kin obligatory	Relationship between kin is a matter of individual choice
Arranged marriage, with an element of choice dependant on interfamilial relationship	Choice of marital partner, determined by interpersonal relationship
Extensive knowledge of distant relatives' lives	Knowledge of close relatives' lives only
Family decision making	Individual autonomy
External locus of control	Internal locus of control
Physician's decision respected and considered holy	Doubt in doctor–patient relationship
Rare suing for malpractice	Common suing for malpractice
Deference to God's will	Self-determination
Healthy doctor–patient relationship	Mistrust in doctor–patient relationship
Individual can be replaced; family should continue and pride is in the family ties	Individual is irreplaceable; pride is in self
Pride in family care of mentally ill patient	Community care of mentally ill patients
Dependence on God regarding health and disease; illness and recovery attributed to God	Self-determined recovery

After Okasha, 2000.

A recent study carried out on 66 patients with schizophrenia above the age of 60 years for 6 months by Ritchie et al. (73) that compared the efficacy and safety of olanzapine and risperidone in the treatment of elderly patients found that both drugs were well tolerated and their use was associated with fewer symptoms of schizophrenia and less side effects than seen when patients received first-generation antipsychotics.

Care of elderly patients differs from culture to culture. In traditional societies, the family takes pride in caring for the elderly, not allowing them to leave their homes; therefore, old peoples homes are not a common feature.

One must first be familiar with the main characteristics that differentiate the position of the individual within his or her community in a traditional society from that in a Western society. Although societies should not to be considered stereotypically, general common attitudes can be assumed (74).

Differences between the two types of societies are listed in Table 29.1. These differences summarized by Okasha (75) are the mainstream norm and not the absolute description of a stereotyped behavior.

CONCLUSION

This chapter briefly reviews the prevalence, burden, and mortality of schizophrenia and first-episode schizophrenia. A recent study by Whitty et al. (76) found that the outcome of schizophrenia may not be as pessimistic on once thought and most patients did not display a downward, deteriorating course of illness, with one systematic review suggesting about 40% experience a favorable outcome (45 Better outcome at follow-up was associated with fewer negative symptoms at baseline, more years in education, and shorter duration of untreated psychosis (DUP).

This means that we are dealing with two different categories between EOS and LOS, as there is a marked difference in genetics, brain pathology and brain imaging, phenomenology, response to treatment, and outcome. As if EOS is a neurodevelopmental disorder with structural and synaptic pathogenesis while LOS is determined more by environmental factors namely the social capital with its social cohesion and trust. Elderly people are more susceptible to isolation, deprivation, and helpless and hopeless expectation. The association by age-related cognitive decline with schizophrenia may confound the diagnosis as early dementia may be associated with schizophrenia-like symptoms. The frequency of visual hallucination may be attributed to the involvement of organic phenomena whether vascular or degenerative in the pathology.

A black box warning shows that there is some cardiovascular disorders and mortality with the use of SGA, especially in the presence of a dementing process apart from the metabolic syndrome manifestations. We should balance between effectiveness and expectations in the management of LOS.

A recent study shows that SGA may have the most notable effects in paranoia anger, including aggression, but not on functioning, cognition, or mood symptoms (77).

Because of the comorbidity of LOS with medical and psychiatric disorders and the possibility of drug–drug interaction and the development of delirium, the psychiatrist should be aware of regular monitoring of his patients and augment his medical knowledge and expertise.

REFERENCES

1. World Health Organization. World Health Report 2001. Mental health – new understanding, new hope. Geneva: World Health Organization, 2001.
2. Melle I, Larsen TK, Haahr U et al. Reducing the duration of intreated first-episode psychosis. Effects on clinical presentation. Arch Gen Psychiatry 2004; 61: 143–50.
3. Lieberman JA and Fenton W. Delayed detection of psychosis: Causes, consequences and effect on public health. Am J Psychiatry 2000; 157: 1727–30
4. Lieberman JA. Neurobiology and the natural history of schizophrenia. J Clin Psychiatry 2006; 67(10): e14.
5. Emsley R, Oosthuizen PP, Kidd M et al. Remission in first-episode psychosis: Predictor variables and symptom improvement patterns. J Clin Psychiatry 2006; 67(11): 1707–12.
6. Swartz. L. Culture and mental health: A southern African view, Oxford University Press; 1998: 204.
7. World Health Organization (WHO). Report of the international pilot study of schizophrenia. Geneva: WHO, 1973.
8. Edgerton RB and Cohen A. Culture and schizophrenia: the DOSMD challenge, Br J Psychiatry1994; 164(2): 222–31.
9. Lucas RH and Barret RJ. Interpreting culture and psychopathology primitivist themes in cross- cultural debate. Cult. Med. Psychiat 1995; 19(3): 287–326.
10. Varma VK. Transcultural perspective on schizophrenia, epidemiology, manifestation and outcome. Report of section of Transcultural Psychiatry, WPA, 2000.
11. Okasha A. Clinical Psychiatry. The Anglo Egyptian Book Shop; 1988: 1131–65.

12. Taleb M, Rouillon F, Petitjean F and Gorwood P. Cross-cultural study of schizophrenia. Psychopathology 1996; 29(2): 85–94.
13. Gawad M, Rakhawy Y, Mahfouz R, Howaidy M. Relative symptom importance in the diagnosis of schizophrenia. The Egypt J Psychiatry1981; 4(1): 39–56.
14. Lehman HE. Clinical features of schizophrenia: Freedman AM and Kaplan HI (Eds), Comprehensive Text Book of Psychiatry. Baltimore: the Williams and Wilkins
15. Willis JH and Bannister D. The diagnosis and treatment of schizophrenia: A questionnaire study of psychiatric opinion. Br J Psychiatry 1965; 111: 1165–71.
16. Edwards G. Diagnosis of schizophrenia: An Anglo – American comparison, Br J Psychiatry 1972; 120: 385–90.
17. Okasha A. A cultural psychiatric study of El- Zar cult in the UAR. Br J Psychiatry 1969; 112: 693.
18. Khalid MS. Symptomatology of schizophrenia in Libya. Psychiatric – Neurol- Med- Psychology Leipz 1977; 29(1): 46–8.
19. Barakat. M. The Arab World: Society, culture, and state, University of California Press, Berkeley and Los Angeles, California, 1993: 97–118.
20. Frindlay AM. The Arab World. Biddles Ltd, Guilford and Kings Lymn, UK, 1994: 126–89.
21. Rakhawy Y, Amin Y, Hamdi E et al. Characteristics of thought disorder in Schizophrenia. Egypt J Psychiatry 1987; 10: 131–50.
22. Murphy HBM and Raman AC. The chronicity of schizophrenia in indigenous tropical people. Br J Psychiatry 1971; 118: 489–97.
23. Ashour A, Okasha A, Hussein M, Sobhi M, Khalil A. The P.S.E.and Social Skills of Chronic Schizophrenics: Descriptions and Correlation. . The Egyptian J Psychiatry 1986; 9: 18–30.
24. Westermeyer J. Some cross-cultural aspects of delusional beliefs. Edited by Othmanns TF, Maher BA, New York, Wiley,1988.
25. El-Sendiony MF. Cultural aspects of delusion: A psychiatric study in Egypt. Aust. N. Z. J. Psychiatry 1976; 10(2): 201–7.
26. Al-Issa I. The illusion of reality or the reality of illusion. Hallucination and culture. Br J Psychiatry1995; 166: 368–73.
27. Sartorius N, Jablensky A and Korten A. Early manifestation and first contact incidence of schizophrenia in different cultures. Psychol Med 1986; 16: 909–28
28. Murphy HBM, Witkower EG and Fried J. Cross cultural survey of schizophrenic symptomatology. Intern J Soc Psychiatry 1963; 9: 237–49.
29. Khalil AH. Psychological assessment of delusional parasitosis in Egypt, A paper presented in the International Congress of Parasitology, ICOPA Paris, Aug 1990: 20–24.
30. Kent G and Wahass S. The content and characteristics of auditory hallucinations in Saudi Arabia and the UK: A cross cultural comparison, Acta Psychiatr Scand 1996; (6): 433–7.
31. Wahass S and Kent G. A cross-cultural study of the attitudes of mental health professionals towards auditory hallucinations. Int. J. Social Psychiatry 1997; 43(3): 184–92.
32. Wahass S and Kent G. Coping with auditory hallucinations: A cross – cultural comparison between Western and non-western patients. J. Nerv. Ment. Dis 1997; 185(11): 664–8.
33. Masloweki J, Rensberg JVD and Mthoko N. A polydiagnostic approach to the symptoms of schizophrenia in different culture and ethnic populations, Acta Psychiatr Scand July1998; 98(91): 46–6.
34. Owaida M, Wilson A, Tawfik M et al. Clinical Assessment of Positive Negative Symptoms. Age of onset and gender in a sample of Egyptian patients having schizophrenia for more than two years. Egypt J Psychiatry 1999; 22: 267–76.
35. Okasha A. Personal communication,2008
36. Okasha A and Maj M. eds. Images in Psychiatry: An Arab Perspective. World Psychiatric Association. Scientific Book House, Cairo.
37. Rakhawy YT, Arafa M, Mahfouz R et al. Schizophrenia: possible characteristics of affective pattern. Egypt J Psychiatry 1985; 8: 41–73

38. Mahfouz R. Patient's Subjective Experiences of Psychotropic Drugs: Can these help gaining new insights in pharmacotherapy. The Egyptian Journal of Psychiatry 1990; 13(2): 247–52.

39. Wig NN, Mendon DK, Bedi H. Expressed Emotions and Schizophrenia in North India: Cross Cultural transfer of ratings of relatives and Expressed Emotions. Br J Psychiatry 1987; 151:156–73.

40. Abol-Magd. S. Psychiatric assessment of families of schizophrenic patients, MD thesis, Cairo University, Faculty of Medicine;1993.

41. Kamal A. Variables in Expressed Emotions associated with relapse: A comparison between depressed and schizophrenic samples in the Egyptian community. Curr Psychiatr 1995; 2(2): 211–5.

42. Moasheng R, Zaijn Hand Mengze X. Emotional expression among relatives of schizophrenic patients. Chin J Psychiatry1998; 31(4): 237–9.

43. Leff J. Contraversal issues and growing points in research on relatives' expressed emotions. Intern J Soc Psychiatry 1989; 35: 133–45.

44. Howard RJ, Rabins PV, Seeman MV, Jeste DV. Late-onset schizophrenia and very late-onset schizophrenia-like psychosis: an international consensus. The International Late Onset Schizophrenia Group. Am J Psychiatry 2000; 157: 172–8.

45. Palmer BW, Heaton SC, Jeste DV. Older patients with schizophrenia: challenges in the coming decades. Psychiatr Serv 1999; 50: 1178–83.

46. Almeida O P, Howard R J, Levy R, David A S. Psychotic states arising in late life (late paraphrenia). The role of risk factors. Br J Psychiatry 1995; 166: 215–28.

47. Howard RJ, Levy R. Late onset schizophrenia, late paraphrenia and paranoid states of late life. In: Jacoby, R. Oppenheimer, C. (Eds.): Psychiatry in the Elderly. 2nd edition. Oxford. Oxford University Press,1996.

48. Harvey PD, Howanitz E, Parrella M etal. Symptoms, cognitive functioning, and adaptive skills in geriatric patients with lifelong schizophrenia: a comparison across treatment sires. Am J Psychiatry 1998; 155: 1080–6.

49. Sachdev P, Brodaty H, Rose N et al. Schizophrenia with age of onset after age 50 years. 2. Neurological, neuropsychological and MRI investigation. Br J Psychiatry 1999; 175: 416–21.

50. Heaton R, Paulsen J, McAdams LA et al. Neuropsychological deficits in schizophrenia: relationship to age, chronicity and dementia. Arch Gen Psychiat 1994; 51: 469–76.

51. Brodaty H, Sachdev P, Koschera A, Monk D, Cullen B. Long term outcome of late-onset schizophrenia: 5-years follow-up study. Br J Psychiatry 2003; 183: 213–19.

52. Purohit DP, Perl DP, Haroutunian V et al. Alzheimer's disease and related neurodegenerative disease in elderly patients with schizophrenia: a postmortem neuropathological study of 100 cases. Arch Gen Psychiatry 1998; 55: 205–11.

53. Brown GW, Birely J and Wing JK. Influence of Family Life on the Course of Schizophrenic Disorders. Br J Psychiatry 1972;.121: 224–58.

54. Harris EC, Barraclough B. Excess mortality of mental disorder. Br J Psychiatry 1998; 173: 11–53.

55. Allbeck P, Rodvall Y, Wistedt B. Incidence of rheumatoid arthritis among patients with schizophrenia, affective psychosis and neurosis. Acta Psychiat Scand 1985; 71: 615–9.

56. Leucht S, Burkard J, Henderson J, Maj M, Sartorius N. Physical illness and schizophrenia: a review of the literature. Acta Psychatr Scand 2007; 116: 317–33

57. Fisher I, Bienskii AV, Fresorova IV. Experience in using serological tests in detecting tuberculosis in patients with severe mental pathology. Probl Tubrek 1996; 1: 19–20.

58. Said WM, Saleh R, Jumaian N. Prevalence of hepatitis B virus among chronic schizophrenia patients. East Mediterr Health J 2001; 7: 526–30.

59. Hummer M, Malik P, Gasser RW et al. Osteoporosis in patient with schizophrenia. Am J Psychiatry 2005; 162: 162–7.

60. Kishimoto T, Watanabe K, Takeuchi H et al. Bone mineral density measurement in female inpatients with schizophrenia. Schizophr Res2005; 77: 113–5

61. Allbeck P. Schizophrenia: a life-shortening disease. Schizophr Bull 1989; 15: 81–9.
62. Lawrence DM, Holman CD, Jablensky AV, Hobbs MS. Death rate from ischaemic heart disease in Western Australian psychiatric patients. 1980-1998. Br J Psychiatry 2003; 182: 31–6.
63. Regier DA, Farmer ME, Rae DS et al. Comorbidity of mental disorders with alcohol and other drug abuse. Results from the Epidemiologic Catchment Area (ECA) Study. JAMA 1990; 264(19): 2511–8.
64. Karatzias T, Gumley A, Power K, O'Grady, M. Illness appraisal and self-esteem as correlates of anxiety and affective comorbid disorders in schizophrenia. Compr Psychiatry 2007; 48: 371–5
65. Kessler RC, Berglund PA, Bruce ML et al. The prevalence and correlates of untreated serious mental illness. Health Serv Res 2001; 36: 987–1007.
66. Black K, Peters I, Rui Q et al. Duration of untreated psychosis predicts treatment outcome in an early psychosis program. Schizoph Res 2001; 47: 215–22.
67. Norman RM, Malla AK. Duration of untreated psychosis: a critical examination of the concept and its importance. Psychol Med 2001; 31: 381–400.
68. Verdoux H, Liraud F, Bergey C et al. Is the association between duration of untreated psychosis and outcome confounded? A two year follow-up of first-admitted patients. Schizoph Res 2001; 49: 231–41.
69. Arunpongpasil S, Ahmed I, Aqeel N, Suchat P. Antipsychotic drug treatment for elderly people with late-onset schizophrenia. Cochrane Database Syst Rev 2003; (2):CD004162.
70. National Institutre for Clinical Excellence. Guidance on the use of newer (atypical) antipsychotic drugs for the treatment of schizophrenia. Issue Date: June 2002 Review Date: May 2005.
71. Jeste DV, Eastham JH, Laroc JP et al. Management of late-life psychosis. J Clin Psychiatry 1996; 57(suppl 3): 39–45.
72. Jin H, Meyer JM, Jeste DV. Phenomenology of and risk factors for new onset diabetes mellitus and diabetes ketoacidosis associated with atypical antipsychotics: an analysis of 45 published cases. Ann Clin Psychiatry 2002; 14(1): 59–64.
73. Ritchie CW, Chiu E, Harrigan S et al A comparison of the efficacy and safety of olanzapine and risperidone in the treatment of elderly patients with schizophrenia: an open study of six months duration. Int J Geriatr Psychiatry 2006; 21: 171–9.
74. Leff J. Psychiatry around the globe: A Transcultural View (Gaskel Psychiatric Series). London, Royal College of Psychiatrists, 1988: 79.
75. Okasha A. The Impact of Arab Culture on Psychiatric Ethics. In Ethics Culture and Psychiatry. International Perspectives. Okasha, A., Arboleda-Florez, J. and Sartorius, N. eds. American Psychiatric Press Inc,2000.
76. Whitty P, Clarke M, Mctigue O et al. Predictors of outcome in first episode schizophrenia over the first 4 years of illness. Psychol Med 2008; 38: 1141–6.
77. Sultzer D, Pavis S, Tariot P et al. Clinical symptoms: responses to a typical antipsychotic medication in Alzheimer's disease- phase of outcomes from the CATIEAD effectiveness Am J Psychiatry. 2008; 165(7): 844–54.

Index

Note: Page references in *italics* refer to tables; those in bold to figures.